Biopharmaceutics and Pharmacokinetics

Biopharmaceutics and Pharmacokinetics

SECOND EDITION

PL Madan PhD
Professor
St John's University
New York, USA

JAYPEE BROTHERS MEDICAL PUBLISHERS
The Health Sciences Publisher
New Delhi | London

Jaypee Brothers Medical Publishers (P) Ltd

Headquarters
EMCA House
23/23-B, Ansari Road, Daryaganj
New Delhi 110 002, India
Landline: +91-11-23272143,
+91-11-23272703
+91-11-23282021, +91-11-23245672
E-mail: jaypee@jaypeebrothers.com

Overseas Office
JP Medical Ltd.
83, Victoria Street, London
SW1H 0HW (UK)
Phone: +44-20 3170 8910
E-mail: info@jpmedpub.com

Corporate Office
Jaypee Brothers Medical Publishers (P) Ltd.
4838/24, Ansari Road, Daryaganj
New Delhi 110 002, India
Phone: +91-11-43574357
Fax: +91-11-43574314
E-mail: jaypee@jaypeebrothers.com

EU GPSR Authorised Representative
Logos Europe, 9 rue Nicolas Poussin
17000, La Rochelle, France
Phone: +33 (0) 6 67 93 73 78
E-mail: Contact@logoseurope.eu

Website: www.jaypeebrothers.com
Website: www.jaypeedigital.com

Inquiries for bulk sales may be solicited at: jaypee@jaypeebrothers.com

Biopharmaceutics and Pharmacokinetics

First Edition: 2000
Second Edition: 2014, Reprint: **2025**

ISBN 978-93-5090-939-3
Printed in India

PREFACE TO THE SECOND EDITION

The second edition of *Biopharmaceutics and Pharmacokinetics* represents a major revision of the book originally published in 2000. This edition has been revised to incorporate new information that has become available since the publication of the first edition a decade ago. Among the major changes that have been made in the second edition, the following are noteworthy. The sequencing of some of the chapters has been revised to attain a logical approach in order to make the flow of material more realistic. For example, the chapter dealing with drug elimination now follows the chapters dealing with drug absorption and drug distribution; and continuous intravenous infusion now follows the chapter dealing with loading dose. A substantial number of solved examples and practice problems have been added to most of the chapters in this edition, and all tables and almost all figures have been formatted to fit the new style of this book.

This edition also contains a new chapter dealing with non-compartmental methods because many research papers report such pharmacokinetic parameters as mean residence time and mean absorption time of the drug using the non-compartment methods without going through the rigorous task to establish the compartment model that will fit the data.

I acknowledge with gratitude the many helpful comments and suggestions received from colleagues, fellow teachers, and students. Wherever possible, these comments and suggestions have been incorporated into this edition, without sacrificing the easy-to-understand format of the book. While every effort has been made to minimize errors, some errors may have been overlooked. As always, your feedback will be highly appreciated.

PL Madan

PREFACE TO THE FIRST EDITION

The primary objective of this book is to present the basic principles of biopharmaceutics and pharmacokinetics for the health professionals. Special emphasis is placed on practical application of the principles that are useful in pharmacy, medicine and other health professions.

The evolution of this book is a result of many years of teaching this subject to the undergraduate and graduate students. It originally began with classroom handouts highlighting important concepts, equations and their use. This was essential because no suitable comprehensive textbook existed at that time. Students were forced to read selected chapter(s) from various books and research articles published in various scientific journals in order to gather some information on the subject. Understandably, it was a hardship on the students because they were experiencing great difficulty not only financially, but also due to inconsistency in the symbols and nomenclature used in various books and journals. Thus, they had to rely largely on notes taken in the classroom, and supplement the information from external sources to the best of their ability and resources. The steadily increasing number of these handouts became increasingly difficult with the increasing number of students enrolled in the course.

The writing of this book was prompted by recent developments in the undergraduate pharmacy curriculum which is now becoming increasingly clinical oriented. The students in most pharmacy schools participate in rounds on the floor of hospitals where knowledge of biopharmaceutics and pharmacokinetics is essential not only for interdisciplinary communication but also for meaningful health care. This knowledge will certainly become more critical as curriculum in the pharmacy schools completes its transition from the traditional 5-year BS degree to the presently proposed 6-year Pharm D degree. The practitioners will then be expected not only to have the basic knowledge of pharmacokinetics, but also apply it in their day-to-day practice. This may require the practitioner to undertake, for example, designing loading dose, maintenance dose, and dosing intervals for individual patients. In clinical situations dealing with severely sick patients and in therapy with life-saving drugs such as antibiotics, anti-coagulants, antidiabetics, etc., the pharmacist will also be called upon to determine dosage regimen adjustments, e.g. in patients with renal failure.

Pharmacokinetics is now taught as a formal course in almost all pharmacy schools in the world. This textbook will hopefully provide the students with the material needed for their degree requirements. The book is also intended for those practitioners who wish to refer to the material for their general use. The material presented in this book is simplified to give the reader a clear and complete understanding of the subject matter. Some of the earlier chapters in this book treat fundamental concepts, since the approach to the subject of biopharmaceutics and pharmacokinetics must be of elementary necessity. These chapters are not merely summaries of the subject matter, but are intended to present a careful treatment of the subject to help the reader apply these concepts in the succeeding chapter. An attempt has been made to keep these discussions brief and direct, but at the same time, clear and complete. Whenever possible, each topic is well illustrated by examples of commonly used drugs, and for the mathematical subjects, by at least one example in the form of a solved problem. These examples have been carefully planned in an effort to illustrate the concepts involved. A set of practice problems is given at the end of each kinetic-related chapter and their answers are provided at the end of the text.

References are not included in the text because only basic information is given in each chapter, and the listing of data (e.g. volumes of distribution, fraction of dose absorbed, extent of protein binding, etc.) are derived from numerous sources. However, a list of suggested reading is provided for each chapter for the interested reader for further information.

Although this book is not intended to create a fully competent clinical pharmacokinetist, it is hoped that it will certainly provide an orientation to the concepts involved and help the practitioner begin learning pharmacokinetic techniques for clinical situations.

The book is organized to provide a smooth flow of the material. The first chapter introduces the reader to the elementary concept of biopharmaceutics and pharmacokinetics, including the off-shoots of pharmacokinetics, e.g. clinical pharmacokinetics and pharmacogenetics. The next two chapters deal with the fundamentals of graphing techniques and linear correlation, and kinetics. It is felt that these two chapters are extremely essential to the understanding of pharmacokinetics for the beginners, although they may be refresher to advanced students. Chapter 4 introduces the concept of drug distribution into various body fluids and tissues, and Chapter 5 deals with mechanisms of drug absorption and the factors influencing absorption of drugs through the gastrointestinal tract. The next two chapters are devoted to the determination and application of bioavailability and bioequivalence.

Chapter 8 introduces the reader to the concept of compartment modeling, and the next two chapters are devoted compartment modeling during intravenous bolus extravascular administration. Chapter 9 deals with one-, two-, and three-compartment models after intravenous bolus injection, and Chapter 10 discusses one- and two-compartment models following extravascular administration.

The next two chapters are devoted to drug excretion. Chapter 11 deals essentially with renal elimination and Chapter 12 includes non-renal mechanisms under the broad concept of clearance. The remaining five chapters are devoted to the applications of pharmacokinetic principles. Chapter 13 details multiple dosing, followed by the concept and determination of loading dose (Chapter 14). Adjustment of dosage regimen in renal insufficiency is discussed in Chapter 15, followed by the concepts of therapeutic drug monitoring (Chapter 16), and the last chapter (Chapter 17) deals with continuous intravenous infusion.

The seventeen chapters of the text are followed by answers to mathematical problems, and three appendices. The first appendix, Appendix A, is a compilation of definitions of terms frequently encountered in pharmacokinetics. The second appendix, Appendix B, is the alphabetical listing of symbols and abbreviations used in this book, and the third appendix, Appendix C, is a compilation of dosage adjustments of drugs in renal failure.

I acknowledges with gratitude the helpful comments and suggestions from colleagues, fellow teachers, and students. While every effort has been made to minimize errors, some errors may have been overlooked. Your feedback will be highly appreciated.

PL Madan

CONTENTS

CHAPTER 1

BASIC CONCEPTS

The concept of biopharmaceutics and pharmacokinetics in pharmaceutical sciences was first introduced in the early 1960s. Since then tremendous advances have been made in this area. At the present time, these concepts have reached such a status that they are now included in almost all textbooks dealing not only with on pharmaceutics, but also in textbooks dealing with pharmacology, medicinal chemistry and other related subjects. Also, these concepts are covered in depth in one or more courses in the curricula of all health-related professions.

The subjects of Biopharmaceutics and Pharmacokinetics are now an important part of curriculum in all schools of pharmacy and other health professions. There are journals exclusively devoted to publishing scientific research papers in this field. While some journals publish research papers and review articles dealing strictly with biopharmaceutics and pharmacokinetics, (e.g. *Journal of Pharmacokinetics and Biopharmaceutics* and *Clinical Pharmacokinetics*), many other journals publish articles concerned with biopharmaceutics and pharmacokinetics (e.g. *Journal of Pharmaceutical Sciences*, *Pharmaceutical Research*, *Journal of Clinical Pharmacology* and *Clinical Pharmacology and Therapeutics*). This chapter will introduce the reader to the fundamental concepts of biopharmaceutics and pharmacokinetics.

The term Biopharmaceutics and Pharmacokinetics was coined in 1960 to include topics relating to dosage form factors and physiological factors that affect the release of drug from the manufactured products. Soon after the introduction of the term, some pharmacy schools began exploring the merit of introducing this subject in their curriculum as a free-standing course.

Several significant events and factors were conducive in generating initial interest in development of the course. Some of these were:

a. During the latter part of 1940s and early 1950s, a significant number of very important antibiotics were discovered. These included chlortetracycline, oxytetracycline and chloramphenicol.
b. The microbiological assays developed for antibiotics in the physiological fluids were specific and highly sensitive.
c. Competing drug companies claimed superiority for their antibiotic on the basis of attaining higher plasma levels of the antibiotic following oral administration of their product.
d. The significance of adding an adjuvant on enhancing oral absorption of the drug was heavily promoted by the pharmaceutical companies. For example, Bristol Laboratories added the adjunct sodium hexametaphosphate to their tetracycline capsules, Pfizer Laboratories added glucosamine hydrochloride and Lederle Laboratories added citric acid.
e. Phenoxymethylpenicillin (Penicillin V) was marketed as a penicillin, which produced higher plasma levels than Benzylpenicillin (Penicillin G) after oral administration. It was shown that the greater acid-stability of the antibiotic Penicillin V accounted for the higher plasma concentration of this penicillin.
f. The significance of rapid disintegration of dry oral dosage forms was recognized. A country doctor, WE Upjohn observed that in many cases pills manufactured during the 1880s passed

through the gastrointestinal tract of patients. He conceived the idea of preparing friable pills. Instead of starting from a paste, friable pills were built up in a revolving pan. His method consisted of spraying a granular diluent with moistening agent and then sifting powdered drug onto them. His pills needed no adhesive or gums to hold them together; therefore they could be easily crumpled with the thumb.

g. After the development of the Stoll and Gershberg disintegration apparatus, the official compendia recognized the significance of disintegration rate for tablets and capsules.
h. The inclusion of an official dissolution test for a few drugs first appeared in the United States Pharmacopeia (USP) in 1970.

Thus, it is seen that the concept of biopharmaceutics is a result of combination of various disciplines. During the early 1960s when research in drug product development became highly active, it was recognized that a great deal of background knowledge is required for studying the relationship among the many factors that influence biological activity of the administered dosage form. Soon it was realized that formulation factors used in the fabrication of dosage form also played an important role in biological activity of the administered dose.

BIOPHARMACEUTICS

The term Biopharmaceutics and its detailed definition first appeared in print in a review article:

> *Biopharmaceutics encompasses the study of relationship between nature and intensity of biological effects observed in animals and man and the following factors: simple chemical modification of drugs such as formation of esters, salts and complexes; modification of physical state, particle size and/or surface area of the drug available to absorption sites; presence or absence of adjuvant in the dosage form with the drug; type of dosage form in which drug is administered; and pharmaceutical processes by which the dosage form is manufactured.*

Therefore, the term Biopharmaceutics may be defined as the study of relationship between physicochemical properties of drug in a dosage form and various effects (pharmacologic, toxicological or therapeutic) observed after administration of dosage form. In other words, the study of biopharmaceutics encompasses all possible effects of dosage form on biological response and all possible physiological factors, which may affect the drug contained in dosage form and the dosage form of the drug itself.

Initially, the study of biopharmaceutics was limited essentially to a descriptive discipline, but with the development of pharmacokinetics, the study of biopharmaceutics has been extended to encompass relationship between the nature and intensity of biological effects observed as well as physical and chemical properties of drug in the dosage form.

To prevent possible confusion of the term biopharmaceutics with other rapidly growing and closely related fields, biopharmaceutics is best defined as: *"the study of factors influencing bioavailability of a drug (in humans and animals) and the use of this information to optimize pharmacologic or therapeutic activity of drug products in clinical application"*.

Factors Influencing Drug Availability

There are many and varied pharmaceutical factors that may influence the availability of the drug from its dosage form. Obviously, depending upon the formulation variables used in the preparation of various dosage forms of a given drug, the drug may exhibit different degrees of availability when given by the same route, but in a different dosage form (e.g. orally administered tablet, capsule, solution or suspension, etc.). For example, the drug may exhibit different onset of action or achieve different plasma concentrations depending on whether it is administered orally in a solution, suspension, tablet or capsule dosage form. Similarly, differences in the availability of drug from the same dosage form manufactured by different manufacturers may be observed depending on the different process variables used in the method of manufacture employed by different manufacturers. There is always the possibility of variation in the biological availability of drug from one batch to another even when the dosage form is made by the same manufacturer. This is because the biological availability of a drug is greatly affected by its physical state and by the various pharmaceutical factors including the dosage form in which it is administered.

Many factors may influence the availability of a drug from its dosage form. For example, the steps involved in the release of drug from an extravascularly administered dose (oral, intramuscular, subcutaneous, rectal, etc.) being made available for absorption influence the availability of drug to the biological system. The intravascularly administered dose is not included because intravascular administration places the drug directly into the systemic circulation. The factors influence availability of drug from its dosage form may therefore be classified into two categories. These are:

i. Physicochemical properties of the drug substance.
ii. Formulation factors that may affect release of drug from the dosage form.

Physicochemical Properties of the Drug

From the chemical structure of a drug molecule one can deduce many physicochemical properties of the drug. For example, the presence of an amino group on the molecule means that one can prepare salts with acids and therefore enhance water-solubility of the drug. Similarly, the presence of a carboxyl group can be used to prepare salts with sodium, potassium, calcium and amino compounds. The presence of both, an amino group and a carboxylic group, means that the molecule can exist in zwitterionic form. When a zwitterionic form of a drug molecule is possible (e.g. ampicillin), one can expect that pH versus solubility profile of the compound will reveal minimal solubility of the compound at a particular pH (the pH where concentration of zwitterionic form is at a maximum). The physicochemical properties of drug, which affect absorption include aqueous solubility, particle size, polymorphic form, salt form, pK_a and/or pK_b and partition coefficient of the drug.

Aqueous Solubility: In order for a drug to be absorbed, it must first be dissolved in the fluid at the absorption site. For example, the solid drug administered orally must dissolve in aqueous fluids of the gastrointestinal tract prior to absorption. Hence, aqueous solubility of the drug is an important consideration influencing drug absorption. As a general rule, aqueous solubility greater than 1 percent (1 g of drug per 100 mL of solution) usually indicates that no potential problems are expected in the absorption of drug due to solubility characteristics of a compound. This solubility limit is an arbitrary guideline based essentially on experience and does not in any way represent a universal limitation in terms of solubility and absorption relationships.

Particle Size: For a drug to be absorbed, it must dissolve in the fluid at the absorption site. Therefore, the particle size of the drug powder used in the formulation of a solid, semi-solid or suspension dosage form can have a significant effect on the availability of drug from the dosage form, especially in those cases where the drug is poorly water soluble. This is because although the particle size of a powder does not influence the extent of solubility of the drug, it does influence the rate at which the particles dissolve in the dissolution medium. When a drug particle is reduced to a large number of smaller particles, the total surface area created is increased. The surface area of spherical particles is related to particle diameter (particle size) by the relationship:

$$\text{surface area} = (\pi)(\text{diameter})^2 \qquad (1\text{-}1)$$

Thus, when a large drug particle is reduced to a large number of smaller particles, the total surface area created is increased and smaller particles dissolve at a faster rate than larger particles. Drugs that are poorly or slowly soluble can generally be dissolved at a faster rate by reducing their particle size. Faster dissolution of poorly water-soluble drugs can be expected to improve their therapeutic response at lower doses with reproducible results. Higher blood levels due to smaller particle size have been reported with such drugs as dicumerol, spironolactone and tolbutamide. Also, increased therapeutic response due to smaller particle size of orally administered drug has been reported for many drugs, notably, griseofulvin, nitrofurantoin, sulfisoxazole and theophylline. Griseofulvin was first marketed to be administered at a dose of 500 mg, but was soon followed by a micronized form with a dose of 250 mg. Inadequate particle size was one cause of relatively poor availability of some generic chloramphenicol capsules, which were recalled several years ago.

The smaller particle size of a drug will not automatically assure faster and better absorption of all drugs. For example, tetracycline hydrochloride can be administered in two different particle sizes and no difference in the concentration of tetracycline in the plasma is obtained. This is because the drug is soluble enough, so that, particle size has no influence on absorption. Smaller particle size can also be disadvantageous for some drugs, e.g. erythromycin base and benzylpenicillin are rapidly destroyed in gastric fluids. Particle size reduction of these drugs will increase their rate of dissolution thereby causing greater inactivation in gastric environment. In this instance, a coarse particle size would slow dissolution rate and thus rate of inactivation and thereby favor improvement in absorption. The size of drug particles is sometimes deliberately increased (e.g. nitrofurantoin is marketed as macrodantin) in order to decrease dissolution rate and hence reduce side effects of the drug.

Polymorphic Form: The occurrence of polymorphic forms with organic compounds is relatively common. Since most drugs are organic compounds, they can exist in more than one polymorphic form. It has been estimated that approximately 70% of drugs exhibit polymorphism. For a large number of drugs, the crystalline or amorphous form of the drug substance has a profound effect on the stability of the drug and its dissolution rate after the drug is ingested. The polymorphic forms of a drug, referred to as the metastable forms, usually differ in their physicochemical properties as compared to the thermodynamically stable crystalline form. In general, polymorphic forms are less stable and have greater solubility and faster dissolution than the crystalline forms. Also, one of the polymorphic forms of a drug may be more suitable for formulation than the other polymorphic forms of the drug. For example, the availability of cortisone acetate and novobiocin is altered by changes in their crystalline forms. Different polymorphic forms exhibit different solubilities, which may differ significantly. Since a more soluble compound has faster rate of dissolution, a product formulated with the metastable polymorphic form of the compound will likely exhibit faster dissolution rate and therefore more predictable and reproducible absorption. Hence, the more soluble polymorphic form is a better candidate for marketing as a drug product, if it is stable at least during the shelf-life of dosage form. The more stable polymorph is marketed because of fear that a less stable one may revert to the less soluble and more stable entity on standing. An example of oral absorption efficiency of polymorphic forms is chloramphenicol, which can exist in three polymorphic forms. Absorption of two of these forms (faster dissolving polymorph B and slower dissolving polymorph A) was studied by comparing mean serum levels of chloramphenicol obtained after oral administration of chloramphenicol palmitate suspension (equivalent to 1.5 g of chloramphenicol) containing either polymorph A or polymorph B. Mean peak levels obtained with these polymorphic forms were: 3 μg/mL from polymorph A and 22 μg/mL from polymorph B. Although polymorph B is less stable than polymorph A, its stability is adequate to permit marketing of an oral suspension. Not all polymorphs of a drug exhibit such dramatic differences in peak plasma concentrations. For example, mefenamic acid exists in two polymorphic forms (polymorph I and polymorph II), but there is no significant difference between *in vivo* absorption characteristics of polymorphs I and II. Cocoa butter is widely used as a suppository base because it melts between 30°C and 35°C. Cocoa butter is a triglyceride (combination of glycerin and one or more different fatty acids) obtained from the roasted seeds of *Theobroma cacao*. When cocoa butter is hastily and carelessly melted at a temperature greatly exceeding its melting point and then quickly chilled, it results in a metastable form (alpha form) with a melting point of about 15°C, which is lower than the melting point of original cocoa butter. This renders the metastable form unsuitable for the preparation of suppositories, because the metastable alpha form does not congeal at room temperature. Although the metastable form eventually converts to the more stable form, the transition may require several days.

Salt Form: Most drugs are either weak organic acids or weak organic bases and are poorly water soluble. They are rarely marketed as in the form of either a weak acid or a weak base. The salt forms of these drugs possess much greater solubility than their respective free acids or bases. Therefore, they are often marketed as salts, because dissolution and absorption rates of monovalent salts of weakly acidic drugs (e.g. sodium or potassium salt) or strong acid salts of weakly basic drugs (e.g. sulfates, hydrochlorides or phosphates) will usually be faster than their corresponding free acids or bases. Examples of acidic and basic drugs, which are marketed as salts include tetracycline hydrochloride, phenobarbital sodium, phenytoin sodium and propoxyphene hydrochloride. The plasma levels of novobiocin (a weakly acidic compound) after oral administration of the drug as a free acid, as a calcium salt or as sodium salt was reported to be 1.5, 10 and 25 μg/mL, respectively. It is not surprising because novobiocin as free acid has a water solubility of 50 μg/mL and the solubility of its monosodium salt is 100 μg/mL. In the case of some drugs, complexation of the drug with ethylenediamine moiety produces a compound, which is more soluble than the free drug. For example, addition of the complexing agent ethylenediamine moiety to theophylline results in a 5-fold increases in the water solubility of theophylline. The use of ethylenediamine salt of theophylline has allowed development of oral aqueous theophylline solutions and therefore avoids the need to use hydroalcoholic mixtures (e.g. elixirs) to formulate pediatric dosage forms of theophylline.

Dissociation Constant: Dissociation constant of a drug (K_a for acidic drugs and K_b for basic drugs) is a parameter commonly used in the pH-partition theory. The dissociation constant is indicative of the extent to which a compound will dissociate into its ionized form and hence this parameter is indicative of drug absorption. The usefulness of dissociation constant is important in assessing the permeability potential of a compound, usually in relation to a series of chemically related compounds, because in most instances, gastrointestinal mucosa generally permits passage of drugs in their unionized (undissociated) form, but restricts entry of the dissociated (ionized) form of the drug. Because dissociation constant is only one of several parameters relating to drug absorption, its value cannot be related directly to absorption of a compound.

Partition Coefficient: Absorption of drug by passive diffusion through a lipoidal barrier and the rate of absorption of drug in solution is a function of partition coefficient (C_{oil}/C_{water}) of drug. Therefore, partition coefficient of drug becomes another important parameter in pH-partition theory of drug absorption. Many investigators have shown a correlation between partition coefficient and rate of absorption of compounds in a homologous series. However, a correlation between partition coefficient and rate of absorption of compounds that are not in a homologous series, is less than satisfactory.

Formulation Factors

Depending on formulation variables used in the preparation of dosage forms of a given drug, the drug may exhibit different degrees of availability, different onsets of action or achieve different plasma concentrations when given by the same route, but in different dosage form. Similarly, differences in the availability of drug from the same dosage form manufactured by different manufacturers may be observed depending on the process variables used in the manufacturing method employed by different manufacturers. As mentioned earlier, there is always the possibility of variation in biological availability of a drug from one batch to another even when the dosage form is made by the same manufacturer.

One of the early decisions that the manufacturer of a new drug product makes is the choice of dosage form in which to formulate the drug. Every effort is made to market the product in a dosage form that will have high acceptance by the patient, the prescriber and the pharmacist. Although solid dosage forms are the dosage forms of choice, some drugs must be formulated as liquid dosage forms, e.g. for infants and young children. Also, some drugs may not be available as a powder, but exist only as a liquid or gas.

A solid dosage form will generally be either a tablet or a capsule. The preparation of an emulsion or suspension dosage form may be limited by stability or taste considerations. In some cases, the ultimate decision in selection of dosage form may have a significant effect on clinical performance of a drug. For example, the dramatic influence of dosage form on drug availability has been demonstrated in the case of indoxole, a low water soluble anti-inflammatory agent. The reported peak plasma concentration of the drug after oral administration in various dosage forms was as follows: soft gelatin capsule is 4.5 μg/mL, emulsion is 4 μg/mL, suspension is 1.5 μg/mL and hard gelatin capsule is 0.5 μg/mL. Hard gelatin capsules performed poorest, perhaps because the drug particles released from hard gelatin capsule must first disperse, become wetted and finally dissolve in the gastrointestinal fluids before becoming available for absorption. Some important formulation factors that may influence the release of drug from the dosage form include: nature of excipients used in the formulation of dosage form, disintegration and hardness of tablet dosage forms and the type of polymer used in the coating of a tablet dosage form.

Excipients: Pharmaceutical dosage forms containing active ingredients also contain a variety of so-called inactive or inert ingredients, commonly referred to as the adjuncts or excipients. These excipients are usually necessary in the formulation of the final product. Each inert ingredient serves a specific function in the formulation of the finished product.

The nature of excipients used in the dosage form that may affect release of drug from the dosage form include: binders, diluents and disintegrants, presence or absence of surface active agents, colorants, preservatives, antioxidants, buffering agents, suspending agents and sweetening agents. These adjuncts can affect bioavailability of drug from the dosage form. For example, some excipients are known to form a complex with some drugs, rendering a portion or the entire administered dose unavailable for absorption. For example, if calcium salts, such as dicalcium phosphate, are used as diluents in tetracycline dosage forms, much lower plasma levels of the drug are obtained after oral administration, because tetracycline forms an insoluble complex with calcium, which prevents drug dissolution and therefore absorption of tetracycline. Hence, tetracycline products should not be ingested with dairy products (milk, cheese, etc.) and other materials containing such metals as Al^{+++}, Fe^{++} or Fe^{+++}. Another example of drug-excipient interaction is amphetamine. Amphetamine interacts with sodium carboxymethylcellulose with a resulting decrease in drug availability. Studies have reported that phenobarbital absorption is reduced when tablets are formulated with polyethylene glycol 4000.

The most common example of an essential excipient in the formulation of tablets and capsules, which has been shown to influence drug availability is the widely used lubricant magnesium stearate. It is perhaps the best lubricant available for use in the tablet and capsule dosage forms, but it is very hydrophobic in nature. Although used in a very small quantity (for most tablet formulations, between 0.5% and 0.75% of the total formulation), if used in a slightly larger quantity, magnesium stearate literally coats drug particles. This coating is water-repellent and renders particles impermeable to dissolution medium. A few other excipients used in tablet and capsule dosage forms (e.g. diluents and binders) have also been reported to affect water permeability, therefore, affecting dissolution, absorption and availability of drug from these dosage forms.

In liquid dosage forms, aqueous solutions provide the fastest absorption of drug, because the drug in this dosage form is available in an absorbable form. Absorption from suspensions is usually slower than from solution dosage forms because absorption from a suspension is a function of dissolution rate of suspended particles in the biological environment. Suspensions contain solid particles, which are not soluble in the medium in which they are placed and because suspension formulations administered orally are prepared in an aqueous medium, therefore, suspended particles are not readily soluble in biological fluids. In emulsion dosage forms, although the drug is present as a solution in water or in oil, absorption of drug depends on partitioning of drug between the aqueous and the lipid phases of the emulsion, i.e. on the relative solubility of drug in the aqueous and lipid media. Drugs, which possess a reasonably good partition coefficient (relatively good solubility in both the lipid as well as the aqueous medium) partition readily and are absorbed relatively faster than drugs, which have poor partition coefficient.

Tablet Hardness and Disintegration: For most conventional tablets, the disintegration time of the tablet depends on compression used during the manufacture of the tablet dosage form (tablet hardness). Generally speaking, higher compressional force tends to produce hard tablets that often disintegrate slowly and lower compressional force tends to produce softer tablets that disintegrate relatively rapidly. Faster disintegration usually results in smaller drug particles producing faster drug dissolution of the drug, resulting in better availability of the drug. In a study, correlating absorption efficiency of a phenoxymethylpenicillin tablet with disintegration time, it was found that disintegration times greater than 10 minutes had significant effect on the availability of drug. The average plasma levels of penicillin in 10 fasted subjects following administration of 400,000 units of potassium phenoxymethylpenicillin tablets having four different disintegration times followed the order:

$$1 \text{ minute} > 10 \text{ minutes} > 30 \text{ minutes} > 75 \text{ minutes}$$

In recent years, some manufacturers have developed disintegrating agents that can cause the tablet to disintegrate completely in just a few seconds regardless of tablet hardness. These disintegrants, (generally referred to as 'super disintegrants') are polymers in nature, which absorb water very rapidly by a capillary action. The absorbed water creates almost instantaneous swelling of the polymer causing the tablet to literally explode into smaller particles. Thus, not only hardness of the tablet, but also the type, quality and the quantity of the disintegrating agent used in the formulation of the tablet may affect the availability of drug from the tablet dosage form.

During the processes of tablet disintegration, drug dissolution and drug absorption, the rate at which the drug reaches systemic circulation is determined by the slowest step in the sequence of these dynamic processes. The slowest step in this sequence is called the rate-limiting step, because the slowest step poses the greatest hurdle in the absorption of drug. Disintegration of a conventional tablet is usually more rapid than drug dissolution and drug absorption. For poorly water-soluble drugs, the dissolution rate is often the slowest step and for drugs that are highly water-soluble, the rate at which the drug crosses the cell membrane is usually the rate-limiting step.

Tablet Coating: Most tablet and capsule manufacturers coat their tablets and capsules (generally with a polymer) for many reasons. Film coating is very popular for conventional dosage forms. The two most common reasons for coating tablets are aesthetic appeal and ease of identification of product. Other less common reasons for coating tablets or capsules are: covering manufacturing defects in a tablet (e.g. mottling and speckling) and masking unpleasant odor or taste. Some tablet and capsule dosage forms are coated with suitable polymers to prevent release of drug from the dosage form in the gastric environment mainly for two reasons:

i. Instability of drug in the acidic medium (enteric coating) or
ii. To provide delayed release of drug from the dosage form.

Some coating solutions used in tablet coating and/or methods used in the application of coating solution have been shown to release drugs incompletely, unevenly or not at all.

In addition to the three most relevant formulation factors discussed above, there are various other formulation factors that may influence the release of drug from given dosage form. Some of these factors may be specific to the specific dosage form, while others may be specific to the specific method of product fabrication. Figure 1-1 is a schematic of release of drug from the popular extravascularly administered dosage forms.

The final step in each of the solid dosage forms is availability of drug in a solution form at the site of absorption. While tablets need disintegration for rapid dissolution of drug, the shell in capsule dosage forms must dissolve before the drug is released for dissolution. Once the drug is released from the capsule or tablet dosage form, it may produce aggregates of powder particles, which must be deaggregated to produce fine particles.

It should be mentioned that in addition to the pharmaceutical factors mentioned above, the availability of drug from the administered dose is also affected by various other factors, including pharmacological factors, physiological factors and biochemical factors.

PHARMACOKINETICS

The term Pharmacokinetics is derived from Greek words, *Pharmakon* (drug) and *Kinesis* (motion, change of rate) and deals with application of kinetics in the study of drug absorption, drug distribution, drug metabolism and drug elimination. This study is sometimes abbreviated as **KADME**, which stands for **K**inetics of **A**bsorption, **D**istribution, **M**etabolism and **E**limination. Essentially, the purpose of pharmacokinetics is to study the time course of amounts and concentrations of drug as well as its metabolites in different tissues in the body and to construct suitable models to interpret the data.

Pharmacokinetics is interrelated with many disciplines, e.g. biopharmaceutics, therapeutics and pharmacology. Although the origin of pharmacokinetics can be traced back to papers

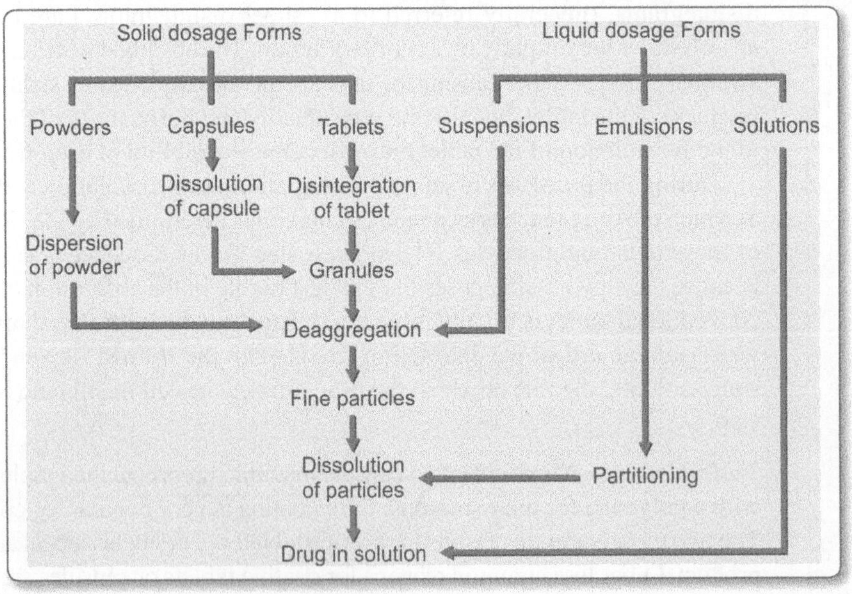

Fig. 1-1 Schematic of release of drug from extravascularly administered dosage forms

published by Professor Theorell in late 1930s, most of its foundation was laid in late 1950s and early 1960s. It continues to be a comparatively young discipline among the health sciences. Two of Professor Theorell's papers were:

1. "Kinetics of distribution of substances administered to the body: I. The extravascular modes of administration," *Arch Int Pharmacodyn*, **56**, 205 (1937), and
2. "Kinetics of distribution of substances administered to the body: II. The intravascular modes of administration, *Arch Int Pharmacodyn,* **57**, 226 (1937).

The first textbook on the subject of pharmacokinetics was published in 1953 ("*Der Blutspeigel*" by Professor FH Dost, Leipzig, Thieme) and the first review of pharmacokinetics in the English language was published 8 years later: "Kinetics of drug absorption, distribution, metabolism and excretion," by E Nelson, *J Pharm Sci.* **50**, 181 (1961). The application of pharmacokinetics in the health sciences, however, made great advances in the seventies, particularly in drug product development and in the treatment of patients in the clinical setting. The development of strong correlations between drug concentrations and their pharmacologic response has enabled clinicians to apply the principles of pharmacokinetics to actual patient situations. An off-shoot of the wide application of this discipline is seen in the evolution of a specialty in the field of pharmacokinetics, which is now recognized as Clinical Pharmacokinetics.

The knowledge of pharmacokinetics can be used for a variety of purposes. These may be clinical in nature, or may be of interest from an industrial and/or formulation stand point. Examples of importance of pharmacokinetics include the following:

a. Estimation of absorption, distribution, metabolism and elimination rates of drug in body.
b. Estimation of bioavailability of drug from multisource products marketed by various manufacturers containing the same drug (bioequivalence).
c. Estimation of bioavailability of drug from different formulations of the same drug.
d. Prediction of concentration of drug in various body tissues, organs and fluids at any time.
e. Optimizing dosage regimen of drugs.
f. Calculation of appropriate dosage regimen for individuals.
g. Determining effect of plasma protein binding of drug on its distribution in the body.
h. Determining effect of food on absorption of drugs.
i. Determining effect of concomitant administration of other drugs on absorption and elimination of drugs.
j. Designing optimal dosage regimen in individual patients.
k. Estimation of accumulation and elimination of drug during renal impairment.
l. Designing of improved drugs and drug products.
m. Estimation of fraction of extravascularly administered dose absorbed by the body.
n. Calculation of pharmacokinetic parameters of drug to describe its time-course in the body.

Pharmacokinetics is a step further towards rational and optimal drug therapy. The goal of application of pharmacokinetics is to assure maintenance of therapeutic drug concentration in the body while preventing danger of toxicity. This is particularly important not only in the severely sick patients, but also during therapy with such life-saving drugs as antibiotics, anticoagulants, antidiabetics and chemotherapeutics.

Pharmacokinetic Parameters

There are many pharmacokinetic parameters, which relate to the kinetics of drug absorption, drug distribution, drug metabolism and drug elimination. Depending on the drug in question and the route of administration of that drug, some pharmacokinetic parameters of the drug may be more relevant than other pharmacokinetic parameters. For example, biological half-life is an important parameter for all drugs, but steady-state plasma concentration of a drug is a more relevant pharmacokinetic parameter for a drug that is administered on a chronic basis than when the same drug is administered for a very short period of time, e.g. as a single dose treatment.

Listed below (in alphabetical order) are some important pharmacokinetic parameters that may be generated following the administration of a drug:

1. Area under the plasma concentration versus time curve (AUC), commonly referred to as area under the curve, is a measure of the extent of drug absorption from the administered drug dose into the systemic circulation.
2. Biological half-life of the drug ($t_{1/2}$) is an indicator of time needed for the plasma drug concentration to decline by 50 percent.
3. Clearance (Cl) is a theoretical concept. This concept is used for describing elimination of drug from the body without identifying the specific mechanism of the process of drug elimination.
4. Fraction of administered dose absorbed (F) is a measure of the extent of administered dose that actually reaches systemic circulation. Sometimes the fraction of dose absorbed is referred to as relative bioavailability or simply bioavailability.
5. Maximum concentration of drug in plasma (C_{max}) is the peak concentration of drug plasma concentration attained after the administration of a given dose.
6. Mean absorption time (MAT) describes the average time for all the drug molecules to be absorbed from the site of administration. Mean absorption time applies only to extravascularly administered drugs.
7. The mean residence time (MRT) of a drug describes the average time for all the drug molecules of a given dose to reside in the body.
8. Rate constant of absorption of drug (K_a) is a measure of the rate at which the drug is absorbed after it has become available for absorption.
9. Rate constant of metabolism of drug (K_m) is a measure of the rate at which the drug is metabolized or biotransformed in the body.
10. Rate constant of elimination of drug (K_e) reflects the rate at which the drug is removed from the body by an excretory process.
11. Rate constants of transfer of drug between plasma and tissues (K_{12}, K_{21}, etc.) indicate rates at which drug moves between plasma and body fluids or tissues.
12. Steady state concentration of drug (C_{ss}) indicates that, upon chronic administration of the drug dose, the concentration of drug in plasma attains a plateau level.
13. Time of maximum concentration of drug in plasma is the time when peak plasma concentration of the drug (C_{max}) occurs.
14. Apparent volume of distribution of the drug (V_d) represents a hypothetical volume of body fluid in which the drug appears to be dissolved or distributed.

The intravascular administration of drug places the drug directly into the systemic circulation. Administration of drug by any one of the extravascular routes (e.g. oral, intramuscular, rectal, subcutaneous, sublingual and transdermal routes) involves an absorption step before the drug can reach systemic circulation. Since a rapidly absorbed drug also exhibits higher concentration in plasma soon after administration, therefore, in extravascular administration, rate of drug absorption also determines the extent to which a drug may reach systemic circulation. Once the drug becomes available in systemic circulation, it reaches biophase, or the site of action to produce its therapeutic action. The site of action is the generic term used by professionals in health care industry, although medicinal chemists and pharmacologists prefer the term receptor site.

From a pharmacokinetic standpoint, biophase is accessible through plasma and drug in plasma is assumed to be in equilibrium with drug in biophase. Therefore, concentration of drug in plasma is often used as an indicator for concentration of drug in biophase. The plasma volume and tissues/fluids with which drug attains instant equilibrium is known as central compartment.

Figure 1-2 is a schematic of pathways of distribution that a drug may take after it has been made available for absorption.

The principles of pharmacokinetics are used in many disciplines. These include: toxicology, drug metabolism, clinical pharmacology, toxicokinetics and clinical pharmacy. This is because scientists in different disciplines look at pharmacokinetics from different view points. For example, some may consider pharmacokinetics as an academic study of relationship between pharmacologic response of a drug dose and the levels of drug and drug metabolite in various body fluids. To some others, the study of pharmacokinetics is important to improve and optimize drug therapy for the therapeutic management of each individual patient. However, pharmacokinetics has been viewed as the field dealing with plasma (or serum) concentration of drug upon administration of a therapeutic drug dose to the human or animal body. This concept is held partly because the major research interest of the pharmaceutical industry is in the development of new drug delivery systems rather in the discovery and synthesis of new chemical compounds. Thus, the synthesis of new prodrugs is aimed at the chemical modification of the compounds which, upon administration, will convert to the active moiety at a desired rate, that is, drug moiety (active ingredient) will be released (or delivered) at the desired rate. The principle of desired rate of release is the basis for research in various drug delivery systems, e.g. prodrugs, osmotic pumps, transdermal drug delivery systems, coated dosage forms, etc.

The pharmacokinetic approach to analyze experimental data obtained from plasma or serum concentration of the drug and to derive pharmacokinetic parameters of the drug is based on the type of pharmacokinetics exhibited by the drug in question. Two types of pharmacokinetics are recognized: linear pharmacokinetics and non-linear pharmacokinetics. Although many drugs exhibit linear pharmacokinetics, some important drugs follow non-linear pharmacokinetics.

Linear Pharmacokinetics

A drug is said to follow linear pharmacokinetics, if the maximum plasma concentration of the drug is directly proportional to the size of drug dose administered. For example, if 50 mg dose of the drug produces a maximum plasma drug concentration of 10 μg/L, then one would expect that by doubling the dose, the maximum plasma drug concentration will also become two-fold, i.e. 100 mg dose of the drug would be expected to produce a maximum plasma drug concentration of 20 μg/L. Similarly, 200 mg dose of the drug would produce a maximum plasma drug concentration of 40 μg/L and 25 mg dose of the drug would produce maximum plasma

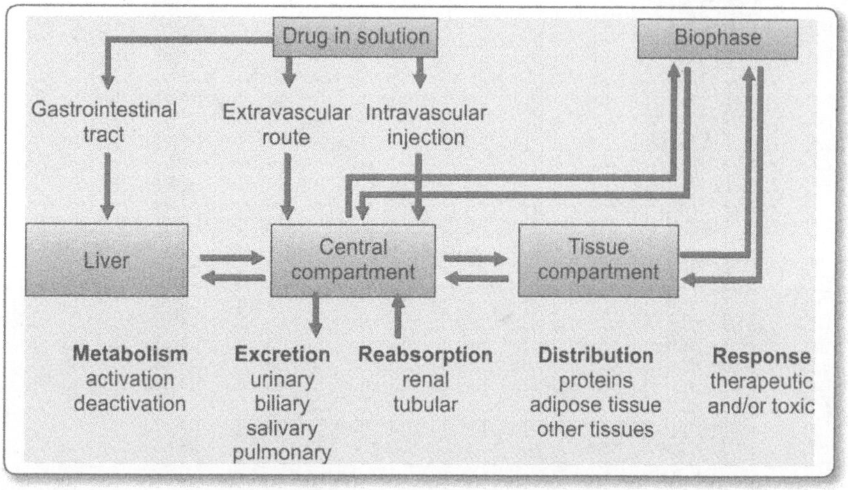

Fig. 1-2 Schematic of pathways of distribution of drugs (*Courtesy:* WH Barr. "Principles of Biopharmaceutics." *Am J Pharm Educ.* 52, 958-81, 1968)

drug concentration of 5 μg/L. That is, the maximum plasma drug concentration will increase or decrease in direct proportion to the size of drug dose administered.

Figure 1-3 is a schematic of linear pharmacokinetics.

If the same drug was given to different patients at different dose levels, the maximum plasma concentration of drug may not necessarily be identical in all patients (due to individual variations), but the maximum drug concentration levels will be expected to change by the same degree as the change in the size of the drug dose. Hence, a plot of the maximum concentration of drug in plasma (or serum) as a function of the size of drug dose administered would be a linear relationship, indicating that the maximum plasma concentration of the drug increases or decreases proportionally according to the size of dose administered. It is due to this linear relationship (between the maximum concentration of drug in plasma and the size of drug dose administered) that the drug is said to follow linear pharmacokinetics.

Non-linear Pharmacokinetics

Most drugs follow linear pharmacokinetics, i.e. they exhibit a change in the maximum plasma drug concentration, which is proportional to the change in the size of the administered dose. However, there are some drugs that do not exhibit a change in the maximum plasma drug concentration with a proportional change in the size of the administered dose. In such cases, a plot of maximum concentration of drug in plasma as a function of size of the dose is not linear and the drug is said to follow non-linear pharmacokinetics or *dose-dependent pharmacokinetics*. Non-linear pharmacokinetics has also been termed *capacity-limited pharmacokinetic* or *saturation pharmacokinetics*. Due to the non-linear kinetic character of drugs that exhibit non-linear pharmacokinetics, it is often very difficult to dose these drugs correctly and efficiently.

Box 1-1 is an alphabetical listing of examples of some drugs, which exhibit non-linear pharmacokinetics.

The main observation in drugs that exhibit non-linear behavior is a change in the value of apparent rate constant of elimination. In addition, non-linear pharmacokinetics also exhibits the following characteristics:

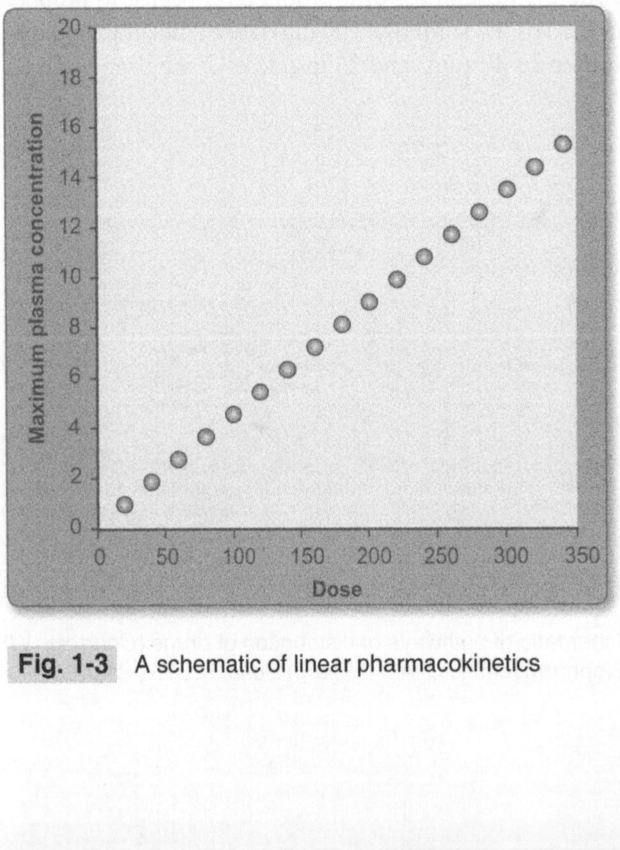

Fig. 1-3 A schematic of linear pharmacokinetics

Box 1-1 Examples of drugs that exhibit non-linear pharmacokinetics

Acetaminophen	Griseofulvin
Alcohol	Iodipamide
p-Aminohippuric acid	Isotretinoin
Ascorbic acid	Lidocaine
Baclofen	Methotrexate
Benzylpenicillin	Mezlocillin
Carbamazepine	Omeprazole
Ceftibuten	Penicillin G
Ceftriaxone	Phenylbutazone
Cephapirin	Phenytoin
Chlorothiazide	Propranolol
Cimetidine	Riboflavin
Danazol	Salicylamide
Dextroamphetamine	Saquinavir
Diazepam	Salicylic acid
Diazoxide	Theophylline
Disopyramide	Valproic acid
L-dopa	Verapamil
Gabapentin	Warfarin

1. Elimination of drug does not follow simple first-order kinetics. Elimination kinetics is non-linear and difficult to predict. Drugs that follow non-linear pharmacokinetics may demonstrate zero-order elimination at very high drug concentration, mix of zero and first order at intermediate drug concentration and first-order elimination at very low drug concentration.
2. The amount of drug excreted in the urine is not proportional to the dose administered.
3. The biological half-life of the drug changes with a change in the dose. Usually, the biological half-life increases with increasing dose, but in some cases, the biological half-life may decrease with increasing dose (e.g. carbamazine).
4. The extent of absorption of drug (area under the curve) is not proportional to the amount of drug available for absorption.
5. The maximum concentration of drug in plasma is not proportional to the size of drug dose administered.
6. The presence of other drugs during treatment with the drug that exhibits non-linear behavior may affect pharmacokinetic parameters of the drug in question. For example, the saturation of capacity-limited processes may be affected by other drugs that require the same enzyme or carrier systems for the transport of drug in question.
7. The composition of the metabolites of the drug in question may be affected by a change in the dose of the drug.

Because drugs that exhibit non-linear pharmacokinetics have a changing value of apparent rate constant of elimination with larger doses of the drug, it becomes very difficult to predict plasma drug concentrations obtained at higher doses of the drug based on plasma drug concentrations obtained at lower dose of the drug. This is due to the fact that plasma drug concentration can increase rapidly once the elimination process gets saturated. If the pharmacokinetic data were estimated only from blood levels obtained with a lower dose of the drug, one would considerably underestimate a variety of other pharmacokinetic parameters, such as the plasma drug concentration, area under the curve and the duration of action of the drug. The disproportional change in the maximum plasma concentration with change in dose can exhibit the following:

Increase in Plasma Concentration: The maximum plasma concentration of the drug does increase with increase in the dose administered, but the increase is more than that would be expected if the drug followed linear pharmacokinetics. The most likely explanation for this type of outcome is that the process of removal of drug from the body has become saturated. Therefore, the removal of drug from the body does not increase with corresponding increase in the concentration of drug in plasma. This phenomenon is known as *saturable pharmacokinetics* or *Michaelis-Menten pharmacokinetics*. Examples of drugs that exhibit this phenomenon include phenytoin and salicylic acid.

Decrease in Plasma Concentration: In some cases, increase in dose of the drug does exhibit an increase in the maximum plasma concentration of the drug, but the increase is less than that would be expected if the drug followed linear pharmacokinetics. When the maximum concentration increases less than that expected after a dosage increase, there are two typical explanations:

i. The drug tends to saturate plasma protein binding sites, so that as the dose is increased, the maximum plasma concentration of drug increases less than expected. Examples of drugs that exhibit this behavior are valproic acid and disopyramide.
ii. Some drugs increase their own rate of metabolism as the drug dose is increased, so that the maximum plasma concentration increases less than anticipated. This process, known as autoinduction of drug metabolism, is exhibited by carbamazepine.

The occurrence of non-linear pharmacokinetics, whether due to the saturation of a process involving drug absorption, binding, first-pass effect or renal excretion of the drug, can have significant clinical consequences. However, non-linear pharmacokinetics may not be noticed in drug studies that use a narrow dose range in patients. In this case, estimation of the dose of a drug based upon narrow dose range studies may result in disproportionate increases in adverse reactions, but insufficient therapeutic benefits. It should be mentioned that non-linear pharmacokinetics can occur anywhere, i.e. above, below or within therapeutic window of the drug.

Figure 1-4 is a schematic exhibiting the typical behavior of linear pharmacokinetics, saturation of binding sites and autoinduction of drug metabolism.

Clinical Pharmacokinetics

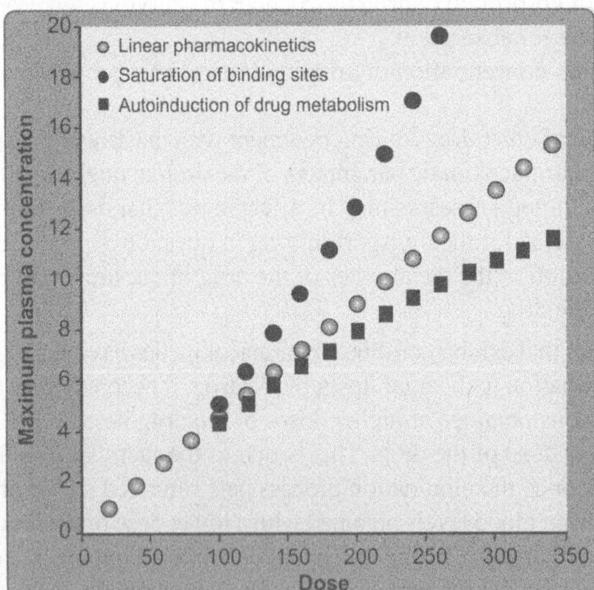

Fig. 1-4 A schematic exhibition of linear pharmacokinetics, saturation of binding sites and autoinduction of drug metabolism

Although the term pharmacokinetics was first used in the 1930s, the discipline of clinical pharmacokinetics had already been introduced in the 1920s by Torsten Theorell, who published many research articles dealing with the kinetics of distribution following extravascular administration. Clinical pharmacokinetics is a rapidly growing area within medical and pharmaceutical fields. It deals with the application of pharmacokinetic principles to therapeutic management of individual patients. The term therapeutic management as used here implies safe and effective therapeutic management.

The study of clinical pharmacokinetics of drugs in disease states requires input from medical as well as pharmaceutical research. Age, gender, obesity, genetic and ethnic differences have been reported to result in pharmacokinetic differences that may ultimately affect the outcome of drug therapy in individual patients. The study of pharmacokinetic differences of drugs in various population groups has been referred to as Population Pharmacokinetics.

A principal application of clinical pharmacokinetics is to optimize drug therapy, i.e. increase effectiveness and/or decrease toxicity of the drug during a patient's drug therapy. Since the magnitudes of both the desired response and toxicity of drug are functions of drug concentration at the site of action, therapeutic failure results when either drug concentration is too low (ineffective therapy) or too high (unacceptable toxicity). In order to achieve therapeutic success, one must maintain plasma drug concentration within therapeutic limits, i.e. greater than minimum effective concentration, but less than toxic levels. While this region (therapeutic window) is wide enough for some drugs, it is often relatively narrow for others. Since, the concentration of drug at site of action can rarely be measured directly, one determines concentration of drug at an alternative and more accessible site, which happens to be plasma for almost all drugs. This is based on the premise that the concentration of drug in plasma is directly related to the concentration of drug at the site of action.

When the therapeutic window of a drug is narrow, the drug has to be administered in small accurate doses for fear that a larger dose may cause unwanted effects or toxic concentrations. If the drug is eliminated rapidly (short half-life), e.g. theophylline, doses are repeated more frequently, but when the drug is eliminated relatively slowly (longer half-life), e.g. digoxin, the drug is administered at less frequent time intervals. Also, if orally administered drug is rapidly metabolized by the liver before it enters general circulation (e.g. morphine), then oral administration would not be the preferred route of administration of these drugs. That is why morphine is administered intramuscularly because it is rapidly metabolized in the liver before entering general circulation. Similarly, the preferred route of self-administration of insulin is subcutaneous injection.

An important problem in drug therapy is variability in drug response, i.e. different individuals responding differently to the same drug administered in the same dose and dosage form by the same route. Some sources of this variability may be patient related (patient's age, weight, degree of obesity, genetic make-up, etc.) or may be due to such factors as the type and degree of severity of disease, other drugs concurrently administered and environmental factors. Thus, the therapeutic response of each individual patient to a given drug dose is not necessarily the same. The therapeutic concentration of drug in the plasma may therefore be different for different people. The drug manufacturers usually publish values of maintenance dose, biological half-life, volume of distribution and therapeutic drug plasma concentrations based on studies on a large population of human subjects. These data reflect an average value for these parameters, which is accompanied with a wide range because individual patient response to a treatment often plays an important role in determination of therapeutic and/or toxic concentrations of drug. Therefore, there may be substantial overlap in values of these concentrations, i.e. therapeutic concentration in one individual may prove to be subtherapeutic or toxic in another. Hence, toxic, therapeutic and subtherapeutic drug concentrations are not necessarily divided by absolute boundaries.

For example, theophylline is recommended at a dose of 100 to 200 mg every 6 hours and its therapeutic concentration has been reported to range between 10 μg/mL and 20 μg/mL. For most patients the concentration of theophylline at levels less than 8 μg/mL is generally considered inadequate for therapeutic effect and concentrations greater than 20 μg/mL are associated with side effects such as nausea and vomiting, nervousness and tachycardia. This means that some patients will respond to the treatment when theophylline concentration in plasma is 10 μg/mL, while others may need as much as 20 μg/mL of theophylline before the drug shows therapeutic effect and yet some may report toxic symptoms even before the concentration of theophylline approaches 20 μg/mL. Hence, determination of optimum dose needed to provide the required therapeutic concentration of theophylline in an individual patient becomes very important.

Similarly, in the case of the antiepileptic drug, phenytoin, although the average plasma concentration of the drug tends to increase with the increase in the rate of drug dosing, there is considerable variation in the individual values of plasma concentration of the drug. In a clinical study, which dealt with a substantially large group of patients, the average steady state concentration of phenytoin in the plasma was determined at a daily dose of 5 mg/kg of body weight. In about 50 percent of the patients in this study, the average steady state concentration of phenytoin in the plasma was found to range between 1 mg/L and 10 mg/L, while in the other 50 percent of the patients, the average steady state concentration of phenytoin in plasma ranged between 10 mg/L and 50 mg/L. In the latter group, a large number of patients had the average steady state phenytoin plasma concentration ranging between 20 mg/L and 30 mg/L. The importance of this study can be appreciated when one considers the fact that the therapeutic window of phenytoin is very narrow, (between about 7 mg/L and about 20 mg/L).

PHARMACODYNAMICS

Pharmacodynamics is defined as the study of biochemical and physiological effects of drugs and their mechanisms of action. This discipline deals with the relationship between concentration of the drug at the site of action and the magnitude of effect produced by the drug. The term magnitude of effect as used here is defined as the intensity and time course of effects (adverse as well as therapeutic) produced by the administered drug dose.

Clearly, there are fundamental differences between the concepts of pharmacodynamics and pharmacokinetics. Pharmacokinetics is primarily concerned with the relationship between concentration of drug in plasma and such variables as the size of dose, dosage form, frequency of administration and route of administration. While pharmacokinetics and pharmacodynamics are complementary, the two terms are not identical. Some practitioners explain the difference as follows: pharmacokinetics deals with the study of concentration of drug and its metabolites in the body fluids and pharmacodynamics deals with the relationship between drug concentration at the site of action and pharmacologic response including biochemical and physiologic effects that influence interaction of drug with the receptor. Another way to differentiate the two terms is to consider differences in their variability. Pharmacokinetic variability means that the same dose of a drug produces different concentrations at the site of pharmacologic effect in different individuals due to interpatient variability in drug absorption, distribution, metabolism and excretion. The pharmacodynamic variability, on the other hand, means that some individuals are more sensitive or more resistant to the effects of the drug than other individuals.

Although pharmacokinetics and pharmacodynamics are complementary, the two terms are not identical in many respects. Some practitioners have used the following statement to explain the difference between pharmacokinetics and pharmacodynamics: If pharmacokinetics is the study of what the body does to the drug, then pharmacodynamics is the study of what the drug does to the body. That is, pharmacokinetics deals with the study of concentration of drug and its metabolites in the body fluids and the study of pharmacodynamics deals with the relationship between drug concentration at the site of action (or the receptor site) and pharmacologic response, including biochemical and physiologic effects that influence the interaction of drug with the receptor. Early pharmacologic research had demonstrated that the pharmacodynamic response produced by the administered dose of a drug was dependent upon the chemical structure of the drug molecules. This research indicated that receptors interacted only with the drugs of specific chemical structure and therefore receptors were classified according to the type of pharmacodynamic response induced.

Figure 1-5 is a schematic of the relationship between the disciplines of pharmacokinetics and pharmacodynamics. While the two disciplines are clearly delineated and are concerned with specific concepts, there is some degree of overlap. Specifically, concentration of drug at receptor site is concerned with both disciplines.

Pharmacodynamics is concerned with interaction between drug and receptors responsible for drug activity. To produce therapeutic or toxic effect, the drug interacts with receptors in the body. A substance that binds to receptors to initiate a response and produces a maximum effect is called a *full agonist*. The term agonist is normally used for a drug, which combines with a receptor to initiate a response, e.g. norepinephrine produces vasoconstriction when it acts upon vascular alpha-adrenergic receptors. A drug, which binds to the receptor and produces less than a maximal effect is called a *partial agonist*. A drug, which binds to the receptor but does not activate second messenger systems to produce biochemical or physiological effect is called an *antagonist*.

An antagonist has the capability to antagonize or oppose the agonist. For example, Atropine has a high affinity for some of the receptor sites responsive to acetylcholine and Atropine competitively prevents acetylcholine from reaching receptor sites. Therefore, Atropine effectively prevents the activity of acetylcholine due to competitive inhibition. Other drugs, which share with Atropine the ability to block access of acetylcholine to its receptors include antihistamines, antiparkinsonian agents, phenothiazines and tricyclic antidepressants (imipramine group). The term antagonist is also used for the drug, which has the capability to antagonize or oppose the agonist.

PHARMACOGENETICS

The term pharmacogenetics describes an area concerned with unusual drug responses that have a genetic or hereditary basis. Much of an individual's pharmacogenetic response reflects genetic difference in foreign chemical metabolism, i.e. a drug may be either detoxified more rapidly or converted to toxic intermediates more efficiently in some individuals than in majority of

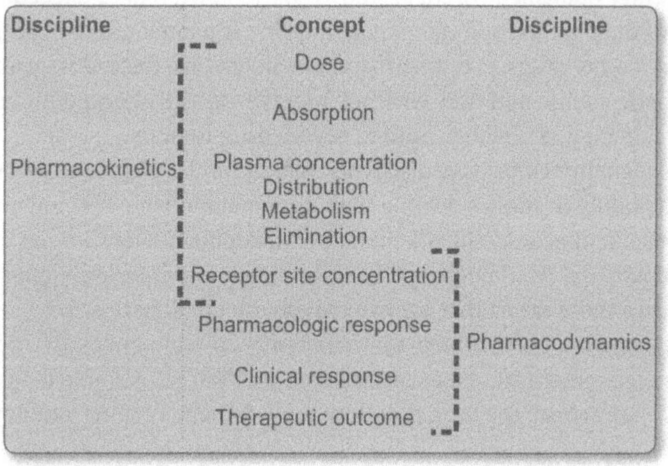

Fig.1-5 Relationship between pharmacokinetics and pharmacodynamics

patients. The difference is referred to as genetic polymorphism. In other words, the differences in response to a drug by different individuals are always modulated by the genetic predisposition of the patient. This observation implies that genes encoding enzymes or proteins that play a role in drug response differ in some respect from one individual to the next.

Drugs which have been shown to exhibit genetic differences include those which exhibit polymorphic acetylation and those which exhibit polymorphic oxidation. Examples of drugs, which exhibit polymorphic acetylation (i.e. undergo N-acetylation), include p-aminosalicylic acid, amrinone (a positive inotropic agent with vasodilatory properties used to a limited extent in the treatment of congestive heart failure), caffeine, dapsone (used in the treatment of leprosy and dermatitis herpetiformis), hydralazine, isoniazid, procainamide (used orally for the treatment of ventricular arrhythmias), sulfadiazine, sulfamethazine and sulfapyridine. Examples of drugs, which exhibit polymorphic oxidation include alprenolol, debrisoquine (an adrenergic blocker used in the treatment of hypertension), diazepam, encainide (a class I antiarrhythmic agent), flecainide (an orally effective antiarrhythmic agent), guanoxan (antihypertensive drug chemically related to debrisoquine and guanethidine), imipramine, metoprolol, phenacetin, phenytoin, propafenone (a new antiarrhythmic agent currently under clinical testing) and timolol.

In the case of isoniazid, the metabolism of the drug is exclusively by the pathway of N-acetylation. The metabolite formed is acetylisoniazid, which is rapidly excreted through the urine. The N-acetylation of the drug has been found to be genetically determined with at least two identifiable groups: those who metabolize it rapidly (rapid acetylators) and those who metabolize it slowly (slow acetylators). Individuals with slow acetylation are prone to isoniazid-induced neurotoxicity. Interestingly, the acetylation rate seems to have an ethnic component. The slowest acetylators are Chinese, Eskimos and Japanese, while rapid acetylators are Egyptians, Finns, Israelis and Scandinavians. Similarly, glucose-6-phosphate-dehydrogenase deficiency has been observed in approximately 10 percent of black American population. Another drug, which exhibits differences in metabolism due to ethnic background is phenytoin. In the case of phenytoin, two phenotypes are identified—efficient metabolizers (extensive metabolizers or rapid metabolizers) and poor metabolizers. The poor metabolizing frequency in caucasians is about 4 percent and among Japanese about 16 percent.

The exceedingly fast action and short duration of skeletal muscle relaxant succinylcholine is attributed to its rapid hydrolysis by plasma esterase. In some patients (about 0.03%), succinylcholine has a prolonged effect that appears to be due to the presence of a genetically determined 'abnormal' plasma esterase that degrades the drug slowly and inefficiently.

A recently published Swedish study reported differences exceeding 100-fold in the plasma half-life of the psychotropic agent nortriptyline in a large group of patients. Since this drug, like a number of other drugs, is ordinarily administered on a fixed-dosage schedule, fast-metabolizers will be undermedicated and will not receive its full therapeutic advantage, whereas slow metabolizers may experience mild to severe drug toxicity.

It is evident from the above discussion that examples of genetic variability in pharmacokinetics are found mainly in studies dealing with drug metabolism. This indicates that renal excretion of drugs does not appear to show genetic polymorphism. Hence renal clearance of drugs that are predominantly excreted unchanged exhibit much less interindividual variability in metabolism kinetics than those drugs that are extensively metabolized.

Genetics also contributes to variability in the senses of individuals. For example, approximately one-third of the caucasian population are not able to taste thiocyanate groups and therefore, fail to taste the drug polythiouracil, which contains a thiocyanate groups.

TOXICOKINETICS

Toxicokinetics, as the name suggests is the kinetics of toxicity. The term toxicokinetics refers to the study of kinetics of absorption, distribution and excretion of drugs at high doses, in other words, it is the application of pharmacokinetics to toxicology. Toxicokinetic studies are conducted to determine how blood levels of a drug relate to toxicity. The main distinction between toxicokinetics and the more traditional pharmacokinetics is the doses used in these studies. In pharmacokinetic studies the size of dose used is determined by the pharmacologic response and in toxicokinetic studies the dose used is substantially greater than that likely to be administered to humans.

Toxicokinetic data are usually obtained during the course of toxicology studies using the best available animal models. If performed early in the development of a new drug, toxicokinetic data can provide valuable information in testing the safety of a drug. For example, these studies can help predict whether or not the unexpected toxicity is due to excessive doses and also determine whether the lack of toxicity is due to lack of drug absorption. It is believed by some that properly designed toxicokinetic studies may help reduce the numbers of test animals required for safety evaluation of the drug.

Toxicokinetic studies play a vital role both during the preclinical phase of drug development as well as in chronic toxicological evaluation of the drug. The importance of toxicokinetic studies at early preclinical stage is to determine the effect of administered dose of the drug on systematic exposure in test animals. In chronic toxicology studies, toxicokinetic procedures are used to monitor the dose-related continuous exposure of animals to the drug. This also helps to relate any unusual drug accumulation with the aging process.

Many toxicological methods used for assessing the safety of a drug during the preclinical stages of drug development may possibly be limited in their usefulness. This is due to the fact that a large number of these studies are based on many assumptions. Of the various assumptions, the following two assumptions are the major assumptions:

i After administration of the dose, drugs are completely absorbed
ii Test animals handle high and low doses of the drug in a similar manner.

In addition to these and other assumptions made in toxicological methods used for assessing drug safety at the preclinical stages, these studies fail to take species differences into account.

Sometimes the development of a new drug is abandoned when an unusual toxicity is encountered. In some of these cases the toxicity may very well have been due to the exaggerated dose, or perhaps due to the formation of a toxic metabolite specific to the species being tested.

It is a known fact that most experimental animals and humans differ to some extent in size and weight. This disparity can result in significant species differences in the metabolism of certain drugs. For example, different metabolites might be formed, or similar metabolites might be formed at different rates in different animals (i.e. species differences). It has been reported that the metabolism of drugs usually occurs at higher rates in rodents than in humans. This is due to a number of factors, but notably due to higher ratio of liver to body weight in rodents, larger relative amount of liver cytochrome P450, more rapid circulation time and oxygen tension, which affects enzyme activity. Therefore, these differences, which can modify the effects of toxic metabolites in rodents, must be considered when data from animals studies are extrapolated for interpretation in humans.

Similarly, rodents tend to clear drugs more rapidly than humans. Such rapid clearance of the drug can lead to a failure to maintain adequate exposure of drug in the test animals during the dosing interval. The data thus generated therefore should not be extrapolated to humans because human therapy is generally designed to provide continuous drug exposure. Similarly, when interpreting toxicity data from data obtained from animal studies and extrapolating these data to humans, species differences in such areas as protein building, receptor properties and metabolic profiles should be considered. For example, some drugs bind extensively to plasma proteins and thereby become inactive pharmacologically since the activity of the drug is related to the availability of free drug at the receptor site. In some drugs the extent of binding may decrease as the dose is increased and when that happens a disproportionately higher concentration of the biologically active compound (drug) may be in circulation at higher dose levels than at lower doses. This drug may therefore be more toxic than suggested by data based on dose levels alone.

Another term frequently encountered in toxicokinetic studies is clinical toxicology. Clinical toxicology is the study of adverse effects of drugs and toxic substances (usually poisons) in the body. The pharmacokinetics of a drug in an over-medicated (or intoxicated) individual may be very different from the pharmacokinetics of the same drug administered in therapeutic doses. At very high doses, the concentration of drug in the body may saturate enzymes involved in the processes of absorption, biotransformation or renal secretion mechanisms. This may change the pharmacokinetics from linear to non-linear pharmacokinetics. Drugs frequently involved in toxicity cases include acetaminophen, salicylates, morphine and tricyclic antidepressants.

LEGAL DEFINITIONS

The commonly used terms such as drug, cosmetic, food, vitamins and device mean different things to different people. For example, many believe that a drug is a substance prescribed by a physician and is used to treat an infection or a disease. Similarly, many people do not consider a non-prescription product as a drug, even though almost all non-prescription products contain drugs. The logic used by most people is that since these products are sold over-the-counter and do not require a prescription, these are not drugs. This is especially true for the elderly, who are most susceptible to take many prescription and non-prescription products for a variety of ailments. Therefore, this segment of our human population is at a greater risk of drug interactions because in most cases their physicians may have no knowledge as to the types and/or quantities of other products that the patient may be consuming. Also, most elderly usually do not follow recommended dosage regimen of non-prescription product, perhaps because they do not consider over-the-counter products as a drug product.

Drug interaction is a phenomenon, which occurs when the effect of one drug is modified by the presence of another drug. A study published in 1964 reported that hospitalized patients receive an average of 14 different medications during their stay in the hospital. Fortunately, there has been an increasing awareness of drug interactions in recent years.

The over-usage of drug products in the 1960s was the topic of a presentation made in 1968 by Dr Knyvett of Australian Royal Brisbane Hospital. In his presentation, Dr Knyvett addressed the status of over-usage of drug products in 1960s as follows: He pointed out that the decade of the 1960s were the era of symptomatic therapy in medicine. According to him, this was the basic factor underlying modern drug usage. He stated that the over-usage of drug products was not only because of the fact that the physicians were prescribing enormous amounts of drugs, but also because some patients were also self-medicating themselves heavily. It was his view that apparently many people seemed to have some sort of a psychological need for taking medication for every ailment, regardless of whether the ailment was real or imaginary. Dr Knyvett cited an example of treatment for common cold. He stated that if a person has common cold, the best treatment is to take aspirin, drink plenty of fluids, ingest a good dose of vitamin C and take complete bed rest. But a physician is not likely to give the same advice because the patient would not be happy.

Experience indicates that a patient treated at a physician's office or in a hospital would be prescribed a regimen entirely different than self-medication and likely to be much more intensive than that used in a typical patient self-treatment. Treatment by a physician may include some or all of the drugs shown in Table 1-1.

Although each one of the preparations prescribed by the physician can be justified based upon their symptomatic value, every one of these may on some occasions produce side effects and many of these drugs, if administered concurrently, may give rise to drug interactions. Many patients do not inform their health provider that they may be self-medicating themselves with over-the-counter products for pain or mild arthritis (Aspirin, acetaminophen or Ibuprofen), anti-allergy products (antihistamines, e.g. diphenhydramine hydrochloride) or a stool softener. The risk of excessive medication intake by the patient and possible drug interactions is increased without the knowledge of the physician or pharmacist.

It is only in recent years that people have become aware of the fact that caffeine in soft drinks and nicotine in cigarettes are addictive drugs. However, consumers of alcoholic drinks do not associate ingestion of alcoholic drinks as ingestion of the addictive drug alcohol.

The term cosmetic is generally associated with products marketed and advertised by the cosmetic industry. They are generally considered beautifying agents. These products are used primarily by younger generation, although many elderly also use these products. Most consumers do not consider a bar of soap as a cosmetic product, but if a cosmetic company markets a bar of soap, some people would consider it a cosmetic product. Similarly, talcum powder is generally not considered a cosmetic except when a talcum body powder is marketed by a cosmetic company, is vigorously advertised and is sold at a higher price.

The term food, to most people is something solid that is eaten when one is hungry. The use of this term is usually limited to solids only because ingestion of liquid preparations is generally associated with thirst-quenching. Thus, almost all liquid preparations are not perceived as food, although some liquid preparations may contain nourishing ingredients, which are in reality foods (e.g. liquid food preparations and nourishment supplements used in geriatric and pediatric population and intravenous infusion of total parenteral nutrition). Chewing gum, according to legal definition, is considered a food, but the general concept of a chewing gum was that it is a harmless and inert chewable, chewed merely as a habit, or something used simply to exercise gums. Some will label chewing gum as a breath-freshening device or a substitute for mouthwash.

Vitamins have always been previously considered as essential ingredients for growth. In the past many people were afraid to admit that they were taking vitamins, because it was generally believed that anybody taking vitamin was unhealthy or suffering from deficiency or malnourishment. Vitamins are now considered food supplements by some and an essential health resource by others. The intake of vitamins is considered a healthy practice for maintaining good health, improving vitality and assuring better quality of life.

Table 1-1 Self-treatment versus physician treatment

Possible self-treatment	*Possible physician treatment*
1. Aspirin	1. Compound codeine tablets (for aches and pain)
2. Plenty of fluids	2. Nose drops (to free nasal airways)
3. Favorite alcoholic beverage	3. Antihistamine (to reduce nasal "allergic" congestion)
4. Bed rest	4. An inhalant (to reduce nasal "allergic" congestion)
	5. Antitussive syrup (to ease present or anticipated cough)
	6. Antibiotic (to prevent "secondary" infection)
	7. Sleeping pills (to ensure restful nights)
	8. Laxative (for constipating effects of codeine and fever)

The term device appears to have no meaning to a majority of people. Some may believe that the term device is used to indicate some kind of a machine or an instrument, which is used by certain specialists essentially for diagnostic or treatment purposes.

From a legal standpoint, the terms drug, cosmetic, food and vitamin, have specific meaning, use and applications. The legal definitions of these terms are:

Drug

The legal definition of the term drug includes the following:

A. *Articles recognized in USP, NF, official Homeopathic Pharmacopeia or supplements thereof.*
B. *Articles intended for use in the diagnosis, cure, mitigation, treatment or prevention of disease in man or other animals (mammals understood).*
C. *Articles (other than food) intended to affect the structure or any function of the body of man or other animals.*
D. *Articles intended for use as a component of any article specified in A, B or C above, but does not include any of their components, accessories, or parts.*

According to the official definition, therefore, the term *drug* is not limited to the common belief that a drug is a chemical entity manufactured by a pharmaceutical firm for the treatment of a disease or condition (for example, aspirin, acetaminophen or ibuprofen) or used to alleviate a certain undesirable condition, or used in the prevention of a disease (for example, a vaccine). As can be seen from the definition of the term *drug*, the term *drug* also includes those substances which may in one way or another affect body function and structure. Substances and articles, which may be used for diagnostic purposes are also included in the legal definition of the term *drug*.

Food

The term food includes:

Articles used for food or drink for man or other animals, chewing gum and articles used for components of food, drink or chewing gum.

Thus, the term *food* includes a large variety of substances and is not limited to what is considered food *per se*, as most people would think. The term *food* also includes substances, which are usually not considered food by a large majority of people. For example, the term *food* includes substances used not only for humans, but also for animals and articles used not only for food, but also for drink. Also included in the term *food* are substances, which are not food *per se*, but are used as components in the preparation of food. It should be mentioned, however, that although chewing gum is considered food, chewing gums containing therapeutic agents (e.g. the popular chewing gum containing aspirin) are not considered food, but are treated as a drug. This is because the chewing gum used with these products signifies that the gum is simply the delivery system for the therapeutic agent contained on the chewing gum.

Device

The term device includes:

Instruments, apparatus, contrivances including components, parts and accessories used in B or C above.

According to the official definition, the term *device* excludes chemical entities used in the diagnosis of disease because such entities are included in the definition of *drug* and therefore are considered as drugs. The term device, however, certainly includes non-chemical entities and articles used in the diagnosis, cure, treatment, or prevention of disease, or affect body function or structure. These non-chemical articles may be physical, mechanical or electronic in nature.

Cosmetic

The term cosmetic includes:

> *Articles intended to be rubbed, poured, sprinkled or sprayed on, introduced into or otherwise applied to the human body or any part thereof for cleansing, beautifying, promoting attractiveness or altering the appearance (excluding soap) and articles intended for use as components.*

As can be noticed from this definition, the term *cosmetic* covers a broad spectrum of substances, which are used for a variety of purposes and treatment. According to the definition, the term cosmetic does not use the word treatment in its definition because cosmetics are not considered as treatment in the sense of treatment with a drug, although some cosmetic products are advertised as 'treatments', e.g. wrinkle remover, etc. Such claims should not be made by the manufacturer unless the product is approved as drug. The definition also excludes soaps, because common soaps serve hygienic functions and medicated soaps are used essentially for therapeutic purposes.

Vitamin

Vitamins are generally regarded as organic compounds that are essential for the maintenance of normal metabolic functions, growth and maintenance of life. While some vitamins are used in larger doses (e.g. vitamin C), many vitamins, especially those belonging to the family of vitamin B-complex group, are used in relatively smaller amounts. Vitamins, as a rule, do not furnish energy (as advertised by many misguided health-food providers), but they are essential for the transformation of energy and for regulation of metabolism of structural units. This view is supported by researchers who have shown a relationship between maintenance of an optimal state of health and good nutritional practices.

Recent years have seen tremendous growth and popularity of 'health-food stores' specializing in selling nutritional supplements and herbal medications. Most of these stores are operated by merchants who are not knowledgeable and are not very well versed in the science of nutrition. They promote vitamins and minerals not only as dietary supplements, but also for the treatment of various diseases and conditions that are not approved by the official regulatory agencies. Presently, the Food and Drug Administration (FDA) has very little, if any, regulatory authority over the manufacturers of vitamin supplements and that is perhaps the reason that these manufacturers are able to make substantial claims concerning the effectiveness of their products in the treatment and/or prevention of disease or disease condition.

Since, vitamins are freely available over-the-counter. A large majority of people take vitamins as per the directions on the label of these products, without regard to the amount of a particular vitamin that should be taken per dose or per day. Until a few years ago, physicians were reluctant to recommend, much less prescribe vitamins .as a nutritional supplement. As one friendly physician graciously confided, "physicians do not prescribe vitamins for a variety of reasons: first of all, the role of vitamins in nutrition or prevention of disease is not adequately covered in the curriculum of medical schools. Although a large majority of physicians recognize the importance of vitamins, they are reluctant to prescribe vitamins because most people come to a physician looking for a prescription for a drug. Physicians recommend acetaminophen or ibuprofen as an analgesic rather than Aspirin, because most people may have taken aspirin on their own before coming to the physician and expect the physician to recommend something other than what they have already taken. People do not think that vitamins can also work as drugs in the treatment of a disease or condition. Physicians would start prescribing vitamins the day they are allowed to charge a fee for a prescription of vitamins."

With the exception of vitamin K and high doses of vitamins A and D, vitamins are considered by the FDA to be food supplements. Although the term high doses of vitamin A and vitamin D is not specifically defined, but it is understood to mean a dose much greater than the usual daily recommended dose as a food supplement.

Vitamin K is excluded from the term *vitamin* because of lack of information concerning its human intake. The primary activity, which makes vitamin K essential in human metabolism is its involvement in the blood-clotting system, since vitamin K is a pre-cofactor in the synthesis of prothrombin and other clotting factors. The dietary allowance for vitamin K is relatively small. It is believed that an average diet contains adequate amounts of vitamin K making it unnecessary to administer supplemental quantities. This is based on the fact that few (if any) malnourished humans have presented findings of dietary lack of vitamin K. However, if deficiency of vitamin K does occur, the deficiency appears to be primarily due to two reasons—malabsorption or lack of bile. Malabsorption is associated with such conditions as celiac disease, steatorrhea, spru, extensive resection of small intestine, etc. Lack of bile is associated with obstructive jaundice, biliary fistulae. Such a deficiency is unlikely to occur because intestinal bacteria synthesize vitamin K. Also, vitamin K is relatively non-toxic even in extremely high doses. High doses of vitamins A and D are excluded from the term *vitamin* because of potential toxicity caused by these vitamins at high doses.

Vitamin A is an over-the-counter product, available in varying strengths, but most popularly as 5,000 IU tablets and 10,000 IU capsules. It is also a prescription item in 25,000 IU and 50,000 IU capsules. Although vitamin A is essential for vision (it plays an essential role in the function of the retina), dental development and for growth and reproduction, acute and chronic vitamin A toxicity is well recognized in adults. Acute poisoning may occur after a single dose in excess of 1,000,000 units. The chronic toxicity of vitamin A is determined by the dose and duration of ingestion. Chronic administration of 25,000 to 50,000 IU daily for several months has shown to induce pathologic changes in bone and periosteal tissues, liver, skin and mucous membrane and changes in behavior. Other common symptoms from chronic use of vitamin A include fatigue, dizziness, nausea, vomiting, drying and/or cracking of skin and/or lips, inflammation of tongue and/or gums, loss of hair, night sweats and irritability. Recent studies indicate that excessive intake of vitamin A during pregnancy could be a teratogenic risk. However, a daily dose of less than 10,000 IU is believed to be non-teratogenic.

Vitamin D is considered a hormone rather than a vitamin, although it is not a natural hormone. It is available over-the-counter. Vitamin D is essential for the absorption and utilization of calcium and phosphate, normal calcification of bone and regulation of serum calcium concentration. Absorption of calcium in the duodenum is an active process facilitated by vitamin D, with calcium absorption as much as four times more than that in vitamin D deficiency states. It is believed that calcium-binding protein, which increases after vitamin D administration, binds calcium in the intestinal cell and transfers it out of the base of the cell to the blood circulation. Vitamin D has been used for the prevention and treatment of rickets or osteomalacia and in the management of hypocalcemia associated with hypothyroidism.

Tolerance to vitamin D varies widely. Large doses of vitamin D (more than 50,000 IU/day) have the potential to result in toxicity. Symptoms of vitamin D toxicity include anorexia, diarrhea, vomiting, weakness, mental changes and proteinuria. The early signs of over dosage

Table 1-2 Dietary allowance for vitamins A, D and K

Age	*Vitamin A (IU)*	*Vitamin D (IU)*	*Vitamin K (IU)*
Infants	625	300–400	5–10
Children	700–1200	400	40–45
Adults			
Males	1,700	400–200	45–80
Females	1,300	400–200	45–65
Pregnant	1,300	400	65
Lactating	2,000	400	65

of vitamin D are manifested as weakness, headache, somnolence, nausea, vomiting, dry mouth, constipation, muscle and bone pain and metallic taste sensation. Later signs of over dosage of vitamin D are evidenced by anorexia, weight loss, nocturia, photophobia, pruritus, disorientation, hallucinations, hyperthermia, hypertension and cardiac arrhythmias.

High doses of vitamin D ingested over a long period of time (long-term consumption of 1,000 IU/kg per day) have resulted in hypertension, anorexia and hypercalcemia and attendant complications, such as metastatic calcification and renal calculi. Prolonged hypercalcemia may result in calcification of soft tissue including renal tubules, lungs, heart and blood vessels, resulting in death due to cardiovascular or renal failure.

Table 1-2 shows dietary allowance for vitamins A, D and K for various age groups. These recommendations were published by the National Academy of Sciences.

SUGGESTED READING

1. Ariens E, ed. Drug Design. Academic Press; 1971.
2. BE. Ballard. Teaching Biopharmaceutics at the University of California. Amer J Pharm Ed. 1968;32:939-57.
3. Batra VK, Yacobi A. An overview of toxicokinetics. In: Yocobi A, Skelly JP, Batra VK (Eds). Toxicokinetics and New Drug Development. Pergamon Press; 1989.
4. Cluff LE, Thouton GF, Seidl LG. Studies on the epidemiology of adverse drug reactions. J Am Med Assoc. 1964;188:976-83.
5. Dost FH. Der Blutspiegal. Leipzig: Thieme; 1953.
6. Nelson E. Kinetics of drug absorption, distribution, metabolism and excretion. J Pharm *Sci.* 1961;50:181-92.
7. Theorell T. Kinetics of distribution of substances administered to the body: I. The extravascular modes of administration. Arch Int Pharmacodyn. 1937;57:205.
8. Theorell T. Kinetics of distribution of substances administered to the body: II. The intravascular modes of administration. Arch Int Pharmacodyn. 1937;57:226.
9. Wagner J. Biopharmaceutics and Relevant Pharmacokinetics. Drug Intelligence Publications. 1971.
10. Wagner JG. Biopharmaceutics: Absorption Aspects. J Pharm Sci. 1961;50:359-89.
11. Wagner J. Fundamentals of Clinical Pharmacokinetics. Drug Intelligence Publications. 1979.
12. Wagner J. Pharmacokinetics. Annual Review Pharmacol. 1968;8:67-94.

CHAPTER 2

MATHEMATICAL CONCEPTS

As defined in Chapter 1, the study of pharmacokinetics involves the application of principles of kinetics. The principles of kinetics, in most cases, involve rather extensive use of logarithms, as well as construction of graphs with the data in order to obtain a clear and comprehensive picture of the data. This is important, because in most cases raw data are difficult to comprehend. Even in a tabular form, the raw data do not present a clear picture. When it is very difficult to comprehend raw data, any conclusions drawn from the raw data are a gross approximation at best.

In constructing graphs, an effort is made to obtain a linear relationship between the variables. Sometimes, a linear relationship can be obtained with data as presented, but at other times, a linear relationship can be obtained only if logarithms of concentration terms are used. If it is not possible to obtain a straight line, one may settle for a smooth curve, because even a smooth curve permits a much better understanding of relationship between the variables than looking at raw data in a tabular form. Constructing a graph to obtain a linear relationship between variables under study offers several advantages. For example, a graph expressing the concentration of drug or the amount of drug as a function of time can be used to predict the value of one variable (e.g. concentration of drug in plasma) at a given value of the other function (e.g. time after administration of the dose). More importantly, a linear relationship affords the opportunity to express the relationship between variables as a mathematical equation, which can then be used to predict the connection between variables in a scientific manner.

LOGARITHMS

Logarithms were invented more than 3 centuries ago. The invention of logarithms was more of a necessity than a luxury. At that time, calculators were not available to carry out difficult calculations and logarithms provided a relatively simple means of conducting time-consuming lengthy and complicated calculations. Logarithms were also used as a convenient means of expressing very large or very small numbers in a simple fashion. For example, a small number, such as concentration of hydronium ions in a dilute solution may be expressed as a decimal fraction, e.g.,

0.000032 moles/L may be expressed as (or 3.2×10^{-5} moles/L)

or one can express this in logarithmic fashion on the pH scale as a solution having a pH of 4.5;

$$-\log[H_3O^+] = pH$$

$$-\log 3.2 \times 10^{-5} = 5 - 0.5 = 4.5$$

Because logarithms convert a relatively very small number into a more conveniently expressible number, logarithms have no units and are considered as real numbers. Logarithms are exponential functions. Logarithms play an important role in pharmacokinetic calculations, because the pharmacokinetics of various rate processes, such as absorption, metabolism, distribution and elimination, etc. tends to be exponential in nature.

Definition

The logarithm of a number is defined as the exponent of the power to which a given base must be raised in order to equal that number. For example, in the equity

$$a^b = x \tag{2-1}$$

a = base, b = exponent and x = the number

Therefore, by definition, this equity is expressed in the logarithmic notation as

$$\log_a x = b \tag{2-2}$$

The exponent b to which the base a is raised to give x in equation (2-1) is referred to as the logarithm of x.

Since the logarithm of x is b, therefore, b is known as the antilogarithm of x. For example, the equity $10^2 = 100$ is expressed in the logarithmic notation as $\log_{10} 100 = 2$ and as before, the exponent 2 to which the base 10 is raised to give the value 100 is referred to as the logarithm of 100. Since the logarithm of 100 is 2, therefore 2 is known as the antilogarithm of 100. Similarly, the equity $4^3 = 64$ can be expressed in the logarithmic notation as $\log_4 64 = 3$. The exponent 3 to which the base 4 is raised to give the value 64 is therefore the logarithm of 64. As above, since the logarithm of 64 is 3, therefore 3 is the antilogarithm of 64.

Origin

Logarithms were invented by John Napier of Scotland more than 300 years ago. He used natural log number, 2.718281828..... as the base for his logarithms. The natural log number is the quantity a in equation (2-2). A few years later, Henry Briggs used Napier's discovery and instead of using the natural log number, Briggs introduced 10 as the base for his logarithms. Napier's system of logarithms is called Napierian logarithms or natural logarithms, because it uses the natural log number as the base. Napier's system is favored by Physical Chemists and is used extensively in pharmacokinetics. Briggs' system is favored by Biological Scientists and is widely used for computation purposes. It is known as the Briggsian logarithms or common logarithms.

Common Logarithms

Common logarithms, also known as Briggsian logarithms use 10 as the base. The base 10 is the quantity a in equation (2-2). Therefore, equation (2-2) in common logarithms is:

$$\log_{10} x = b \tag{2-3}$$

As a general practice, when common logarithms are written as log, it is understood that the term *log* represents common logarithms and therefore, base 10 is not written. Equation (2-3) is generally written as,

$$\log x = b \tag{2-4}$$

Thus, in common logarithms, $\log_{10} 100 = 2$ is frequently written as $\log 100 = 2$ and this would indicate that $10^2 = 100$. Since $10^0 = 1$, therefore, $\log 1 = 0$.

Natural Logarithms

Natural logarithms are also known as Napierian logarithms. Since the base used in natural (or Napierian) logarithms is the irrational = number 2.7182818.., (designated e), equation (2-2) in natural logarithms is written as,

$$\log_e x = b \tag{2-5}$$

As a general practice, the base e must be written if natural logarithms are abbreviated as log. If one does not want to write the base e, then instead of writing log, one writes ln. Thus, equation (2-5) may be written as:

$$\ln x = b \tag{2-6}$$

Equation (2-6) indicates that $e^b = x$. Thus, ln 100 = 4.605 means $e^{4.605} = 100$ and $e^{4.605}$ means $(2.71828.....)^{4.605}$. Therefore, $(2.71828.....)^{4.605} = 100$.

Since $e^0 = 1$, therefore, ln 1 = 0.

The natural log number, (the quantity e used as the base in natural logarithms), is defined as the limit of the series $\{1 + (1/n)\}$, where n is made larger and larger. The value of this series, as the value of n is increased has been calculated to be 2.718281828...... from the sum of the following series:

$$1+\frac{1}{1}+\frac{1}{1\times 2}+\frac{1}{1\times 2\times 3}+\frac{1}{1\times 2\times 3\times 4}+\frac{1}{1\times 2\times 3\times 4\times 5}+\ldots$$

When n is equal to 1, $\{1 + (1/n)\}^n = \{1 + (1/1)\}^1 = 2.000$

When n is equal to 100, $\{1 + (1/n)\}^n$ is equal to $\{1 + (1/100)\}^{100} = 2.70481$

The value of $\{1 + (1/n)\}^n$ becomes larger as the value of n is increased and when n approaches infinity, the value of $\{1 + (1/n)\}^n$ reaches its limiting value of 2.71828.

Table 2-1 shows how the value 2.71828.... is calculated.

Table 2-1 Calculations of $\left(1+\frac{1}{n}\right)^n$ for increasing values of *n*

n	$\left(1+\frac{1}{n}\right)^n$	*Numerical value*
1	$\left(1+\frac{1}{n}\right)^1$	2.00000
2	$\left(1+\frac{1}{n}\right)^2$	2.25000
5	$\left(1+\frac{1}{n}\right)^5$	2.48832
10	$\left(1+\frac{1}{n}\right)^{10}$	2.59374
100	$\left(1+\frac{1}{n}\right)^{100}$	2.70481
1,000	$\left(1+\frac{1}{n}\right)^{1,000}$	2.71692
10,000	$\left(1+\frac{1}{n}\right)^{10,000}$	2.71815
50,000	$\left(1+\frac{1}{n}\right)^{50,000}$	2.71825
100,000	$\left(1+\frac{1}{n}\right)^{100,000}$	2.71827
500,000	$\left(1+\frac{1}{n}\right)^{500,000}$	2.71828
1,000,000	$\left(1+\frac{1}{n}\right)^{1,000,000}$	2.71828
Infinity	$\left(1+\frac{1}{n}\right)^{\infty}$	2.71828

Rules

As mentioned earlier, logarithms were invented at a time when sophisticated calculators were not available for difficult and time-consuming calculations. Logarithms provided a relatively simple means of conducting time-consuming, lengthy and complicated calculations. Using logarithms, one could convert calculations dealing with multiplications into simple additions, calculations dealing with divisions into simple subtractions and calculations dealing with exponential terms into simple multiplication of terms. As with any other science, logarithms follow specific rules. These rules are similar for natural logarithms, as well as for common logarithms. The more important rules are given in Table 2-2.

Example 2-1 Calculate the common logarithm of $\frac{1}{5.932}$

Solution

This problem can be solved in two ways:

a. Apply the rule:

$$\log\frac{1}{a} = -\log a$$

$$\log\frac{1}{5.932} = -\log(5.932) = -0.7732$$

b. Apply the rule:

$$\log\frac{a}{b} = \log a - \log b$$

$$\log\frac{1}{5.932} = \log(1) - \log(5.932) = 0 - 0.7732 = -0.7732$$

Example 2-2 Calculate the natural logarithm of $\frac{(5.893)(2.716)(5.932+1.187)}{(4.893)(2.875)}$

Solution

Two rules apply in solving this problem:

Rule # 1: $\ln\frac{a}{b} = \ln a - \ln b$

Table 2-2 Important rules of logarithms

Common logarithms		*Natural logarithms*	
log (a)(*b*)	= log a + log b	ln (a)(b)	= ln a + ln b
log (*a*/b)	= log a – log b	ln (a/b)	= ln a – ln b
log (1/a)	= – log a	ln (1/a)	= – ln a
log a^b	= b log a	ln a^b	= b ln a
log $a^{1/b}$	= (1/b) log a	ln $a^{1/b}$	= (1/b) ln a
log a^{-b}	= – b log a	ln a^{-b}	= – b ln a
	= b log (1/a)		= b ln (1/a)
log (a + b)	= log (a + b)	ln (a + b)	= ln (a + b)
log (a – b)	= log (a – b)	ln (a – b)	= ln (a – *b*)
log 10	= 1	ln e	= 1
log 10^a	= a	ln e^a	= a
log 10^{-a}	= –a	ln e^{-a}	= – a

Rule # 2: ln(a)(b)(c) = ln a + ln b + ln c

Either one of these two rules may be used first. Since there are no divisions either in the numerator or in the denominator, it will be prudent to use rule # 1 first and then apply rule # 2.

1. Applying the first rule:

$$\ln = \frac{(5.893)(2.716)(5.932+1.187)}{(4.893)(2.875)} \text{ (ln numerator)} - \text{(ln denominator)}$$

(ln numerator) = ln(5.893)(2.716)(5.932 +1.187) and (ln denominator) = ln(4.893)(2.875)

2. Now applying the second rule to the numerator as well as to the denominator:

$$\begin{aligned}\text{ln numerator} &= \ln(5.893)(2.716)(5.932+1.187)\\ &= \ln 5.893 + \ln 2.716 + \ln(5.932+1.187)\\ &= \ln 5.893 + \ln 2.716 + \ln 7.119\\ &= 1.7738 + 0.9992 + 1.9628\\ &= 4.7357\end{aligned}$$

$$\begin{aligned}\text{ln denominator} &= \ln(4.893)(2.875)\\ &= \ln 4.893 + \ln 2.875\\ &= 1.5878 + 1.0561\\ &= 2.6439\end{aligned}$$

$$\ln \frac{(5.893)(2.716)(5.932+1.187)}{(4.893)(2.875)} = \text{(ln numerator)} - \text{(ln denominator)}$$

$$\ln \frac{(5.893)(2.716)(5.932+1.187)}{(4.893)(2.875)} = 4.7358 - 2.6439 = 2.0919$$

Example 2-3 Calculate the common logarithm of $\frac{(7.532)(1.873)^{-1.37}(2.895)}{(5.983)^{1.4}}$

Solution

$$\begin{aligned}\ln \frac{(7.532)(1.873)^{-1.37}(2.895)}{(5.983)^{1.4}} &= \log(7.532)(1.873)^{-1.37}(2.895) - \log(5.983)^{1.4}\\ &= \log 7.532 + (-1.37)(\log 1.873) + \log 2.895 - (1.4)(\log 5.983)\\ &= 0.8769 - 0.3734 + 0.4616 - 1.0877 = -0.1226\end{aligned}$$

Relationship Between Common and Natural Logarithms

The relationship between common and natural logarithms is as follows:

$$\text{If } \log x = b \tag{2-7}$$

$$\text{then, } x = (10)^b \tag{2-8}$$

Now, if we take natural logarithms on both sides of equation (2-8) then,

$$\ln x = \ln(10)^b \tag{2-9}$$

$$\ln x = (b)(\ln 10) = (b)(2.303) \tag{2-10}$$

$$\text{therefore, } b = \frac{\ln x}{2.303} \tag{2-11}$$

Substituting the value of b from equation (2-11) into equation (2-7), we have

$$\log x = \frac{\ln x}{2.303} \quad (2\text{-}12)$$

$$\ln x = (2.303)\log x \quad (2\text{-}13)$$

Example 2-4

What is the common logarithm of 300, if natural logarithm of 300 is 5.704?

Solution

According to equation (2-12),

$$\log x = \frac{\ln x}{2.303}, \text{ therefore,}$$

$$\log 300 = \frac{\ln 300}{2.303}$$

$$\log 300 = \frac{5.704}{2.303} = 2.477$$

Example 2-5

If common logarithm of 40 is 1.602, calculate the natural logarithm of 40.

Solution

From equation (2-13),

$$\ln x = (2.303) \log x$$

$$\ln 40 = (2.303)(\log 40)$$

$$\ln 40 = (2.303)(1.602) = 3.689$$

GRAPHIC METHODS

Data in some studies are presented in a tabular form, so that the reader may comprehend salient points being presented. In pharmacokinetic studies, data in a tabular form may not necessarily provide important and vital information sought from the study. Therefore, instead of tabulating data collected during the course of the study, the data must invariably be plotted on a graph paper, so as to provide a better understanding of information desired from the study. Graphs are convenient and important way of picturing functions geometrically by means of a rectangular coordinate system. Since a linear relationship between variables being investigated provides a more meaningful picture, the data are often plotted in such a manner that a linear relationship between variables can be obtained. The equation of the straight line thus obtained also enables expression of connection between variables in the form of a mathematical equation, which can then be used to calculate various parameters associated with the study.

Graph

Graphs used in pharmacokinetic studies are plotted on a two-dimensional graph paper. The horizontal line (x-coordinate or abscissa) is referred to as x-axis and the vertical line (y-coordinate or ordinate) is known as y-axis. Convenient units of length are selected to lay off distances to the right and left and upwards and downwards from the point of origin. Distances to the right and upward of origin are called positive distances and those to the left and downward are called negative distances.

In a two-dimensional graph, the independent variable is measured along the horizontal coordinate scale and dependent variable is measured along vertical coordinate scale. In plotting a two-dimensional graph, it is important to select units of measurement along the axes in order to maximize graph on graph paper. To draw the graph of a linear function (equation of a straight line), it may be sufficient to plot two of its points and draw a straight line through them. However, plotting more than two points serves as a check against errors.

The axes of a two-dimensional graph divide the plane into four segments or quadrants, which are counted counter clock-wise starting with top right-hand quadrant and represent the following.

First quadrant: Positive x and positive y. This is the upper right-hand quadrant and is also known as the first quadrant.

Second quadrant: Negative x and positive y. This is the upper left-hand quadrant and is also known as the second quadrant.

Third quadrant: Negative x and negative y. This is the lower left-hand quadrant, also known as the third quadrant.

Fourth quadrant: Positive x and negative y. This is the lower right-hand quadrant and is also known as the fourth quadrant.

In a two-dimensional graph, any point in any of the four quadrants may be located by its distance from the two axes. Any point on the x-axis has its ordinate equal to 0 and any point on the y-axis has its abscissa equal to 0. The coordinates of origin are: x = 0 and y = 0. Figure 2-1 is a graphic representation of the four quadrants of a graph.

In all pharmacokinetic studies, negative values are not encountered. The most common situation is when both x and y have positive values. Therefore, in almost all studies, only the first quadrant (the upper right-hand quadrant) is used.

Equation of a Straight Line

The simplest relationship between the two variables is described by a first-degree equation. A first-degree equation is an equation in which the value of exponent of the variables is equal to one. A plot of first-degree equation on a rectangular (two-dimensional) graph yields a straight line described by the following equation, known as the equation of a straight line:

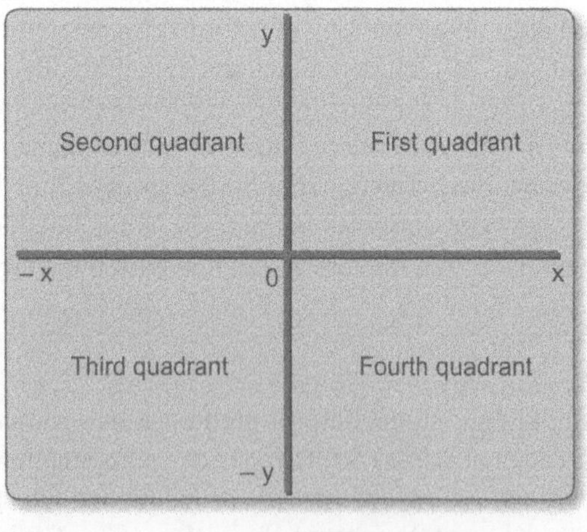

Fig. 2-1 The four quadrants of a graph

$$y = b + mx \tag{2-14}$$

where, y = dependent variable, b = y-intercept, m = slope of straight line and x = independent variable.

Y-Intercept

The y-intercept, b, signifies the point at which the straight line intersects y-axis, i.e. y-intercept is the value of y when x = 0. If y-intercept is positive, the point of intersection is above the x-axis. If y-intercept is negative, then the point of intersection is below x-axis. If the value of y-intercept is 0, then the straight line passes through origin and equation (2-14) becomes

$$y = 0 + mx = mx \tag{2-15}$$

Slope

The slope of the straight line is represented by symbol m in equation (2-14) and is expressed as a numerical change in the value of y with a corresponding numerical change in the value of x, that is ($m = \Delta y/\Delta x$). The slope of a straight line may be negative or positive and may have a value equal to zero, equal to 1, less than 1, or more than one.

A negative slope indicates decrease in change in the value of y with increasing change in the value of x and positive slope indicates increasing change in the value of y with increasing change in the value of x. When slope = 0, the value of y does not change with change in the value of x. When slope = 1, it indicates that change in the value of y exactly equals change in the value of x. If the scales used on the two axis are identical, the straight line will make an angle of 45° with the two axes, but if scales on the two axes are not identical, then depending upon the scales used on x- and y-axis, the angle of the straight line will be either greater or smaller than 45°. Without calculating the actual value, one can visually determine if slope is positive, negative, or equal to 0. The slope is positive (greater than 0) if the line slants upward to right. The slope is negative (less than 0) if the line slants downward to the right.

Figure 2-2 shows variations in the slope of a straight line. In these graphs, the y-axis (dependable variable) is usually the amount of drug or the concentration of drug and the x-axis (the independent variable) is time.

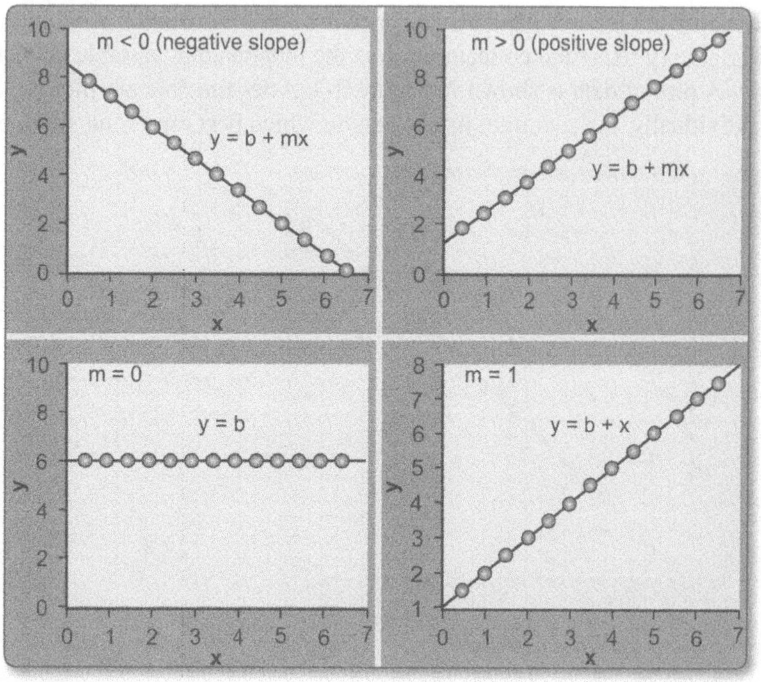

Fig. 2-2 Variations in slope

Steeper slope indicates a large value of m and a less-steeper slope indicates a small value of m. When the ratio $(\Delta y/\Delta x) = 1$, the value of m equals 1 and equation (2-14) becomes

$$y = b + x \tag{2-16}$$

When the ratio $(\Delta y/\Delta x) = 0$, the value of m equals zero and the straight line is horizontal and parallel to x-axis. In this case equation (2-14) is reduced to

$$y = b \tag{2-17}$$

Plotting the Graph

To plot a graph on rectilinear graph paper, the x-axis is used to represent the independent variable. The dependant variable is represented on the y-axis. For example, if one plots degradation of drug as a function of time, then time is independent variable and the amount of drug degraded is the dependent variable (amount of drug degraded depends on the time). Similarly, in a plot of concentration of drug in plasma as a function of time, time will be represented on the x-axis (independent variable) and the concentration of drug in plasma will be represented on the y-axis (concentration of drug in plasma changes with time). In the analytical procedures, e.g. during the spectrophotometric analysis, the absorbance or transmission of light is a function of concentration of substance in the solution. Hence, absorbance is the dependent variable (y-axis) and concentration is the independent variable (x-axis).

The following example illustrates the technique of plotting the graph and deriving the equation which describe the data:

Example 2-6 Spectrophotometric absorbance as a function of concentration of a compound is shown below. Plot the data and determine y-intercept, slope and equation of the straight line.

Concentration (mg/L)	10	20	30	40	50	60	70
Absorbance	0.13	0.25	0.39	0.52	0.65	0.80	0.92

Solution

Because absorbance depends on concentration of substance in solution, absorbance is dependent variable (y-axis) and concentration is the independent variable (x-axis).

A plot of data is shown in Figure 2-3. After the data are plotted, data points are not joined individually, but a straight line is drawn, which best represents these points. Since the points do

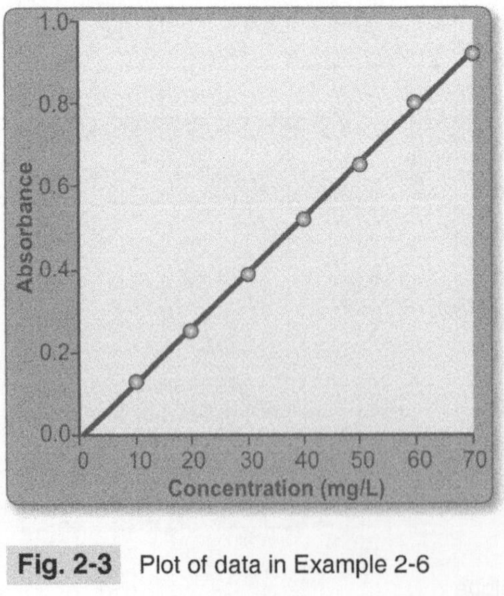

Fig. 2-3 Plot of data in Example 2-6

not exhibit heavy scatter, eyeball judgment is used to draw a straight line. Some points may fall under the line and some points may fall above the line.

Y-intercept: The y-intercept is obtained by back-extrapolating the straight line toward y-axis and determining the point of intersection of the straight line with y-axis at x = 0. Back-extrapolating the straight line toward y-axis shows that the straight line intersects y-axis at 0, i.e., the y-intercept = 0.

Slope: It is change in the value of y with corresponding change in the value of x. In this Example, the straight line drawn shows a positive slope. To calculate slope, one selects two widely separated points on the straight line. If actual data points do not fall on this straight line, then one creates two points on the straight line drawn. If the straight line intersects y-axis and/or x-axis, then one chooses that point of intersection as the points to calculate the slope of the straight line. If the straight line intersects only one axis, then this point of intersection may be chosen as one of the two points to calculate the slope.

In Example 2-6, the straight line passes through the origin. This point (x = 0, y = 0) can be used as one of the two points to calculate the slope of the straight line. For the second point, suppose we choose a point at the other end of the straight line: x = 70, y = 0.91. Therefore,

$$\text{slope} = \frac{y_2 - y_1}{x_2 - x_1}$$

$$= \frac{0.91 - 0}{70 - 0} = \frac{0.91}{70} = 0.013$$

Equation of the Straight Line: Substituting the values of y-intercept (= 0) and slope (= 0.013) into equation (2-14) gives the general equation of the straight line:

$$y = 0 + 0.013x$$

$$y = 0.013x$$

Example 2-7 From the data given in Example 2-6, determine absorbance when concentration is 45 mg/L.

Solution

Substituting the value of concentration (x = 45 mg/L) into equation of the straight line gives

$$y = (0.013)(45) = 0.585$$

$$y = 0.585$$

Therefore, absorbance when concentration is 45 mg/L = 0.585 units.

LINEAR REGRESSION ANALYSIS

An examination of the plot in Figure 2-3 shows that the data produced a straight line and every single data point fell on this straight line. In actual practice, all data points do not necessarily fall on the straight line and the data may exhibit a scatter around the straight line. In such cases, a straight line is drawn to best represent the data points. When data points do not show too much scatter eyeball judgment is used to draw a straight line, which represents all the points. When the scatter begins to increase, then it becomes difficult to know, whether or not the data can be represented by a linear relationship. Even if all indications appear to suggest that the data may be represented by a linear relationship, an eyeball judgment may not produce the straight line, which best represents the data. Also, depending upon how the line is drawn, one may find that the values of the slope and y-intercept are not exactly what the data reflect. A straight line drawn with a slight tilt to the right or a slight tilt to the left will provide different values of both, the y-intercept and the slope. Thus, the equation of the straight line obtained from these values will not reflect the actual equation of the straight line. In situations of this nature, the data are subjected to a technique, known as linear regression analysis to determine correlation coefficient, *r*, to see if the data fit a straight line. If the analysis suggests a linear relationship then this method (regression analysis) is used to determine the slope, the y-intercept and the equation of the straight line.

Correlation Coefficient

The correlation coefficient, *r*, is calculated using the following equation:

$$r = \frac{\sum\{(x-\bar{x})(y-\bar{y})\}}{\left\{\left[\sum(x-\bar{x})^2\sum(y-\bar{y})^2\right]\right\}^{1/2}} \tag{2-18}$$

In this equation, x and y are the x- and y-values provided in the data. The term x (pronounced, x-bar) is the arithmetic mean of the x-values and the term y (pronounced, y-bar) is the arithmetic mean of the y-values. The symbol Σ (pronounced sigma) denotes the sum of the values of the terms included within the brackets.

The value of the correlation coefficient, *r*, can vary between + 1 and 0 if the slope is positive and between – 1 and 0 if the slope is negative. If the value of the correlation coefficient is equal to + 1, it indicates a perfect fit (100% correlation) between the variables with a positive slope. In this case, all data points will lie on the straight line and the straight line will slant upwards to the right. Similarly, if the value of the correlation coefficient is –1, it indicates perfect correlation between the variables with a negative slope. In this case also, all data points will lie on the straight line and the straight line will slant downward towards the left. If the value of the correlation coefficient is found to be equal to zero, the variables are not correlated, meaning that there is no linear correlation between the two variables (i.e. between the x- and the y-values) and none of the data points are likely to fall on the straight line (if a straight line was drawn to represent these points).

If the value of correlation coefficient is less than 1 (i.e. is not a perfect fit between the x- and the y-values, as is usually the case in actual collection of the data), regression analysis of the data is performed at a chosen probability level (also known as the confidence level). The probability level is the level of confidence with which one can claim that the data are linearly correlated or not correlated. Depending on the number of observations in a given set of data and the chosen probability level, one can calculate the value of *r.* If the calculated value of *r* is greater than the published value of *r* at the chosen level of probability, one may conclude that the correlation between the two variables is significant and,a linear relationship (straight line) can represent the data. If the calculated value of *r* at the chosen level of probability indicates lack of correlation, then the data do not fit a straight line at that probability level and a straight line to represent the data is not warranted.

The theoretical values of correlation coefficient, *r* for the various N's (numbers of observations) at the most frequently used levels of probability or confidence (90, 95, 98 and 99% probability levels) are shown in Table 2-3.

Usually, a probability (confidence) level of 95% or greater is used for demonstration of good evidence (a strong correlation) that a linear relationship exists between the two variables. It should be pointed out that the values shown in Table 2-3 are absolute values. These values should be read as positive values for positive slopes and as negative values for negative slopes, i.e. for straight lines having a positive slope, these values are read as positive values and for straight lines having a negative slope, these values should be read as negative values.

Table 2-3 Theoretical values of the correlation coefficient*

Observations	Percent probability level			
N − 2	*90*	*95*	*98*	*99*
1	0.988	0.997	0.9995	0.9999
2	0.900	0.950	0.980	0.990
3	0.805	0.878	0.934	0.959
4	0.729	0.811	0.882	0.917
5	0.669	0.754	0.833	0.874
6	0.622	0.707	0.789	0.834
7	0.582	0.666	0.750	0.798
8	0.549	0.632	0.716	0.765
9	0.521	0.602	0.685	0.735
10	0.497	0.576	0.658	0.708
11	0.476	0.553	0.634	0.684
12	0.458	0.532	0.612	0.661
13	0.441	0.514	0.592	0.641
14	0.426	0.497	0.574	0.623
15	0.412	0.482	0.558	0.606
16	0.400	0.468	0.542	0.590
17	0.389	0.456	0.528	0.575
18	0.378	0.444	0.516	0.561
19	0.369	0.433	0.503	0.549
20	0.360	0.423	0.492	0.537
21	0.352	0.413	0.482	0.526
22	0.344	0.404	0.472	0.515
23	0.337	0.396	0.462	0.505
24	0.330	0.388	0.453	0.496
25	0.323	0.381	0.445	0.487
26	0.317	0.374	0.437	0.479
27	0.311	0.367	0.430	0.471
28	0.306	0.361	0.423	0.463
29	0.301	0.355	0.416	0.456
30	0.296	0.349	0.409	0.449
35	0.275	0.325	0.381	0.418
40	0.257	0.304	0.358	0.393
45	0.243	0.288	0.338	0.372
50	0.231	0.273	0.322	0.354
60	0.211	0.250	0.295	0.325
70	0.195	0.232	0.274	0.302
80	0.183	0.217	0.256	0.283
90	0.173	0.205	0.242	0.267
100	0.164	0.195	0.230	0.254

*The values shown are for positive slopes. For negative slopes, these values should be read as negative values.

If, at a chosen probability level, the calculated value of *r* is greater than its theoretical value, then one can say, at the chosen probability level, that there is a significant correlation between the two variables. If, on the other hand, the published theoretical value of *r* is greater than the calculated value of *r*, then the correlation between the two variables is not significant, i.e. the correlation is questionable.

As an example, for a set of data consisting of 20 values or observations (20 values of x and the corresponding 20 values of y), if the calculated value of *r* is found to be 0.395, then we can say that there is a significant correlation between the two variables at a 90% probability level, because the theoretical (published) value of *r* at 90% probability level in Table 2-3 for (N – 2) = (20 – 2) = 18 observations is 0.378, which is less than the calculated value of *r*. However, if we had set our probability level at 95% level instead of at 90% level, then the correlation between the variables will be declared 'not significant' because the theoretical or published value of *r* at the 95% probability level is 0.444, which is greater than the calculated value of *r*.

In pharmacokinetic procedures, the probability level used for regression analysis is usually set higher than 95%. Depending on the type of analysis, one may choose to set the probability level even significantly higher than 95%. For example, if one wanted to differentiate, whether the data fit a zero-order kinetics (linear relationship between concentration and time), or first-order kinetics (non-linear relationship between concentration and time), one would set the probability level as high as possible. This is because, in some situations, the data in both cases (zero-order and first-order kinetics) may appear linear at the lower probability level. Since the decline in concentration as a function of time differs by a wide margin in these kinetic processes (linear in zero-order kinetics and exponential in first-order kinetics), it may be essential to determine which of these two processes is really operative in a given situation. By setting the probability level higher than usual, one makes the requirement for linearity more stringent and is actually able to detect differences in the two cases.

Equation of the Straight Line

If the calculated value of the correlation coefficient, *r*, shows a good correlation between the variables, then a straight line can be drawn to represent the data accurately. To draw the straight line, one needs to know the equation of this straight line, for which one needs to determine the values of the slope (also known as regression coefficient, m) and the y-intercept.

The slope and the y-intercept are calculated as follows:

Slope: The slope of the straight line, m, is determined using the following equation:

$$\text{slope, m} = \frac{\sum(x-\bar{x})(y-\bar{y})}{\sum(x-\bar{x})^2} \tag{2-19}$$

Y-Intercept: The general equation for determining y-intercept, b, is:

$$b = \bar{y} + m(x - \bar{x}) \tag{2-20}$$

Since, by definition, y-intercept is the value of y when x = 0, equation (2-20) becomes

$$b = \bar{y} - m\bar{x} \tag{2-21}$$

Equation of the Straight Line: Substitution of values of slope, m and y-intercept into equation (2-14) gives the equation of the straight line.

$$y = \bar{y} - \frac{\sum(x-\bar{x})(y-\bar{y})}{\sum(x-\bar{x})^2}(\bar{x}) + \frac{\sum(x-\bar{x})(y-\bar{y})}{\sum(x-\bar{x})^2}(x) \tag{2-22}$$

In equation (2-22), the quantity $\frac{\sum(x-\bar{x})(y-\bar{y})}{\sum(x-\bar{x})^2}$

is common to two terms on the right-hand side of the equation. Equation (2-22) it is simplified to give

$$y = \bar{y} - \frac{\sum(x-\bar{x})(y-\bar{y})}{\sum(x-\bar{x})^2}(x-\bar{x}) \qquad (2\text{-}23)$$

Evaluation of Data

To evaluate the data, one calculates the correlation coefficient *r* to determine if the relationship between the variables is linear at the proposed confidence level. If the value of the correlation coefficient indicates a good linear relationship, then one calculates the slope and the y-intercept. These two parameters define the equation of the straight line.

The following Example illustrates the determination of correlation coefficient, the slope, the y-intercept and the equation of the straight line.

Example 2-8 Plasma concentration after a 300 mg intravenous (IV) dose of a drug is shown below. Calculate correlation coefficient and if *r* indicates linearity, calculate slope, y-intercept and equation of the straight line.

Time (h)	1	2	3	4	5	6	7
Concentration (mg/L)	80	72	56	44	28	24	11

Solution

Figure 2-4 shows a plot of the data.

To determine whether the relationship between the variables may indeed be represented by a linear relationship, the first step is to calculate the correlation coefficient, *r*. If the calculated value of correlation coefficient *r* indicates a good probability of a linear relationship, then slope (m) and the y-intercept (b) can be calculated as follows:

1. Create a table with 7 columns.
2. In column 1, enter the values of x. Add these values and calculate the mean (average). The mean of the x-values is $\bar{x}$.

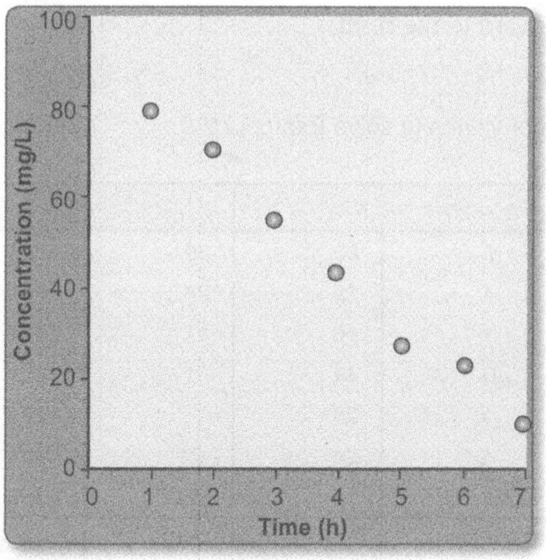

Fig. 2-4 Plot of data in Example 2-8

3. Column 2 is $(x - \bar{x})$. These values are obtained by subtracting the arithmetic mean, $\bar{x}$, from each value of x. After subtraction, some values obtained would be positive and some values would be negative. The total of all values in column 2 must add up to zero.
4. Column 3 is $(x - \bar{x})^2$. These values are obtained by squaring each value of $(x - \bar{x})$. The sum of the values of this column is $\Sigma (x - \bar{x})^2$.
5. Column 4 is similar to column 1, except that instead of tabulating the x-values, the values tabulated are the y-values. The value of $\bar{y}$ is obtained by adding all the values of y and calculating the arithmetic mean of these values.
6. Column 5 is $(y - \bar{y})$. This column is similar to column 2, except the values of y and $\bar{y}$ are used instead of using the values of x and $\bar{x}$. Some values obtained would be positive and some values would be negative. The sum of values in column 5 should be equal to 0.
7. Column 6 is $(y - \bar{y})^2$. The values of $(y - \bar{y})^2$ are obtained by squaring each value in column 5. The sum of the values in this column is $\Sigma(y - \bar{y})^2$.
8. Column 7 is $(x - \bar{x})(y - \bar{y})$. These values are obtained by multiplying each value in column 2 with the corresponding value in column 5. The sum of the values in this column is $\Sigma (x - \bar{x})(y - \bar{x})$.

The calculations involved in the determination of these values are shown in Table 2-4. By substituting the relevant values into the appropriate equations one can calculate the correlation coefficient, the slope and the y-intercept. From the slope and the y-intercept, the equation of the straight line can be developed.

Correlation Coefficient: It is calculated by substituting relevant values from Table 2-4 into equation (2-18):

$$r = \frac{\Sigma\{(x-\bar{x})(y-\bar{y})\}}{\{[\Sigma(x-\bar{x})^2][\Sigma(y-\bar{y})^2]\}^{1/2}}$$

$$r = \frac{-331}{[(28)(3{,}962)]^{1/2}}$$

$$r = \frac{-331}{(110{,}936)^{1/2}} = \frac{-331}{333.07}$$

$$r = -0.9938$$

A correlation coefficient of 0.9938 indicates strong linear relationship between variables. The negative sign in the value of correlation coefficient indicates that slope is negative, i.e. the straight line slants downward to the right.

Table 2-4 Calculation of values to solve Example 2-8

x	$(x - \bar{x})$	$(x - \bar{x})^2$	y	$(y - \bar{y})$	$(y - \bar{y})^2$	$(x - \bar{x})(y - \bar{y})$
1	−3	9	80	35	1,225	− 105
2	−2	4	72	27	729	− 54
3	−1	1	56	11	121	− 11
4	0	0	44	− 1	1	0
5	+1	1	28	− 17	289	− 17
6	+2	4	24	− 21	441	− 42
7	+3	9	11	− 34	1,156	− 102
$\Sigma = 28$ $\bar{x} = 4$	$\Sigma = 0$ $y = 45$	$\Sigma = 28$	$\Sigma = 315$	$\Sigma = 0$	$\Sigma = 3962$	$\Sigma = -331$

Slope: Substituting relevant values from Table 2-4 into equation (2-19) gives slope of the straight line:

$$\text{slope} = m = \frac{\sum(x-\bar{x})(y-\bar{y})}{\sum(x-\bar{x})^2}$$

$$= \frac{-331}{28} = -11.82 \text{ (mg/L)/h}$$

The negative value of slope indicates negative slope, i.e. straight line points downward to the right. The value, 11.82 means decrease in concentration at a rate of 11.82 mg/L per hour.

Y-Intercept: The y-intercept b is calculated using equation (2-21). Substituting the values of $\bar{y}$ (= 45) and $\bar{x}$ (= 4) found in Table 2-4 and the calculated value of slope, m (= –11.82), into equation (2-21) one obtains:

$$b = \bar{y} - m\bar{x}$$

$$= 45 - (-11.82)(4)$$

$$= 92.28 \text{ mg}/L$$

Thus, the straight line intersects y-axis at 92.28 mg/L.

Equation of Straight Line: Substituting values of y-intercept and slope into equation (2-14),

$$y = b + mx$$

$$y = 92.28 - 11.82x$$

Equation (2-23) may also be used to determine the equation of the straight line: – 331

$$y = 45 + \frac{-331}{28}(x - \bar{x})$$

$$= 45 + (-11.82)(x - 4)$$

$$= 45 + (-11.82x + 47.28)$$

$$= 92.28 - 11.82x$$

Plotting the Straight Line: To draw a straight line represented by the equation y = 92.28 – 11.82x, one calculates two points from this equation. The data points are not used because one does not know, which one of the data point falls on the straight line. The two points (x_1, y_1) and (x_2, y_2) to draw the straight line are selected as follows. The y-intercept serves as one point. This is (x_1, y_1) = (0 hour, 92.28 mg/L). For the second point (x_2, y_2) one uses the equation of the straight line by substituting any value of x, say, x = 7 hours and solving for y:

$$y = 92.28 - 11.82x$$

$$= 92.82 - 11.82(7)$$

$$= 92.28 - 82.74$$

$$= 9.54 \text{ mg/L}$$

The second point (x_2, y_2) is x_2 = 7 hours, y_2 = 9.54 mg/L.

These two points are plotted on the graph paper and joined with a straight line.

A plot of the data and the straight line, which best represents the data given in Example 2-8 is shown in Figure 2-5.

This plot shows that all data points do not lie on the straight line. The data points appear o be scattered around the straight line, although the scatter is very small.

The straight line touches only three point, one point is below the straight line and the remaining points are above the straight line. This happened because the straight line was developed using

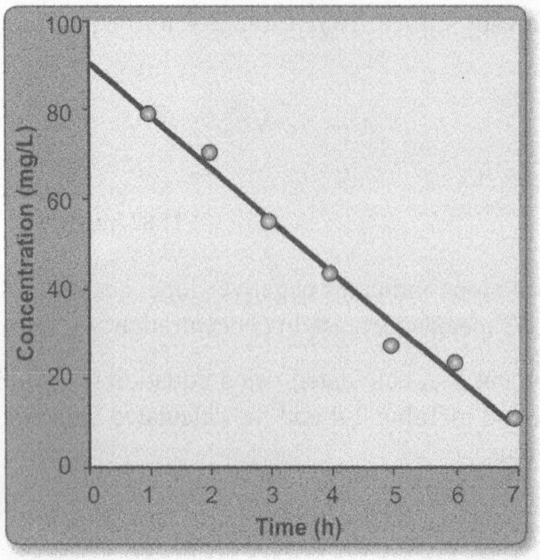

Fig. 2-5 Linear relationship between the data in Example 2-8

statistical methodology. In this technique, the path of the straight line is determined using least-square method. According to this method, the sum of square of perpendicular distance of each point above the straight line cancels the sum of square of perpendicular distance of each point below the straight line.

Application of Equation of a Straight Line

The equation of a straight line derived from a data can be used to predict the connection between the variables. There are several practical applications of the equation of a straight line, especially in the absence of availability of data. For example, suppose degradation of a product is studied over a 6-month period and the amount of drug degraded is determined every 2 weeks. The data are plotted on a regular coordinate graph paper and let us suppose that a linear relationship is found between time and amount of product degraded. From this linear relationship, one determines the equation of the straight line in the form:

$$y = mx + b$$

where,

m = the slope of the straight line

b = the y-intercept.

The equation of straight line thus obtained can be used to obtain useful information even when the actual data or a plot of the data is not available and only the equation of the straight line representing the data is given.

The following five examples illustrate applications of the equation of a straight line in order to obtain useful information.

Reconstruction of the Graph

The graph showing linear relationship between time and amount of drug degraded is reconstructed by generating two points (x_1, y_1) and (x_2, y_2) from the equation of the straight line. The first point (x_1, y_1) is obtained by substituting a value of x, say 0 and solving the equation of straight line for the value of y. The second point, (x_2, y_2), is obtained by similarly substituting a larger value of x into the equation of straight line and obtaining a corresponding value of y. These two values are (x_2, y_2). These two values are then plotted on a rectilinear coordinate graph paper and joined with a straight line.

Example 2-9 The equation describing degradation of a product as a function of time is: y = 0.028x. The graph was generated by plotting amount of drug degraded (in mg) on y-axis and time (in months) on x-axis. Reconstruct the graph, which is described by this equation of the straight line.

Solution

To draw a straight line, one needs two points on the graph. Since there is no y-intercept, the straight line passes through the origin. Therefore, the origin (x = 0 month, y = 0 mg) can be used as one point. If the equation of the straight line exhibited a y-intercept, then the y-intercept (at x = 0 month) would have served as one of the two points. To obtain the second point, one substitutes any value of either x or y (but not both) into the equation of straight line and solves for the corresponding other value. For example, substituting the value of x = 7 months into equation of the straight line, y = 0.028 x:

$$y = (0.028)(7)$$

$$y = 0.196 \text{ mg}$$

This gives a second point (x = 7 months, y = 0.196 mg). These two points (x_1, y_1 = 0 month, 0 mg) and (x_2, y_2 = 7 months, 0.196 mg) are plotted on a rectilinear coordinate graph paper and are connected with a straight line. Figure 2-6 shows these two points plotted on a rectilinear coordinate graph paper and the straight line, which is described by the equation: y = 0.028x.

To assure that the straight line drawn by connecting the two points does in fact reflect the straight line predicted by the equation, it is advisable that one should not depend only on two points, but the straight line should be drawn after a few more points are calculated from the equation of the straight line.

Predict Degradation at any Time

To predict degradation of drug product at any time, one substitutes the value of time (x value) for degradation of drug product into equation of the straight line and solves the equation for y, which gives the amount of drug product degraded.

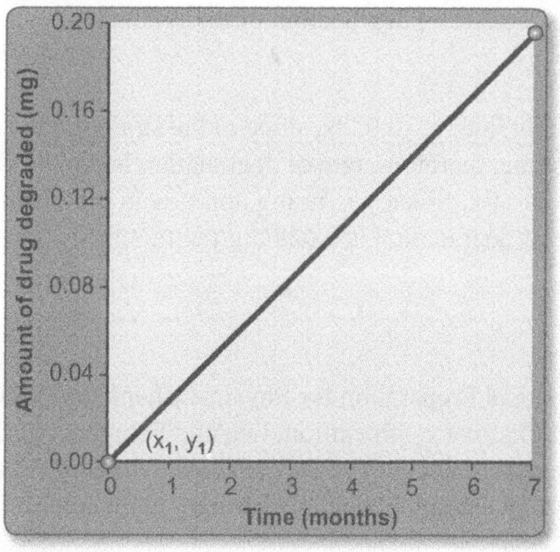

Fig. 2-6 Reconstruction of graph in Example 2-9.

Example 2-10 The equation of straight line describing degradation of a drug product (mg) as a function of time (months) is y = 0.028x. Calculate amount of product degraded after 24 months.

Solution

In this equation of straight line, y = 0.028x, there is no intercept, because there is no degradation of drug product at time 0. The slope of the straight line is 0.028 and the units of slope are units of y divided by the units of x. Since y is in mg and x is in months, the units of slope are mg/month. Substituting the value of x = 24 months into the equation of the straight line and solving for y, we get

$$y = (0.028)(24) = 0.672 \text{ mg}$$

amount of drug degraded after 24 months = 0.672 mg

Estmating Time of Degradation

To predict time when a certain amount of drug product would have degraded, one substitutes the value of amount of drug product being estimated to have degraded (y value) into equation of the straight line and solves the equation for x value.

Example 2-11 The equation describing degradation of a drug product (in mg) as a function of time (in months) is y = 0.028x. Calculate the time when amount of drug degraded would be 0.575 mg.

Solution

To calculate time when 0.575 mg of drug will be degraded, one substitutes y = 0.575 mg into the equation. Substitution gives:

$$0.575 \text{ mg} = (0.028 \text{ mg/month})(x)$$

$$\text{Therefore, } x = \frac{0.575 \text{ mg}}{0.028 \text{ mg/month}} = 20.54 \text{ months} = \text{time for degradation of } 0.575 \text{ mg of product}$$

Determination of Rate of Degradation

Rate of degradation is the amount of drug degraded as a function of time. This is the same as slope of the straight line. Hence, slope of the straight line determines the rate of degradation.

Example 2-12 The equation describing degradation (in mg) as a function of time (in months) is y = 0.028x. What is the rate of degradation of the product?

Solution

In this equation of straight line, y = 0.028x, slope of the straight line is 0.028. Since slope of the straight line represents rate, therefore, rate of degradation is 0.028. The units of slope are units of y divided by the units of x. Since y is in mg and x is in months, the units of slope are mg/month. Therefore, rate of degradation is 0.028 mg per month.

SUGGESTED READING

1. Daniels F. Mathematical Preparation for Physical Chemistry. McGraw-Hill; 1956.
2. Martin A. Physical Pharmacy, 4th edition. Lea and Febiger, 1993.
3. Pagano M, Gauvreau K. Principles of Biostatistics. Duxbury Press. Belmont; 1993.
4. Remington: The Science and Practice of Pharmacy, 21st edition. Mack Publishing, 2005.

PRACTICE PROBLEMS

2-1. Degradation of a chemical compound exhibited the following data. Assuming linear relationship, calculate: (a) correlation coefficient, (b) slope, (c) y-intercept and (d) equation of the straight line.

Time (month)	*Percent degraded*
3	1.3
6	2.6
9	4.0
12	5.5
15	7.0
18	8.8
21	10.7

2-2. Plasma concentration of a drug following intravenous administration of a 100 mg dose gave the following data. Plot the data on a coordinate graph paper. Assuming linear relationship, calculate the following values: (a) *r*, (b) slope (c) y-intercept and (d) equation of the straight line.

Time (hour)	*Concentration (μg/mL)*
0	8.5
1	8.0
2	7.5
3	6.0
4	4.0
5	3.5
6	1.5
7	1.0

2-3. If natural logarithm of 3.8 is 1.335, calculate the common logarithm of 3.8.

2-4. If common logarithm of 42.38 is 1.627, what is the natural logarithm of 42.38?

2-5. If common logarithm of 0.18 is – 0.745, what is the natural logarithm of 0.18?

2-6. If ln 0.13 = – 2.04, calculate log 0.13.

2-7. Calculate common logarithm of $\dfrac{(2.15)(7.98)^{-1.3}}{(5.95)^{-2.5}}$

2-8. Calculate natural logarithm of $\dfrac{(5.87)(2.35)^{0.5}(1.5+2.7)^{1.5}}{(2.9+3.5)(4.83)^{-2.7}}$

2-9. The equation of a straight line y = 135 – 0.137x describes the amount of drug (in mg) remaining to be degraded as a function of time (in months). Calculate the amount of drug remaining to be degraded after 48 months.

2-10. The equation ln C = ln 300 – 0.1155*t* describes a linear function between concentration of drug in plasma (μg/L) and time (hours). Calculate (a) concentration of drug in plasma at 10 hours and (b) time when concentration of drug would be 150 μg/L.

2-11. The equation ln C = ln 135 – 0.135*t* describes a linear function between concentration of drug in plasma (μg/L) and time (hours). Construct the graph showing concentration of drug in plasma as a function of time.

2-12. The following data describe stability of a drug product over a 14-month period. Assuming linear relationship between concentration and time, calculate: (a) Correlation coefficient,

(b) Slope of the straight line, (c) The y-intercept of the straight line and (d) The equation of the straight line.

Time (hour)	Concentration (μg/L)
2	95
4	82
6	68
8	60
10	45
12	43
14	27

2-13. Degradation of a chemical compound was followed over a period of several months and the relationship between time and amount of compound remaining to be degraded was found to be linear. The equation of straight line describing degradation was: $y = 100 - 0.029t$. If the amount of drug product degraded is in mg and time is in weeks, calculate the amount of product expected to degrade in 75 weeks.

2-14. The following equation describes a linear function between concentration of drug in plasma (μg/L) and time (hours): $\ln C = 6.91 - 0.135t$. From this equation, calculate concentration of drug in plasma at 10 hours.

2-15. The following equation describes a linear function between concentration of drug in plasma (μg/L) and time (hours): $\log C = 2.7 - 0.15t$. Calculate the time when concentration of drug in plasma would be 50 μg/L.

2-16. Plot the following data and calculate slope of the straight line.

Time (week)	Amount (mg)
1	4
2	13
3	15
5	25
6	31
7	32

2-17. The following data were obtained when stability of a drug product was evaluated over a 30-month period. Calculate (a) correlation coefficient, (b) slope of straight line and (c) y-intercept of the straight line.

Time (month)	Units degraded
10	1,003
15	1,005
20	1,010
25	1,008
30	1,014

2-18. Plot the following data and determine equation of the straight line.

Time (month)	Concentration (mg/5 mL)	Time (month)	Concentration (mg/5 mL)
0	482	40	350
10	465	45	335
15	445	50	315
20	425	55	295
25	405	60	280
30	390	70	240
35	370		

2-19. Degradation of a chemical compound was followed over a period of several months and the relationship between time and amount of compound remaining to be degraded was found to be linear. The equation of straight line describing degradation was: $y = 200 - 0.3t$. If the amount of drug product degraded is in mg and time is in months, calculate the amount of product remaining to be degraded in 12 months.

2-20. Degradation of a new drug was followed over a period of several months and the relationship between time and amount of drug remaining to be degraded was found to be linear. The equation of straight line describing degradation was: $y = 300 - 0.05t$. If the amount of drug degraded is in mg and time is in days, calculate the amount of drug expected to degrade in 365 days.

2-21. The following equation describes a linear function between the concentration of drug in plasma and time: $\ln C = 6.91 - 0.135t$. If concentration is in μg/L and time is in hours, calculate the concentration of drug in plasma at time zero.

2-22. The following equation describes a linear function between the concentration of drug in plasma and time: $\ln C = 5.7 - 0.1577t$. If concentration is in μg/L and time is in hours, calculate the concentration of drug in plasma at time zero.

2-23. The equation $\ln C = \ln 300 - 0.1155t$ describes a linear function between concentration of drug in plasma and time. If concentration is in μg/L and time is in hours, calculate the concentration of drug in plasma at time zero.

2-24. The equation $\ln C = \ln 300 - 0.1155t$ describes a linear function between concentration of drug in plasma and time. If concentration is in μg/L and time is in hours, calculate the time when concentration of drug in plasma would be 150 μg/L.

CHAPTER 3

RATE PROCESSES

Rate processes in pharmacokinetic studies follow the principles of kinetics. The term kinetics refers to 'motion' or 'movement'. Since these terms connote velocity, rate or rate of change, the term kinetics, therefore deals with the study of rate of change.

The fundamental rate equation describes the rate of change or the rate of a reaction as:

$$\frac{dC}{dt} \propto -(C)^n \tag{3-1}$$

In equation (3-1), dC is change in concentration (or amount), dt is change in time, therefore, dC/dt is change in concentration (or amount) with change in time, i.e. rate of reaction, C is concentration (or amount) and n is the order of reaction.

The negative sign on the right-hand side of equation (3-1) implies that, the concentration decreases as reaction progresses. Sometimes, the negative sign is placed on the left-hand side of equation (instead of the right-hand side), but it is customary to place the negative sign on the right-hand side of the equation. The exponent n (order of reaction) can be any positive number. For example, when n = 0, it is a zero-order reaction, when n = 1, it is a first-order reaction and when n = 2, it is a second-order reaction, etc.

The proportionality sign in equation (3-1) can be changed into equality sign by introducing a constant, so that equation (3-1) becomes

$$\frac{dC}{dt} = -(K)(C)^n \tag{3-2}$$

Where, K is a constant, known as the reaction rate constant. In zero-order reaction, equation (3-2) becomes

$$\frac{dC}{dt} = -(K)(C)^0 \tag{3-3}$$

since, $C^0 = 1$, equation (3-3) is written as dC

$$\frac{dC}{dt} = -K \tag{3-4}$$

And in a first-order reaction (i.e. when n = 1), equation (3-2) becomes

$$\frac{dC}{dt} = -(K)(C)^1 \tag{3-5}$$

$$\frac{dC}{dt} = -KC \tag{3-6}$$

Equation (3-4) shows that rate of reaction in zero-order kinetics is independent of amount of reactant or concentration of reacting species. Equation (3-6) shows that rate of reaction in first-order kinetics depends on concentration, i.e. rate of reaction is a function of concentration or amount of the reactant species.

ZERO-ORDER KINETICS

Equation (3-4) shows that the rate of a zero-order reaction does not depend on concentration of the reactant, but proceeds at a fixed rate, i.e. concentration decreases at a fixed rate irrespective of the amount of reactant. This fixed rate is K, the rate constant of reaction. If a drug product degrades at the rate of 0.5 mg/day (K = 0.5 mg/day), then the rate of degradation of the product will be 0.5 mg/day regardless of the initial amount of product. For example, if the initial amount of active ingredient in the formulation was 50 mg, then the active ingredient in the product will degrade completely in 100 days and if the initial amount of active ingredient in the product was 200 mg, then it will take 400 days for complete degradation of the product.

Mathematical Treatment

Equation (3-4) may be written as

$$dC = -(K)(dt) \tag{3-7}$$

Equation (3-7) can be integrated between the limits of concentration and time as follows: If $C = C_1$ at $t = t_1$ and $C = C_2$ at $t = t_2$ (where $C_1 > C_2$ and $t_2 > t_1$), then integration yields

$$C_1 - C_2 = -K\,(t_1 - t_2) \tag{3-8}$$

Equation (3-8) contains five quantities. If four of these are known, the fifth can be calculated. For example, equation (3-8) can be rearranged to calculate K, if two concentrations at 2 times are known:

$$K = -\frac{C_1 - C_2}{t_1 - t_2}\,;\; K = \frac{C_1 - C_2}{t_2 - t_1} = \frac{C_2 - C_1}{t_1 - t_2} \tag{3-9}$$

Equation (3-8) can also be used to calculate the following:

a. Concentration at any given time provided zero-order rate constant and concentration at another time is known or
b. Time when a given concentration will occur provided zero-order rate constant and concentration at another time is known.

Equation (3-8) can also be written in a form which includes concentrations at time 0 and at any given time t. Concentration at time 0 is initial concentration, i.e. at $t_1 = 0$, $C_1 = C_0$ and concentration at any other time t is C_t, i.e. $C_2 = C_t$ at $t_2 = t$. Thus, equation (3-8) becomes

$$C_0 - C_t = -K(0 - t) \tag{3-10}$$

$$C_0 = C_t + K(t) \tag{3-11}$$

or

$$C_t = C_0 - K(t) \tag{3-12}$$

Equation (3-12) describes zero-order kinetics as a function of concentration, time and reaction rate constant. This equation indicates that concentration in a zero-order reaction at any time t is equal to the initial concentration minus the product of reaction rate constant and time. Equation (3-12) contains four quantities. If three are known, the fourth can be determined.

Use of Equation

In some instances, the solution to a given problem may require the use of equation (3-8) more than once. For example, the information provided in the problem may not lend itself to obtaining the answer by directly substituting the values into the equation. In these instances, equation (3-8) is used twice: first, to obtain the information needed to solve the problem and then to obtain the answer.

The following examples illustrate the use of equations (3-8) and (3-12).

Example 3-1 The amount at 4 and 12 months after preparation of a product was 365 mg and 341 mg, respectively. If degradation follows zero-order kinetics, calculate the rate constant of degradation.

Solution

Since amount at two different times is known (C_1 at t_1 and C_2 at t_2), we use equation (3-9) to calculate K. Substituting into equation (3-9) values of $C_1 = 365$ mg at $t_1 = 4$ months and $C_2 = 341$ mg at $t_2 = 12$ months:

$$K = \frac{C_1 - C_2}{t_2 - t_1} = \frac{365 \text{ mg} - 341 \text{ mg}}{12 \text{ months} - 4 \text{ months}};\ K = \frac{24 \text{ mg}}{8 \text{ months}} = 3 \text{ mg/month}$$

Example 3-2 A product degrades by zero-order kinetics. When prepared, the amount was 23 µg. After 5 months, the amount was 21 µg. Calculate the time, when amount will be 17.5 µg.

Solution

In order to use equation (3-12) to find t, when $C_t = 17.5$ µg, one needs to know K. Since the value of K is not provided, it must be determined by substituting the available data into equation (3-12) as follows:

$$C_t = C_0 - K(t)$$

$$21\ \mu g = 23\ \mu g - K\ (5 \text{ months})$$

$$K(5 \text{ months}) = 23\ \mu g - 21\ \mu g = 2\ \mu g$$

$$K = 2\ \mu g/5 \text{ months} = 0.4\ \mu g/\text{month}$$

After calculating the value of K, equation (3-12) is used once again to get the value of time, t. This time one uses $C_0 = 23$ µg at t = 0, K = 0.4 µg/month and solve for t, when C_t = 17.5 µg.

$$C_t = C_0 - K(t)$$

$$17.5\ \mu g = 23\ \mu g - (0.4\ \mu g/\text{month})(t)$$

$$t = \frac{23\ \mu g - 17.5\ \mu g}{0.4\ \mu g/\text{month}} = \frac{5.5\ \mu g}{0.4\ \mu g/\text{month}} = 13.75 \text{ months}$$

Alternatively, one can use two known amounts and the rate constant of degradation to solve for time that elapses between these two amounts. Knowing the amount at 5 months ($C_1 = 21$ µg, $t_1 =$ 5 months) and the rate constant K = 0.4 µg/month, one can calculate the time (t_2) for the amount to reduce from 21 µg to 17.5 µg ($C_2 = 17.5$ µg). Substituting these values into equation (3-8):

$$C_1 - C_2 = -K(t_1 - t_2)$$

$$21\ \mu g - 17.5\ \mu g = -(0.4\ \mu g/\text{month})(5 - t)$$

$$5 - t = \frac{21\ \mu g - 17.5\ \mu g}{0.4\ \mu g/\text{month}} = 8.75 \text{ months}$$

$$t = 8.75 \text{ months} + 5 \text{ months} = 13.75 \text{ months}$$

Example 3-3 A product is ineffective after it has decomposed 10 percent. At the time of preparation, the amount of active ingredient was 500 mg. After 12 months, the amount of active ingredient was 491 mg. What should be the expiration date, if degradation follows zero-order kinetics?

Solution

Degradation of 10% means that the amount of active ingredient remaining in the product is 90% of initial concentration. In this question, C_0 = 500 mg and one needs to calculate t, when C_t = 90% of 500 mg = 450 mg. Although equations (3-8) or (3-12) can be used to find time, when C_t = 450 mg, one cannot use either equation unless the value of degradation rate constant, K is known. The value of K can be determined by substituting C_0 = 500 mg, C_t = 491 mg and t = 12 months into equation (3-12):

$$C_t = C_0 - K\,(t)$$

$$491\text{ mg} = 500\text{ mg} - K\,(12\text{ months})$$

$$K\,(12\text{ months}) = 500\text{ mg} - 491\text{ mg}$$

$$K = \frac{500\text{ mg} - 491\text{ mg}}{12\text{ months}} = \frac{9\text{ mg}}{12\text{ months}} = 0.75\text{ mg/month}$$

Having calculated the value of K, one can use either equation (3-8) or equation (3-12) to calculate time, when C_t will be 450 mg. Substituting into equation (3-12), the values of C_0 = 500 mg, C_t = 450 mg, K = 0.75 mg/month and solving for t, one gets:

$$450\text{ mg} = 500\text{ mg} - (0.75\text{ mg/month})(t)$$

$$(0.75\text{ mg/month})(t) = 500\text{ mg} - 450\text{ mg}$$

$$t = \frac{500\text{ mg} - 450\text{ mg}}{0.75\text{ mg / month}} = \frac{50\text{ mg}}{0.75\text{ mg / month}} = 66.667\text{ months}$$

Graphical Representation

Equation (3-12) is equation of a straight line: y = $mx + b$. Here, y = C_t, x = t, the y-intercept, b = C_0 and the slope, m = –K. Therefore, a plot of concentration (C_t) as a function of time (t) on a regular coordinate graph paper should yield a straight line having y-intercept = C_0 and slope = –K. The concentration terms are plotted on the y-coordinate (ordinate) and time is plotted on the x-axis (abscissa).

The graph paper selected for plotting the data should assure that the data points are plotted as accurately as possible. A good rectangular graph paper should have a minimum of 10 divisions per linear inch, although a better graph paper should have no less than 20 divisions per linear inch. These divisions are important for the y-coordinate, because this axis is used for concentration terms. Since concentration terms tend to be in decimal fractions rather than in whole numbers, the larger number of divisions on the ordinate scale (y-axis) minimizes estimation in plotting concentration terms on the y-axis.

The following example illustrates the application of equation (3-12) for the graphical determination of parameters in zero-order kinetics.

Example 3-4 The amount of active ingredient in a cough syrup as a function of time is shown below. Plot the data on a rectangular graph paper and calculate parameters associated with the data.

Time (day)	5	10	20	30	40	50
Amount (µg)	84	76	60	44	32	16

Solution

A plot of the data in Figure 3-1 shows a linear relationship between the x and y variables. A straight line is drawn to represent the data points and this straight line is back-extrapolated to obtain the y-intercept.

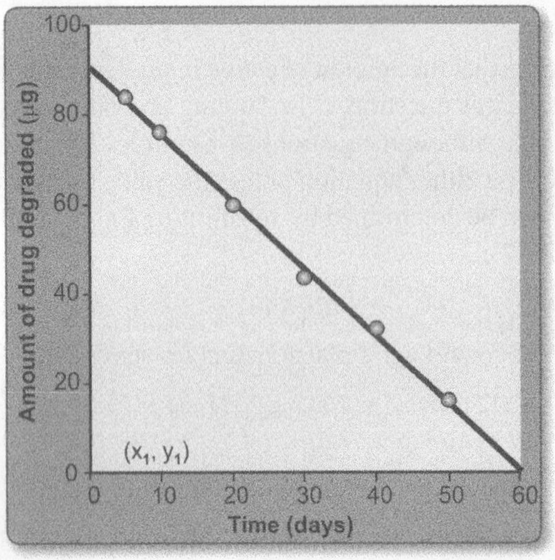

Fig. 3-1 Plot of concentration as a function of time

As can be seen from the graph, the relationship between the x and the y variables is linear. A straight line is drawn to represent the data points in a linear fashion and this straight line is back extrapolated to time 0 to obtain the y-intercept. According to the graph, the y-intercept (the value of y at time 0) is 90 µg. This is C_0. The slope of the straight line is change in y with a corresponding change in x, i.e.

$$\text{slope} = \frac{\text{change in y}}{\text{change in x}} = \frac{y_2 - y_1}{x_2 - x_1}$$

Now we use two points, as far apart from each other as possible, to calculate slope of the straight line. It is important that the two points used for calculating the slope should be as far apart from each other as possible, because this would help to minimize possible errors due to estimation in reading points from the graph.

Using the following two points as (x_1, y_1) and (x_2, y_2):

$$x_1 = 0 \text{ days}, y_1 = 90 \text{ µg and } x_2 = 60 \text{ days}, y_2 = 0 \text{ µg}$$

the slope is calculated as follows:

$$\text{slope} = \frac{0 \text{ µg} - 90 \text{ µg}}{60 \text{ days} - 0 \text{ day}} = \frac{-90 \text{ µg}}{60 \text{ days}} = -1.5 \text{ µg/day}$$

Since slope = – K, therefore, K = – slope = – (– 1.5 µg/day) = 1.5 µg/day. Thus, the active ingredient degrades at the rate of 1.5 µg per day.

This graph can also be used to find concentration at any time or to find time for a given concentration. For example, if one wanted to know time, when concentration will be 22.5 µg, one reads time from the graph (on the x-axis), when concentration (on the y-axis) corresponds to 22.5 µg. The graph shows that concentration is 22.5 µg on day 45. Similarly, if one wishes to know tje concentration on day 15, one reads y-axis corresponding to 15 days on x-axis. The graph concentration on day 15 will be 67.5 µg.

The time for a given concentration or the concentration at a given time can also be found using equation (3-12). For example, having known that C_0 = 90 µg and K = 1.5 µg/day, one can calculate t for C_t = 22.5 µg, as follows:

$$C_t = C_0 - K(t)$$

$$22.5 \text{ µg} = 90 \text{ µg} - (1.5 \text{ µg/day})(t)$$

$$(1.5 \text{ µg/day})(t) = 90 \text{ µg} - 22.5 \text{ µg} = 67.5 \text{ µg}$$

$$t = \frac{67.5\ \mu g}{1.5\ \mu g/days} = 45 \text{ days}$$

Similarly, to find C_t on day 15:

$$C_t = C_0 - K\ (t) = 90\ \mu g - (1.5\ \mu g/day)(15\ day) = 67.5\ \mu g$$

Half-Life

The half-life of a reaction, indicated by such symbols as $t_{½}$, $t_{0.5}$ or $t_{50\%}$, is defined as the time when original concentration (or amount) is reduced to one-half of the original concentration (or amount). For example, if a product was formulated to contain 5 mg of the active ingredient per mL of solution, then half-life of the product would be the time, when the concentration of active ingredient in the product is reduced to one-half of the original concentration, i.e. 2.5 mg per mL. The half-life in zero-order reaction can be calculated using an equation obtained by rearranging the zero-order rate equation as follows:

According to equation (3-12),

$$C_t = C_0 - K(t)$$

Half-life ($t_{½}$) is time, when C_t is equal to ½C_0. Substituting ½C_0 for C_t and $t_{½}$ for t into equation (3-12):

$$(1/2)C_0 = C_0 - K(t_{1/2})$$

which, upon rearrangement gives

$$t = \frac{C_0 - (1/2)C_0}{K} = \frac{(1/2)C_0}{2K} = \frac{C_0}{2K} \qquad (3\text{-}13)$$

It should be pointed out that the half-life of a zero-order reaction is based upon the initial concentration or concentration at time zero, C_0 and not concentration at any other time. The half-life calculated using concentration at any other time, C_t, would obviously reflect the half-life of reaction from that particular point in time and would not be indicative of the half-life of the reaction itself. Thus, if the initial concentration and the rate constant of reaction are known, equation (3-13) can be used to calculate the half-life. It is important to remember that half-life in a zero-order reaction is dependant on zero-order rate constant and initial concentration, i.e. concentration at time zero. For two products having the same zero-order rate constant, the product with larger initial concentration will have a longer half-life than the product made with a smaller initial concentration.

Example 3-5 Calculate the half-life of cough syrup using the data given in example 3-4.

Solution

Two methods can be used to determine half-life of the cough syrup:

i. The graphical method
ii. Using the zero-order equation.

Graphical Method

In the graphical method, the half-life is read directly from the graph. By definition, half-life is the time for the initial concentration (concentration at time zero) to be reduced to one-half the initial concentration (one-half the concentration at time zero). Hence, one reads the graph for the time, when initial concentration is reduced to 50%. From the graph shown in Figure 3-1, it is seen that the initial concentration (concentration at time 0) is 90 µg. Half-life is, therefore, time when this concentration (90 µg) is reduced to 50% (one half of 90 µg = 45 µg). Reading the graph to determine time, when $C = 45$ mg (45 µg on y-axis), one finds that this happens on day 30.

Therefore, the half-life of the cough syrup is 30 days.

Use of the Equation

Since $C_0 = 90$ μg and K was found to be 1.5 μg/day, half-life of the cough syrup can be determined by substituting these values into equation (3-13):

$$t_{1/2} = \frac{C_0}{2K} = \frac{90\ \mu g}{(2)(1.5\ \mu g/day)} = \frac{90\ \mu g}{3\ \mu g/day} = 30\ days$$

Therefore, the half-life of the cough syrup is 30 days. Thus, both methods yield the same answer.

Example 3-6 A drug in a suspension degrades according to zero-order kinetics. If half-life of the suspension is 400 days and K = 0.2 mg/day, calculate time, when suspension will contain 75 mg of the drug.

Solution

To calculate t, when C_t = 75 mg, one can use either equation (3-8) or equation (3-12). To use these equations, one needs to know initial amount of drug (C_0) in the suspension. Since K and $t_{1/2}$ are known, C_0 can be calculated by substituting the given values into equation (3-13):

$$t = \frac{C_0}{2K}$$

Therefore, $C_0 = (t_{1/2})(2K)$ = (400 days)(0.4 mg/day) = 160 mg

Substituting the values of C_0 = 160 mg, C_t = 75 mg and K = 0.2 mg/day into equation (3-12),

$$75\ mg = 160\ mg - (t)(0.2\ mg/day)$$

$$(t)(0.2\ mg/day) = 160\ mg - 75\ mg$$

$$(t)(0.2\ mg/day) = 85\ mg$$

$$t = \frac{85\ mg}{0.2\ mg/day} = 425\ days$$

Example 3-7 An antibiotic in its 100 mL suspension formulation, undergoes degradation according to zero-order kinetics. If the half-life of the suspension is 400 days and the zero-order rate constant of degradation is 0.1 mg/day, calculate the time, when the suspension will contain 75 mg of the antibiotic.

Solution

To calculate time (t), when concentration (C_t) will be 75 mg, one can use either equation (3-8) or equation (3-12). To use these equations, we need to know the initial amount of antibiotic (C_0) in the suspension. Since K and $t_{1/2}$ are known, C_0 can be calculated using the zero-order equation (3-13).

Substituting the given values into equation (3-13),

$$t_{1/2} = \frac{C_0}{2K}\text{, therefore,}$$

$$C_0 = (t_{1/2})(2K) = (400\ days)(0.2\ mg/day) = 80\ mg$$

Now substituting the values of C_0 (= 80 mg), C_t (= 75 mg) and K (= 0.2 mg/day) into equation (3-12),

$$C_t = C_0 - K(t)$$

$$75\ mg = 80\ mg - (0.1\ mg/day)(t)$$

$$t = \frac{5\ mg}{0.1\ mg/day} = 50\ days$$

FIRST-ORDER KINETICS

As shown in equation (3-6),

$$\frac{dC}{dt} = -KC$$

That is, the rate of a first-order reaction depends on the concentration of the reacting species. Thus, if the concentration of the reacting species is high, the reaction proceeds at a faster rate and if the concentration of the reacting species is small, the reaction proceeds at a slow rate. It will be recalled that the rate of reaction in zero-order kinetics was independent of the concentration of the reactant and the reaction proceeded at a constant rate, irrespective of the concentration of the reacting species. This is the basic difference between zero-order and first-order reactions.

Mathematical Treatment

The first-order rate equation is $\frac{dC}{dt} = -KC$

which may be written as $dC = -KC(dt)$ (3-14)

Or $$\frac{dC}{C} \; -K(dt) \qquad (3\text{-}15)$$

Equation (3-15) can be integrated between the limits of: $C = C_1$ at $t = t_1$ and $C = C_2$ at $t = t_2$ (where $C_1 > C_2$, and $t_2 > t_1$). Integration yields

$$\ln C_1 - \ln C_2 = -K(t_1 - t_2) \qquad (3\text{-}16)$$

Equation (3-16) contains five quantities. If four of these are known, the fifth quantity can be calculated. For example, equation (3-16) can be used to calculate the concentration at any given time provided the first-order rate constant and concentration at another time is known or to calculate time, when a given concentration will occur provided the first-order rate constant and concentration at another time is known.

Equation (3-16) can be rearranged to calculate the first-order rate constant of reaction if two concentrations at two different times are known:

$$K = \frac{\ln C_1 - \ln C_2}{t_1 - t_2} \qquad (3\text{-}17)$$

$$K = \frac{\ln C_1 - \ln C_2}{t_2 - t_1} \qquad (3\text{-}18)$$

Equation (3-16) can also be written in a form, which includes concentrations at time 0 and at any given time t. Concentration at time 0 is initial concentration, i.e. at $t_1 = 0$, $C_1 = C_0$ and concentration at any time t is C_t, i.e. $C_2 = C_t$ at $t_2 = t$. Thus, equation (3-16) becomes

$$\ln C_0 - \ln C_t = -K(0 - t) \qquad (3\text{-}19)$$

$$\ln C_0 = \ln C_t + K(t) \qquad (3\text{-}20)$$

or $$\ln C_t = \ln C_0 = -K(t) \qquad (3\text{-}21)$$

The natural logarithms in equation (3-21) can be converted into common logarithms using the relationship between the natural and common logarithms in Chapter 2 and given by equation (2-13). Multiplying equation (3-21) with the conversion factor 2.303, one gets

$$2.303 \times \log C_t = 2.303 \times \log C_0 - K(t) \qquad (3\text{-}22)$$

dividing both sides of equation (3-22) with the factor 2.303 gives K(t)

$$\log C_t = \log C_0 - \frac{K(t)}{2.303} \qquad (3\text{-}23)$$

Equation (3-23) is an equation of a straight line: y = b + mx.

In this equation, $y = \log C_t$, $b = \log C_0$, x = t and m = –K/2.303.

Equations (3-21) and (3-23) are similar to equation (3-12) of zero-order kinetics, the difference being that the concentration terms in first-order kinetics are logarithmic, while in zero-order kinetics, the concentration terms are not logarithmic. Logarithmic concentration terms in first-order reaction indicate exponential decrease in concentration with time, as opposed to linear decline in zero-order.

Equation (3-21) may be converted into an exponential form as follows:

$$\ln C_t = \ln C_0 - K(t)$$

$$\ln C_t - \ln C_0 = -K(t) \tag{3-24}$$

$$\ln \frac{C_t}{C_0} = -K(t) \tag{3-25}$$

taking inverse logarithms on both sides of equation (3-25),

$$\frac{C_t}{C_0} = e^{-K(t)} \tag{3-26}$$

$$C_t = C_0(e^{-K(t)}) \tag{3-27}$$

or

$$C_0 = C_t(e^{K(t)}) \tag{3-28}$$

Use of Equation

Equations (3-21) and (3-23) are equations of a straight line: y = mx + b. Similar to the zero-order equation (3-12), equations (3-21) and (3-23) contain four quantities; if three of these four quantities are known, the fourth quantity can be calculated.

Example 3-8 The amount of active ingredient in a tablet at 4 and 12 months after preparation of a product was found to be 365 mg and 341 mg per tablet, respectively. If degradation follows first-order kinetics, calculate, rate constant of degradation of the active ingredient.

Solution

Since amount of active ingredient at two different times is known, equation (3-17) can be used to calculate the rate constant K. Although equation (3-17) is written in terms of concentration (not amount), the amount of active ingredient in each tablet may be translated to mean concentration of active ingredient per tablet. Substituting the values C_1 = 365 mg/tablet at t_1 = 4 months and C_2 = 341 mg/tablet at t_2 = 12 months into equation (3-17), one gets

$$K = \frac{\ln C_1 - \ln C_2}{t_1 - t_2}$$

$$K = -\frac{\ln 365 - \ln 341}{4 \text{ months} - 12 \text{ months}} = \frac{0.06801}{8 \text{ months}} = 0.0085/\text{month}$$

Example 3-9 A product degrades according to first-order kinetics. When prepared, the concentration of active ingredient was 23 μg/mL and after 5 months, the concentration of active ingredient was 21 μg/mL. Calculate time, when concentration of active ingredient in the product will be 17.5 μg/mL.

Solution

To use equation (3-21) to find t, when C_t = 17.5 μg/mL, one needs to know the value of K. The value of K is determined by substituting the available data (C_0 = 23 μg/mL, C_t = 21 μg/mL and t = 5 months) into equation (3-21):

$$\ln C_t = \ln C_0 - K\,(t)$$

$$\ln 21\ \mu g/mL = \ln 23\ \mu g/mL - (K)(5\ months)$$

$$K\,(5\ months) = \ln 23\ \mu g/mL - \ln 21\ \mu g/mL$$

$$K = \frac{\ln 23\ \mu g/mL - \ln 21\ \mu g/mL}{5\ months} = 0.01819/months$$

Equation (3-21) is used again. Now C_0 = 23 μg/mL, when t = 0 and K = 0.01819/month. Solving for t, when C_t = 17.5 μg/mL, we have

$$\ln C_t = \ln C_0 - K(t)$$

$$\ln 17.5\ \mu g/mL = \ln 23\ \mu g/mL - (0.01819/month)(t)$$

$$t = \frac{\ln 23\ \mu g/mL - \ln 17.5\ \mu g/mL}{0.01819\ /\ months} = 15\ months$$

Alternatively: One can use the rate constant of degradation and either one of the two concentrations (23 μg/mL at time 0 or 21 μg/mL at 5 months) to solve for time that will elapse for the concentration to be reduced to 17.5 μg/mL.

Using concentration at time 0 (= 23 μg/mL), one can calculate time for concentration to be reduced from 23 μg/mL to 17.5 μg/mL or using concentration at 5 months (= 21 μg/mL), one can calculate time for concentration to be reduced from 21 μg/mL to 17.5 μg/mL.

To calculate t for concentration to reduce from 21 μg/mL to 17.5 μg/mL, one substitutes the values into equation (3-16).

$$\ln C_1 - \ln C_2 = -K(t_1 - t_2)$$

$$\ln 21\ \mu g/mL - \ln 17.5\ \mu g/mL = -(0.01819/month)(5 - t)$$

$$0.18232 = -(0.01819/month)(5 - t)$$

$$0.18232 = -0.09095 + 0.01819t$$

$$0.18232 + 0.09095 = 0.01819t$$

$$0.01819t = 0.27327$$

$$t = \frac{0.27327}{0.01819/month} = 15\ months$$

To calculate t for concentration to reduce from 23 μg/mL to 17.5 μg/mL, one substitutes the relevant values into equation (3-16).

$$\ln 23\ \mu g/mL - \ln 17.5\ \mu g/mL = -(0.01819/month)(0 - t)$$

$$0.27329 = -(0.01819/month)(0 - t)$$

$$0.27329 = 0.01819t$$

$$0.01819t = 0.27327$$

$$t = \frac{0.27327}{0.01819/month} = 15\ months$$

Example 3-10 A product is ineffective after it has decomposed 10%. At the time of preparation, the concentration of active ingredient in the product was 500 mg/mL. After 12 months, the concentration of active ingredient was 491 mg/mL. What should be the expiration date, if degradation follows first-order kinetics?

Solution

The product is ineffective after the active ingredient has decomposed 10%, therefore, it should not be used, when concentration of active ingredient remaining in the product is equal to or less than 90% of initial concentration. In this problem, C_0 = 500 mg/mL and one needs to find t when C_t is 90% of C_0, i.e.

$$90\% \text{ of } C_0 = 90\% \text{ of } 500 \text{ mg/mL} = (0.9)(500 \text{ mg/mL}) = 450 \text{ mg/mL}$$

One can use either equation (3-21) or (3-23), but one will need to know the value of K. To find the value of K, one can use equation (3-21).

Since two concentrations at two time periods are known (C_0 = 500 mg/mL at t = 0 month, and C_t = 491 mg/mL at t = 12 months), this information is used to calculate K.

The value of K is determined by substituting these data into equation (3-21) as follows:

$$\ln C_t = \ln C_0 - K(t)$$

$$\ln 491 \text{ mg/mL} = \ln 500 \text{ mg/mL} - K(12 \text{ months})$$

$$K(12 \text{ months}) = \ln 500 \text{ mg/mL} - \ln 491 \text{ mg/mL}$$

$$K = \frac{\ln 500 \text{ mg/mL} - \ln 491 \text{ mg/mL}}{12 \text{ months}} = \frac{0.0816}{12 \text{ months}} = = 0.0015/\text{ month}$$

Substituting into equation (3-21), C_0 = 500 mg/mL, K = 0.0015/month, and C_t = 450 mg/mL,

$$\ln C_t = \ln C_0 - K(t)$$

$$\ln 450 \text{ mg/mL} = \ln 500 \text{ mg/mL} - (0.0015/\text{month})(t)$$

$$(0.0015/\text{month})(t) = \ln 500 \text{ mg/mL} - \ln 450 \text{ mg/mL} = 0.1054$$

$$t = \frac{0.1054}{0.0015/\text{months}} = 70.3 \text{ months}$$

Graphical Representation

Equations (3-21) and (3-23) are equations of a straight line.

In equation (3-21), the values of y, b, m and x are: y = ln C_t, b = ln C_0, m = –K and x = t and in equation (3-23), the values of y, b, m and x are: y = log C_t, b = log C_0, m = –K/2.303 and x = t.

A plot of logarithm of concentration at any time t as a function of time will yield a straight line, with y-intercept = logarithm of C_0. The first-order rate constant can be determined from the slope of the straight line. The graphical representation of first-order equations is best illustrated using an example.

Example 3-11 A product is prepared by reconstitution. The degradation of the product as a function of time gave the following data (time is in months and concentration is in mg/product). From these data, calculate the rate constant of degradation.

Time(months):	1	2	4	6	8	10	12	14
Concentration (mg/product):	300	260	200	150	115	85	65	50

Solution

Figure 3-2 shows a plot of concentration of product remaining to be degraded as a function of time according to zero-order kinetics.

The data in Figure 3-2 do not exhibit a linear relationship. A non-linear relationship between concentration and time indicates that degradation does not follow zero-order kinetics. Therefore, the data should be plotted according to first-order kinetics to see, if degradation proceeds according to first-order kinetics.

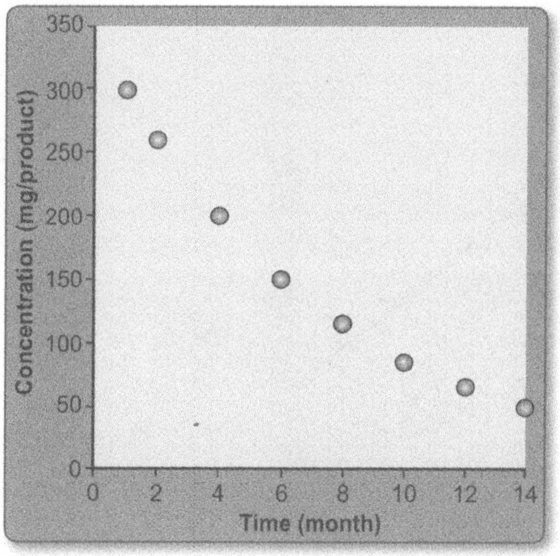

Fig. 3-2 Zero-order plot of data in Example 3-11

In order to plot the data according to first-order kinetics, one may plot either the natural logarithms of concentration terms as a function of time or the common logarithms of concentration terms as a function of time. To do this, all concentration terms need to be converted into their corresponding (natural or common) logarithmic terms. Table 3-1 lists the common logarithms as well as the natural logarithms of the concentration terms provided in the data.

Plot of ln C versus t: In this plot, the natural logarithms of concentration terms (ln C) are plotted on the y-axis and the corresponding time terms (t) are plotted on the x-axis. Figure 3-3 shows the plot of ln C versus t.

A linear relationship indicates first-order kinetics. Since the data do not exhibit too much scatter, a straight line that best represents the data is drawn using eye-ball judgment. The straight line is back extrapolated to read the y-intercept. The y-intercept is in C_0. The y-intercept reads 5.86. This means that:

$$\ln C_0 = 5.86$$

$$\text{therefore, } C_0 = \text{inverse } \ln 5.86$$

$$\text{inverse } \ln 5.86 = 350 \text{ mg}$$

$$\text{Therefore, } C_0 = 350 \text{ mg}$$

Table 3-1 Logarithms of concentration terms for data shown in Example 3-11

Time (month)	*Concentration (mg/product)*	*ln concentration*	*log concentration*
1	300	5.70	2.477
2	260	5.56	2.415
4	200	5.30	2.301
6	150	5.01	2.176
8	115	4.75	2.061
10	85	4.44	1.929
12	65	4.17	1.813
14	50	3.91	1.699

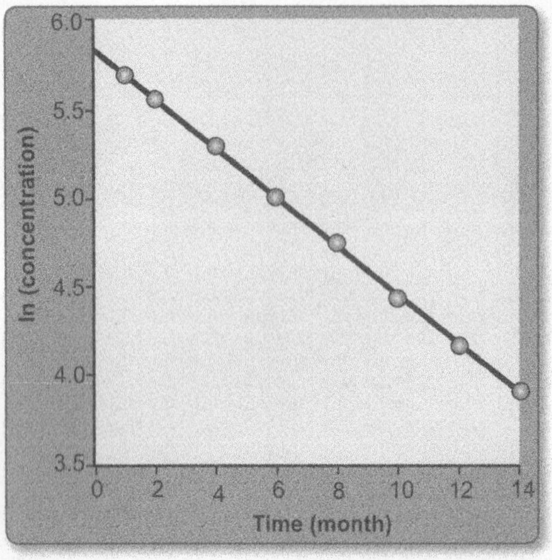

Fig. 3-3 Plot of 'ln C versus Time' for data in Example 3-11

The slope of straight line = –K. To determine K (rate constant), one finds the slope of the straight line by choosing two points. If the points chosen are: (x_1 = 0 month, ln y_1 = 5.86 mg) and (x_2 = 14 months, ln y_2 = 3.91 mg), then

$$\text{slope} = \frac{\Delta y}{\Delta x} = \frac{\ln y_2 - \ln y_1}{x_2 - x_1}$$

$$K = -\text{slope} = -\frac{3.91 - 5.86}{14 - 0} = -\frac{-19.5}{14 \text{ months}} = 0.14/\text{month}$$

This graph can also be used to determine the concentration at a given time or time for a given concentration. For example, to find C at 9 months, one reads y-axis corresponding to t = 9 months.

From the graph, In C at 9 months = 4.6, therefore,

C at 9 months = inverse ln 4.6 = 99.5 mg

Similarly, to know t for, say, a concentration of 220 mg, one reads t for ln 220

ln 220 = 5.39; according to Figure 3-3 t for ln 220 (5.39) = 3.2 months

Therefore, concentration 220 will be at 3.2 months.

Equation (3-21) can also be used to determine C_t at any time t or t for a given C_t when C_0 and K are known.

Since C_0 = 350 mg, and K = 0.14/month, one can calculate C_t at 9 months as follows:

$$\ln C_t = \ln C_0 - K\,(t)$$

$$\ln C_t = \ln 350 \text{ mg} - (0.14/\text{month})(9 \text{ months}) = 5.858 \text{ mg} - 1.26 = 4.598 \text{ mg}$$

$$C_t = \text{inverse} \ln 4.598 \text{ mg} = 99 \text{ mg/product}$$

Similarly to determine t for a concentration of 220 mg,

$$\ln 220 \text{ mg} = \ln 350 \text{ mg} - (0.14/\text{month})(t)$$

$$t = \frac{\ln 350 - \ln 200}{0.14/\text{month}} = \frac{0.4643}{0.14/\text{month}} = = 3.3 \text{ months}$$

Plot of log C versus t: This plot is similar to the plot of natural logarithms of concentration as a function of time, except common logarithms of concentrations are plotted as a function of time. Figure 3-4 shows this plot. The straight line is back extrapolated to time 0. The y-intercept reads 2.544, i.e. log C_0 is 2.544.

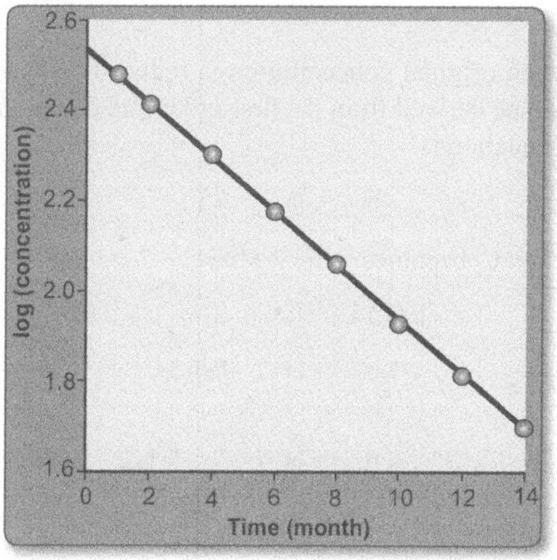

Fig. 3-4 Plot of 'log C versus Time' for data in Example 3-11

$$\log C_0 = 2.544$$

$$\text{therefore, } C_0 = \text{inverse log } 2.544 = 350 \text{ mg}$$

The slope of the straight line is –K/2.303. To determine K, one finds slope by choosing two points on the straight line. If one chooses ($x_1 = 0$, $\log y_1 = 2.54$) and ($x_2 = 14$, $\log y_2 = 1.7$):

$$\text{slope} = \frac{\Delta y}{\Delta x} = \frac{\log y_1 - \log y_1}{x_2 - x_1} = \frac{1.7 - 2.54}{14 - 0} = -0.06 \text{ months and}$$

$$K = (-2.303)(\text{slope}) = (-2.303)(-0.06/\text{month}) = 0.14/\text{month}$$

This graph can also be used to determine concentration at a given time or time for a given concentration. For example, to find C at 9 months, one reads y-axis corresponding to t = 9 months. From the graph, log C at 9 months = 2.0, therefore, C = inverse log 2.0 = 100 mg/product.

Similarly, to know time when C = 220 mg, one reads t for log 220 = 2.34. From Figure 3-4, t = 3.2 months. Equation (3-23) can also be used to determine C_t at any time t or t for a given C_t (when C_0 and K are known). For example, C_t at 9 months is calculated as follows:

$$\log C_t = \log C_0 - \frac{K(t)}{2.303}$$

$$\log C_t = \log 350 - \frac{(0.14/\text{month})(9 \text{ months})}{2.303}$$

$$\log C_t = 2.544 - 0.541 = 2.003 \text{ mg}$$

$$\text{therefore, } C_t = \text{inverse log } 2.003 \text{ mg} = 100 \text{ mg/product}$$

And, to determine t for C = 220 mg/product:

$$\log C_t = \log C_0 - \frac{K(t)}{2.303}$$

$$\log C_t = \log 350 - \frac{(0.14/\text{month})(t)}{2.303} = 2.5441 - 0.00608\ t$$

$$\log 200 \text{ mg} = 2.5441 - 0.0608\ t$$

$$\text{therefore, } 2.3424 = 2.5441 - 0.0608\ t$$

$$0.0608t = 2.5441 - 2.3424 = 0.202$$

$$t = \ = 3.3 \text{ months}$$

Half-Life

Half-life is the time when original concentration is reduced 50%, i.e., when $C_t = ½C_0$. The equation for half-life can be derived from the first-order rate equation as follows:

The first-order rate equation is

$$\ln C_t = \ln C_0 - K(t)$$

Substituting $t_{1/2}$ for t when C_t becomes $½C_0$, we have

$$\ln(0.5)C_0 = \ln C_0 - K(t_{1/2}) \quad (3\text{-}29)$$

$$K(t_{1/2}) = \ln C_0 - \ln(0.5)C_0 \quad (3\text{-}30)$$

$$K(t_{1/2}) = \ln \frac{C_0}{(0.5)C_0} = \ln 2 = 0.693 \quad (3\text{-}31)$$

$$t_{½} = \frac{0.693}{K} \quad (3\text{-}32)$$

The equation for half-life can also be derived from equation (3-23), the first-order rate equation in common logarithms. Equation (3-32) shows that half-life in first-order kinetics is independent of initial concentration (whereas in zero-order kinetics, half-life is a function of original concentration). Thus, half-life of a product, which follows first-order kinetics would be the same regardless of initial concentration of the product. The half-life in first-order kinetics can be either read from the graph or it can be determined by using equation (3-32) as long as K is known.

Example 3-12 Calculate half-life of the reconstituted product in Example 3-11.

Solution

Half-life of the reconstituted product can be determined either by using equation (3-32) or by reading from the graph.

1. *Using Equation*: Since rate constant, K was found to be 0.14/month, half-life is obtained by substituting the value of K into equation (3-32):

$$t = \frac{0.693}{K} = \frac{0.693}{0.14/\text{month}} = 4.95 \text{ months}$$

2. *Graphical Method*: A graph can be plotted using either log concentration or ln concentration as a function of time. Two graphs were constructed to plot the data in Example 3-11.

Plot of ln C Versus t: Since, the y-intercept in Figure 3-3 is ln C_0, therefore, C_0 = inverse ln 5.858 = 350 mg. Since half-life is the time for 50% of the product to be degraded, one reads the time when the concentration becomes 50% of the initial concentration, i.e. when C = 50% of C_0 = 50% of 350 mg = 175 mg. Since y-axis is ln C, one reads the time for ln 175 (= 5.165). From Figure 3-3, the time corresponding to 5.165 on the y-axis is about 5 months. Therefore, half-life is approximately 5 months.

Plot of log C Versus t: The y-intercept in Figure 3-4 is log C_0. Therefore, C_0 = inverse log 2.544 = 350 mg. Half-life is time when concentration is 50% of C_0. 50% of $C_0 = ½C_0 = ½(350)$ = 175 mg. Since y-axis is log C, one reads the time for log 175 = 2.243. From Figure 3-4, the time corresponding to 2.243 on the y-axis is about 5 months; therefore half-life is approximately 5 months.

SEMI-LOGARITHMIC GRAPH PAPER

To construct a plot of natural logarithm of concentration as a function of time (Fig. 3-3) or a plot of common logarithm of concentration as a function of time (Fig. 3-4), one needs to convert concentration terms into either natural logs or common logs before it is possible to plot concentration terms on the graph paper. To avoid the time-consuming process of converting each concentration term into its logarithmic form, a semi-logarithmic graph paper is used. As the name suggests, one axis of this graph paper is in the log scale and the other axis is in coordinate scale. The semi-log paper used to plot data in pharmacokinetic studies has y-axis in the logarithmic scale and the x-axis in regular coordinate scale.

Plotting the data on a semi-log graph paper differs from plotting the data on a regular coordinate graph paper in several respects because a semi-log graph paper differs from a regular coordinate graph paper in several respects. The following features distinguish a graph paper having a regular coordinate scale on one axis and a log scale on the other axis from a graph paper having regular coordinate scale on both of its axis:

1. In a rectangular two-dimensional coordinate graph paper, both axis of graph paper are in rectilinear coordinate scale. In a semi-logarithmic graph paper one axis is in the logarithmic scale and the other is in regular coordinate scale. Since, in pharmacokinetic studies, a semi-log graph paper is used to plot concentration of drug in plasma as a function of time, it is traditional that the y-axis of the semi-logarithmic graph paper is used in the logarithmic scale.
2. Negative numbers cannot be plotted on the logarithmic scale because one cannot take either natural logarithm or common logarithm of a negative number. Also, the concentration of drug in plasma cannot be negative.
3. The logarithmic scale (y-axis) of a semi-logarithmic graph paper is divided into 9 main divisions and each main division is further divided into smaller subdivisions. Depending on the space available between the main divisions, the main divisions may be sub-divided into 5, 10 or 20 subdivisions.
4. The 9 main divisions are pre-set and cannot be changed. These divisions are neither equally spaced nor equally subdivided, but are spaced and subdivided in a logarithmic fashion. The nine main divisions on the logarithmic scale constitute one cycle of semi-logarithmic graph paper. The y-axis on a rectangular graph paper is generally divided into 10 equally spaced main divisions and each main division is subdivided into 10 or 20 equally spaced subdivisions. No specific rules govern the assignment of numerical values on y-axis as long as each division and subdivision is treated in an identical manner.
5. There is no zero on the y-axis of logarithmic scale, because logarithm of zero does not exist. The lowest or highest point on the y-axis of a semi-logarithmic graph paper cannot have any arbitrary numerical value. It must have a numerical value equal to 1×10^n, where n can be any positive or negative whole number. On a rectangular coordinate paper, the lowest or highest point on the y-axis can be assigned any positive or negative numerical value.
6. A semi-logarithmic graph paper having 9 main divisions on its entire y-axis is called one cycle semi-logarithmic graph paper. The highest point on the y-axis of this graph paper has a numerical value equal to 10 times the numerical value of the lowest point, i.e. if the lowest point on a semi-logarithmic graph paper has a numerical value of 1×10^n, then the numerical value of highest point on this graph paper will be $1 \times 10^{(n+1)}$.
7. Figure 3-5 shows the difference in spacing on the y-axis on a rectangular and semi-logarithmic graph paper.
8. In both cases the highest point on y-axis has a numerical value of 10 and the entire length of the y-axis is used. In rectangular graph paper the numerical values range from 0 to 10 (10 main divisions represent 10 unit). On a semi-log paper, the numerical values range from 1 to 10 and

9 divisions represent the values from 1 through 10. The same amount of space that describes 10 units on a rectangular paper describes 9 units on a semi-log paper, but the space allotted to each unit is different. Each unit on y-axis of a rectangular paper is assigned an identical numerical value (the same amount of space is occupied by each unit of numerical values). On the other hand, each unit on the y-axis of a semi-log paper differs in value greatly. For example, on the y-axis of a semi-log paper the distance between the numerical values of 1 and 2 (1 unit) occupies the same amount of space as is occupied by 3 units on a rectangular paper (between the numerical values of 0 and 3). The distance between the numerical values of 5 and 10 (5 units) on a semi-log paper occupies the same amount of space as is occupied by 3 units on a rectangular graph paper (between the numerical values of 7 and 10). The amount of space needed to describe a given distance on the y-axis of a semi-log graph paper decreases as the numerical values of the point being plotted increases (exponential change). Figure 3-6 shows one-cycle semi-logarithmic graph paper.

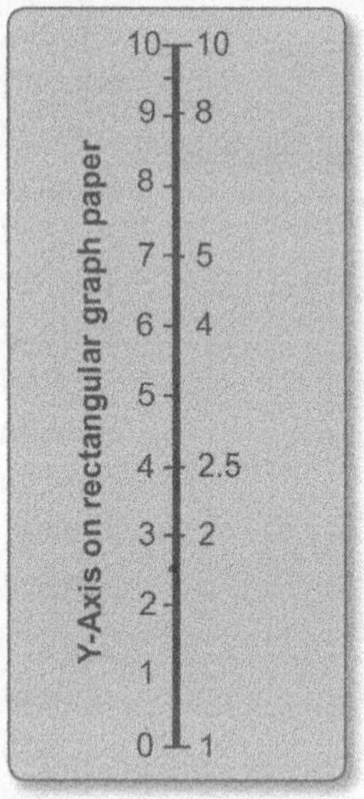

Fig. 3-5 Difference in spacing on y-axis of rectangular and semi-logarithmic graph papers
* The spacings on the semi-logarithmic scale are approximate

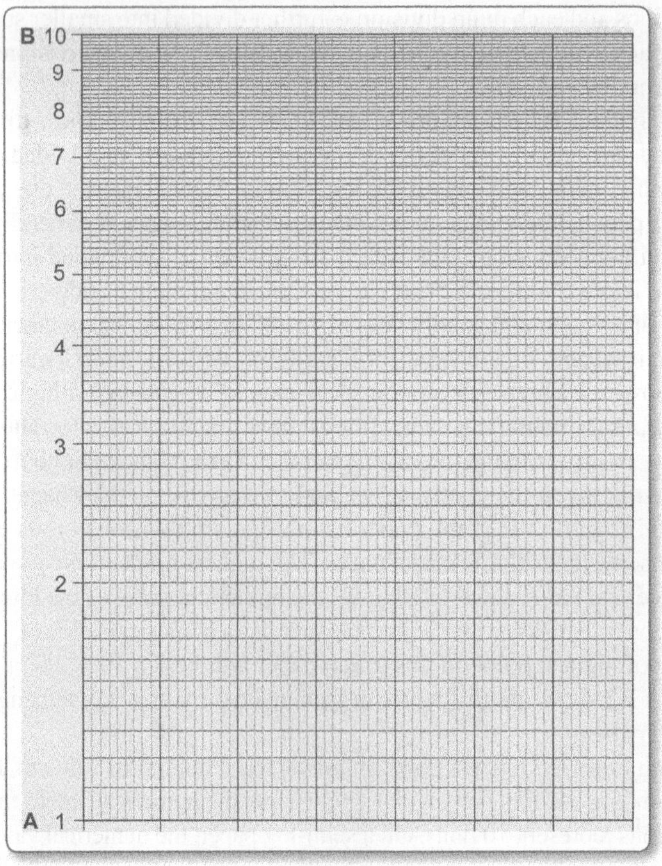

Fig. 3-6 One-cycle semi-logarithmic graph paper

9. When the highest point on the y-axis of a semi-logarithmic graph paper has a numerical value equal to 10 times the numerical value of the lowest point, then this graph paper is called one cycle semi-logarithmic graph paper. Figure 3-6 shows one-cycle semi-logarithmic graph paper. Thus, if point A on the y-axis of this graph paper = 1, then point B must be 1 × 10 = 10. Similarly, if point A is 0.01, then point B = 0.1 and if point A is 100 then point B = 1,000 and so on.
10. One-cycle semi-logarithmic graph paper should only be used if the highest term on y-axis (usually, concentration term) is expected to be equal to or less than 10 times the smallest term, which starts the cycle on logarithmic scale or if the lowest term is expected to be equal to or more than one-tenth the concentration term, which ends the logarithmic scale. If the highest concentration term is expected to be greater than 10-times the concentration term, which starts the logarithmic cycle, then one cycle semi-log paper should not be used, because points greater than 10 times the lowest concentration term which starts the logarithmic cycle cannot be plotted on this cycle. Similarly, if lowest concentration term is less than one-tenth the highest concentration term which ends the logarithmic cycle, then one would not be able to plot points, which are less than one-tenth the highest concentration term on this cycle. Thus, one would need a two or more than a two cycle semi-log paper.
11. A two cycle semi-logarithmic graph paper contains two logarithmic cycles on y-axis. The two cycles are placed one on top of the other. The two cycles combined occupy the same space as is occupied by a single cycle on one cycle semi-log paper. The lowest point on a two cycle semi-log paper has a numerical value of 1×10^n and the highest point has a numerical value of $1 \times 10^{(n+2)}$.
12. Figure 3-7 shows a two cycle semi-logarithmic graph paper. Here, if point A on y-axis is 1, then point B on y-axis would be 10 times the numerical value of point A or 1 × 10 = 10,

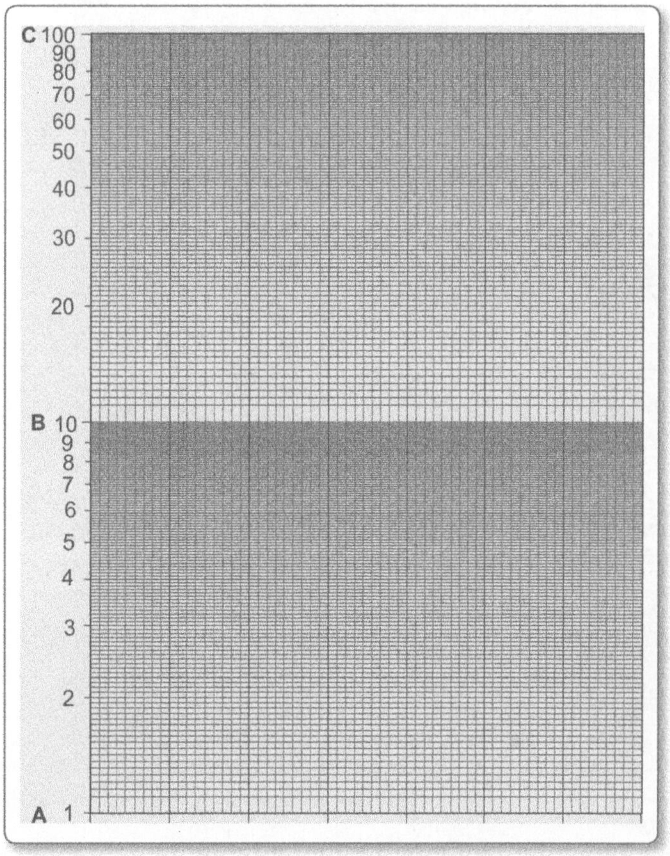

Fig. 3-7 Two-cycle semi-logarithmic graph paper

and the numerical value of point C will be 10 × 10 = 100. Similarly, if the numerical value of point A on y-axis is 0.01, then the numerical value of point B will be 0.01 × 10 = 0.1 and the numerical value of point C will be 0.1 × 10 = 1.0. That is, from point A to point B constitutes one cycle, therefore numerical value of point B is 10 times the numerical value of point A. Similarly, from point B to point C is second cycle and the numerical value of point C is 10 times the numerical value of point B (or 100 times the numerical value of point A). A two-cycle semi-logarithmic graph paper is used when the highest concentration term to be plotted is expected to have a numerical value equal to or less than 100 times the numerical value of the lowest concentration term on y-axis or when the lowest concentration term is expected to have a numerical value equal to or greater than 100th the numerical value of the highest concentration term on y-axis.

13. A three cycle semi logarithmic graph paper contains three logarithmic cycles on the y-axis, each cycle repeating one after another. These three cycles combined occupy the same space on the y-axis as is occupied by two logarithmic cycles on the y-axis of a two cycle semi-logarithmic graph paper or by one cycle of the one cycle semi-logarithmic graph paper.
14. If the lowest concentration, which starts the three cycle semi-logarithmic graph paper has a numerical value of 1×10^n, then the highest concentration, which ends the third cycle on the three-cycle semi-logarithmic graph paper will have a numerical value of $1 \times 10^{(n+3)}$, or 1,000 times the numerical value of the concentration which started the first cycle of the 3-cycle paper. Figure 3-8 shows a three cycle semi-logarithmic graph paper. Here, if the numerical value of point A is 1, then the numerical value of point B will be 1 × 10 = 10, the numerical value of point C will be 10 × 10 = 100 and the numerical value of point D should be 100 × 10 = 1,000. Similarly, if the numerical value of the lowest point, point A, on this paper is 0.01, then the numerical value of point B will be 10 times the numerical value of point A, i.e. 10

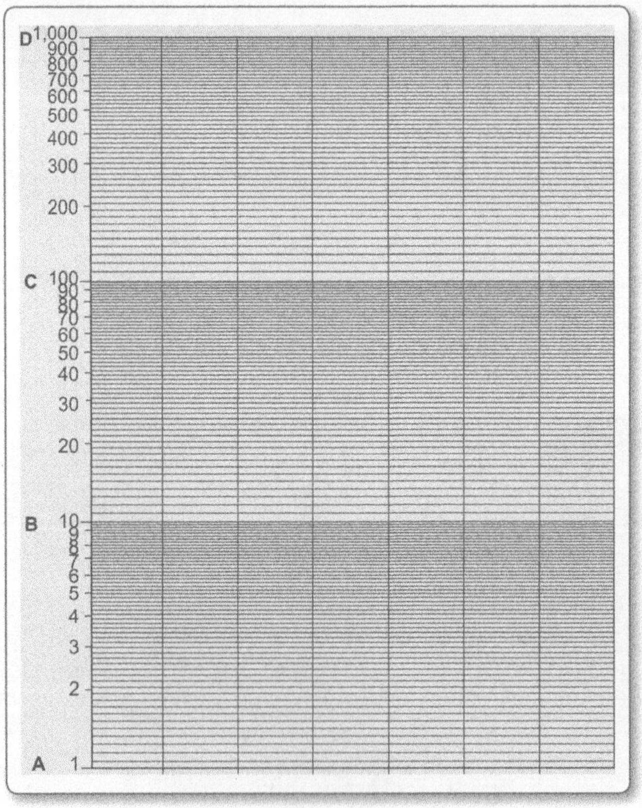

Fig. 3-8 Three-cycle semi-logarithmic graph paper

× 0.01 = 0.1. The numerical value of point C will be 10 times the numerical value of point B or 10 × 0.1 = 1.0 and the numerical value of point D should be 10 times the numerical value of point C_0 or 10 × 1.0 = 10.

15. A three-cycle semi-logarithmic graph paper is used when the numerical value of the highest concentration term is expected to be equal to or less than 1,000 times the numerical value of the lowest concentration term, which starts the first-logarithmic cycle or when the lowest numerical value, which starts the first cycle of logarithmic scale is expected to be equal to or greater than one thousandth the numerical value of highest concentration term, which ends the third logarithmic cycle.
16. Semi-logarithmic graph papers containing more than three cycles (e.g. four, five or more than five cycles) are also available. These graph papers are used when the concentration terms to be plotted on the y-axis exhibit a range that cannot be accommodated on a semi-log graph paper containing fewer cycles.
17. One must be careful in choosing the right type of semi-logarithmic graph paper to plot the data. One should not use the one-cycle semi-logarithmic graph paper when the data suggest that more than one logarithmic cycle will be needed to plot the graph, because the data (concentration points) that do not fit the one logarithmic cycle on the y-axis cannot be plotted. Similarly, one should not use a multi-cycle semi-logarithmic graph paper when one-cycle semi-logarithmic graph paper would do the job, because the space allotted to one logarithmic cycle on the y-axis in the multi-cycle semi-logarithmic graph paper is much less than the space allotted to one-cycle on the y-axis of the one-cycle semi-logarithmic graph paper. If a much smaller space (than that needed) is used to plot the data on the y-axis, the accuracy of plotting the data decreases as the number of logarithmic cycles increases.
18. When the data are plotted on one logarithmic cycle of a multi-cycle semi-logarithmic graph paper, the concentration terms get "squeezed" into a very small segment of the y-axis. This makes it very difficult to assess whether or not the relationship between the variables under study is linear or not. More often than not, the data which do not exhibit linearity may mistakenly be considered linear when a much smaller space is used to squeeze the concentration points.

Advantage of Using a Semi-log Paper

1. The main advantage of using semi-log graph paper is that one does not convert concentration terms into their individual logarithmic terms. The concentration terms are plotted as "real" numbers because divisions on the logarithmic y-axis plot these numbers as if logarithms of these numbers were being plotted.
2. If one wants to know the concentration at a specific time, the concentration corresponding to that time is "read" directly from the graph.
3. Similarly, if one wanted to determine the time for a given concentration, the concentration is read directly on the graph without conversion to inverse logarithms and the corresponding time is read from the graph.
4. The only drawback of plotting the data on the semi-logarithmic graph paper is that, if slope of the straight line needs to be determined, one must convert concentration points on the y-axis chosen for calculating the slope into logarithms of concentration in order to reflect the change in the y-values.

Example 3-13 From the data given in Example 3-11, calculate the rate constant of degradation of the reconstituted product using a semi-logarithm graph paper.

Solution

Figure 3-9 shows a plot of the data on a two-cycle semi-logarithmic graph paper. Because the concentration terms range from 300 to 50, a two-cycle semi-log graph paper is used. One cycle will accommodate concentration terms between 10 and 100 and the second cycle will accommodate concentration terms between 100 and 1000.

Although the concentration terms were plotted without conversion to logarithms, the y-axis plotted these terms as if logarithms of these concentration terms were being plotted.

A linear relationship between the concentration terms and time indicates first-order kinetics, and the y-intercept = C_0, not log C_0 or ln C_0.

To determine the slope, we choose two points on the straight line:

$x_1 = 0$ month, $y_1 = 350$ mg; and $x_2 = 14$ months, $y_2 = 50$ mg

$$\text{slope} = \frac{\log y_2 - \log y_1}{x_2 - x_1} \quad \text{or} \quad \text{slope} = \frac{\ln y_2 - \ln y_1}{x_2 - x_1}$$

$$\text{slope} = \frac{\log 50 - \log 350}{14 - 0} \quad \text{or} \quad \text{slope} = \frac{\log 50 - \log 350}{14 - 0}$$

$$\text{slope} = \frac{-0.845}{14} = -0.06035/\text{ month} \quad \text{or} \quad \text{slope} = \frac{-1.95}{14} = -0.14/\text{month}$$

The slope is related to the rate constant K as follows:

K = – slope, if natural logarithms are used and

K = (–2.303)(slope) if common logarithms are used.

When common logarithms are used:

Rate constant K = (–2.303)(slope)

Rate constant K = (–2.303)(–0.06035/month) = 0.14/month.

When natural logarithms are used:

Rate constant K = –slope

Rate constant K = –(–0.14/month) = 0.14/month.

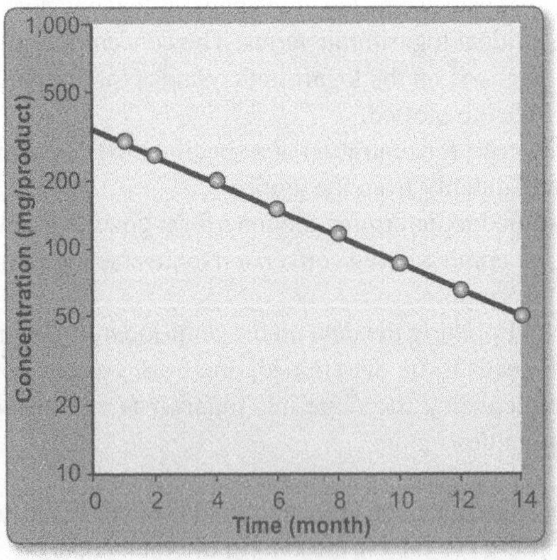

Fig. 3-9 Semi-logarithmic plot of data given in Example 3-11

Thus, the value of rate constant K is the same, whether one uses natural or common logarithms.

Determination of concentration at any time or finding time for a given concentration is also much simpler when a semi-logarithmic graph paper is used because concentration terms on the y-axis are "real terms," not the logarithmic terms. For example, to find time for a concentration of 220 mg in the product, the concentration on the y-axis is read directly. Figure 3-9 shows that the time corresponding to the concentration/product of 220 is 3.2 months.

Similarly, to know what will be the concentration at 9 months, one reads the graph for concentration (on the y-axis) corresponding to 9 months (on the x-axis) and the graph in Figure 3-9 shows that at 9 months the concentration = 99 mg/product.

Half-Life: The y-intercept in Figure 3-9 is concentration at time 0 or C_0, because in this plot "real" numbers are plotted on the y-axis. Therefore half-life is when C_0 (= 350 mg) becomes one-half of C_0 = one-half of 350 mg = 175 mg. The time corresponding to 175 mg is about 5 months; therefore, the half-life is approximately 5 months.

Example 3-14 The amount of active ingredient in a pharmaceutical product (degrading by first-order kinetics) 3 months and 10 months after preparation was found to be 26 and 18 mg, respectively. Calculate half-life of the product.

Solution

To determine half-life of the product one needs to know K, the rate constant of degradation. From the data available, K can be calculated using equation (3-18) as follows:

$$K = \frac{\ln C_1 - \ln C_2}{t_1 - t_2}$$

$$K = \frac{\ln 26 - \ln 18}{10\,\text{months} - 3\,\text{months}}$$

$$K = \frac{3.258 - 2.890}{7\,\text{months}}$$

$$K = \frac{0.368}{7\,\text{months}}$$

$$K = 0.0526/\text{month}$$

The rate constant of degradation, K, can also be calculated using the equation dealing with common logarithms shown in Example 3-13:

$$\text{slope} = \frac{\log C_1 - \log C_2}{t_2 - t_1}$$

$$\text{slope} = \frac{\log 26 - \log 18}{3\,\text{months} - 10\,\text{months}}$$

$$\text{slope} = \frac{1.415 - 1.255}{-7\,\text{months}} = -0.0229/\text{month}$$

$$K = -(2.303)(\text{slope})$$

$$K = -(2.303)(-0.0229/\text{month}) = 0.0526/\text{month}$$

therefore,

$$t_{1/2} = \frac{0.693}{0.0526/\text{months}} = 13.2\ \text{months}$$

SUGGESTED READING

1. Daniels F. Mathematical Preparation for Physical Chemistry. MGraw-Hill; 1956.
2. Martin A. Physical Pharmacy. 4th edition. Lea and Febigerl; 1993.
3. Remington. The Science and Practice of Pharmacy. 21st edition. Mack Publishing; 2005.
4. Steinbach O, King C. Experiments in Physical Chemistry. American Book Co; 1950.

PRACTICE PROBLEMS

3-1. Plot the following data and determine: (a) order of reaction, (b) initial concentration, (c) half-life, and (d) concentration at 24 months.

Time (month)	*Concentration (mg/mL)*
2.0	7.0
4.0	5.3
6.0	4.2
8.0	3.3
10.0	2.6
12.0	2.0

3-2. Plot the following data and determine the following: (a) order of reaction, (b) initial amount, (c) rate constant of degradation, (d) half-life, and (e) amount on day 5.

Time (day)	*Amount (mg)*
10	690
20	575
30	470
40	350
50	250
60	125

3-3. From the following data calculate initial concentration, rate constant of degradation and time when concentration will be 130 mg/L

Time (day)	*Concentration (mg/L)*
10	310
20	300
40	285
60	275
100	250
140	225
180	210
260	175

3-4. From the following data calculate concentration on day 70.

Time (day)	*Concentration (µg/L)*
5	3.3
10	2.6
15	2.0
20	1.6
25	1.3
30	1.0
35	0.8

3-5. After rapid intravenous bolus administration of 250 mg dose of a drug at 6 am, the concentrations of drug in plasma at 10 am and 1 pm were 290 and 195 μg/mL respectively. If the drug is eliminated according to first-order kinetics, what will be the concentration of drug in plasma at 6 am the following morning?

3-6. Plot the following data and calculate C_0, K and $t_{1/2}$ (assume zero-order kinetics).

Time (week)	*Concentration (mg/mL)*
1	131
2	124
4	122
6	117
10	103
12	96

3-7. From the following data calculate half-life:

Time (week)	*Concentration (μg/mL)*
4	5.2
8	4.6
12	4.0
20	3.1
28	2.5
40	1.7

3-8. When prepared, a product contained 500 mg of active ingredient. After 12 months, the amount of active ingredient was found to be 392 mg. If degradation follows zero-order kinetics, calculate:
(a) half-life, and (b) the amount of active ingredient at 36 months.

3-9. A product is ineffective after it has decomposed 20%. At the time of preparation, the concentration of active ingredient was 500 mg per fluid ounce. After 6 months the concentration of active ingredient was found to be 450 mg per fluid ounce. What should be the expiration date if degradation follows zero-order kinetics?

3-10. A dye in a product fades according to zero-order kinetics. When manufactured, intensity of the dye was 620 units. After 10 months intensity was reduced to 510 units. When will intensity be 180 units?

3-11. The concentration of active ingredient in a product at 4 and 12 months after preparation was found to be 365 mg per fluid ounce and 100 mg per fluid ounce, respectively. If the product degrades according to first-order kinetics, calculate the concentration of active ingredient per fluid ounce at the time of preparation of the product.

3-12. The active ingredient in a product degrades according to zero-order kinetics. When prepared, the amount of active ingredient was 100 mg/tablet. After 2 months the amount of active ingredient was found to be 97.5 mg/tablet. When will the amount of active ingredient be 85 mg/tablet?

3-13. Calculate the half-life of a product if concentrations on day 10 and day 40 after preparation of the product were determined to be 28 mg/mL and 16 mg/mL, respectively. Assume the product undergoes degradation according to zero-order kinetics.

3-14. The manufacturer of a product wants to assure that each tablet contains at least 300 mg of drug throughout the shelf-life of the product. If expiration date on the product is 4 years and first-order rate constant of degradation is 0.001/month, calculate the amount of drug that should be present in each tablet at the time of preparation of the product.

3-15. An oral antibiotic suspension should not be used after the antibiotic has degraded 15%. A hospital pharmacist reconstituted the suspension and put an expiration time of 14 days. Calculate the rate constant of degradation if concentration of antibiotic at reconstitution time was 125 mg/5 mL and degradation follows zero-order.

3-16. A product is ineffective after it has decomposed 30%. At the time of preparation, the concentration of active ingredient was 5 μg/teaspoonful. After 3 months concentration of active ingredient was reduced to 4.5 μg/teaspoonful. What should be expiration date on the label if degradation follows zero-order kinetics?

3-17. The rate constant of degradation of a product degrading by first order kinetics is 0.25 per year. What is its half-life?

3-18. The manufacturer of a product wants to assure that each tablet contains 300 mg of the active ingredient throughout the shelf-life of the product. If expiration date on the product is 4 years and zero-order rate constant of degradation is 0.5 μg/h, calculate amount of active ingredient that should be present in each tablet when the product is made.

3-19. From the following data calculate: Initial amount, rate constant of degradation and half-life of the product. Degradation follows zero-order kinetics.

Time (hour)	*Amount (μg)*
0.5	12.0
1.0	11.5
1.5	11.0
2.0	10.5
3.0	9.5
4.0	8.5
5.0	7.5

3-20. The following data were obtained after administration of a single 500 mg intravenous bolus dose of a drug to a 32-year male patient:

Time (hour)	*Concentration (μg/mL)*
2	32.749
3	29.633
4	26.813
6	21.952
8	17.973
10	14.715
12	12.048
14	9.864

Calculate the following: (a) Concentration immediately after administration of the dose, (b) Rate constant of elimination, (c) Biological half-life, and (d) Concentration at 30 hours.

3-21. A product is ineffective after it has decomposed 20 percent. At the time of preparation, the concentration of active ingredient was 500 mg per fluid ounce. After 6 months the concentration of active ingredient was found to be 450 mg per fluid ounce. What should be the expiration date if degradation follows first-order kinetics?

3-22. The following data were obtained after administration of a 50 mg intravenous bolus dose of a drug to a 52-year male patient:

Time (hour)	Concentration (μg/L)
2	95
4	82
6	68
8	60
10	45
12	43
14	27
16	20

If elimination follows zero-order kinetics, calculate: (a) initial concentration, (b) rate constant of elimination, and (c) half-life.

3-23. Calculate the half-life of a product if concentrations on day 10 and day 40 after preparation of the product were determined to be 28 mg/mL and 16 mg/mL, respectively. Assume the product undergoes degradation according to first-order kinetics.

3-24. The rate constant of degradation of a pharmaceutical product degrading according to first-order kinetics is 0.25 per year. Calculate the fraction of drug that will degrade in 2 years.

3-25. An oral antibiotic suspension should not be used after the antibiotic has undergone 15% degradation. A hospital pharmacist reconstituted the suspension and put an expiration time of 14 days. Calculate the rate constant of degradation if the concentration of antibiotic at the time of reconstitution was 125 mg/5 mL and degradation follows first-order.

3-26. Calculate the concentration of active ingredient on day 30 in a product if concentrations on day 15 and day 60 after preparation of the product were determined to be 80 mg/mL and 16 mg/mL respectively. Assume the product undergoes degradation according to first-order kinetics.

3-27. Calculate the concentration of active ingredient on day 30 in a product if concentrations on day 15 and day 60 after preparation of the product were determined to be 80 mg/mL and 16 mg/mL respectively. Assume the product undergoes degradation according to zero-order kinetics.

3-28. A pharmacist prepared 60 mL of a drug solution containing 300 mg of the drug. The half-life of the drug in solution is 3 days and the drug degrades according to first-order kinetics. Calculate the amount of drug in solution 2 days after the solution was prepared.

3-29. A product is ineffective after it has decomposed 30%. At the time of preparation, the concentration of active ingredient was 5 μg/teaspoonful. After 3 months concentration of active ingredient was reduced to 4.5 μg/teaspoonful. What should be expiration date on the label if degradation follows first-order kinetics?

CHAPTER 4

DRUG ABSORPTION

The availability of an administered dose for its systemic effect depends, among other factors, on the route of administration of the drug. For example, an intravenously administered dose is available in the blood stream at its maximum concentration immediately after administration, but an orally administered dose must release its contents in the gastrointestinal tract (e.g. from a capsule dosage form) and the drug must dissolve in the gastrointestinal fluids before it becomes available for absorption. Since absorption is not an instantaneous process, the administered dose does not appear in the plasma all-at-once immediately after administration. Thus, the peak plasma concentration of the drug is delayed. Also, the peak plasma concentration during extravascular administration, is expected to be less than that obtained after intravenous administration because appearance of drug in plasma is not as rapid as during intravenous administration. Similarly, in other extravascular routes, e.g. buccal, extravascular parenteral (intramuscular, subcutaneous, etc.) or transdermal route, the drug must diffuse through the biological membrane(s) before it can reach systemic circulation. The plasma profile in all these cases exhibits an absorption phase, very similar to the plasma profile obtained after oral administration.

In the case of orally administered drugs, the situation can become very complex. Some drugs are unstable in gastrointestinal environment and part of the administered dose is 'lost' before absorption can take place. There are instances where the drug is quite stable, but the entire administered dose is not available for absorption, i.e. the extent of absorption for these drugs is less than 100 percent. This may be due to many reasons. The main reasons for the lack of availability of drug for absorption are:

i. Incomplete dissolution of drug from the dosage form or
ii. Partial and/or slow inactivation of drug in the gastric environment.

Some drugs are absorbed completely, but their systemic availability is small because these drugs undergo enterohepatic circulation. Presystemic elimination of drugs due to first-pass effect may reduce systemic availability, even after the drug has been completely absorbed. Thus, even though the drug may have been absorbed 100 percent from the dosage form, the fraction of dose reaching systemic circulation is less than 1.

Some drugs, however, cannot be administered orally for absorption through the gastrointestinal tract because they are either not absorbed at all or they undergo rapid degradation in the environment of the gastrointestinal tract. Therefore, these drugs must be administered by routes other than the gastrointestinal tract and liver. Common routes, which bypass gastrointestinal tract are—intravenous, intramuscular or subcutaneous injection, sublingual or rectal administration or through the skin, as a transdermal patch. The choice of route of administration in these cases is dictated by the nature and physicochemical properties of the drug. When immediate response of nitroglycerin is desired, sublingual route is preferred because the drug reaches systemic circulation rapidly by this route. Unpleasant and bitter tasting drugs are not administered by sublingual route for obvious reasons. Although nitroglycerin is administered transdermally (nitroglycerin patch) for sustained release of the drug, drugs having a large molecular weight cannot be administered transdermally because they are difficult to diffuse through the skin.

Similarly, those drugs, which are insoluble in suitable aqueous solvents, such as, water for injection, dextrose solution, normal saline, cannot be administered intravenously, but may be given as a suspension either subcutaneously or intramuscularly and drugs unstable in a solution form must be reconstituted just before administration.

A partial listing of some examples of drugs, which are administered by routes other than the gastrointestinal route is shown in Table 4-1. These drugs are either not absorbed or are very poorly absorbed through the gastrointestinal tract.

The most direct route of placement of drug in the systemic circulation is the intravascular (intravenous) route of drug administration. All other routes of drug administration, including the oral route and other extravascular routes (e.g. subcutaneous, transdermal and intramuscular routes), involve an absorption step. This step is essential for the appearance of drug into the systemic circulation.

The potential sites for drug absorption following oral administration are:

i. The buccal cavity
ii. The gastrointestinal tract.

Absorption of drugs from the gastrointestinal tract can occur from the stomach, small intestines, large intestines and the rectum.

The small intestine is a common area for drug absorption. Once absorbed in the gastrointestinal tract, the drug is channeled through the portal vein to the liver and then gains access to the systemic circulation for delivery to the site of action. Because the liver and the intestinal walls are the major sites of biotransformation of the drug, all or part of the administered dose may undergo degradation at these sites. That is, a portion of the extravascularly administered dose may not reach systemic circulation. In these situations, the fraction of the administered dose absorbed (referred to as the F value) is less than 1.0. If the F value of an extravascularly administered drug is very low (much less than 1.0), it indicates poor bioavailability of the drug.

It should be mentioned, however, that not all drugs are biotransformed into inactive metabolites. The metabolites of some drugs are active and exert pharmacologic effects. For example, the antianxiety drug prazepam (Centrax) metabolizes in part, to oxazepam (Serax), which also has antianxiety effects. Similarly, in some instances, a pharmacologically inactive drug (usually referred to as the prodrug) may be administered for the known effects of its metabolites.

A relatively high proportion of drug administered in the buccal cavity and rectum is absorbed and drained into the venous circulation, thereby avoiding (bypassing) the initial biotransformation

Table 4-1 Examples of drugs administered by routes other than the oral route

Drug	*Usual Route of Administration*	*Drug*	*Usual Route of Administration*
Amikacin	IV, IM	Dopamine	IV
Azlocillin	IV	Gentamicin	IM
Aztreonam	IV, IM	Insulin	IV, IM, SC
Cefazolin	IM	Kanamycin	IM
Cefotaxime	IV, IM	Methicillin	IV, IM
Cefoxitin	IV, IM	Mezlocillin	IV, IM
Ceftizoxime	IV, IM	Moxalactam	IV, IM
Cefuroxime	IV, IM	Netilmicin	IV, IM
Cephacetrile	IV, IM	Sisomicin	IV, IM
Cephalothin	IV, IM	Streptomycin	IV, IM
Dobutamine	IV	Ticarcillin	IV, IM

IV = intravenous, IM = intramuscular, SC = subcutaneous

step. In general, low bioavailability of drugs administered by oral route is caused not only by the poor water-solubility and poor intestinal permeability of the drug, but also due to biodegradation of drug in the upper portion of the digestive tract.

Many drugs are absorbed completely, i.e. 100 percent of the extravascularly administered dose is absorbed and is able to appear in systemic circulation. These drugs have an F value equal to 1.0. The symbol F stands for—fraction of dose absorbed. However, a large number of drugs exhibit F values, which range from almost zero to slightly less than 1.

Table 4-2 lists examples of some drugs and their F values following oral administration. The data presented in this Table have been extracted from a large number of publications and listed as the mean data. As can be seen from this Table, while some drugs are absorbed completely, others are absorbed to a very small extent.

Table 4-2 Fraction of dose absorbed (F) of some important drugs

Drug	F	Drug	F	Drug	F
Acetazolamide	1.0	Clonazepam	0.9	Fenfluramine	0.65
Amobarbital	1.0	Digitoxin	0.9	Methotrexate	0.65
Amodiaquine	1.0	Disopyramide	0.9	Atenolol	0.6
Amphetamine	1.0	Disulfiram	0.9	Digoxin	0.6
Antipyrine	1.0	Ethosuximide	0.9	Furosemide	0.6
Butobarbital	1.0	Isoniazid	0.9	Haloperidol	0.6
Carbenoxolone	1.0	Levodopa	0.9	Hydromorphone	0.6
Cefadroxil	1.0	Meprobamate	0.9	Nortryptine	0.6
Cephradine	1.0	Minocycline	0.9	Penicillin V	0.6
Chloroquine	1.0	Penbutalol	0.9	Ranitidine	0.6
Chlorpropamide	1.0	Phenobarbital	0.9	Prazocin	0.57
Clofibrate	1.0	Phenytoin	0.9	Nifedipine	0.56
Desipramine	1.0	Secobarbital	0.9	Papaverine	0.53
Diazepam	1.0	Sulfadiazine	0.9	Ampicillin	0.5
Diazoxide	1.0	Sulfaethidole	0.9	Cloxacillin	0.5
Glutethimide	1.0	Sulfamerazine	0.9	Codeine	0.5
Hexobarbital	1.0	Sulfamethazine	0.9	Diphenhydramine	0.5
Hydrocortisone	1.0	Valproate	0.9	Flucloxacillin	0.5
Ibuprofen	1.0	Warfarin	0.9	Griseofulvin	0.5
Indomethacin	1.0	Acetaminophen	0.85	Imipramine	0.5
Lithium	1.0	Flucytosine	0.85	Meperidine	0.5
Methocarbamol	1.0	Lorazepam	0.85	Nafcillin	0.5
Naproxen	1.0	Procainamide	0.85	Pentazocine	0.5
Oxazepam	1.0	Acetyldigoxin	0.8	Metoprolol	0.45
Pentobarbital	1.0	Cimetidine	0.8	Oxprenolol	0.45
Phenprocoumon	1.0	Clonidine	0.8	Chlorpheniramine	0.4
Phenylbutazone	1.0	Dicloxacillin	0.8	Erythromycin	0.4
Probenecid	1.0	Dicumarol	0.8	Lincomycin	0.4
Protriptyline	1.0	Doxycycline	0.8	Nadolol	0.4
Pseudoephedrine	1.0	Ethambutol	0.8	Propranolol	0.35
Pyrimethamine	1.0	Flunitrazepam	0.8	Chlorpromazine	0.32

Contd...

Contd...

Quinine	1.0	Methadone	0.8	Metformin	0.32
Rifampin	1.0	Methaqualone	0.8	Azidocillin	0.3
Sotalol	1.0	Methenamine	0.8	Fentanyl	0.3
Sulfisoxazole	1.0	Metronidazole	0.8	Mianserin	0.3
Theophylline	1.0	Nitrazepam	0.8	Penicillin G	0.3
Tolbutamide	1.0	Primidone	0.8	Tolamolol	0.3
Trimethoprin	1.0	Sulfisomidine	0.8	Vincamine	0.3
Dapsone	0.9	Tetracycline	0.8	Zimelidine	0.3
Pindolol	0.9	Oxytetracycline	0.8	Doxepin	0.27
Practolol	0.9	Atropine	0.75	Hydralazine	0.22
Sulfinpyrazone	0.9	Oxtriphylline	0.75	Verapamil	0.22
Tocainide	0.9	Quinidine	0.75	Propoxyphene	0.2
Zomiprac	0.9	Timolol	0.75	Mebendazole	0.17
Amoxicillin	0.9	Guanethidine	0.7	Ketamine	0.16
Carbamazepine	0.9	Methacycline	0.7	Chlorothiazide	0.14
Cefaclor	0.9	Oxacillin	0.7	Phenacetin	0.13
Cephalexin	0.9	Thyroxine	0.7	Propantheline	0.1
Clindamycin	0.9	Amitriptyline	0.65	Alprenolol	0.01

ROUTES OF DRUG ADMINISTRATION

Drugs intended for systemic circulation are administered by various routes of administration. Broadly speaking, the various routes of drug administration may be classified into the following two major categories. i. intravascular route and ii. extravascular route. In the intravascular route of administration, the drug is placed directly into the blood stream. In the extravascular route, the drug undergoes an absorption process before it reaches systemic circulation. Although intravascular route has the advantage that the drug is placed directly into the blood stream, its main disadvantages are that besides causing discomfort to the patient, the dosage form must be sterile, pyrogen-free and free of particulate matter. Also, these dosage forms are relatively more expensive (because of stringent requirements for the manufacture of parenteral products) and require a physician or a trained health-care professional for administration. The most common intravascular route is intravenous administration. The drug may be given as a single bolus dose, or as continuous infusion over a period of time, which may range from a few hours to more than 24 hours. The most popular and common extravascular route of administration is the oral route. The oral route suffers from the disadvantage of potential first-pass effect, which causes a portion of the drug not being available for absorption. Other commonly used extravascular routes include intramuscular, subcutaneous and transdermal routes. The various routes of drug administration and the types of dosage forms commonly used for these routes are shown in Table 4-3.

Choice of Route of Administration

Of the various routes of drug administration, the most common routes of drug administration are the intravenous route and the extravascular route. The intravenous route is preferred when the drug must be placed directly into the systemic circulation for immediate effect (e.g. in emergency situations), because administration of drugs by extravascular route involves absorption of drug into the systemic circulation. If the drug is absorbed slowly, then there would be a possible delay in the onset of action. Even if the drug is absorbed relatively rapidly, one would expect some

Table 4-3 Dosage forms and routes of drug administration

Route	*Site*	*Commonly* used dosage forms*
Parenteral		
Intra-arterial	Artery	Solutions
Intra-articular	Joint	Solutions, suspensions
Intra-cardiac	Heart	Solutions
Intradermal	Skin\	Solutions, suspensions
intramuscular	Muscle	Solutions, suspensions
intrasynovial	Joint-fluid	Solutions
Intrathecal	Spine	Solutions
Intravenous	Vein	Solutions
Subcutaneous	Under skin	Implants, solutions, suspensions
Aural	Ear	Solutions, suspensions, ointments
Conjunctival	Conjunctiva	Ointments
Intranasal	Nose	Inhalants, ointments, solutions, sprays
Intraocular	Eye	Solutions
Intrarespiratory	Lung	Aerosols
Oral	Mouth	Capsules, elixirs, emulsions, gels, lozenges, magmas, powder, solutions, suspensions, syrups, tablets
Rectal	Rectum	Ointments, solution, suppositories, tablets
Sublingual	Under the tongue	Lozenges, tablets
Transdermal	Skin	Aerosols, creams, lotions, ointments, patches, powders
Urethral	Urethra	Solutions, suppositories
Vaginal	Vagina	Inserts, ointments, solutions, suppositories, tablets

*Only the most commonly used dosage forms are listed here.

delay before the plasma concentration of drug reaches the minimum effective concentration of drug in order to exhibit its therapeutic action.

Among the many extravascular routes of drug administration, the oral route is preferred by everybody involved in the treatment with the drug. This includes the pharmaceutical manufacturer, the wholesale distributor, the patient, the physician, the pharmacist and the health care attendant. The reason for the preference of oral route is that this route of administration offers many advantages. Some of these advantages include the following:

a. Patients prefer oral route because of ease of administration of drug and self-medication with the drug.
b. The pharmacists prefer dosage forms intended for oral administration because it offers convenience in storage, handling and dispensing.
c. The prescribers favor this route because orally administered dosage forms offer relative accuracy of dose and patient compliance.
d. The manufacturers like it because these dosage forms are less expensive to manufacturer and are more economical in packaging, storage and shipping than other dosage forms.

Among the dosage forms available for oral administration, the solid dosage forms are most preferred. Liquid dosage forms are more popular with those who are not comfortable with solid dosage forms, e.g. pediatric and geriatric patients (for obvious reasons). Liquid dosage forms are not popular with adult patients because of inconvenience in carrying the day's supply, handling and measuring the dose and administration of the dose.

The many extravascular routes of drug administration may be classified into two major groups:

i. Parenteral route
ii. Non-parenteral route.

The more popular extravascular parenteral routes are intramuscular and subcutaneous injections and the more popular non-parenteral routes include oral, rectal, vaginal and more recently, topical administration. In general, the non-parenteral extravascular routes are preferred because dosage forms intended for administration by a non-parenteral extravascular route offer the following advantages:

a. They are relatively less expensive because all parenteral dosage forms must be sterile, free of particulate matter and pyrogen and manufacturing conditions for these dosage forms are stringent.
b. They are relatively painless during administration because skin-penetration is not required.
c. They exhibit better patient compliance because they offer the advantage of ease of administration.
d. They afford feasibility of self-administration.

Although oral route has been and continues to be the most preferred route of drug administration for systemic action, the rectal and vaginal routes are used for both systemic as well as topical effect of the drug. Not too long ago, topical application of drugs was intended exclusively for local effect of drug at the site of application. For example, topical application of analgesic creams, ointments, liniments and lotions has been a standard practice for local effect of the drug, although it has also been known for some time that topical application of a drug does not necessarily mean that the drug will not be absorbed through skin. For example, rectal absorption of glucocorticoids (hydrocortisone, prednisolone or betamethasone) following their administration as an enema or suppository has been reported to range from 25% to 50%. In recent years, traditional topical route (skin) of administering drugs for local effect has gained popularity as a route of administering drugs for systemic effect (transdermal delivery) due to successful administration of such drugs as nitroglycerin, clonidine, estradiol, nicotine and scopolamine. Transdermal delivery of other drugs is being investigated by many companies as an alternative to optimizing drug therapy.

TOPICAL ABSORPTION

Compared to absorption by other routes of administration, topical absorption of drugs is limited mainly due to anatomical structure of the skin. Historically, skin has seldom been regarded as a suitable route for systemic absorption of drugs, because it has always been thought of as the most impenetrable tissue of the body, serving the primary function of a protective barrier. Recent studies have shown that although not all drugs permeate through the skin, those that do exhibit skin permeation differ in their rate and extent of permeation. The rate and extent of permeation of drugs through the skin appears to depend primarily upon two factors:

i. The physico-chemical properties of the drug and
ii. The anatomical nature of the skin.

Studies have demonstrated that the differences observed in the rate and extent of skin permeation are not only drug-related, but these differences are also related to the specific absorption sites. For example, several studies have shown that the rate and extent of absorption of nitroglycerin is more predictable and reproducible when the drug is applied on the chest area. Similarly, the earlobe appears to be a better site for the transdermal delivery of scopolamine and the upper arm is suggested for the application of nicotine patch. Based on the various studies involving transdermal delivery of drugs the following observations have been made:

a. Skin permeability is a passive process rather than a biologically active property,
b. Permeation of drugs through intact skin can be regarded as a process of dissolution and molecular diffusion of drug,
c. The principle barrier to permeation is stratum corneum, which is 3 to 5 orders of magnitude less permeable than dermis, making permeability of the entire epidermis more or less indistinguishable from that of stratum corneum *per se*,
d. Stratum corneum is the rate-limiting layer of skin penetration and may be regarded as a two phase lipid/protein heterogeneous membrane in which lipid is continuous and

e. The membrane permeability of drug correlates with aqueous solubility and lipid/protein partition coefficient of the specific drug.

From a comparative stand-point and in order to distinguish drug absorption through the skin and through the gastrointestinal mucosa (lining of the gastrointestinal tract, mouth and rectum), the following observations can be made:

a. The skin is much less permeable to drugs than the mucosa.
b. Absorption of drugs through gastrointestinal mucosa depends on lipid/water partition coefficient, but permeation of drugs through skin is a function of lipid/protein partition coefficient of the drug.
c. The surface area of the entire skin in an adult is only 1.73 m^2 compared to the absorbing surface area of lung (about 70 m^2) or surface area of the gastrointestinal tract (120–200 m^2). Table 4-4 lists the surface area of various anatomical sites and parts of the human body.

The relatively large absorbing surface area of the gastrointestinal tract and the ease of oral administration of drugs is perhaps the reason for the popularity of oral administration of drugs. Compared to oral drug therapy, transdermal application of drugs for systemic effect has the following potential advantages: avoiding biochemical degradation in gastrointestinal tract, avoiding presystemic metabolism in the gut wall and liver and provide long periods of drug action for relatively short-acting drugs. The transdermal route is also recommended for potent, lipophilic drugs with short half-lives.

Rate and Extent of Absorption

The rate and extent of absorption of a drug from a topically applied dosage form (transdermal delivery system) depends on many factors. Some of these factors may be related to the site of application of the delivery system, while some of the factors may be related to the delivery system itself. The following is a listing of some of these factors:

1. Concentration of drug in the delivery system.
2. Nature of vehicle containing the drug. If the vehicle used for the delivery of drug has greater affinity for the drug, it will have a tendency to retard the rate of release of drug from the delivery system.
3. Surface area of the film of drug applied to the skin. Larger the surface area of film containing the drug, greater is the rate and extent of release of drug from the delivery system.

Table 4-4 Surface area of body parts and anatomical sites

Site	*Surface area (m^2)*	*Body part*	*Surface area (m^2)*
Skin	1.73	Index finger	0.006
Head	0.1	Hand + 5 fingers	0.05
Trunk	56	Lower arm (includes hand, but does not include fingers)	0.07
Lung	70	Upper arm	0.1
Mouth cavity	0.02	Thigh	0.2
Stomach	0.1 – 0.2	Lower leg	0.1
Small intestine	120 – 200	Foot	0.05
Large intestine	0.5 – 1		
Rectum	0.05		
Glomeruli (both kidneys)	1.16		

4. Thickness of film of drug applied to the skin. A thicker film of drug acts like a reservoir, thereby prolonging release of drug from the delivery device.
5. Presence or absence of occlusion over drug reservoir.
6. Presence or absence of permeation enhancers in the dosage form. Permeation enhancers are used to increase permeability of drug through the skin.
7. Nature of skin to which dosage form is applied. Nature of skin includes the following factors:
   a. Anatomical region of body. Different regions of the body offer different types of resistance to transport of drug and therefore affect the rate and extent of absorption of drug.
   b. Age of the patient. Skin permeability changes with age due to physiological changes.
   c. Sex of the patient. It has been reported that there are differences in drug permeability from identical sites of application in males and females.
   d. Thickness of skin. Greater the thickness of skin, slower the rate of permeability of drug, because the drug has to travel a longer distance to permeate.
   e. Multiple applications at the same site. The permeability of a drug tends to increase if the same site is used for multiple applications, probably due to occlusion and/or due to inflammation caused by adhesive used in the fabrication of delivery system.
   f. Miscellaneous factors. These include: presence of skin pigmentation, psoriasis, dermatitis and hydration. These factors are equally important in considering transdermal absorption of drugs, because permeation of drugs changes in the presence of these factors.

In addition to the factors listed above, there are other factors, which also affect rate and extent of transdermal absorption of drugs. These include the following:

1. Metabolism of drug in skin. Some drugs undergo rapid metabolism in the skin, while others do not.
2. Binding of drug to epidermis. In the case of drugs, which bind to epidermis, initial applications of drug are lost in the epidermis. Since binding is a reversible process, the bound drug is ultimately released after application of drug is terminated.
3. Blood supply affected by the presence of drug. Drugs, which affect blood supply will also affect their rate and extent of absorption soon after their first application.
4. Effect of first dose on absorption of subsequent doses. Some drugs influence their own absorption once they appear in systemic circulation, e.g. by enzymes induction.

ORAL ADMINISTRATION

Although oral ingestion of a dosage form not only represents the most popular route, it also represents the most frequently used route of administration. However, the oral route of drug administration also poses many problems to efficient drug therapy. Most of these problems are primarily due to two main reasons:

i. Dosage form considerations or
ii. Physiological variables.

In order to achieve the best therapeutic results, a rapid rate of absorption of drug from the administered dose is of utmost importance (except in the case of modified release dosage forms). Some of the reasons for the desirability of rapid rate of drug absorption are as follows:

1. Rapidly absorbed drugs provide maximal concentration in plasma, assuring rapid onset of action and maximum pharmacologic response.
2. Rapid absorption means less time for exposure of drug to the gastrointestinal fluids, thereby reducing drug interactions with the components of these fluids and minimizing drug degradation.
3. Rapid absorption generally assures uniform and predictable pharmacologic response, thus reducing undesirable variability.

In order for a drug to be absorbed through a biological membrane and reach systemic circulation, it must be released from the dosage form and be available as an aqueous solution at the absorption site. The release of drug from the dosage form depends on three major factors:

1. Physicochemical properties of the drug
2. Physicochemical properties of the dosage form and
3. Physicochemical factors of the human body at the site of administration or absorption.

The formulation of dosage form is the most important factor in obtaining proper release of drug from the dosage form. The drug released from a dosage form may not necessarily be absorbed if drug molecule is bound to mucosa. If the drug is bound to the surface of mucosa by hydrogen bonding, ion binding or van der Waals forces, the process is termed adsorption and if the drug permeates through capillary walls and enters systemic circulation, the process is called absorption. In oral administration, the drug usually must permeate more than one membrane (e.g. in lumen of gastrointestinal tract) before the drug molecule passes from outside into a capillary. However, the only rate controlling factor appears to be the rate of permeation through epithelial cells. Other factors the which affect, rate of drug permeation include vascularity and rate of blood flow at absorption site. This is also true for drugs administered rectally and topically.

ABSORPTION MECHANISMS

There are six accepted mechanisms of drug absorption. These, in order of their importance are:

1. Passive diffusion
2. Active transport
3. Facilitated transport
4. Convective transport
5. Ion-pair transport and
6. Pinocytosis.

A prerequisite for absorption is that the drug must be present in a solution form at the absorption site. This is valid for all absorption mechanisms, except absorption by pinocytosis.

Passive Diffusion

Passive diffusion is transport through a semi-permeable membrane. In this transport mechanism, drug molecules diffuse through a membrane by first dissolving in the aqueous portion of the membrane and then by dissolution in the lipid portion of the membrane. The solubility of a drug in the aqueous portion and in the portion of the membrane is governed by the partition coefficient of the drug. After entering the membrane, the drug molecules leave the lipid portion of the membrane and dissolve again in the aqueous portion of the membrane, but this time on the other side of the membrane and according to the concentration gradient. Once the drug enters the blood stream, it is now available for elimination. Since, the concentration of drug at the absorption site is almost always greater than its concentration in the blood stream, the concentration gradient always favors absorption. The rate of absorption by passive diffusion is given by the following relationship:

$$\text{Rate of Absorption} = \frac{DAK\Delta C}{h} \tag{4-1}$$

In equation (4-1), D = diffusion coefficient of drug, A = surface area of absorbing membrane, K = partition coefficient of the drug, ΔC = concentration gradient and h = thickness of absorbing membrane.

Thus, the rate of drug transport via passive diffusion is directly proportional to diffusion coefficient of the drug, partition coefficient of the drug, surface area of the absorbing membrane, and concentration gradient of the drug. As seen in equation (4-1), the rate of drug transport is inversely proportional to the thickness of absorbing membrane. Because transport via passive diffusion is limited to the non-ionized or undissociated species of the drug, therefore, the rate of absorption also depends on dissociation constant of the drug and the pH of the biological fluids on either side of absorbing membrane. Thus, the extent of drug diffusion through the absorbing membrane is a function of the degree or the extent of ionization of the drug. The fraction of drug non-ionized in a given pH environment can be estimated using Henderson-Hasselbalch equation. The equation relating pH, dissociation constant and ratio of ionized to non-ionized species of an acidic drug is given by the following Henderson-Hasselbalch equation:

$$pH = pK_a + \log \frac{[\text{ionized}]}{[\text{non-ionized}]} \tag{4-2}$$

The corresponding equation for basic drugs is:

$$pH = pK_w - pK_b + \log \frac{[\text{non-ionized}]}{[\text{ionized}]} \tag{4-3}$$

In these equations, the brackets indicate that concentrations of the ionized and the non-ionized species are expressed in the units of moles per liter, not in the units of milligrams per milliliter, or milligrams per liter, etc. Examples of drugs, which undergo passive diffusion include those drugs that are weak organic acids and weak organic bases, organic non-electrolytes (e.g. alcohol, urea and aminopyrine) and some cardiac glycosides.

Example 4-1 The pK_a of aspirin is 3.5. Calculate fraction of dose available for absorption at pH = 1.0.

Solution

Because aspirin is an acidic drug, equation (4-2) should be used. From equation (4-2)

$$pH = pK_a + \log \frac{[\text{ionized}]}{[\text{non-ionized}]}$$

Substituting the value of pH = 1.0 and pK_a = 3.5 into equation (4-2),

$$1.0 = 3.5 + \log \frac{[\text{ionized}]}{[\text{non-ionized}]}$$

This, upon rearrangement yields the following relationship:

$$\text{Log} \frac{[\text{ionized}]}{[\text{non-ionized}]} = 1.0 - 3.5 = -2.5$$

$$\frac{[\text{ionized}]}{[\text{non-ionized}]} = \text{Inverse log of} - 2.5 = - 0.00316 = \frac{0.00316}{1}$$

Since the ratio [ionized]:[non-ionized] = 0.00316:1, therefore

$$\text{Percent [ionized]} = \frac{\text{Fraction}[\text{ionized}]}{\text{Fraction}[\text{ionized}] + \text{Fraction}[\text{non-ionized}]} \times 100\%$$

$$\text{Percent [ionized]} = \frac{0.00316}{0.00316 + 1} \times 100\% = 0.32\%$$

Similarly,

$$\text{Percent [non-ionized]} = \frac{\text{Fraction}[\text{non-ionized}]}{\text{Fraction}[\text{ionized}] + \text{Fraction}[\text{non-ionized}]} \times 100\%$$

$$\text{Percent [non-ionized]} = \frac{1}{0.00316 + 1} \times 100\% = 99.68\%$$

$$\text{Fraction available for absorption} = \text{Fraction [non-ionized]} = \frac{99.68\%}{100\%} = 0.9968$$

Example 4-2 The pK_b of a drug is 6.9. Calculate fraction of dose available for absorption at pH = 7.0.

Solution

Because the drug is a basic drug, equation (4-3) should be used. From equation (4-3)

$$pH = pK_w - pK_b + \log \frac{[\text{non-ionized}]}{[\text{ionized}]}$$

Substituting the value of pH = 7.0 and pK_b = 6.9 into equation (4-3),

$$7.0 = 14 - 6.9 + \log \frac{[\text{non-ionized}]}{[\text{ionized}]}$$

This, upon rearrangement gives

$$\log \frac{[\text{non-ionized}]}{[\text{ionized}]} = 7.0 - 14 + 6.9 = -0.1$$

$$\frac{[\text{non-ionized}]}{[\text{ionized}]} = \text{inverse log}(-0.1) = 0.7943 = \frac{0.7943}{1}$$

$$\text{Percent [ionized]} = \frac{\text{Fraction}[\text{ionized}]}{\text{Fraction}[\text{ionized}] + \text{Fraction}[\text{non-ionized}]} \times 100\%$$

$$\text{Percent [ionized]} = \frac{1}{0.7943 + 1} \times 100\% = 55.73\%$$

$$\text{Percent [non-ionized]} = \frac{\text{Fraction}[\text{non-ionized}]}{\text{Fraction}[\text{ionized}] + \text{Fraction}[\text{non-ionized}]} \times 100\%$$

$$\text{Percent [non-ionized]} = \frac{0.7943}{1 + 0.7943} \times 100\% = 44.27\%$$

$$\text{Fraction available for absorption} = \text{Fraction [non-ionized]} = \frac{44.27\%}{100\%} = 0.4427$$

Active Transport

This mechanism utilizes carriers under expenditure of energy, i.e. utilization of adenosine triphosphate (ATP). To be absorbed by active transport, each drug or a group of drugs needs a specific carrier. The carriers are located on the external surface of the membrane and appear to be enzymes or at least proteinaceous materials. The carriers bind to the drug molecules to form a complex and this complex moves across the membrane utilizing energy provided by ATP. Once transported, the drug-carrier complex dissociates, releasing drug molecules and the carrier thus released from the complex returns to the original site of the absorbing membrane to continue the transport process. The binding of carrier and drug molecules follow drug-receptor theory. When more than one drug is present at the site of absorption, the drug, which possesses relatively higher affinity for the carrier can competitively inhibit or displace the drug, which has a relatively lower affinity for the carrier (competitive inhibition). Similarly certain substances, which interfere with cell metabolism (e.g. cyanides, fluorides, etc.) can also non-competitively inhibit active transport of drugs.

Absorption of drug by active transport becomes saturated, if more drug molecules are present than the carriers available for transporting the drug. Since this transport mechanism requires expenditure of energy, it can proceed against a concentration gradient and in the case of ions, against an electrochemical potential. This means that the drug can be transported from regions of low concentration to regions of high concentration. The process of active transport occurs in unidirectional manner across the membrane. In the case of intestines, active transport proceeds from the mucosal side to the serosal side. Some of the important characteristics of absorption by active transport may be summarized as follows:

a. Transport process shows specificity for a particular type of chemical structure, i.e. a carrier molecule may be highly selective for a specific drug molecule. For example, L-amino acids and monosaccharides are actively absorbed by different carrier systems.
b. Carriers can be poisoned.
c. If two structurally similar substances are transported by the same carrier mechanism, they (the drugs) may compete with each other for adsorption sites on the carrier, i.e. one will competitively inhibit the transport of the other.
d. Carrier can be saturated if the concentration of drug molecules exceeds the number of carriers available for transport.
e. Actively absorbed substances are usually absorbed from a specific site in the gastrointestinal tract, which is located in a limited segment of the small intestine. For example, bile acids are actively absorbed from ileum.

The rate of absorption by active transport can be determined by applying the equation used for Michaelis-Menten kinetics:

$$\text{Rate of drug absorption} = \frac{[C] \times V_{max}}{K_m + [C]} \tag{4-4}$$

In this equation,

$[C]$ = Concentration of drug available for absorption,

V_{max} = Maximal rate of absorption at high drug concentration and

K_m = Affinity constant of drug for the carrier.

Hence, the rate of drug absorption by active transport depends on three factors. These are:
a. Concentration of drug at the site of absorption
b. Affinity constant of drug for the carrier, and
c. Maximal rate of absorption of drug at high drug concentration.

Because the maximal rate of drug absorption at high drug concentration may be considered constant, therefore, the two factors that govern the rate of drug absorption by active transport are:
i. Concentration of drug at the site of absorption and
ii. Affinity constant of drug for the carrier.

Relationship between K_m and C

The effect of drug concentration and affinity constant of drug on the rate of drug absorption by active transport can be considered based on the following two possibilities:
i. The affinity constant of the drug is much greater than the concentration of drug at the site of absorption and
ii. The concentration of drug at the site of absorption is much greater than the affinity constant of drug for the carrier.

K_m>>>C: (Affinity constant of the drug is greater than the concentration of drug at the site of absorption).

There are two probable situations when the affinity constant of drug for the carrier may be much greater than the concentration of drug at the site of absorption. These are:
i. When a drug is administered at a very low dose providing a relatively low concentration at the site of absorption, and
ii. If the affinity constant of drug for the carrier is inherently much greater than the concentration of drug available at the site of absorption.

When the affinity constant of the drug is much greater than the concentration of drug available at the site of absorption (i.e. when K_m>>>C), the numerical value of the term (K_m + [C]) in the denominator of equation (4-4) approaches a numerical value equal to the numerical value of affinity constant of the drug for the carrier (K_m) and the term (K_m + [C]) may be considered approximately equal to the term K_m.

Equation (4-4) now becomes:

$$\text{Rate of drug absorption} = \frac{[C] \times V_{max}}{K_m} \quad (4\text{-}5)$$

By definition, V_{max} and K_m are constant for a given drug-carrier complex. Therefore, these two constants may be combined as a single constant (K') and equation (4-5) now becomes

$$\text{Rate of drug absorption} = K' \times [C] \quad (4\text{-}6)$$

Equation (4-6) is similar to the equation of first-order kinetics given in Chapter 3 and therefore, absorption of drug should proceeds according to first-order kinetics. Thus, when the affinity constant is much greater than the concentration of drug at the site of absorption, absorption of drug proceeds according to first-order kinetics.

C>>>K

$C >>> K_m$: (Affinity constant is smaller than concentration of drug at site of absorption).

This situation may exist when a drug is administered at a very high dose and/or if concentration of drug at the site of absorption is much greater than affinity constant of drug for the carrier.

When C>>>K_m, the numerical value of the term (K_m + [C]) in equation (4-4) approaches the numerical value of the term [C] and equation (4-4) becomes

$$\text{Rate of drug absorption} = \frac{[C] \times V_{max}}{[C]} \quad (4\text{-}7)$$

Canceling the common term, [C], in the numerator and in the denominator of equation (4-7), one obtains the following relationship:

$$\text{Rate of drug absorption} = V_{max} \quad (4\text{-}8)$$

According to equation (4-8), when the concentration of drug at the site of absorption is much greater than the affinity constant of the drug, the rate of drug absorption is constant (equal to the maximal rate of transport of drug at high drug concentration) and further increase in drug concentration does not result in the proportional increase in the rate of drug absorption.

Equation (4-8) is similar to the equation for zero-order kinetics given in Chapter 3. Therefore, the absorption of drug proceeds at a constant rate according to zero-order kinetics.

Examples of drugs, which undergo absorption by active transport include B-vitamins, cardiac glycosides, monosaccharides, amino acids, strong organic acids and strong organic bases.

Example 4-3 Acetaminophen exhibits Michaelis-Menten absorption kinetics. A patient was administered a single 1 g dose of the drug and plasma concentration at 0.5 hr after dosing indicated that the instantaneous rate of absorption was 6 mg/min and 250 mg of the drug had been absorbed. The affinity constant of drug for the carrier is 400 (in the same units as those for the drug dissolved in lumen of gastrointestinal tract). Calculate the maximal rate of drug absorption.

Solution

The rate of absorption of drugs, which follow Michaelis-Menten kinetics is determined using the following the equation:

$$\text{Rate of drug absorption} = \frac{[C] \times V_{max}}{K_m + [C]}$$

Here,

Rate of absorption = 6 mg/min,

[C] = 1,000 mg – 250 mg = 750 mg (dissolved in certain volume of lumen of gastrointestinal tract) and K_m = 400 (same units as those for C).

Substituting these values into equation (4-4), we have:

$$6\ (\text{mg/min}) = \frac{(750)\times V_{max}}{(400)+(750)}$$

$$6\ (\text{mg / min}) = \frac{(750)\times V_{max}}{1150}$$

$$V_{max} = \frac{(6\ \text{mg / min})\times(1150)}{750} = 9.2\ \text{mg/min}$$

Facilitated Transport

Facilitated transport is also a carrier-mediated system. In principle, the mechanism of drug absorption by facilitated transport is very similar to the mechanism of drug absorption by active transport, except that facilitated transport does not proceed against a concentration gradient, i.e. the drug moves only from a region of high concentration to a region of low concentration. It is perhaps for this reason that the mechanism of facilitated transport is sometimes considered as a sub-group of the mechanism of active transport.

The classical example of absorption by facilitated transport is absorption of vitamin B_{12}. Vitamin B_{12} molecules form a complex with the intrinsic factor produced by the stomach wall. The B_{12}-intrinsic factor complex then combines with a carrier for transport across the membrane. Up to 1.5 μg of vitamin B_{12} are absorbed by facilitated transport.

Convective Transport

Convective transport is also known as pore transport because in this transport mechanism, the transport of drug molecules takes place through the pores of biological membrane.

In this transport mechanism, drug molecules dissolve in the aqueous medium of the pores at the site of absorption and move along with the solvent through the aqueous pores. The movement of drug with the solvent through the pores is termed 'shifting of the solvent'.

The rate of absorption via convective transport depends on the number and size of aqueous pores available for the transport of the drug and is given by the following equation:

$$\text{Rate of drug absorption} = \frac{(N)(R^2)(A)(\Delta C)}{(\eta)(h)} \qquad (4\text{-}9)$$

In equation (4-9), N = number of pores, R = radius of pores, A = surface area of pores, ΔC = concentration gradient, η = viscosity of fluid in the pore and h = thickness of the membrane.

The aqueous pores in the biological membrane are cylindrical in shape and are filled with water. Since the diameter of aqueous pores is usually in the range of 7 to 10 Angstrom (Å) units, only those substances and drug molecules, which have a relatively low molecular weight can pass through the aqueous pores. Some ions (if they have a charge opposite of the charge on pore lining) and neutral molecules may pass also through the pores. The upper limit of molecules transported via convective transport is a molecular weight of about 150 for spherical compounds and about 400 for compounds, which are chain-like. Organic and inorganic electrolytes up to a molecular weight of about 400 are absorbed by convective transport. Examples of compounds absorbed by convective transport are dextrose, fructose, organic electrolytes, urea and water.

Ion-Pair Transport

Ion-pair transport is transport of charged molecules due to the formation of a neutral complex with another charged molecule carrying an opposite charge. If the neutral ion-pair (molecule) thus formed has an adequate partition coefficient, it can be transported across the biological membrane by passive diffusion. The mechanism of ion-pair transport is believed to be responsible for the absorption of some compounds that are highly ionized and maintain their charge (ionization) at all physiologic pH values. It has been shown by *in vitro* experiments that a large organic anion can combine with a relatively large organic cation to form an electrically neutral ion-pair. This ion-pair is essentially a neutral complex, which possesses both, water solubility as well as lipid solubility, thus providing the desired partition coefficient. Hence the electrically neutral complex is easily transported by passive diffusion. A schematic of ion-pair formation is shown in Figure 4-1.

Thus, highly ionized organic compounds (ions) appear to combine with endogenous substances of gastrointestinal tract, which carry an opposite charge. The combination forms an ion-pair. Once transported, the complex then breaks up releasing the drug and endogenous substance, which formed the complex. The endogenous substance is again available to form complex with more drug for transport across biological membrane.

Quaternary ammonium compounds and sulfonic acids are examples of drugs absorbed by ion-pair transport mechanism.

Two basic drugs have been shown to form ion-pair complexes for absorption:

i. Quinine forms an ion-pair complex with hexyl salicylate, and
ii. Propranolol forms an ion-pair complex with oleic acid.

Pinocytosis

Pinocytosis is thought to be the transport process in the absorption of small fat or oil droplets and small solid particles. It is the only transport mechanism where a drug or a compound does not have to be in aqueous solution to be absorbed. It has been suggested that absorption of the compound (solid particles or liquid substance) takes place in a manner very similar to phagocytosis where bacteria are engulfed and taken up by leukocytes. It is perhaps for this reason that pinocytosis has often been referred to by various other terms such as corpuscular absorption, vesicular absorption or particulate absorption.

Absorption by pinocytosis occurs from lumen of intestinal tract across intestinal epithelium into lymphatic or venous capillaries. Non-aqueous liquid droplets or solid particles are engulfed by processes formed by epithelial cell thereby forming a vacuole or vesicle. These vesicle vary in size and may be as large as 75 nm in diameter, indicating that fairly large solid particles or liquid (oil) droplets may undergo absorption by this mechanism.

The mechanism of absorption by pinocytosis is not fully understood and may not play an important role in the absorption of drugs. However, this process is important in the absorption of oil soluble vitamins, e.g. vitamins A, D, E and K and in uptake of nutrients, such as fatty acids, fats and amino acids. Also, particulate matter, such as parasite eggs, starch, hair and plastic fragments may enter systemic circulation by this process. Absorption by pinocytosis probably explains those absorption phenomenons, which cannot be explained by other absorption processes, e.g. oral efficacy of Sabin polio vaccine, poisoning by botulinus toxin and allergic reactions resulting from ingestion of offending proteins. Pinocytosis activity has been reported to be rather marked at other biologic barriers, such as alveoli of lungs and walls of blood vessels.

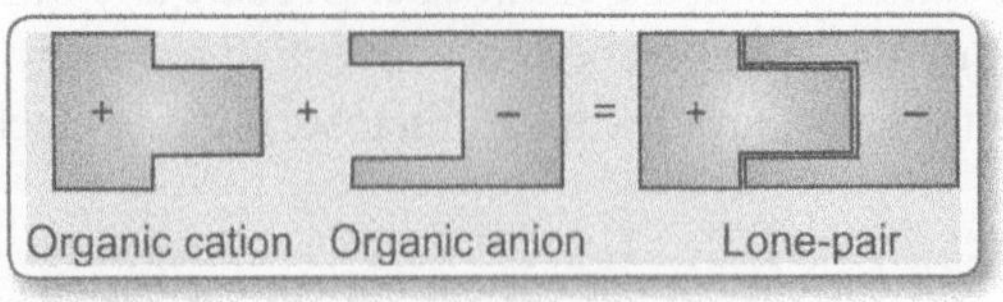

Fig. 4-1 Ion-pair formation

GASTROINTESTINAL TRACT

Although gastrointestinal route of drug administration is the most popular, some of its features can affect rate of drug absorption and therefore duration of action of the administered dose. Anatomically, the gastrointestinal tract is a continuous, coiled, hollow, muscular tube that winds through the ventral body cavity and is open to external environment at both ends. Physiologically, three major processes occur in gastrointestinal tract. These are:

a. Secretion
b. Digestion and
c. Absorption.

From the perspective of absorption of drugs from the gastrointestinal tract, five major organs may be involved in drug absorption:

1. Mouth
2. Esophagus
3. Stomach
4. Small intestine and
5. Large intestine.

Following ingestion of a dosage form, as the drug proceeds through the length of the gastrointestinal tract, the dosage form encounters different environments in different segments of the gastrointestinal tract. These environments differ in various aspects, such as: acidity and pH of the fluid in the particular segment, the presence or absence of enzymes, the types of enzymes, fluidity and consistency and the gastrointestinal surface characteristics. Some characteristics of selected segments of the gastrointestinal tract are shown in Table 4-5. However, only stomach and small intestine play a major role in the rate and extent of drug absorption of majority of orally administered drugs.

Stomach: The stomach is looked upon as a temporary storage house where chemical breakdown of proteins begins and in which food is converted into a creamy paste called the chyme. It is the major digestive organ of the body. The human stomach is the most dilated part of the gastrointestinal tract, having a capacity of about 1 L when filled. The surface area for absorption of drugs is relatively small in the stomach due to the absence of macrovilli and microvilli. Although relatively fixed at both ends (the esophageal end and the small intestinal end), the stomach is quite movable in between. Anatomically, the stomach tends to lie high and run horizontally in short and stout people (known as steer-horn stomach) and is often elongated vertically in tall and thin people.

Intestines: The intestinal tract is considered as comprising of small and large intestines. The length of the intestinal tract is usually about seven times the sitting height of individuals who

Table 4-5 Characteristics of the gastrointestinal tract

Anatomical unit	*Length x diameter (cm)*	*Villi*	*pH*
Mouth cavity	(15 – 20) x 10	Absent	6.4
Esophagus	25 x 2.5	Absent	5.0 – 6.0
Stomach	20 x 15	Absent	1.0 – 3.5
Duodenum	25 x 5	Present	6.5 – 7.6
Jejunum	300 x 5	Present*	6.3 – 7.3
Ileum	300 x (2.5 – 5)	Present*	7.6
Cecum	(10 – 30) x 7	Present	7.5 – 8.0
Colon	150 x 5	Absent	7.9 – 8.0
Rectum	(15 – 19) x 2.5	Absent	7.5 – 8.0

*The villi are most abundant in the jejunum and ileum portions of the gastrointestinal tract

usually eat a diet of mixed food. The intestines of individuals who eat primarily vegetable food diet are about 20 percent longer than those who usually eat a diet of mixed food.

Small Intestine: The small intestine is the longest part of the gastrointestinal tract. It is the site of absorption of most orally administered drugs. Small intestine follows pylorus. Anatomically, the small intestine is a convoluted tube, 6 to 7 meters in length, with variations of between 4.5 and 9.5 meters. The small intestine extends from pyloric sphincter to the ileocecal valve and its mucosa is covered by macrovilli and microvilli. The villi are finger-like projections of mucosa, more than 1 mm high. The villi enhance absorptive surface area of small intestine enormously. In the absence of the villi, the total surface area of small intestine would be approximately 3.5 m^2, but the macrovilli and microvilli increase its surface area enormously. If only macrovilli were present, the surface area of small intestine would increase about 10-fold. The presence of microvilli and macrovilli increases the surface area of the small intestine about 30-fold, giving the small intestine an effective surface area of about 120 m^2. Absorption of drugs occurs mostly in the proximal part of the small intestine.

The small intestine consists of duodenum, jejunum and ileum. Duodenum is the smallest segment of the small intestine. Jejunum and ileum are almost similar in all respects. There is no division between these segments and one segment passes gradually into the other, maintaining generally the same structure with very small differences. The major difference in these three structures is abrupt change in pH from duodenum to jejunum.

Large Intestine: The large intestine frames the small intestine on three sides and extends from the ileocecal valve to the anus. Its diameter is greater than that of small intestine, but its length is much shorter. The major function of large intestine is to absorb water from ingestible food residues, which are delivered to the large intestine in a fluid state and eliminate them from the body as semisolid feces. The large intestine consists of three regions—cecum, colon and rectum. Cecum is a sac-like region, which lies below ileocecal valve. The colon has several distinct regions. First, it travels up the right side of the abdominal cavity as ascending colon, then makes a right-angle turn and travels across abdominal cavity as transverse colon, and then turns acutely at the left colic (splenic) flexure and continues down the left side as descending colon. Finally, the colon enters pelvis, where it becomes the S-shaped sigmoid colon.

What is finally delivered to the large intestine has another 12 to 24 hours to spend there. The large intestine harvests vitamins made by the bacterial flora and reclaims most of remaining water and some of electrolytes (mainly sodium and chloride). Absorption is not the major function of large intestine, mainly due to:

i. The absence of microvilli and
ii. The more viscous and somewhat semisolid nature of lumen contents. Although some drugs are absorbed in this region, the primary function of large intestine is propulsive activity to force fecal matter toward anus and then eliminate it from the body.

The colon is lined with mucin, which serves two functions—lubrication and protection. Only a few drugs (e.g. theophylline and metoprolol) are absorbed in this region. Crohn disease affects colon and thickens the bowel wall. With this disease, the absorption of clindamycin and propranolol is increased, but absorption of other drugs is reduced. The rectum is about 15 cm long and in the absence of fecal material it has about 2 mL of fluid. Absorption of drugs after rectal administration may be variable due to length of stay of dosage form in the rectum (retention) and depending on placement of dosage form (suppository or drug solution) within the rectum.

As the gastrointestinal content passes through small intestine to large intestine, it changes from a fluid into a pasty consistency making it difficult for the drug to diffuse to large intestinal mucosa. The portion of drug that did not dissolve in stomach or small intestine may not dissolve in this region because of lack of fluids. Thus, changes in surface area, availability of aqueous fluids, consistency of intestinal contents and pH account for differences in the extent and rate of absorption from not only large intestine but also other regions of the gastrointestinal tract.

Extent of Drug Absorption

The extent of drug absorption depends on the variable nature of chemical environment found throughout the gastrointestinal tract, especially if the controlling mechanism for the release of drug from its dosage form relies on the environmental pH and/or on the gastrointestinal enzymes. Absorption, degradation or inactivation of drug also depends on its interaction with substances it encounters during its transit through the gastrointestinal tract. Significant loss of drug prior to its appearance in the systemic circulation can occur through many processes. There are various processes that are responsible for degradation or inactivation of a drug as the drug passes through the gastrointestinal tract. These include, but are not limited to the following:

a. Metabolism by intestinal flora
b. Hydrolytic degradation in the gastrointestinal tract, and
c. Metabolism as the drug crosses the gastrointestinal wall.

The processes involved in absorption, degradation and inactivation of an orally administered drug during its passage through the gastrointestinal tract are shown in Table 4-6.

The extent of drug absorption is also affected by variations in the time it takes the stomach to empty its contents. Obviously, acid-labile drugs must not be in contact with the acidic environment of the stomach. It is generally believed that acidic drugs are absorbed better from the stomach than from the intestinal tract (due to reduced ionization in the acidic environment of the stomach). Therefore, increased residence of acidic drugs in the stomach would be expected to result in better absorption. Similarly, basic drugs dissociate more in stomach than in the intestinal tract and hence early emptying of basic drugs from the stomach assures early onset of action.

Stomach emptying applies more to solid dosage forms because the drug has to dissolve in the gastrointestinal fluids before it is available for absorption. Since, solubility and dissolution rate of most drugs is a function of pH, a delivery system carrying a drug that is predominantly absorbed from the stomach, must stay in the stomach for a longer period to assure maximum dissolution of drug and therefore maximum extent of absorption. Various techniques have been used to keep the dosage form in the stomach for prolonged periods and prevent or delay its emptying along with gastric contents. For example, tablets containing bioadhesives have been formulated so that the tablet may stick to stomach lining.

Another approach to retain tablet dosage form in the stomach involves formulating the tablet with materials, which reduce tablet density so that the tablet floats in the gastric fluids (floating tablet). The tablet stays away from pyloric sphincter and emptying of tablet from stomach is delayed. Similarly, tablets that swell in stomach and assume dimensions larger than those of pyloric sphincter have been formulated. Success of these techniques (still in experimental stage) to achieve intended goal is somewhat mixed.

The most important site for drug absorption is small intestine. The transit time of dosage form is a major determinant of the extent of absorption of drugs that are absorbed predominantly through small intestines. Studies using indirect methods based on detection of hydrogen after oral dose of lactulose (fermentation of lactulose by colon bacteria yields hydrogen in the breath) placed the average transit time through small intestine at about 7 hours. Newer studies using gamma scintigraphy suggest a transit time of 3 to 4 hours. Thus, if transit time in the small intestine for most adults is between 3 and 4 hours, a drug may take 4 to 8 hours to pass through stomach and small intestine during the fasting state. During the fed state, transit time through the small intestine may be anywhere between 8 to 12 hours. Therefore, if absorption is not completed by the time a drug leaves the small intestine, then absorption of the drug may be incomplete or erratic.

Table 4-6 Processes involved in the absorptive and degradative pathways of orally administered drugs

Gastrointestinal Segment	*Processes Involved In*		
	Absorption	*Degradation*	*Inactivation*
Mouth	Passive diffusion Convective transport	-	-
Stomach	Passive diffusion Convective transport Active transport	Hydrolytic Enzymatic	Complexation and mucin binding
Duodenum	Passive diffusion Convective transport Active transport Facilitated transport Ion-pair transport Pinocytosis	Hydrolytic Enzymatic	Complexation, mucin Binding, enterohepatic recycling
Jejunum	Passive diffusion Convective transport Active transport Facilitated transport	Hydrolytic Enzymatic	Complexation, mucin binding, enterohepatic recycling
Ileum	Passive diffusion Convective transport Active transport Facilitated transport Ion-pair transport Pinocytosis	Microbial Enzymatic	-
Cecum	Passive diffusion Convective transport Active transport Pinocytosis	Microbial	-
Colon	Passive diffusion	Microbial	-
Rectum	Passive diffusion Convective transport Pinocytosis	Microbial	-

Duration of Drug Absorption

The duration of action of orally administered drugs is affected by the length of time that the dosage form is exposed to the absorbing membrane. In contrast to other routes of administration (transdermal or intramuscular route) by which a dosage form can be placed at the absorption site for extended periods, the gastrointestinal tract offers a relatively brief transit time during which the drug may be absorbed.

The transit time of a drug in the gastrointestinal tract depends on pharmacologic properties of the drug, type of dosage form and various physiologic factors. Studies to determine the gastrointestinal transit time show that the time it takes a balloon to pass through various segments of the gastrointestinal tract is:

Duodenum = 5 minutes
Jejunum = 2 hours
Ileum = 3 to 6 hours
Large intestine = 12 to 24 hours

However, the total time for certain types and certain quantities of food to pass through the entire length of gastrointestinal tract varies enormously in different individuals. Therefore, the time required before food is emptied from stomach and reaches small intestine may be as little as less than 1 hour to as much as more than 5 hours. Considering the variability in gastrointestinal transit time, a drug or food may reach colon (where practically no absorption of drug occurs) in only 2 or 3 hours in the most rapid passage, to more than 8 hours where transit is very slow. Food or drug is stored in colon for several hours, so that the total time spent between intake and rectal excretion may be between 16 and 24 hours or even longer. The effective transit time, i.e. time during which drug is in proximity of absorbing gastrointestinal surface (from the stomach to the end of small intestines) is approximately 12 hours.

Factors Influencing Drug Absorption

Various factors influence absorption of drug from orally administered dosage forms, the more important being: gastrointestinal motility, gastric emptying, pH of gastrointestinal tract, gastrointestinal secretions, food, blood flow and gut flora.

Gastrointestinal Motility: Gastrointestinal motility is an important factor in consideration of transit time of drugs through gastrointestinal tract. Transit of a drug through gastrointestinal tract depends upon many factors, including whether the gastrointestinal tract contains recently ingested food (known as the digestive or fed state) or the gastrointestinal tract is in the fasted (or interdigestive) state. Various gastrointestinal motility patterns have been classified into two general modes:

a. **Digestive Motility Pattern:** Digestive motility pattern takes place when food is present in the stomach. It is characterized by regular, frequent contractions and lasts as long as food remains present in the stomach. The frequency of these contractions is about 4 to 5 contractions per minute and the contractions have the effect of mixing intestinal contents and advancing the contents toward colon in short segments.
b. **The Interdigestive Motility Pattern:** The interdigestive motility (fasted) pattern is also known as migrating motor complex (MMC). It takes place as alternating cycles of non-activity and activity. Each cycle lasts about 30 to 60 minutes and acts as a propulsive movement that empties the upper gastrointestinal tract to the cecum.
   Cycle 1: Cycle 1 is the non-activity cycle. The gastrointestinal tract is quiescent. This cycle lasts approximately 30 to 60 minutes and is followed by the activity cycle.
   Cycle 2: Cycle 2 is the activity cycle. This cycle starts with irregular contractions and is followed by regular contractions to push residual contents further down the gastrointestinal tract. It also lasts about 30 to 60 minutes.

Typically, interdigestive motility sequence begins in the stomach or in the jejunum. Not all interdigestive motility traverse the entire length of small intestines, because gastrointestinal motility depends on various other biological and physiological factors. In general, it takes about 2 hours for the motility wave to migrate from the stomach to the ileum. Gastrointestinal motility is minimal in the large intestine because the musculature of large intestine is inactive much of the time. When it is mobile, its contractions are sluggish or very short lived. The most frequent movements seen in the colon are very slow segmenting movements that typically occur about every 30 minutes.

Gastric Emptying: Gastric emptying plays a major role in the absorption of acidic and basic drugs. Because most drugs are largely absorbed by passive diffusion, it is generally believed that due to larger extent of unionization, acidic drugs are absorbed more from the stomach than from the intestines and basic drugs are absorbed more from the intestines than from the stomach. However, small intestine is also the major site of absorption of acidic drugs, because small intestine offers a much larger surface area of the absorbing membrane than that offered by the stomach. Thus, factors that decrease movement of drug form from the stomach to the small intestine (delayed stomach emptying) will generally delay drug absorption.

Factors influencing gastric emptying. There are several factors that influence emptying of gastric contents. These include the following:

a. pH of stomach
b. Volume of the ingested meal
c. Viscosity of the ingested meal
d. Caloric content of the ingested meal
e. Temperature of the ingested meal
f. Osmolarity of the stomach
g. Emotional state of the person
h. Exercise
i. Presence or absence of other drugs in the gastrointestinal tract
j. Physical state of the person, and
k. Presence of disease.

The stomach usually empties completely within about 4 hours after a normal meal. Larger the volume of meal (the greater the distension) and more liquified its contained food, the faster the food empties from stomach. The volume of the ingested material also affects gastric emptying. Gastric emptying appears to follow first-order kinetics, therefore, as the volume of ingested material increases; there is an initial increase in the rate of emptying of gastric contents (especially when more fluid is present in the stomach). The initial increase in the rate of emptying of gastric contents is then followed by a decrease in the rate of gastric emptying as the volume of gastric contents decreases.

Gastric emptying of bulky and/or solid material tends to be much slower than emptying of liquids. Emptying of liquids in the fasted state is a function of volume. When the volume of liquid is small (less than 100 mL), gastric emptying is controlled by the interdigestive motility pattern. When the volume of liquid is large (greater than 200 mL), the gastric contents empty according to first order kinetics with a half-life of about 10 minutes. Also, presence of large volume of liquids in the stomach helps dissolution of drugs.

Increase in the viscosity of gastric contents reduces the rate of gastric emptying. As a rule, fluids pass through the stomach very quickly and solids remain in the stomach until they are well mixed with the gastric juices and converted into a liquid state. Increased viscosity not only delays stomach emptying, but it also hinders dissolution of the drug.

The rate of gastric emptying depends primarily on the caloric content of the ingested meal, i.e. the extent of delay in gastric emptying is the same for proteins, fats and carbohydrates as long as their caloric content are the same. Since, on a molar basis, the caloric content of carbohydrates, proteins and fats is different, therefore, the rate of emptying of carbohydrates, proteins and fats is also different. In general, carbohydrates empty faster than proteins and proteins empty faster than fats. Slower emptying of fats is also due to the fact that fats form an oily layer at the top of chyme and therefore are digested more slowly by the intestinal enzymes. Thus, when chyme entering the duodenum is high in fats, food may remain in the stomach longer before the stomach is emptied. Some reports indicate that the residence time of fats in the stomach may be as much as 6 hours or more. The delay in gastric emptying by fatty acids appears to increase with the chain length of the fatty acids.

The temperature of the ingested material also affects gastric emptying. Generally speaking, warm food empties faster from the stomach than does cold food. However, as the temperature of cold ingested food increases in the stomach to body temperature, the rate of emptying also increases.

Stress, depression, exercise and aggression have a pronounced effect on the rate of gastric emptying. In general, stress and aggression tend to increase gastric motility and therefore increase emptying rate, although the extent of increase is highly dependant on individual's ability to handle stress and aggression. Depression and vigorous exercise reduce gastric emptying and the extent of reduction here is also highly dependant on the individual's ability to handle depression.

The effect of body posture on the rate of gastric emptying is not clear. Some researchers found faster gastric emptying in supine position, while others found faster emptying in the upright position. Lying on the left side of the body appears to delay gastric emptying because gastric contents have an uphill task to empty from the stomach. Similarly, lying on the right side of the body tends to accelerate gastric emptying, because in this position gravity helps in emptying process.

The presence of drugs in the stomach has been reported to affect gastric emptying. Some drugs increase the rate of gastric emptying, some drugs reduce the rate of gastric emptying and some drugs have no influence on the rate of gastric emptying. Aspirin, anticholinergics, narcotic analgesics and ethanol have been reported to reduce the rate of gastric emptying, while metoclopramide increases the rate of gastric emptying. Acids, in general, reduce the rate of gastric emptying. The extent of reduction depends on the concentration and molecular weight of the acid. Low molecular weight acids appear to be more effective in reducing gastric emptying rate than high molecular weight acids. Alkalies (e.g. sodium bicarbonate) increase the rate of gastric emptying at lower concentrations, but decrease it at higher concentrations. Bile salts reduce the rate of gastric emptying.

There are many disease states and physiological conditions that affect gastrointestinal motility and rate of gastric emptying. Some disease states and physiologic conditions increase the time for transit of gastrointestinal contents through the length of gastrointestinal tract, giving the drug longer time to stay in the gastrointestinal tract. Hence, administration of a drug in the presence of these conditions allows greater time for absorption.

A partial listing of factors other than drugs (disease states and physiological conditions) that increase gastric emptying time is shown in Box 4-1.

There are other disease states and/or physiological conditions that increase the rate of passage of the gastric contents through the small intestinal tract. This therefore reduces the emptying time of the gastric contents. When a drug is administered in the presence of these conditions, the time for drug absorption is reduced.

A partial listing of factors other than drugs (disease states and physiological conditions) that reduce gastric emptying time is shown in Box 4-2.

Box 4-1 Factors other than drugs that increase gastric emptying time

Achlorhydria	Myxedema
Amino acid ingestion	Parkinsonism
Autonomic neuropathy	Particles > 0.5 cm
Constipation	Pernicious anemia
Diabetes mellitus	Postlaporotomy
Diverticulitis	Postoperative
Gastric cancer	Postvagotomy
Gastric ulceration	Pseudo-obstruction
Gastro-esophageal reflux	Pyloroduodenal Stenosis
High-fat meals	Raised intracranial pressure
High osmolality	Steatorrhea
Hypercalcemia	Systemic sclerosis
Hyperkalemia	Thyroid disease
Immobilized patients	Viral gastroenteritis
Migraine	Water > 200 mL

Box 4-2 Factors other than drugs that reduce gastric emptying time

Chronic pancreatitis	Jejunoileal bypass
Colostomy	Pancreatic insufficiency
Crohn disease	Peptic ulcer disease
Diarrhea	Post gastrectomy
Duodenal ulcer	Scleroderma
Gastritis	Thyrotoxicosis
High acidity	Ulcerative colitis
Ileal resection	Vagotomy and pyloroplasty
Irritable bowel syndrome	Zollinger-Ellison Syndrome

pH of the Gastrointestinal Tract: The pH of the gastrointestinal tract is important for drug absorption from two aspects:

i. Extent of ionization of drug in the gastrointestinal tract, and
ii. Chemical stability aspect of the drug in the gastrointestinal tract.

A low pH of the gastric contents has important consequences for drug absorption because low pH can dramatically affect the degree of ionization of many drugs. For example, diazepam, a weak base having a pK_b of 3.3 will be highly protonated (ionized) in the gastric fluids. Consequently, its absorption across the lipid membranes of the stomach will be slow. On the other hand, acetaminophen, a weak acid having a pK_a of 9.5 will exist mainly non-ionized in the stomach and will easily diffuse from stomach into systemic circulation.

Drug molecules absorbed across the gastric mucosa are rapidly removed from their site of absorption by blood flow, thus avoiding establishment of equilibrium condition and therefore, favoring continued absorption. Strong acids, e.g. cromolyn ($pK_a = 2.0$) and benzyl-penicillin ($pK_a = 2.8$) and strong bases, e.g. isoniazid ($pK_b = 10.8$) and mecamylamine ($pK_b = 11.3$) are poorly absorbed from the stomach because they are almost completely ionized at all body pH values.

In the fasting state, the pH of the stomach may vary between 2 and 6. In the beginning of digestion, the range of stomach pH narrows between about 4 and 6 due to the buffering effect of food. During digestion, the pH decreases again to between 1.5 and 2 because the gut secretes hydrochloric acid and enzymes to promote digestion. These gastric secretions overcome the buffering effect of food and reduce the gastric pH to make it more acidic. Because more acid is present at or near the time of eating, if a drug or a compound, which is unstable in the acidic environment of the stomach is ingested at this stage, the compound, will have a greater chance of being degraded than if it had been ingested on an empty stomach. Also, since gastric emptying is delayed in the presence of food, the drug stays in the acidic environment longer than if it had been ingested at or near the time of eating (on an empty stomach). Either one or both of these effects will have a tendency to increase degradation of an acid-labile drug.

The pH of the intestinal tract is not constant throughout its length, but varies with each segment of the intestinal tract. The pH of fluids through the entire intestinal length (from the duodenum to the large intestines) varies between 6 (or slightly less than 6) and about 8. Starting with the duodenum, the duodenal pH is the most acidic in the intestinal tract. The gastric contents experience an abrupt change in pH upon being emptied from the stomach into the duodenum. This is due to the presence of bicarbonate in the duodenum that neutralizes the acidic chyme emptied from the stomach. The pH in the duodenum varies between about 6 and 6.5 and the pH in jejunum varies between about 6 and 7. In ileum (the terminal part of small intestine), the pH is close to neutral (about 7), with the distal part having a pH as high as 8. In the large intestine, the pH is usually between 7.5 and 8.

Gastrointestinal Secretions: Functionally, the gastric mucosa is divided into three areas of secretion. These are:

i. The cardiac gland area secrets mucus and pepsinogen
ii. The oxyntic (parietal) gland area (corresponds to funds and body of stomach) secretes hydrogen ions, pepsinogen and bicarbonate, and
iii. The pyloric gland area (located in the antrum) secretes gastrin and mucus.

Acid secretion by the stomach can be modulated by smell, taste, sight or discussion of food. After food is ingested, gastric distension increases acid secretion. Proteins present in the ingested meals also stimulate acid secretion. Evidence from animal studies suggests that after protein amino acids are converted to amines, gastrin is released. The secretions in the gastrointestinal tract are produced by glands, which are found throughout its entire length of the gastrointestinal tract. These secretions, most of which are enzymatic in nature, mix with food by means of peristalsis and help in the digestion process. Table 4-7 lists secretions in gastrointestinal tract and the average daily amount secreted.

The secretions of the gastrointestinal may be considered as consisting of two components: an aqueous component and a mucus component. The functions of the aqueous and mucus components of the gastrointestinal tract are as follows:

i. **Aqueous Component** The aqueous component of gastrointestinal secretions consists mainly of enzymes which help in the digestion process by breaking large chemical compounds in food into simpler and smaller compounds.
ii. **Mucus Component** Mucus is secreted primarily by goblet cells located throughout the gastrointestinal tract. Mucus is thick and in gel form at the surface of membrane, but becomes more dilute and less viscous towards the lumen. Gastrointestinal mucus serves many functions. Some of the more important functions served by the gastrointestinal mucus include the following:
   a. The primary function gastrointestinal mucus is protection. Mucus protects the surface of mucosal cells.
   b. The outer layer of mucus lubricates and protects mucosal epithelium from mechanical damage during passage of solid food and fecal material.
   c. Mucus serves as a barrier to proteolytic enzymes (e.g. pepsin).
   d. Due to its presence as a stagnant layer, mucus can provide hydration to the underlying tissue since it can retain and immobilize water.
   e. Because of its presence as a stagnant diffusion layer, mucus serves as an absorptive barrier and hinders absorption of drugs.

The thickness of the mucus layer varies in the various segments of the gastrointestinal tract. In the stomach the mucus layer is about 200 nm thick.

Food: The effects of food on drug absorption are not always predictable. However, the presence of food in the gastrointestinal tract can affect the availability of some drugs. Digested foods contain amino acids, fatty acids, electrolytes and many nutrients that may affect not only the gastrointestinal

Table 4-7 Daily gastrointestinal secretions

Gastrointestinal Segment	*Secretion*	*Amount (mL/day)*
Mouth	Ptyalin, Maltase, Mucin	500–1,500
Stomach	Pepsin, Lipase, Rennin, Hydrochloric acid	2,000–3,000
Duodenum	Bile, Trypsin, Amylase, Chymotrypsin	Bile: 250–1,100, Pancreatic juice: 300–1,500
Jejunum	Erepsin, Amylase, Maltase, Lactase, Sucrase	3,000
Ileum	Lipase, Nuclease, Nucleotidase, Enterokinase	?

pH, but also the solubility of many drugs. The effect of food on drug absorption depends largely on two factors: the nature of the drug and to some extent on the type of food ingested. For some drugs, the presence of food has no effect on their absorption, while absorption of other drugs is greatly affected by the presence of food in the gastrointestinal tract. For example, the presence of food delays absorption of amoxicillin and reduces its extent of absorption. Decamethonium and tetracyclines are highly ionized and can complex with calcium ions leading to a reduction in their rate of absorption. The calcium ions may be present in the membrane of the gastrointestinal tract, food or milk. The presence of calcium in the dosage form (e.g. dicalcium phosphate, a common excipient in solid dosage forms) or presence of calcium-containing food (such as milk, cheese and other dairy products) in the gastrointestinal tract will interfere with the absorption of these drugs. The presence of food in the gastrointestinal lumen stimulates the flow of bile. Bile contains bile acids, which are surfactants; therefore, bile acids increase the solubility of fat-soluble drugs through micelle formation, thereby increasing absorption of fat-soluble drugs.

Table 4-8 is a partial listing of examples of drugs whose absorption is affected by the presence of food in the gastrointestinal tract.

The absorption of most drugs is better and more predictable when the drug is administered in the fasted state and with a large volume of water. Some drugs (e.g. griseofulvin) are better absorbed with food rich in fat-content, while absorption of some drugs (e.g. penicillin and tetracycline) is decreased when given with food. Some drugs (e.g., iron salts, erythromycin and some non-steroidal anti-inflammatory agents) are irritating to the gastrointestinal mucosa. Therefore these drugs are generally administered with food, not so much to improve the extent of absorption of the drug, but to minimize gastrointestinal irritation.

As mentioned above, digested foods contain amino acids, fatty acids and many nutrients that may affect intestinal pH and/or drug solubility. Also, presence of food in the stomach stimulates secretion of hydrochloric acid, which lowers the pH of stomach, causing faster dissolution of basic drugs (cinnarizine) and therefore better absorption of these drugs.

Blood Flow: Blood flow to the gastrointestinal tract is an important factor in gastrointestinal absorption, because blood flow to the gastrointestinal tract is responsible in carrying the absorbed drug to the systemic circulation. Absorption of compounds with high intestinal permeability is affected by changes in blood flow to the gastrointestinal tract. Blood vessels serving the digestive system include hepatic portal circulation and those arteries that serve the digestive organs. A large network of capillaries and lymphatic vessels perfuse duodenal region and peritoneum. The arterial supply of celiac trunk that serve stomach and superior and inferior mesenteric arteries that serve small and large intestines, normally receive about one quarter of total cardiac output. This percentage of blood volume is not constant and increases after a meal has been eaten. After absorption from the small intestine, the drug enters liver via mesenteric vessels prior to reaching systemic circulation. Any decrease in mesenteric blood flow (e.g. congestive heart failure), will decrease the rate of drug removal from intestinal tract, i.e. decrease rate of absorption.

Table 4-8 Examples of drugs whose absorption is affected by presence of food

Increased	*Delayed*	*Delayed*	*Not affected*
Dicoumarol	Amoxicillin	Acetaminophen	Cephradine
Griseofulvin	Ampicillin	Amoxicillin	Chlorpropamide
Hydralazine	Ethanol	Cefaclor	Melperone
Metoprolol	Isoniazid	Cephalexin	Metronidazole
Oxazepam	Levodopa	Cephradine	Prednisone
Phenytoin	Oxytetracycline	Sulfadiazine	Sulfasomidine
Propoxyphene	Propantheline	Sulfanilamide	Sulfonylurea
Propranolol	Rifampin	Sulfisoxazole	Theophylline

Absorption of drugs through the lymphatic system (lymphatic vessels under the microvilli) eliminates first-pass effect due to liver metabolism, because absorption through the hepatoportal vein is avoided. Examples of drugs whose intestinal absorption is dependant on blood flow include aminopyrine, antipyrine, benzoic acid, ethanol and salicylic acid.

Gut Flora: The entire length of human gastrointestinal tract contains a large population of viable bacteria and a large number of microorganisms are ingested with food. Microorganisms also enter the gastrointestinal tract through various other sources, e.g. environment and oral dosage forms (tablets, capsules and liquid dosage forms). The total bacterial population (viable count per gram of wet sample) in various regions of gastrointestinal tract generally increases as one traverses the gastrointestinal tract. The smallest bacterial population, about 1 million, is found in the mouth and stomach, although the population may be less than 1 million in the stomach due to strongly acidic environment. From the stomach to small intestine, bacterial population increases to about 10 million and reaches about 1 billion in the rectum and feces. It should be remembered, however, that the intestinal flora also plays a major role in metabolism of drugs, e.g. acetylsalicylic acid, L-dopa, methyldigoxin, morphine and sulfasalazine.

SUGGESTED READING

1. Delgado J, Rermers W (eds). In: Wilson and Gisvold's Textbook of Organic Medicinal and Pharmaceutical Chemistry, 9th edition. Lippincott; 1990.
2. Goodman and Gilman's Pharmacological Basis of Therapeutics, 9th edition. Macmillan; 1995.
3. Marieb E. Human Anatomy and Physiology, 2nd edition. Benjamin/Cummings Publishing Company; 1991.
4. Pratt W, Taylor P. (eds). In: Principles of Drug Action: The Basis of Pharmacology, 3rd edition. Churchill Livingstone; 1990.
5. Remington: The Science and Practice of Pharmacy, 21st edition. Mack Publishing; 2005.
6. Tortora GJ. Principles of Anatomy and Physiology, 7th edition. Harper Collins; 1993.
7. Wagner J. Biopharmaceutics and Relevant Pharmacokinetics. Drug Intelligence Publications; 1971.

PRACTICE PROBLEMS

4-1. The pK_a of salicylic acid is 3.0. Calculate the percentage of dose ionized in the stomach if pH of the stomach is 2.0.

4-2. The pK_b of a drug is 12.7. Calculate the percentage of dose ionized in the stomach if pH of the stomach is 2.5.

4-3. The usual dose of an acidic drug is 300 mg twice a day before meals. If pK_a of the drug is 2.5, calculate the percent dose available for absorption if the pH of gastric fluids is 2.0.

4-4. The usual dose of an acidic drug is 300 mg twice a day before meals. If pK_a of the drug is 2.0, calculate the percent dose available for absorption if the patient is in the habit of taking antacids before meals, which raises the stomach pH to 3.0.

4-5. Calculate pH of the resultant solution if pKb of an amine is 6.6 and the ratio of non-ionized to ionized species is 10:1.

4-6. Acetaminophen exhibits Michaelis-Menten absorption kinetics. A patient received a single 1 g dose of the drug and plasma concentration of drug at 0.5 hour after dosing indicated that the instantaneous rate of absorption was 5 mg/min and 225 mg of the drug had been absorbed. The affinity constant of drug for the carrier is 410 in the same units as those for the drug dissolved in the lumen of gastrointestinal tract. Calculate the maximal rate of drug absorption.

4-7. If the pK_a of an acidic drug is 3.5, calculate fraction of dose ionized in the stomach at pH = 2.5.

4-8. The pK_b of a basic drug is 6.6. Calculate the fraction of dose ionized in the intestinal tract at a pH of 6.5.

4-9. The pK_a of an acidic drug is 3.5. What should be the pH of gastric fluids if it is desired that 50 percent of the administered dose should in the non-ionized form?

4-10. The pKa of an acidic drug is 4.5. Calculate the pH of gastric fluids if approximately 24 percent of the administered dose is found to be in the non-ionized form in the gastric fluids.

4-11. The usual dose of an acidic drug is 250 mg twice a day before meals. If pK_a of the drug is 2.5, calculate the percent dose available for absorption if the pH of gastric fluids is 3.0.

CHAPTER 5

DRUG DISTRIBUTION

After the administration of a drug dose, the following events occur: drugs which are administered intravascularly are placed directly into the blood stream and therefore appear in the blood stream as soon as the drug is administered. In the case of drugs, which are administered by an extravascular route, the drug undergoes release and/or dissolution from the dosage form and the drug now becomes available for absorption. Regardless of the route of administration, after its appearance in the blood stream, part of the drug starts undergoing elimination via an excretory mechanism and part of the drug begins distributing into the various body fluids and tissues. The extent of distribution of drug into the various body fluids and tissues depends on the affinity of the drug for the particular body fluid and/or tissue.

The distribution of a drug into various body fluids and tissues is an important determinant of the therapeutic effect of the drug. Although there are some exceptions, the large majority of drugs is not distributed in the plasma fluid alone, but appears to be distributed in the plasma as well as in some other body fluid and/or tissues. Examples of body fluids, in which drugs appear to be distributed include extracellular body water, total body water, etc. and examples of tissues in which drugs distribute include the adipose tissue, muscles, bones, hair, etc. A large variety of drugs are distributed in the plasma as well as in the proteins. The distribution of drugs is not limited to one tissue or one body fluid alone. Some drugs may be distributed in the plasma, in the adipose tissue, as well as in the proteins. However, the extent of distribution of drug in the body fluids or each tissue (adipose tissue, protein, bones, etc.) depends on relative affinity of drug for the particular tissue. Therefore, concentration of drug in plasma depends on:

1. Whether or not the drug distributes into other body fluids (other than plasma) and tissues.
2. The extent of distribution in these tissues.

This is, because the distribution of drug in other body fluids and/or tissues will decrease the concentration of drug in plasma. Thus, for drugs which exhibit extensive tissue distribution, a higher dose may be needed to achieve the desired therapeutic concentration of drug in the plasma.

Following the appearance of drug in the plasma, some drugs distribute rapidly between plasma and other body components, while others do not. In the case of those drugs that do not distribute in other body fluids and/or tissues, the concentration of drug in the plasma declines due to the process of elimination only. If, on the other hand, the distribution of drug into body fluids and/or tissues is rapid, then the concentration of drug in plasma exhibits a rapid initial decline because the drug is removed from the plasma by two processes:

1. Distribution into other body components
2. Elimination.

When distribution of drug in the body is slow, the decline in the concentration of drug in the plasma is not as rapid and the drug tends to reside in the component(s) with which it has an affinity. The rapid initial decline of concentration of drug in plasma due to distribution and elimination follows a relatively slow decline due to equilibration of drug between plasma and tissues involve in drug distribution.

Most drugs have a tendency to bind reversibly to one or more macromolecules in plasma. The main plasma components involved in associating with drugs are plasma proteins. These include albumin, globulins, glycoproteins, α- and β-lipoproteins and transferrin. Binding of drugs to plasma proteins depends on the nature of drug (acidic or basic character). Acidic drugs bind principally to albumin and basic drugs will generally bind to albumin, lipoproteins and α1-acid glycoproteins (α-AGP). Certain disease states and physiological conditions can alter the protein content of the body and can influence associating and/or binding capacity of the drug. There are, however, certain disease states and other physiological conditions that are capable of altering (increasing or decreasing) the protein content of the body and therefore, these conditions influence the associating and/or binding capacity of the drug. A partial listing of these conditions is shown in Table 5-1.

The fraction of administered drug dose that will bind to or form a complex with body components (adipose tissue, protein, minerals, etc.) influences drug distribution and rate of elimination of the drug. This is because only the free fraction of the drug (fraction of drug not bound to the tissues) is able to take part in the biological processes, i.e. diffuse through biological membrane, undergo metabolism or be excreted through the kidney. Since only the unbound fraction of drug is responsible for its therapeutic activity, it follows that therapeutic concentration of drug in the plasma is therefore governed by the extent to which the drug binds to other tissues. There are examples of few drugs that either do not bind to proteins or bind to a very small extent. Table 5-2 lists examples of drugs (and the extent of their binding), which exhibit low (10% or less) protein binding.

Table 5-1 Conditions capable of altering plasma proteins

Decreased plasma protein	*Increased plasma protein*
Albumin	**Albumin**
Burns	Hypothyroidism
Chronic liver disease	
Cystic fibrosis	Alpha1-acid glycoprotein
Protein-losing enteropathy	Celiac disease
Nephrotic syndrome	Crohn disease
Pregnancy	Myocardial infarction
Chronic renal failure	Renal failure
Trauma	Rheumatoid arthritis
	Trauma
Alpha1-Acid Glycoprotein	
Nephrotic syndrome	

Table 5-2 Examples of drugs exhibiting low protein binding

Drug	*EPB**	*Drug*	*EPB*	*Drug*	*EPB*
Antipyrine	10	Tobramycin	<10	Flucytosine	4
Cefadroxil	10	Amikacin	5	Ethinamate	1
Gentamicin	10	Insulin	5	Ethosuccimide	0
Netilmicin	10	Levodopa	5	Kanamycin	0
Sisomicin	10	Viomycin	5	Lithium	0
Timolol	10	Acetaminophen	<5	Meprobamate	0
Vancomycin	10	Atenolol	<5	Metformin	0

*EPB = Extent of protein binding expressed as a percentage

The reversible binding (or complexation) of a drug is governed by the association and dissociation constants of drug-tissue complex. The complex attains dynamic equilibrium with free drug according to the law of mass action, given by the equation:

$$\text{Free drug} + \text{Tissue} \rightleftarrows \text{Drug-tissue complex} \quad (5\text{-}1)$$

Equation (5-1) can be written as:

$$K = \frac{[\text{Drug-tissue complex}]}{[\text{Free drug}] \times [\text{Tissue}]} \quad (5\text{-}2)$$

In equation (5-2), K is association constant of the complex and the terms in the brackets indicate molar concentrations of species involved in complexation. The term tissue is used in a generic sense and indicates any body component, which may be involved in binding or forming a complex with the drug. For example, fatty tissues, proteins, minerals (e.g. calcium), etc. which may bind to the drug are considered as tissues binding to the drug. The numerical value of K is an indicator of affinity between the drug and the tissues involved in the formation of the complex. Larger numerical values of K indicate stronger affinities in the formation of the complex and smaller values of K reflect weaker affinity in the formation of the complex. As the unbound (free) drug leaves circulation (due to biotransformation or elimination, etc.), the complex dissociates so as to maintain the numerically constant value of K and more free (unbound) drug then becomes available for absorption.

Since, only the unbound (free) fraction of the drug can diffuse through the biological membrane, it follows that extensive binding of the drug with the tissues will have a tendency to decrease the intensity of action of the drug. The magnitude of decrease in intensity is usually in direct proportion to the fraction of administered drug dose bound to the tissue(s); because at low drug concentration, a stronger affinity between the drug and the tissues binds a larger fraction of drug to the tissues, thereby removing a large portion of drug from the circulation. This leaves a small fraction of drug, which is not bound and a larger dose must be administered to achieve the desired effective drug concentration of the unbound fraction. As the dose is progressively increased, the binding capacity of tissue may be saturated and additional drug would remain free (unbound).

Tissues and fluids involved in slow distribution of drug may be looked upon as a storage house for the drug. Some drugs may be bound to one tissue (e.g. adipose tissue), while others may have an affinity for more than one tissue (e.g. proteins and/or calcium in addition to the adipose tissue). A drug having affinity for calcium will find its way to tissues, which contain calcium (e.g. bones, teeth, etc.). If the affinity between the drug and tissues is strong, then the release of drug from these tissues will be relatively slow. That is, the drug will be released slowly over a long period of time and the drug will exhibit a depot action and a longer biological half-life. For example, suramin, used in treatment of trypanosomiasis, is bound so strongly to the plasma protein that one intravenous dose produces therapeutic levels for up to 3 months. In this case, the blood serves as a circulating reservoir for the drug.

It should be pointed out that in determining the usual recommended dose that will provide therapeutic plasma levels of the drug; the manufacturer should consider the extent of binding of drug to the tissues in the body. If, during treatment with a drug which binds to tissues, another drug with stronger affinity for these tissues is administered, the second drug would displace the first drug from these tissues. As a consequence, the concentration of the first drug would increase in the plasma (because of release of drug from the tissues), resulting in possibly approaching toxic levels. The pharmacist must consider inherent danger in concomitant administration of drug combinations, which may cause such displacement of one drug by the other drug.

The most common body components known to have a strong affinity for certain drugs are the adipose tissue and the plasma proteins. Those drugs, which are lipophilic in nature (e.g.

barbiturates), will have an inherent affinity for the adipose tissue and those drugs, which possess functional groups that are compatible with the amino groups or carboxylic groups on the protein molecule will have a tendency to bind to the proteins. As mentioned earlier, since the fraction of dose bound to the lipid tissues or the plasma proteins effectively removes a portion of free drug from the systemic circulation, therefore, a good working knowledge of the mechanism and the extent of drug distribution is important in the determination of size of the drug dose, i.e. needed to provide the necessary therapeutic concentration of drug in the systemic circulation. Also, since the fraction of dose bound to the lipid tissue or plasma proteins acts as a storehouse for the drug, the frequency of administration of the drug may also have to be taken into account to prevent accumulation of drug in the body and assure therapeutic plasma levels of the drug.

Only the free-drug, i.e. the fraction of drug not bound to the body tissues is eliminated from the body. The removal of unbound drug from systemic circulation takes place primarily through the kidneys. Some drugs undergo reabsorption to a significant extent. The main processes of reabsorption of drug are renal, tubular or enterohepatic. Drugs, which undergo reabsorption stay in systemic circulation longer than those drugs, which are not reabsorbed but undergo excretion through an excretory mechanism (urinary, biliary, pulmonary, etc.) rapidly.

Table 5-3 lists examples of drugs which exhibit high (60% or more) protein binding.

Most clinical laboratory reports of concentration of drug in plasma usually represent the total concentration of drug in the plasma, i.e. drug that is bound as well as the drug that is free (unbound). The free drug is the pharmacologically active moiety because it is the free drug, i.e. in equilibrium with the receptor sites. Also, it is only the free drug, i.e. capable of undergoing elimination. Therefore, it is important to know what fraction of the administered drug dose is free and what fraction is bound. Based on the total plasma concentration of the drug, the fraction of free drug concentration (α) is given by the following relationship:

$$\alpha = \frac{\text{Plasma drug concentration of free drug}}{\text{Total plasma drug concentration}} \quad (5\text{-}3)$$

$$\alpha = \frac{C_{free}}{C_{total}} \quad (5\text{-}4)$$

$$\alpha = \frac{C_{free}}{C_{free} + C_{bound}} \quad (5\text{-}5)$$

The effective free drug concentration can be calculated by rearranging equation (5-4):

$$C_{free} = \alpha \times C_{total} \quad (5\text{-}6)$$

ROLE OF PROTEINS IN DRUG DISTRIBUTION

Plasma Proteins

Human plasma is composed of about 200 known proteins. The proteins in plasma function in different capacities. Some of these include the following:

a. To maintain osmotic pressure between intracellular and extracellular fluids (albumins).
b. Coagulation of blood (clotting factors, thrombin, fibrinogen, etc.).
c. Immune reactions (antibodies).
d Transport of endogenous and exogenous compounds.
e. Function as enzymes.
f. Function as hormones.

From a clinical standpoint, the proteins that are important in binding to drugs in the plasma include albumin, α1-acid glycoprotein and lipoproteins. The size (molecular weight) and normal concentration range of these proteins is shown in Table 5-4.

Table 5-3 Examples of drugs extensively bound to plasma proteins

Drug	*EPB*	*Drug*	*EPB*	*Drug*	*EPB*
Carbenoxolone	> 99	Amoxapine	91	Methaqualone	81
Thyroxine	> 99	Diazoxide	91	Ceforanide	80
Warfarin	> 99	*Tolamalol*	91	Diltiazem	80
Dicumarol	99	Amodiaquine	90	Doxepin	80
Furosemide	99	Amphotericin B	90	Penicillin V	80
Ibuprofen	99	Aprindine	90	Sulfamethazine	80
Ketoconazole	99	Cefoperazone	90	Methacycline	79
Naproxen	99	Ceftriaxone	90	Dapsone	77
Phenprocoumon	99	Clindamycin	90	Minocycline	76
Phenylbutazone	99	Guanabenz	90	Propoxyphene	76
Sulfadimethoxine	99	Lorazepam	90	Chlorthalidone	75
Sulfaethidole	99	Mianserin	90	Sulfamerazine	75
Sulfinpyrazone	99	Nafcillin	90	Cefamandole	74
Zomepera	99	Oxacillin	90	Erythromycin	73
Diphenhydramine	98	Probenecid	90	Carbamazepine	72
Nifedipine	98	Sulfamethizole	90	Chlorpropamide	72
Deslanoside	97	Valproate	90	Lincomycin	72
Diazepam	97	Verapamil	90	Alprozolam	71
Indomethacin	97	Zimelidine	90	Aspirin	71
Prazosin	97	Phenytoin	89	Fentanyl	70
Amitriptyline	96	Acetohexamide	88	Mexiletine	70
Chlorpromazine	96	Meprotiline	88	Nomifensine	70
Dicloxacillin	96	Droperidol	87	Quinine	70
Flucloxacillin	96	Hydralazine	87	Salicylates	70
Imipramine	96	Papaverine	87	Trimethoprim	70
Oxazepam	96	Rifampin	87	Disopyramide	68
Clofibrate	95	Tolbutamide	87	Sulfamethoxazole	68
Glyburide	95	Cefazolin	86	Amantadine	67
Hydrocortisone	95	Sulfisomidine	86	Lidocaine	66
Mebendazole	95	Sulfisoxazole	86	Para-aminosalicylate sodium (PAS)	65
Nortriptyline	95	Azidocillin	85	Cephalothin	65
Chlordiazepoxide	94	Clonazepam	85	Chlorthiazide	65
Cloxacillin	94	Methadone	85	Penicillin G	65
Acetazolamide	93	Nitrazepam	85	Meperidine	64
Digitoxin	93	Acebutalol	84	Vincamine	64
Nalidixic Acid	93	Dexamethasone	84	Pentazocine	61
Propranolol	93	Doxycycline	82	Chloramphenicol	60
Haloperidol	92	Erythromycin	82	Oxtriphylline	60
Miconazole	92	Phenethicillin K	82	Theophylline	60
Imipramine	92	Quinidine	82	Ticarcillin	60

EPB = Extent of protein binding

Table 5-4 Properties of major plasma proteins

Plasma protein	*Molecular weight (Daltons)*	*Concentration range (mg/mL)*
Albumin	69,000	35–50
α1-Acid glycoprotein	44,000	0.4–1.0
Lipoproteins	200,000–3,400,000	variable

Albumin

As a result of its abundance in plasma, serum albumin is the most important protein in terms of drug binding. It is perhaps for this reason, that almost all *in vitro* protein binding studies have used albumin as the protein and the results of these studies are usually generalized to the whole plasma.

Albumin is an acidic protein having an isoelectric point of 4.8. It is very soluble in water. Albumin is a very stable protein and has an elimination half-life of 17 to 18 days.

The primary function of albumin is to serve as an osmotic agent for the regulation of pressure differences between intracellular and extracellular fluids. It also serves as an important transport protein in the plasma for both endogenous and exogenous compounds.

The most salient aspect of albumin is its ability to bind to many different types of molecules. The interaction of bilirubin (a by-product of heme metabolism) with albumin has been reported to occur at two different sites. One of the binding sites has a very high affinity for bilirubin, while the other site binds bilirubin with slightly lower affinity. Many weakly acidic drugs, such as salicylates and penicillins, interact with albumin.

α1-Acid Glycoprotein

The α1-acid glycoprotein (AGP) is a globular protein. The plasma concentration of α1-acid glycoprotein is very low and it preferentially binds with basic drugs, such as imipramine, propranolol and lidocaine.

Lipoproteins

Lipoproteins are high molecular weight complexes of proteins with lipids. Lipoproteins are classified according to their densities and separation in an ultracentrifuge. Lipoproteins are classified according to their densities as

1. Very low density lipoprotein (VLDL)
2. Low density lipoprotein (LDL)
3. High density lipoprotein (HDL).

Although lipoproteins are primarily responsible for the binding and transport of lipids, they do interact with drugs, especially, when the binding sites on the albumin are saturated.

For most drugs that are bound primarily to albumin, the fraction of drug that is free (α) does not vary with the plasma drug concentration because the number of protein binding sites far exceeds the number of drug molecules available for binding. However, the albumin binding sites can be saturated, when the plasma concentrations for drugs bound to albumin exceed 25 to 50 mg/L. For example, salicylates and valproic acid (Depakene) can saturate plasma protein binding sites and both of these drugs frequently have plasma protein concentrations exceeding 25 to 50 mg/L.

For those drugs that do not reach plasma concentrations capable of saturating protein binding sites, the plasma protein concentration (in many cases, this is albumin) and the binding affinity of the drug for the plasma protein are the two major factors, which control α.

Many other drugs are bound primarily to globulin rather than albumin. It would be inappropriate to make adjustments of plasma drug concentrations for these drugs based upon plasma concentrations of albumin. Unfortunately, adjustments for changes in globulin binding are difficult because drugs usually bind to a specific globulin, which is only a small fraction of total globulin concentration. In general, acidic drugs (e.g. phenytoin and most anti-epileptic drugs) and some neutral compounds bind primarily to albumin and basic drugs (e.g. lidocaine and quinidine) bind more extensively to the globulins.

From a clinical perspective, any factor which alters protein binding may become clinically important, when a drug is protein bound. In the case of drugs that are not highly protein bound, a small change in the fraction bound does not substantially increase or decrease the amount of free drug available to the pharmacologically active sites. But for those drugs that are highly protein bound, a small change in the fraction of dose bound can substantially increase or decrease the amount of free drug available to the pharmacologically active sites. For example, if a drug is bound to the extent of 90%, i.e., 10% of the drug is free ($\alpha = 0.1$) and the value of α is increased from 0.1 to 0.2 because of decreased amounts of protein, the concentration of free drug available for any given value of total drug concentration C_{total} (bound + free) would be double the usual values. Although the increase in the value of α from 0.1 to 0.2 appears to be a small increase, the fact remains that 0.2 is two-fold compared to the original value of 0.1. Therefore, if the value of α is doubled, the amount of free drug is also doubled.

For drugs that are not extensively bound, i.e. drugs having high α values (α values greater than 0.5), small changes in plasma protein binding are not likely to cause significant clinical consequences. For example, if α for a drug is increased from 0.5 (50% free) to 0.6 (60% free) because of decreased protein concentration, the concentration of free drug would actually be increased by only 20%. Here, the increase in the value of α from 0.5 to 0.6 is a change of 20% in the value of α and therefore when α increased from 0.5 to 0.6 (a 20% increase), the amount of free drug will also increase 20%.

Example 5-1 Calculate the concentration of free phenytoin in plasma in a uremic patient with an α of 0.2 and a reported phenytoin concentration of 6 mg/L.

Solution

According to equation (5-6):

$$C_{free} = \alpha \times C_{total}$$

$$C_{free} = (0.2) \times (6 \text{ mg/L}) = 1.2 \text{ mg/L}$$

Example 5-2 The concentration of free phenytoin in plasma in a uremic patient with an α of 0.2 is 1.0 mg/L. Calculate the total phenytoin concentration in this patient.

Solution

According to equation (5-4):

$$\alpha = \frac{C_{free}}{C_{total}}$$

$$C = \frac{C_{free}}{\alpha}$$

$$C_{total} = \frac{1.0 \text{ mg / L}}{0.2} = 5 \text{ mg / L}$$

Example 5-3 The value of α for a drug is 0.1 and the total concentration of drug in the plasma is 8 mg/L. What will be the percent increase in C_{free} if α becomes 0.25?

Solution

$$\text{When } \alpha = 0.1\text{: } C_{free} = (0.1)(8 \text{ mg/L}) = 0.8 \text{ mg/L}$$

$$\text{When } \alpha \text{ becomes } 0.25\text{: } C_{free} = (0.25)(8 \text{ mg/L}) = 2.0 \text{ mg/L}$$

$$\text{Increase in } C_{free} = 2.0 \text{ mg/L} - 0.8 \text{ mg/L} = 1.2 \text{ mg/L}$$

$$\text{Therefore, percent increase in } C_{free} = \frac{1.2 \text{ mg / L}}{0.8 \text{ mg / L}} \times 100\% = 150\%$$

PERFUSION AND DRUG DISTRIBUTION

The term perfusion signifies blood flow or the rate of flow of blood. The tissues and organs in the body receive varying rates of blood flow. Tissues and organs that receive the highest blood flow are termed highly perfused tissues, while organs and tissues that receive poor blood supply are known as poorly perfused tissues.

Perfusion

According to perfusion theory, after the drug molecules enter bloodstream, the pattern of distribution is determined by perfusion to each tissue. Since highly perfused tissues (heart, liver, kidneys, etc.) are in rapid distribution equilibrium with blood, they receive a larger amount of drug in a very short time and equilibrate with the drug most rapidly. Tissues with poor blood supply (muscles, skin tissue, etc.) generally receive a much smaller amount of drug over a long period of time and do not equilibrate with drug rapidly. The relatively slow equilibration of drug with these tissues is essentially because of poor blood supply to these tissues.

Drug Distribution

Although not all drugs distribute into the various body fluids and tissues, some drugs do undergo distribution into one or more tissues and/or fluids in the body. In the case of those drugs that distribute into the tissues, the distribution of the drug into various tissues and fluids of the body is an important consideration. This is because this distribution reflects the rate of uptake of drug into the various body tissues following the administration of the drug dose.

Following administration of the drug dose, the distribution of the drug into the body fluids and tissues is controlled by several factors. Some of the important factors that must be considered in the distribution of drug include the following four factors:

1. Rate of flow of blood through the tissue
2. Partition characteristics of the drug between plasma and the tissue
3. Partition coefficient of the drug into the various tissues
4. The volume or mass of the tissue.

Rate of Flow of Blood Through the Tissue

The rate of flow of blood through various tissues of the human body varies tremendously. On a per gram basis, highly perfused tissues receive higher blood supply than that received by poorly perfused tissues. For example, highly perfused tissues receive blood at the rate of about 500 mL per 100 g of tissue per minute and poorly perfused tissues may receive blood at the rate of less than 2 mL per 100 g of tissue per minute. Since the drug is carried to the tissues by systemic circulation, it follows that a drug will generally distribute rapidly into those tissues, which receive a higher rate of flow of blood (highly perfused tissues) and slowly into those tissues where the rate of flow of blood is poor. Table 5-5 shows the rate of blood flow to major human tissues.

Table 5-5 Approximate blood flow to major human tissues

Tissue	*Body weight (%)*	*Cardiac output (%)*	*Blood flow (mL/100 g tissue/min)*
Adrenal	0.02	1	550
Brain	2.0	15	55
Connective Tissue	7.0	1	1
Fat	15	2	1
Heart (basal)	0.4	4	70
Kidneys	0.4	24	450
Liver	2.0		
Hepatic		5	20
Portal		20	75
Muscle (basal)	40.0	15	3
Portal-drained viscera	2.0	20	75
Skin	7.0	5	5
Thyroid	0.04	2	400

**Courtesy:* T. C. Butler, "The Distribution of Drugs," in "Fundamentals of Drug Metabolism and Disposition," B. N. LaDu, H. G. Mandel, and E. L. Way eds., Williams and Wilkins, Baltimore (1972).

Partition Characteristics of Drug Between Plasma and the Tissue

Partition characteristics of the drug between plasma and tissues determine the extent of drug distribution into the tissues. Drugs, which have poor partition characteristics between plasma and tissues tend to stay in the plasma and therefore do not distribute into the tissue to the same extent as drugs, which have better partition characteristics in favor of the tissue. This is because partitioning of the drug is favored in the plasma than in the tissues.

Partition Coefficient of Drug into the Various Tissues

Partition coefficient of a drug between plasma and the tissue in question determines extent of distribution of drug between plasma and the tissue. Partition coefficient of the drug into the various tissues is affected by many factors, including, relative lipid solubility of drug in plasma and the tissue, complexation of drug to the proteins and binding of drug to the adipose tissue.

Volume or Mass of the Tissue

The extent of distribution of a drug into a tissue depends upon the mass or the volume of the tissue. The greater the mass or volume of the tissue, the larger will be the amount of drug distributed into it. It should be realized, however, that a smaller mass or a smaller volume of a tissue may accumulate a large amount of drug, if the tissue in question has a stronger affinity or better partition coefficient for the drug in question.

Because of the four factors mentioned above, the concentration of drug will be generally different in different tissues. Also, different groups of tissues will accumulate different amounts of drug at different rates. It should be remembered that any change in the flow of blood to the tissue is likely to alter distribution of drug to tissues experiencing change in blood flow. The blood flow to various tissues may be changed due to various reasons, e.g. in many physiologic conditions and during various disease states. For example, under normal conditions, blood flow to muscles is usually very little, but during exercise, blood flow to the muscles increases. The increase depends on the nature and intensity of exercise. Many diabetic patients receiving insulin experience changes in onset of action and duration of activity of insulin, when the general area of injection is subjected to an increase in exercise. For example, a patient who normally injects insulin in the abdominal area is very likely to experience changes in onset and duration of action of insulin, if the drug was injected in the arm or thigh area or in an area, which is subjected to exercise to a greater extent. Similarly, a bed-confined patient, who normally injects insulin in the thigh area is likely to experience changes in onset and duration of action if the patient becomes less bed-confined and more active and starts going for a walk after taking insulin injection.

Perfusion Groups

Since various tissues receive blood at different rates, it is difficult to find many tissues, which exhibit similar blood flow per unit mass (or volume) of tissue per unit time. Thus, various tissues would differ from each other in the rate and extent of distribution of drug. It is for this reason, as well as for the sake of simplicity, that the human body is divided into groups based on perfusion and partition characteristics of the drug. Broadly speaking and based on perfusion and partition characteristics of the drug, the human body may be conceived as being divided into four major groups:

Group I: Highly Perfused Lean Tissue Group

The highly perfused lean tissue group consists of lean tissues, which receive high flow of blood. Included in this group are the heart, hepatoportal system, lungs, kidneys, endocrine glands and under certain instances, brain and spinal system.

Group II: Poorly Perfused Lean Tissue Group

The poorly perfused lean tissue group consists of those lean tissues, which have relatively poor blood flow. Included in this group are the large mass of muscle and the skin tissue. Although the fatty tissue is poorly perfused, fat is not included in this group, because the fatty tissue is considered as a separate group by itself.

Group III: Fat Group

This group consists of tissues, which are essentially made up of fat, e.g. the adipose tissue and marrow.

Group IV: Negligible Perfusion Tissue Group

This group consists of tissues, which receive negligible blood supply. Included in this group are bones (not marrow), teeth, ligaments, tendons, cartilage, contents of the alimentary tract and hair.

DRUG DISTRIBUTION AND BODY WATER COMPARTMENTS

Considering all tissues, fluids and everything else in the body, water is the most abundant substance in the body. The total body water in normal adults and children weighing 10 kg or more is directly proportional to body weight. That is, when body weight increases by 20%, the total body water also increases by 20%. For normal subjects, who have normal lean body mass: fat ratio, one would expect a linear relationship between the volume of total body water and body weight. This relationship does not exist in individuals suffering from dehydration, pathologic fluid deposits or obesity. For example, in the case of patients, who have pathologic fluid deposits one would expect an increase in the volume of total body water per unit body weight and in obese subjects one would expect this ratio to be smaller.

The customary requirement of water is about 2,000 mL to 3,000 mL per day. This is based on the daily production of approximately 1,000 mL to 1,500 mL of urine. The minimum water requirements for fluid balance can be estimated from the sum of urine output necessary to excrete the daily solute load (about 500 mL per day) and the loss of insensible water from the skin and the respiratory tract (between about 500 mL and 1,000 mL per day), minus the amount of water produced from endogenous metabolism (about 300 mL per day). The loss of insensible water depends on a variety of factors, such as, ambient temperature, respiratory rate, relative humidity and body temperature. The loss of fluid from body due to perspiration can vary from almost 0 to 2,000 mL per hour depending on ambient temperature, physical activity and body temperature. The loss of water from body due to body temperature increases by about 100 mL to 150 mL per day for each degree of body temperature over the normal body temperature.

In an average adult male the total body water accounts for approximately 60% of total body weight, while in an average adult female it is about 50% of the body weight. Obesity has a tendency to decrease the percentage of water in the body, sometimes to as low as 45%. In a newborn infant, the total body water may be greater than 75% of body weight, but it progressively decreases as the infant grows in age. The total body water decreases from birth to old age, with most decrease occurring in the first 10 years of life.

Total Body Water in Newborn

In a newborn, the total body water may be greater than 75% of body weight, but it progressively decreases with age, most decrease occurring in the first 10 years of life. Table 5-6 shows decreasing percentage of total body water with increasing age in infants and children.

Body Water Compartments

For the purposes of drug distribution, the fluids in the body are divided into groups or compartments, generally referred to as body water compartments. The total body water in an average adult male is between 58% and 60% of body weight. Since an average adult male is considered to weigh approximately 70 kg, therefore the total body water in an average adult male is considered to be between 58% and 60% of 70 kg = 41 or 42 kg by weight or about 41 to 42 L in volume. Figure 5-1 is a schematic of the body water compartments in an average adult male. The percent body weight and percent body water and the volume (in L) of each body water compartment has been rounded off to the nearest whole number.

The total body water in the body may be divided into two broad categories:

1. The extracellular fluid
2. The intracellular fluid.

Table 5-6 Total body water as a function of age

Age	*Body water as percent body weight*
Birth–11 days	77.6
11 days–6 months	72.2
6 months–2 years	63.1
2 years–7 years	59.5
7 years–16 years	58.4
16 years–adult years	58.0

**Courtesy*: J.G. Wagner, "Biopharmaceutics and Relevant Pharmacokinetics," Drug Intelligence Publications, Hamilton, 1971;261.

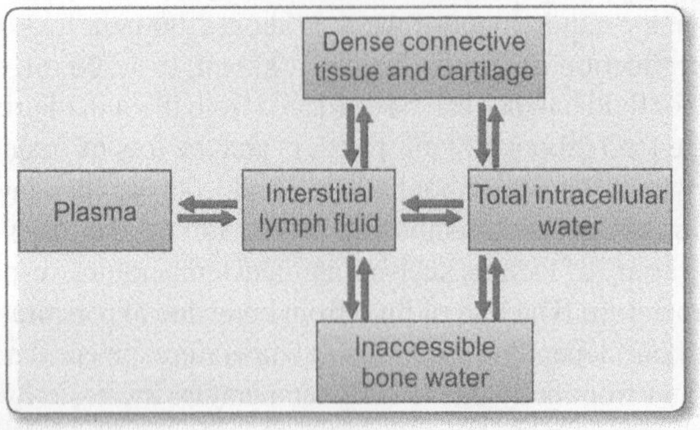

Water compartment	*Volume (L)*	*Body weight (%)*	*Body water (%)*
Plasma	3	5	8
Interstitial-lymph fluid	8	12	19
Dense connective tissue and cartilage	3	5	8
Inaccessible bone water	3	5	8
Total extracellular water	17	27	43
Total intracellular water	**24**	**33**	**57**
Total body water	41	60	100

The values in the last three columns have been rounded off to the nearest whole number. *Courtesy:* Edelman and Leibman, "Anatomy of body water and electrolytes," Amer. J Med. 1959;27,256-277.

Fig. 5-1 Body water compartments in average adult male

The volume of the total extracellular fluid is the sum of fluids in the plasma, the interstitial lymph fluid, dense connective tissue and cartilage and the inaccessible bone water. The volume of the intracellular fluid is the difference between the volume of the total body water and the volume of the total extracellular fluid.

Not included in these fluids are transcellular fluids. The term 'transcellular fluids' was introduced to designate a variety of extracellular fluid connections, which are not simple transudates. Transcellular fluids have the common property of being formed by the transport activity of cells. These fluids are found in various parts of the body, e.g. in the fluid cavity of eye, the cerebrospinal fluid, the intraluminal fluid of the gastrointestinal tract, salivary glands, pancreas, liver and biliary tree, thyroid gland, gonads, skin, mucous membrane of respiratory and gastrointestinal tracts and the kidneys.

The volume of the transcellular fluid is estimated to be about 1.5% of the body weight or about 2.5% of total body water or about 1 L in volume. For all practical purposes the volume of the total body water available for distribution of the drug in an adult male is approximately one liter less than the total body water, i.e. 42 L – 1 L = 41 L. Approximately two-thirds of the total body water is inside the cells in the intracellular fluid and the remaining one-third of total body water is outside the cells, in the extracellular fluid. The intracellular fluid actually consists of about 75 trillion tiny individual compartments, known as the cells.

Total Extracellular Fluid

All fluids outside the cells are collectively known as extracellular fluid (or extracellular water) and these fluids are constantly mixing. The extracellular fluid serves two important functions—it constitutes 'internal environment' of the body and the 'external environment' of each body cell. The volume of total extracellular fluid is about 27% of body weight and constitutes about 43% of total body water or about 17 L in volume. The most important determinant of extracellular fluid

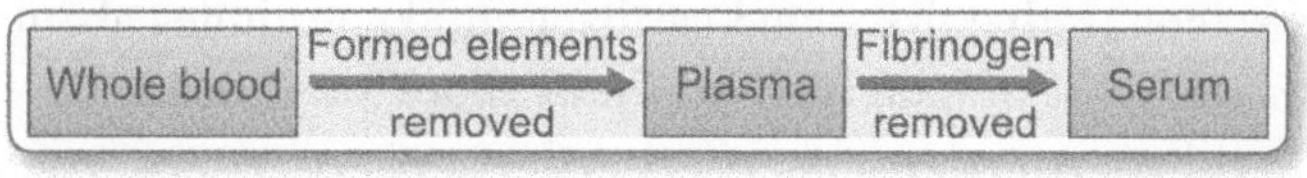

Fig. 5-2 Relationship between whole blood, plasma and serum

is the sodium content. Changes in the extracellular fluid volume are dictated by net gain or net loss of sodium, with accompanying gain or loss of water. The most common causes of depletion of extracellular fluid are associated with the loss of body fluid, e.g. diarrhea, vomiting, diuretics, renal or adrenal disease and blood loss. Similarly, conditions resulting in excessive extracellular fluid volume include edema and excessive renal sodium and water retention as in heart failure, renal failure and cirrhosis. The total extracellular fluid is divided into plasma, interstitial lymph fluid, dense connective tissue and cartilage and inaccessible bone water.

Plasma

In pharmacokinetic studies, the concentration of drug may be expressed in blood or in plasma or in serum. Therefore, it is important to understand the difference between blood, plasma and serum. Whole blood refers to the fluid portion in combination with the formed elements (red cells, white cells and platelets). Plasma refers only to the fluid portion of blood, i.e. plasma is whole blood devoid of solid matter but includes matter dissolved in the blood. Therefore, soluble proteins are included in plasma, but the formed elements are not included in plasma. Serum refers to the product remaining after removal of the soluble protein fibrinogen from the plasma. Figure 5-2 is a schematic showing the relationship between whole blood, plasma and serum.

The boundaries of plasma volume are provided by the cellular elements of blood and heart and blood vessels. Plasma is the non-cellular portion of the blood and is part of the extracellular fluid. It communicates continually with the interstitial fluid through pores in the capillaries. The plasma is about 5% of body weight and constitutes about 8% of total body water. Therefore, its volume is approximately 8% of 41 L or about 3 L. The plasma compartment is reversibly connected to the interstitial-lymph fluid compartment. This means that after the appearance of drug in plasma, the drug must go through the interstitial-lymph fluid compartment before it can appear in the inaccessible bone water or in the dense connective tissue and cartilage.

Interstitial-lymph Fluid

The interstitial-lymph fluid is in close functional and structural relationship to plasma. The interstitial-lymph fluid lies in spaces between the cells. More than 99% of this fluid is held in the gel of interstitial spaces and only a minute portion of it is free in the form of actual flowing fluid. The volume of the interstitial-lymph fluid is determined by the volume of distribution of inulin, mannitol and sucrose, which closely approximates the sum of plasma volume and interstitial lymph fluid volume. The interstitial-lymph fluid is about 12% of body weight and constitutes about 19% of total body water or about 8 L in volume. Pharmacokinetically, interstitial-lymph fluid compartment is reversibly connected to all other fluid compartments of the body. Once the drug reaches interstitial-lymph fluid compartment, it can distribute into all other fluid compartments of the body. Not that it does, only that it can.

Dense Connective Tissue and Cartilage Fluid

The dense connective tissue and cartilage water is distinguished from other body waters not only because of anatomical reasons but also because tracers either do not penetrate this fluid or penetrate it very slowly. Therefore, the volume of this water compartment is not determined directly, but is assessed indirectly.

The dense connective tissue and cartilage fluid constitutes about 5% of total body weight, i.e. approximately 8% of total body water, or about 3 L in volume.

Inaccessible Bone Water

The inaccessible bone water is the skeletal water, which is not readily accessible, hence the name inaccessible bone water. Based on the fact that bones constitute about 16% of total body weight, the total skeletal water has been estimated to be about 3.4 L for a 70 kg man. Of the 3.4 L total skeletal water; only about 10% is readily accessible, leaving the remainder 90% skeletal water (about 3 L) as inaccessible bone water. The inaccessible bone water is estimated at about 5% of total body weight, and constitutes about 8% of total body water or about 3 L in volume.

Total Intracellular Fluid

The total intracellular fluid is considered to be the difference between total body fluids and total extracellular fluids. The total intracellular fluid is about 33% (60 – 27 = 33) of body weight or about 57% (100 – 43 = 57) of total body water or about 24 L (41 L – 17 L = 24 L) in volume. The fluid of each cell contains its own individual mixture of different constituents, but its concentration is reasonably similar in all cells. For this reason the intracellular fluid of all different cells is considered to be one large fluid compartment, although in reality the total intracellular fluid is actually an aggregate of about 75 trillion minute compartments.

VOLUME OF DISTRIBUTION

Few drugs are distributed into exactly the same tissues and fluids of the body. The situation gets complicated, when one considers the fact that a variety of factors affect distribution or concentration of drugs into various tissues, organs or fluids of the body. Some important factors, which have been shown to affect distribution of drugs into various body fluids and tissue include the following:

a. Complexation or binding of drug to such body components as plasma proteins, nucleic acids, and adipose tissues.
b. Some drugs pass into cerebrospinal fluid while others do not.
c. Some drugs are secreted into bile and enter an enterohepatic cycle while others do not.
d. Some drugs enter red blood cells readily while others do not.
e. Some drugs enter and leave bones readily while many drugs do not.

These factors indicate that there are no real volumes of drug distribution that may be applicable to all drugs. The fact that some drugs appear to be distributed in a volume essentially equal to the volume of a given body fluid or tissue may be just coincidental and the conclusion that the drug is distributed only in that particular body fluid (and nowhere else) would not necessarily be accurate.

The volume of distribution, V_d or V_D, more appropriately known as the *Apparent Volume of Distribution* is defined as the volume of fluid, in which the drug appears to be distributed. The volume of distribution is not a true anatomic, physiological or physical volume and therefore, the calculated value of apparent volume of distribution does not have a true physiologic meaning. It represents a hypothetical volume of body fluid, in which the drug appears to be dissolved or distributed. The volume of distribution represents a factor that must be taken into account, when one estimates the amount of drug in the body based on concentration of drug in the sampling compartment.

When the drug is contained (or distributed) only in the vascular space of the body (e.g. blood, plasma or serum), the apparent volume of distribution, V_d, should not be less than the vascular volume (volume of blood, plasma or serum). Since the minimum volume of fluid in the body is plasma and the volume of plasma in an average adult is approximately three liters, therefore, the apparent volume of distribution in an average adult should never be less than 3L. Similarly, when the administered dose is distributed into the extravascular space and tissues, the apparent volume of distribution becomes larger, exceeding not only total body weight, but it may be in hundreds or thousands of liters.

Table 5-7 lists the approximate values of apparent volume of distribution of some drugs. The values listed in this table are approximate, and are indicated for a normal healthy individual. It should be pointed out that in some publications the values of apparent volume of distribution are indicated in terms of liters per kilogram body weight.

Determination of Volume of Distribution

The volume of distribution is determined using the relationship:

$$\text{Volume} = \frac{\text{Amount}}{\text{Concentrationn}} \tag{5-7}$$

Thus, if the amount and concentration of drug in the body at a given time is known, then the volume, in which the drug appears to be distributed can be determined. For example, if the amount of drug in the body of an individual was 70 mg and plasma concentration of drug at that time was found to be 10 μg/mL, then the apparent volume of distribution of drug in this individual can be determined using the relationship shown in equation (5-7):

$$\text{Volume} = \frac{\text{Amount}}{\text{Concentrationn}}$$

$$\text{Volume} = \frac{70 \text{ mg}}{10 \ \mu\text{g} / \text{mL}}$$

$$\text{Volume} = \frac{70{,}000 \ \mu\text{g}}{10 \ \mu\text{g} / \text{mL}} = 7{,}000 \text{ mL} = 7 \text{ L}$$

Since it is difficult to determine the amount of drug in the body at any given time, except immediately after intravenous bolus injection of the dose, this simple approach to determine the apparent volume of distribution is used only, when the drug is administered by rapid intravenous bolus injection. Thus, knowing the size of the dose (amount) and the concentration of drug in plasma immediately after administration but before the start of elimination, one can use equation (5-7) to estimate apparent volume of distribution of the drug.

To determine concentration of drug in the plasma immediately after administration of the dose, one does not take a blood sample immediately after intravenous bolus dose is administered, because one does not know exactly, when the drug distributes or diffuses completely into the plasma volume after the drug is administered by intravenous injection. It has been suggested that rapid intravenous bolus dose takes about three complete cycles or circulations through the blood stream before the administered drug dose fully diffuses into blood circulation. Thus, withdrawal of a blood sample before complete diffusion of the drug dose would yield a lower drug concentration in plasma than actually exists. Also, it is conceivable that blood sample may be drawn at exactly the same time, when the bolus dose in circulation is passing through the point of withdrawal; hence most of the administered dose (or possibly the entire drug dose) is removed from blood circulation at that time. Similarly, if the blood sample is withdrawn just before the bolus dose is about to pass through the point of withdrawal, no concentration of drug will be found in the withdrawn sample. The normal practice to determine apparent volume of distribution of a drug is as follows:

The drug dose is administered by a rapid intravenous bolus injection and blood samples are withdrawn at predetermined time intervals. The concentration of drug in each plasma sample is determined by an appropriate assay method for the drug and concentration of drug in plasma

Table 5-7 Approximate volumes of distribution (vd) of some drugs

Drug	*Vd (L)*	*Drug*	*Vd (L)*	*Drug*	*Vd (L)*
Chloroquine	6500	Glutethimide	150	Digitoxin	40
Metformine	4200	Nitrazepam	150	Erythromycin	40
Hydroxychloroquine	3600	Dapsone	130	Insulin	40
Meprotiline	3600	Oxytetracycline	135	Penicillin G	35
Desipramine	3000	Chlortetracycline	120	Amoxicillin	30
Mianserin	2800	Cimetidine	120	Hetacillin	30
Amodiaquine	2500	Coumarin	120	Lincomycin	30
Methotrimeprazine	2100	Phenacetin	110	Methotrexate	30
Haloperidol	1750	Acetylprocainamide	100	Minocycline	30
Disulfiram	1600	Doxycycline	100	Cefotaxime	25
Chlorpromazine	1500	Griseofulvin	100	Cloxacillin	25
Miconazole	1500	Hexobarbital	100	Oxacillin	25
Doxepin	1400	Lidocaine	100	Cephradine	22
Nortriptyline	1400	Lorazepam	100	Chlordiazepoxide	21
Nortriptyline	1400	Lorazepam	100	Chlordiazepoxide	21
Chloroguanide	1350	Secobarbital	100	Azidocillin	20
Ouabain	1100	Carbamazepine	85	Dicloxacillin	20
Imipramine	1000	Oxazepam	85	Hydrocortisone	20
Levodopa	1000	Oxprenolol	85	Kanamycin	20
Brompheniramine	800	Quinine	85	Methicillin	20
Penbutalol	700	Fentanyl	80	Phenylbutazone	20
Amitriptyline	600	Acetaminophen	80	Cephalexin	18
Digoxin	450	Amobarbital	80	Cephalothin	18
Propoxyphene	400	Clindamycin	80	Ceftizoxime	18
Propranolol	400	Clorazepate	75	Gentamicin	18
Verapramil	370	Dextromethorphan	75	Viomycin	17
Acetyldigoxin	300	Dexamethasone	70	Cefaclor	16
Amphetamine	300	Morphine	70	Cephaloridine	16
Amphotericin B	300	Pentobarbital	70	Acetylsalicylic acid	15
Chlorpheniramine	300	Zomiperac	70	Acetazolamide	15
Chlorthalidone	300	Dopamine	65	Chlorothiazide	15
Meperidine	300	Indomethacin	65	Furosemide	15
Metoprolol	300	Azathioprine	60	Cephacetrile	13
Pentazocine	300	Baclofen	60	Cefazoline	12
Hydralazine	270	Hydrochlorothiazide	60	Cefadroxil	11
Methadone	270	Lithium	60	Cefamanadol	11
Alprenolol	250	Sulfadiazine	60	Chlorpropamide	11
Amantadine	250	Disopyramide	55	Carbenicillin	10
Clonidine	250	Primidone	55	Cefoxitin	10
Codeine	250	Aminopyrine	50	Ceftriaxone	10
Dicyclomine	250	Meprobamate	50	Cephapirin	10
Diphenhydramine	250	Metronidazole	50	Probenecid	10
Timolol	210	Phenobarbital	50	Thyroxin	10
Zimelidine	210	Antipyrine	45	Tolbutamide	10
Acebutolol	200	Ethosuximide	45	Warfarin	10
Atropine	200	Phenytoin	45	Dicumarol	9
Methaqualone	200	Isoniazid	42	Clofibrate	8
Clonazepam	175	Ampicillin	40	Carbenoxolone	7
Diazepam	150	Chloramphenicol	40	Ibuprofen	5
Ethambutol	150	Colistin sulfate	40	Naproxen	5

as a function of time is plotted to obtain plasma profile of the drug. The concentration of drug in plasma immediately after administration of dose is determined by back-extrapolating plasma concentration vs time profile of drug to time 0 and equation (5-7) now becomes:

$$V_d = \frac{\text{Dose}}{C_0} \tag{5-8}$$

Intravenous bolus dose is preferred to determine volume of distribution because the entire drug dose is placed into systemic circulation all at once. Thus, the amount of drug in systemic circulation is known and C_0 is concentration of drug before elimination begins. In extravascular administration, the concentration of drug in plasma immediately after administration of dose is 0. Also, it is difficult to know the exact amount of drug actually absorbed into systemic circulation because an unknown portion of the administered dose may not be absorbed due to several reasons. Some of these reasons include the following.

1. Lack of complete release of drug from the dosage form.
2. Lack of complete dissolution of drug from the dosage form.
3. Inactivation or metabolism of drug at the site of administration or in the environment of absorption.
4. First-pass effect.

Example 5-4 The plasma drug concentration immediately after administration of a 30 mg intravenous bolus dose was found to be 0.732 μg/mL. Calculate the volume of distribution of the drug.

Solution

Using equation (5-8), 30 mg

$$V_d = \frac{30\ \text{mg}}{0.732\ \mu\text{g/mL}}$$

$$V_d = \frac{30{,}000\ \mu\text{g}}{0.732\ \mu\text{g/mL}} = 40{,}948\ \text{mL}$$

$$V_d \cong 41\ \text{L}$$

Significance of Volume of Distribution

The significance of volume of distribution in relation to the concentration of drug in plasma may be appreciated as follows.

Some drugs have a strong affinity for certain tissues or components in the body. When a portion of the dose is attached or bound to these tissues or components, this portion of the dose is 'taken out' of circulation, leaving a relatively smaller amount of free drug in the plasma. Since only the unbound fraction of the drug dissolves in the fluid portion of the body, only a fraction of the administered dose is now distributed in the fluid portion of the body. Therefore, the concentration of drug in the plasma is reduced and the volume of distribution of the drug exhibits a large value.

For example, suppose a 50 mg dose of a drug is given by rapid intravenous injection and this drug is 70% bound to tissues. The unbound (free) fraction of the drug distributes instantaneously in total body fluids. Since 70% of the 50 mg dose (= 35 mg) is bound, therefore, the amount of free (unbound) drug distributed in body fluids is 50 mg–35 mg = 15 mg.

Since the volume of total body fluids in an average adult is about 41 L, therefore, the concentration of drug in the body fluids immediately after administration of dose can be calculated using the following relationship:

$$\text{Concentration immediately after administration of dose} = \frac{15\text{ mg}}{41\text{ L}} = 0.366\text{ mg / L}$$

If one did not know that the drug is bound to tissues and calculated the apparent volume of distribution based on the fact that a 50 mg dose produced a concentration of drug in plasma immediately after administration was 0.366 mg/L, then the volume of distribution would be determined to be: 50 mg.

$$V_d = \frac{50\text{ mg}}{0.366\text{ mg/L}} = 136.6\text{ L}$$

A volume of 136.6 L is much larger than the volume of total body fluids. It cannot be true volume of body fluids but it shows that a portion of the drug is taken out of circulation. This volume of distribution indicates that if the dose were distributed in total body fluids it would require 136.6 L of body fluids to give a concentration of 0.366 mg/L. The value of volume of distribution (V_d) can range from a small number (equal to plasma volume, when drug is distributed only in the vascular space) to an extremely large value (in hundreds of liters, when drug is distributed into extravascular space, tissues and proteins, etc.).

Example 5-5 Following administration of a 60 mg intravenous bolus injection, plasma concentration immediately after injection was found to be 0.17 µg/mL. Calculate the volume of distribution.

Solution

From equation (5-8),

$$V_d = \frac{\text{Dose}}{C_0}$$

$$V_d = \frac{60\text{ mg}}{0.17\ \mu\text{g/mL}} \quad 0.17\ \mu\text{g/mL}$$

$$V_d = \frac{60\text{ mg}}{0.17\text{ mg/mL}} = 353\text{ L}$$

Determination of Amount of Drug in the Body

Once the apparent volume of distribution of a drug is known, it is then possible to estimate the amount of drug in the body at any given time.
Since,

$$\text{Concentration} = \frac{\text{Amount}}{\text{Volume}} \tag{5-9}$$

therefore,

$$\text{Amount} = \text{Volume} \times \text{Concentration} \tag{5-10}$$

This means that the amount of drug in the body at any time can be determined by multiplying the concentration of drug in plasma at that time with the volume of distribution of the drug.

Example 5-6 The apparent volume of distribution of a drug is 37 L. If concentration of drug in plasma at a given time is 3.2 µg/mL, calculate the amount of drug in the body at that time.

Solution

From equation (5-10),

$$\text{Amount} = (3.2\ \mu\text{g/mL}) \times (37\text{ L})$$

$$\text{Amount} = (3.2\ \mu\text{g/mL}) \times (37{,}000\text{ mL})$$

$$\text{Amount} = 118{,}400\ \mu g = 118.4\ mg$$

The amount of drug in the body at that time is 118.4 mg.

Example 5-7 A patient received a 300 mg dose of a drug by intravenous bolus injection at 6 AM. At 10 AM the concentration of drug in the body was 1.5 μg/mL. If the apparent volume of distribution of this drug is 140 L, calculate the amount of drug in the body at 10 AM.

Solution

Since the concentration of drug in the body at 10 AM is known, the amount of drug in the body at 10 AM can be determined using equation (5-10):

$$\text{Amount} = (\text{Volume}) \times (\text{Concentration})$$

$$\text{Amount} = (1.5\ \mu g/mL) \times (140\ L)$$

$$\text{Amount} = (1.5\ \mu g/mL) \times (140{,}000\ mL)$$

$$\text{Amount} = 210{,}000\ \mu g = 210\ mg$$

BODY COMPOSITION

The dose of a given drug may be expressed in various ways. For some drugs, the recommended dose is based on a certain amount (e.g. 25 mg), while the dose of some drugs is based on the body weight of the individual. For example, the manufacturer of Zovirax® (PDR 2002, p. 1710) suggests that for the treatment of herpes infections, a maximum dose equivalent to 20 mg/kg body weight every 8 hours should not be exceeded for any patient. Similarly, the suggested dose of Nebsin® (PDR 2002, p. 1957) for adults with serious infections and normal renal function is 3 mg/kg/day in 3 equal doses. Therefore, although two individuals having the same body weight will receive the same amount of drug, it is conceivable that they may not necessarily exhibit similar concentration of free-drug in the plasma.

The average adult male is considered to weigh about 70 kg and it is generally believed that a person weighing more than 70 kg is overweight. This may not be true, because tall individuals may weigh more than 70 kg and yet may not be considered overweight. Similarly, short people may weigh 70 kg and may be considered overweight.

For the sake of simplicity, individuals are grouped into three categories:

1. An adult individual with average weight is termed normal
2. A person who weighs less than an average adult is termed lean
3. A person who weighs more than an average adult is labeled as an obese adult.

The criteria used to identify individuals based on their weight have changed in the past few years, because the ideal weight corresponding to height has undergone a significant change.

In the past, the terms lean, normal and obese were essentially based on the weight of the individual. Afterwards the terms lean, normal and obese were based on the weight corresponding to the height of the individual. Later, the ideal weight corresponding to the height of males and females were identified to be different. Some believe that this criterion is more arbitrary than it is scientific, because the body of an individual may be a normal frame, a small frame (petite) or a large frame (tall and/or big-boned). Not only this, the normal, petite and large frames in both males and females are different in terms of height and weight. Table 5-8 shows the desired weight of individuals based on the height and type of frame of the individual.

From a pharmacokinetic standpoint and for the purposes of distribution of drugs in the human body, the pharmacokinetist considers the human body as consisting of three major constituents. These are—water, fat and fat-free solids.

Table 5-8 Desired weight based on height and body frame of males and females

MALES					FEMALES				
Height		Frame			Height		Frame		
feet	inch	Small	Medium	Large	feet	inch	Small	Medium	Large
5	2	128–134	131–141	138–150	4	10	102–111	109–121	118–131
5	3	130–136	133–143	140–153	4	11	103–113	111–123	120–134
5	4	132–138	135–145	142–156	5	0	104–115	113–126	122–137
5	5	134–140	137–148	144–160	5	1	106–118	115–129	125–140
5	6	136–142	139–151	146–164	5	2	108–121	118–132	128–143
5	7	138–145	142–154	149–168	5	3	111–124	121–135	131–147
5	8	140–148	145–157	152–172	5	4	114–127	124–138	134–151
5	9	142–151	148–160	155–176	5	5	117–130	127–141	137–155
5	10	144–154	151–163	158–180	5	6	120–133	130–144	140–159
5	11	146–157	154–166	161–184	5	7	123–136	133–147	143–163
6	0	149–160	157–170	164–188	5	8	126–139	136–150	146–167
6	1	152–164	160–174	168–192	5	9	129–142	139–153	149–170
6	2	155–168	164–178	172–197	5	10	132–145	142–156	152–173
6	3	158–172	167–182	176–202	5	11	135–148	145–159	155–176
6	4	162–176	181–187	181–207	6	0	138–151	148–162	158–179

Water

The term 'water' used in the composition of human body is intended to include all aqueous fluids in the human body. Therefore, the term water includes such fluids as plasma water, extracellular fluid, intracellular fluid, etc.

Fat

The term 'fat' used in the composition of human body essentially signifies the fatty tissue or the adipose tissue.

Fat-free Solids

The term 'fat-free solids' used in describing the composition of human body, as the name implies, includes all solids, which do not contain fat. Examples of fat-free solids are proteins and such extracellular solids as collagen, elastin and bone matrix.

The relative proportion of water, fat and fat-free solids in the human body varies not only with the weight of the individual (lean person, normal person or obese person), it also depends on the structure (type of body frame, e.g. small, medium or large) of the individual. Also, the relative proportion of water, fat and fat-free solids is different in females and in males. The composition of these three constituents in young adult males and females is shown in Table 5-9. This composition changes with age because the total body water decreases with age. For example, in the geriatric period, the average body water decreases from 60% to 55% in normal males and from 50% to 45% in normal females. There is an approximately proportional decrease in total body water in lean and obese males as well as in females.

Table 5-9 Body composition of males and females

Constituent	*Lean*	*Normal*	*Obese*
Males			
Fat	4%	18%	32%
Water	70%	60%	50%
Fat-free solids	26%	22%	18%
Females			
Fat	18%	32%	42%
Water	60%	50%	42%
Fat-free solids	22%	18%	16%

The practical implication of variation in fat and protein in obese, normal and lean individuals is that drugs, which have an affinity for fat (or protein) will exhibit smaller plasma concentration in those individuals, who have a larger mass of fat (or protein) than in individuals, who have a smaller mass of fat (or protein).

Those drugs, which are distributed in the body fluids and have an affinity for the adipose tissue have a tendency to accumulate in this tissue, thus exhibiting less plasma concentration than those drugs, which do not accumulate in the fatty tissue and are distributed in the body fluids. The plasma profile of these drugs shows a rapid initial decline in plasma concentration because of removal of drug from the plasma due to two processes

1. Equilibration of drug between the plasma and fatty tissue
2. Elimination of drug through the kidneys.

Since an obese individual has a larger proportion of adipose tissue than a leaner individual, it follows that a larger amount of the drug is bound to fatty tissue of an obese person than in a lean person. The same is true for protein-binding of drugs. Depending on the amount of protein in the body, larger amount of drug is bound if the protein mass is high.

Pediatric Definitions

Pediatric patients (premature through adolescents) exhibit age-related differences in their physiology. For example, the kidneys in a new-born are not fully developed. Therefore, pediatric patients require unique considerations because age-related differences in physiology of pediatric patients alter pharmacokinetics of many drugs. In infants, particularly neonates, there are differences in the absorption, distribution, metabolism and excretion of drugs. These differences affect the plasma concentration of an administered drug dose. Therefore, care and caution must be exercised in the dosing of drugs in these patients. Table 5-10 defines the terminology for different pediatric age groups from birth through adolescent years.

Table 5-10 Pediatric definitions

Category	*Age*
Premature	Fewer than 38 weeks gestation
Neonate	Birth to 1 month
Newborn	Birth to 1 month
Baby	1 – 24 months
Infant	1 – 24 months
Young child	2 – 5 years
Older child	6 – 12 years
Adolescent	13 – 18 years

**Courtesy:* Text book of Therapeutics: Drugs and Disease Management, Chapter 96, Hartfield and Gourley eds, 7th ed., Lippincot Williams & Wilkins, 2000

Table 5-11 Pediatric weights

Age	*Average weight*	
	lb	*kg*
Birth	7.3	3.3
6 months	17.0	7.7
1 year	21.6	9.8
15 months	23.0	10.5
2 years	27.0	12.3
3 years	32.0	14.5
4 years	36.4	16.5
5 years	41.0	18.6
6 years	46.0	20.9
7 years	52.0	23.6
8 years	57.2	26.0
9 years	62.0	28.2
10 years	68.0	30.9

Pediatric Weights

Since most pharmacokinetic parameters are based on age and weight of the patient, it is helpful to define the average weight of pediatric patients. Table 5-11 lists average weight of pediatric patients from birth through adolescent years.

SUGGESTED READING

1. Delgado JN, Rermers W (eds). "Wilson and Gisvold's Textbook of Organic Medicinal and Pharmaceutical Chemistry, 9th edition. Lippincott; 1990.
2. Goodman and Gilman's Pharmacological Basis of Therapeutics, 9th edition. Macmillan; 1995.
3. Marieb E. In: Human Anatomy and Physiology, 2nd edition. Benjamin/Cummings Publishing Company; 1991.
4. Pratt W, Taylor P. In; Principles of Drug Action: The Basis of Pharmacology. 3rd edition. Churchill Livingstone; 1990.
5. Remington: The Science and Practice of Pharmacy, 21st edition. Mack Publishing; 2005.
6. Tortora GJ. Principles of Anatomy and Physiology, 7th edition. Harper Collins; 1993.
7. Wagner JA, Biopharmaceutics and Relevant Pharmacokinetics. Drug Intelligence Publications; 1971.

PRACTICE PROBLEMS

5-1. The apparent volume of distribution of a drug is 27 L. If concentration of drug in plasma at a given time is 3.2 μg/mL, calculate the amount of drug in the body at that time.

5-2. Plasma drug concentration immediately after administration of a 30 mg intravenous bolus dose was found to be 0.32 μg/mL. Calculate apparent volume of distribution of the drug.

5-3. The apparent volume of distribution of a drug is reported to be 2 L/kg body weight and it is desired that concentration of drug immediately after intravenous bolus injection should be 2 mg/L. If the patient weighs 75 kg, calculate the size of dose that should be administered.

5-4. A 200 mg dose of a drug was given by rapid intravenous injection and this drug is known to bind to plasma proteins. If the drug distributes instantaneously in total body fluids and the drug is 40% bound to proteins, calculate the concentration of unbound drug in plasma after administration of the dose.

5-5. Following administration of a 250 mg intravenous bolus dose of a drug, the plasma concentration of drug immediately after injection was found to be 17 μg/mL. Calculate the apparent volume of distribution.

5-6. A patient received a 300 mg dose of an antibiotic by intravenous bolus injection at 6 AM. At 10 AM the concentration of drug in the body was 2.4 μg/mL. If the apparent volume of distribution of this drug is known to be 37 L, calculate the amount of drug in the body at 10 AM

5-7. A 75 kg male patient was given a 60 mg dose of a drug by intravenous bolus injection at 9 AM. At 3 PM the concentration of drug in plasma was found to be 0.28 μg/mL. If the apparent volume of distribution of this drug is known to be 0.22 L/kg, calculate the amount of drug in the body at 3 PM

5-8. The minimum effective concentration of diazepam has been reported to be 300 ng/mL. If the apparent volume of distribution of diazepam in a patient is 90 L, calculate the size of dose that must be given to produce a plasma concentration of 300 ng/mL.

5-9. The apparent volume of distribution of phenobarbital in a patient was found to be 40 L. If a 30 mg dose is given by rapid intravenous bolus injection, calculate the concentration of drug in plasma immediately after administration of the injection.

5-10. A patient received a 500 mg dose of an antibiotic by intravenous bolus injection at 6 AM. At 10 AM the concentration of drug in the body was 2.4 μg/mL. If the apparent volume of distribution of this drug is known to be 37 L, calculate the concentration of drug in the body at 6 AM.

5-11. The apparent volume of distribution of a drug is known to be 2 liters per kilogram of body weight. If a single 30 mg dose is given by rapid intravenous bolus injection to a 65 year old male weighing 165 lbs, calculate the concentration of drug in plasma immediately after administration of the dose.

5-12. The value of α for a drug is 0.1 and the total drug concentration is 10 mg/L. Calculate the concentration of unbound drug

5-13. The value of α for a drug is 0.1 and the total drug concentration is 5 mg/L. What will be the percent increase in the concentration of unbound drug if the value of α becomes 0.25?

CHAPTER 6

DRUG ELIMINATION

The elimination of drugs from systemic circulation can take place through a variety of pathways. For example, the unchanged drug and/or its biotransformed product may be removed into urine via the kidneys and some volatile drugs may be eliminated through the lungs. In pharmacokinetics, two terms have been used interchangeably to indicate the loss of drug from the body. These two terms are:

i. Elimination
ii. Excretion.

The term elimination is usually used to indicate removal (or loss) of drug from the body through kidneys and the term excretion is generally used to mean drug removal from body by all processes including elimination. That is, excretion is the final means of drug elimination, either as a metabolite or as the unchanged parent drug. The definition of these two terms according to the Bantam Medical Dictionary is as follows:

> *Elimination: The term elimination (noun, physiology) indicates the entire process of excretion of metabolic waste products from blood by the kidneys.*
> *Excretion: The term excretion (also a noun) is a generic term and refers to the removal.*

Excretion also includes loss of water, salts and some urea through sweat glands and carbon dioxide and water vapor through the lungs. The term excretion is also used to include the egestion of feces. From a pharmacokinetic standpoint, excretion of drugs is the final elimination (or loss) from the body and many researchers in the field use the terms elimination and excretion interchangeably. Drugs may be eliminated from systemic circulation by different pathways and then excreted through one or more of the excretory processes, e.g. via urine, bile, intestines, saliva, lungs, skin, mother's milk and perspiration.

ELIMINATION OF DRUG

The rate of drug elimination is a critical determinant of rate of change of concentration of drug in the body. This is because the determination of dosage regimen, i.e. the size of dose and the frequency of drug administration required to attain optimal therapeutic activity of a drug is dependent on biological half-life of the drug, which depends on the rate of elimination of drug from the body, which in turn is a function of rate constant for the elimination of the drug. Failure to take into consideration, the concept of biological half-life or the factors which may influence the biological half-life of a drug can lead to under-medication of drug or dangerous drug accumulation in the body.

Drugs are eliminated either in the unchanged form or as metabolites. Excretory organs, (excluding lungs), eliminate polar compounds more efficiently than they do highly lipid-soluble compounds. Lipid-soluble drugs are therefore not readily eliminated until they are transformed into a more polar compound (metabolite). Elimination of a drug can occur either through an excretion mechanism (e.g. renal elimination via kidneys or biliary excretion through bile) or via biotransformation as metabolites. The metabolites of a drug are generally considered inactive compounds as far as therapeutic effect is concerned, but not all metabolites of all drugs are necessarily inactive in nature. For example, morphine, a drug used in a variety of conditions, is also a metabolite of codeine. Although codeine is not used as a substitute for morphine *per se*, administration of codeine will result in the production of morphine in the body. Another example of a drug which forms pharmacologically active metabolite is acetaminophen. Acetaminophen is a metabolite of phenacetin, but acetaminophen is used more extensively than phenacetin itself.

Other examples of drugs which form pharmacologically active metabolites are: salicylic acid is a metabolite of acetylsalicylic acid, nortriptyline is a metabolite of amitriptyline, digoxin is a metabolite of digitoxin, methylepinephrine and methyl norepinephrine are metabolites of methyldopa, amphetamine is a metabolite of methamphetamine, phenobarbital is a metabolite of primidone, caffeine is a metabolite of theophylline and benzodiazepam forms various active metabolites.

Table 6-1 is a partial listing of examples of some drugs and their pharmacologically active metabolites.

The metabolites of some drugs either possess less therapeutic activity than the parent molecule or are inactive compounds, while metabolites of other drugs possess more potent therapeutic activity or toxic properties, which may be equal to or even greater than the activity of the drug itself. These drugs have come to be known as prodrugs, because therapeutic agent in these instances is the metabolite rather than the drug itself. In the case of some drugs, however, the metabolite may not exhibit therapeutic activity as strong as being equal to that of the parent compound, but the metabolite may possess less side-effects than the drug itself. In such cases, it may be desirable to use the metabolite rather than the parent compound as the therapeutic agent (drug).

ROUTES OF DRUG EXCRETION

Drugs can be excreted from the body through many pathways of excretion. These routes, not necessarily in any particular order, include the following: kidneys, lungs, saliva, perspiration (sweat), bile, intestines, hair and skin and milk. However, kidney is the main route for excretion of most drugs from the body, whether as the unchanged (unmetabolized) drug or biotransformed in the form of a metabolite. Some drugs undergo excretion predominantly by routes other than the renal route. Substances excreted in the feces are either mainly unabsorbed orally ingested drugs or metabolites excreted into the bile and not reabsorbed from the intestinal tract. Excretion of drugs in the breast milk is important, not because of the amounts eliminated, but because the excreted drugs are potential sources of unwanted pharmacological effects in the nursing infant. Pulmonary excretion is important mainly for the elimination of anesthetic gases vapors and volatile drugs.

Excretion through Lungs

The removal of drugs through the lungs is called pulmonary elimination. Excretion through the lung is not considered a common route of excretion for most drugs because excretion through lungs involve removal of drug in a vapor state, e.g. pulmonary elimination of anesthetic gases. The odor of alcohol in the breath has been used to detect the presence of alcohol in people, who had ingested alcohol within the last few hours. This test is now used to quantitatively

Table 6-1 Examples of some drugs with pharmacologically active metabolites

Parent drug	*Active metabolite(s)*
Acetaminophen	N-Acetyl-imidoquinone
Acetohexamide	Hydroxyhexamide
Acetylsalicylic acid	Salicylic acid
Allopurinol	Alloxanthine
Aldophosphoramide	Phosphoramide mustard
Amitriptyline	Nortriptyline
Benzodiazepine	Various
Chloral Hydrate	Trichloroethanol
Chloramphenicol	Glycolic acid metabolite
Chlordiazepoxide	Desmethylchlordiazepoxide, Demoxepam
Codeine	Morphine
Cortisone	Cortisol
Dacarbazine	5-Aminoamidazole-4-carboxamide
Dipivefrin	Epinephrine
Diazepam	Desmethyldiazepam, oxazepam
Digitoxin	Digoxin
Digoxin	4-OH-Glutethimide
Enalapril	Enalaprilat
Flurazepam	Desalkylflurazepam
Fluorouracil	Fluorodeoxyuridine phosphate
Glutethimide	4-Hydroxyglutethimide
Imipramine	Desipramine
Lidocaine	Glycinexylidide
Meperidine	Normeperidine
Mephobarbital	Phenobarbital
Methyldopa	Methylepinephrine, methylnorepinephrine
Methamphetamine	Amphetamine
Phenacetin	Acetaminophen
Phenylbutazone	Oxyphenbutazone
Prazepam	Oxazepam
Prednisone	Prednisolone
Primidone	Phenobarbital
Procainamide	N-Acetylprocainamide
Propoxyphene	Norpropoxyphene
Propranolol	4-Hydroxypropanolol
Quinidine	3-Hydroxyquinidine
Spironolactone	Canrenone,Cancrenoate
Sulfasalazine	Sulfapyridine
Tamoxiphen	4-Hydroxytamoxiphen
Theophylline	Caffeine
Trimethadione	Dimethadione
Verapamil	Norverapamil

estimate concentration of alcohol in the blood of an individual suspected of ingesting alcohol. This indicates that the lungs not only excrete volatile substances; the concentration of a volatile compound excreted through the lungs may also be correlated with the concentration of volatile compound in the plasma.

Since volatile substances appear in the lungs in large enough concentration to be excreted, therefore, lungs may be considered a major pathway of excretion of volatile substances. Examples of compounds excreted through lungs include ammonium chloride, camphor, chloroform, ethanol, iodides and sodium carbonate.

Excretion through the lungs usually follows passive diffusion, i.e. only the non-ionized form of the drug is excreted.

Excretion through Perspiration

Perspiration is also not a common route of drug excretion, although some substances are excreted through perspiration. For example, excretion of low-molecular weight, water-soluble electrolytes (e.g. sodium chloride) through perspiration has been known for a long time. Excretion of non-electrolytes (such as garlic), through perspiration on hot summer days is also common knowledge. For most drugs, however, the concentration of drug excreted through perspiration is much smaller than the concentration excreted through the kidneys or feces. However, there is one exception. The anti-leprosy drug, ditophal, is largely excreted through perspiration. Its concentration in sweat equals to or exceeds its concentration in urine and feces.

Except for highly water-soluble add/or low-molecular weight electrolytes, excretion through perspiration follows passive diffusion. Therefore, the extent of dissociation (degree of ionization) of the drug and the partition coefficient of the drug play a major role in its excretion through perspiration. Hence, most weak organic acids and weak organic bases are excreted through perspiration to some degree. Some examples of drugs excreted through perspiration include p-aminohippuric acid (PAH), sulfonamides thiamine and urea.

Biliary Excretion

Bile is an important pathway of drug excretion. Drugs that are mainly excreted in the bile usually require a molecular weight greater than about 300 and a strong polar group. Drugs with molecular weights less than about 300 are almost exclusively excreted via the kidneys and those having molecular weights between about 300 and about 500 are excreted both in the urine as well as in the bile. Drugs with molecular weights exceeding 500 are relatively too large for the kidney to handle and therefore, cannot be excreted by the kidneys. These drugs are mainly excreted in the bile.

Passive diffusion, active transport and pinocytosis are the three major pathways of biliary excretion of drugs.

Examples of drugs excreted through the bile include bile salts, cholesterol, chloramphenicol, diazepam, digitalis glycosides, doxycycline, estradiol, quinine, indomethacin, penicillin, steroids, streptomycin, strychnine and tetracycline.

Drugs and chemicals excreted into the bile enter the intestine and are subsequently either reabsorbed into the blood or eliminated in the feces. Therefore, removal of drugs through the bile is significant only when reabsorption of drug from the gastrointestinal tract is minimal.

Many drugs that are excreted into the bile are excreted as metabolites, mostly as glucuronide conjugates of the parent compound. Since the glucuronide compounds are highly polar in nature, conjugation of the parent compound with the glucuronide makes the metabolites more polar than the parent drug. Also, formation of the glucuronide increases the molecular weight of the parent compound by nearly 200 or so, hence its excretion through bile is favored. The glucuronide conjugates can be hydrolyzed by the intestinal bacteria resulting in reformation of the parent drug or the metabolite and can be readily absorbed into blood. This process of drug excretion into the bile and subsequent reabsorption into intestine is known as enterohepatic circulation.

Some examples of drugs, which have been reported to undergo enterohepatic circulation are listed in Table 6-2.

Table 6-2 Examples of drugs which undergo enterohepatic circulation

Chloral hydrate	*Non-steroidal anti-inflammatory agents*
Colchicine	Phencyclidine
Digitalis preparations	Phenothiazines
Glutethimide	Phenytoin
Isoniazid	Salicylates
Methaqualone	Tricyclic antidepressants

Salivary Excretion

Although the saliva has never been considered as a route of excretion of drugs, the salivary excretion of drugs has been well known for a long time. For example, although unpleasant tasting drugs are traditionally administered orally either as a palatable elixir or as a coated solid dosage form, yet the patient is able to detect the unpleasant taste of drug in the mouth long after the dose had been administered. Such feeling and/or the taste of the administered dose has been reported even, when the drug was administered by the intravenous route or by the rectal route or by routes other than the gastrointestinal route. The presence of the taste of drug in the mouth even when the drug is not administered by mouth is attributed to the excretion of drug in the saliva. If the extent of excretion of drug in the saliva is negligible and/or the drug does not possess markedly unpleasant taste, then one does not suspect the presence of drug in the saliva, even though the drug may be excreted in the saliva. However, if the drug has a very unpleasant taste and/or the drug is excreted in saliva to a relatively large extent, then the presence of drug in the saliva can be felt and it cannot be ignored.

Excretion of drugs through the saliva appears to follow the passive diffusion as well as active transport. The pH of saliva ranges between 5.5 and 7.8 and therefore a large number of drugs can undergo passive diffusion. Drugs excreted in the saliva enter the mouth where they are usually swallowed. In some cases, e.g. bitter dugs, the patient may have a tendency to spit the drug out of the mouth and thus the drug is removed (excreted) from the body. However, if the drug is not bitter and/or the patient swallows his/her saliva, then the fate of drug in the saliva is the same as that of the drugs administered orally.

Although in most cases the concentration of drug in the saliva is less than its concentration in the plasma, the concentration of some drugs in the saliva parallels the concentration of drug in the plasma. In some cases, however, the saliva concentration is many times greater than the concentration of drug in the plasma. A good correlation between the concentration of drug in saliva and the concentration of drug in the plasma has been reported for some drugs. At least in these cases, the saliva may be used as a useful biological fluid for the determination of drug concentration, when it is either difficult or inconvenient to obtain concentration of drug in the plasma.

Table 6-3 lists examples of some commonly used drugs which are excreted in the saliva. This tabulation also lists their relative saliva: plasma drug concentration.

Fecal Excretion

Fecal excretion is excretion of drugs through the intestines. The major pathways of fecal excretion are passive diffusion and unrecycled biliary secretion.

When a drug appears in feces after oral administration, it is difficult to conclude whether the presence of drug in the feces is due to incomplete absorption of the drug or it is due to the biliary excretion of the drug. The presence of drug in the bile due to biliary excretion can be estimated in experimental studies involving animals. In these studies, cannulation of the bile

Table 6-3 Salivary excretion of drugs

Drug	S/P Ratio*	Drug	S/P Ratio*
Ratio >1		Ratio = 0.5–0.1	
Propranolol	12.0	Phenobarbital	0.32
Methylprednisolone	5.2	Sulfamerazine	0.32
Metoprolol	2.9	Sulfadiazine	0.31
Lithium	2.85	Carbamazepine	0.26
Amphetamine	2.76	Chloramphenicol	0.25
Lidocaine	1.78	Sulfathiazole	0.23
Acetaminophen	1.4	Erythromycin	0.21
Trimethoprim	1.26	Streptomycin	0.15
Ethosuximide	1.04	Nortriptyline	0.14
Isoniazid	1.02	Phenytoin	0.11
Ratio = 1.0–0.5		Ratio <0.1	
Primidone	0.97	Lincomycin	0.086
Sulfacetamide	0.92	Sulfamethoxazole	0.074
Sulfanilamide	0.87	Valproic acid	0.06
Sulfapyridine	0.81	Nitrazepam	0.057
Theophylline	0.75	Methotrexate	0.042
Sulfadimidine	0.72	Salicylate	0.033
Digoxin	0.66	Diazepam	0.029
Phenacetin	0.60	Penicillin	0.015
Caffeine	0.55	Tolbutamide	0.012
Quinidine	0.51	Acetazolamide	0.009
Pentobarbital	0.42	Estriol	0.009

*S/P ratio = Salivary/Plasma ratio

duct provides a means of estimating the amount of drug excreted through the bile. However, in human studies, an approximate estimation of biliary excretion may be made from recovery of drug through the feces after parenteral administration of the drug. Studies have shown that ionized organic acids are excreted through intestinal excretion.

Excretion via Milk

A large number of drugs are excreted through mother's milk. Box 6-1 is a partial listing of examples of some commonly used drugs, which are excreted in the milk of nursing mothers.

Although excretion of many drugs through the milk of nursing mothers has been known to the medical profession for a long time, its implication and the possible effects of excretion of a drug through the mother's milk on the nursing child has gained public awareness only in recent years. Also, the awareness of excretion of drugs through mother's milk and its effect on the growing fetus has been publicized only recently.

Excretion of drugs through the milk follows both passive diffusion as well as active transport. This means that the ionized species of the drug can be excreted by active transport and the unionized form of drug is excreted by passive diffusion. The pH of human milk is about 6.6 and the pH of the plasma is 7.4. Because the pH of human milk is more acidic than the pH of plasma, therefore, weak bases will have a tendency to be more ionized in the acidic environment of milk than they would in the more basic environment of the plasma. Due to increased ionization of basic drugs in the milk, the concentration of basic drugs, therefore, may be higher in mother's milk than in mother's plasma. The situation will be reversed for the acidic drugs, meaning that

Box 6-1 Examples of drugs appearing in the milk of lactating mothers

Allergens	Ethanol	Pentobarbital
Ampicillin	Ether	Phenobarbital
Anticoagulants	Folic acid	Phenylbutazone
Antihistaminics	Heroin	Potassium chloride
Aspirin	Hexachlorobenzene	Primidone
Atropine	Hydrochlorothiazide	Propoxyphene
Bishydroxycoumarin	Imipramine	Propylthiouracil
Bromides	Isoniazid	Pyrilamine maleate
Caffeine	Kanamycin	Pyrimethamine
Calomel	Lincomycin	Quinine sulfate
Carbamazepine	Lithium carbonate	Reserpine
Cascara	Meperidine	Rifampin
Chloral hydrate	Mephenesinic acid	Salicylic acid
Chloramphenicol	Mercury	Scopolamine
Chloroform	Methadone	Sex hormones
Chlorpromazine	Methotrexate	Sodium chloride
Chlorthalidone	Methotrimeprazine	Sodium iodide
Colistin sulfate	Metronidazole	Sodium salicylate
Corticosteroids	Morphine	Streptomycin sulfate
Cycloserine	Nalidixic acid	Sulfonamides
Diazepam	Nicotine	Tetracyclines
Dioxin	Nitrofurantoin	Theophylline
Diphenylhydantoin	Novobiocin	Thiouracil
Ergot alkaloids	Oral contraceptives	Thyroxine
Erythromycin	Penicillin	Tolbutamide

acidic drugs will tend to be more ionized in the plasma than in the milk. The implication of the difference in the pH of mother's milk and the pH of mother's plasma is that nursing mothers will tend to excrete basic drugs in the milk more than they would excrete acidic drugs in the milk.

Thus, following ingestion of a drug dose by the mother, the nursing child may receive higher doses of basic drugs (from the mother's milk) than acidic drugs. It should be mentioned, however, that for those drugs which exhibit their pharmacologic activity at low doses, ingestion of even small amounts of these drugs may cause possible toxicity in the newborn.

As a rule, nursing mothers should avoid all drugs and mothers, who must take such drugs as chloramphenicol, lithium, sulfonamides, anticancer and antithyroid drugs should preferably not nurse at all. Also, special care must be exercised, when drugs with an extremely low therapeutic index are used. Some examples of drugs which have a relatively very low therapeutic index include kanamycin, gentamicin and streptomycin. Similarly, excretion of tetracyclines into the mother's milk may lead to the deposition of tetracycline in the bones and teeth of the newborn. Special attention should also be given to drugs that bind to proteins. Newborns have less concentration of albumin and cannot metabolize bilirubin. Therefore, those drugs which have an affinity for proteins may displace bilirubin from its protein binding sites, thus causing hyperbilirubinemia in the newborn. A very common example of a drug that has an affinity for protein is sulfonamides.

Box 6-2 Drugs principally eliminated through the kidneys

Acetazolamide	Furosemide
Acetohexamide	Gentamicin
Aminoglycosides	Hetacillin
Amoxicilin	Hydrochlorothiazide
Amphetamine	Isoniazid
Amphotrecin B	Kanamycin
Ampicillin	Lithium
Carbenicillin	Methamine salts
Cefaclor	Methotrexate
Cefadroxil	Nitrofurantoin
Cefazoline	Oxytetracycline
Cephalexin	Penicillin G
Cephaloridine	Phenobarbital
Cephalothin	Phenytoin
Chloramphenicol	Procainamide
Chlorpropamide	Pseudoephedrine
Chlorothiazide	Sulfamethizole
Cimetidine	Tobramycin
Dexamethasone	Vancomycin
Dexamethasone	Viomycin
Digoxin	Warfarin
Ethambutol	

RENAL EXCRETION

Renal excretion (excretion of drugs through the kidneys) plays a major role in the elimination of most drugs, especially those that are water soluble and/or undergo biotransformation relatively slowly. Some examples of drugs that are principally eliminated through the kidneys are listed in Box 6-2.

As a rule, polar, highly ionized water-soluble compounds are excreted relatively unchanged by the kidney. Penicillins and aminoglycosides are common examples of polar compounds that are excreted relatively unchanged through the kidney. Also, many antibiotics are eliminated significantly unaltered by the kidney and therefore, renal excretion becomes the major pathway of elimination of these antibiotics. It is for this reason that kidney function is an important factor that must be given due consideration in pharmacokinetic evaluation of a drug.

Kidney Function

Kidney function is an important factor in the pharmacokinetic evaluation of drugs, because renal excretion of drugs (whether eliminated unchanged or eliminated as a metabolite) is highly dependant on the kidney function. Kidney function is also important because acute renal failure in a patient presents with a sudden decline in the ability of the kidney to maintain homeostasis. This sudden failure results in the failure of kidney to clear metabolic waste, as well as failure of kidney to correct electrolyte, acid-base and volume disturbances. Although a variety of tests can be used to measure kidney function, the following two tests are most commonly used to evaluate kidney function:

i. Excretion ratio (ER)
ii. Effective renal plasma flow (ERPF).

Excretion Ratio (ER)

Excretion ratio describes the fractional decrease in concentration of drug in the plasma due to removal of the drug by the kidney. Thus, the difference between the arterial concentration and renal concentration of a drug as a function of the arterial concentration of the drug can be used as an indicator of ER. Since drugs are excreted by filtration as well as by secretion, one can use those compounds, which are filtered as well as secreted by the tubular cells to measure excretion ratio.

Excretion ratio is defined as follows:

$$\text{ER} = \frac{\text{Arterial concentration} - \text{Renal concentration}}{\text{Arterial concentration}} \tag{6-1}$$

Since ER is a ratio, it has no units. Also, because ER is a fraction, its value may range from a lowest value of 0 to a highest value of 1. When the value of ER is zero, it means that the renal concentration of drug is equal to the arterial concentration of drug (indicating that no drug is excreted through the kidneys). When the value of the numerator is equal to the value of the denominator, the excretion ratio is then equal to 1. This can only happen when renal concentration of the drug is zero (indicating that 100% of the drug is excreted through the kidneys). For example, an excretion ratio of 0.35 indicates the renal concentration of the drug is 65 that of the arterial concentration, meaning that 35 of the arterial drug concentration is excreted renally as the drug passes

$$0.35 = \frac{\text{Arterial concentration} - \text{Renal concentration}}{\text{Arterial concentration}}$$

$$\text{Renal concentration} = \text{Arterial concentration} - (0.35)\text{Arterial concentration}$$

$$\text{Renal concentration} = (0.65)\text{Arterial concentration}$$

Effective Renal Plasma Flow (EPRF)

Effective renal plasma flow is also known as clearance. ERPF is calculated using the following relationship:

$$\text{ERPF} = \frac{(\text{Concentration of drug in urine}) \times (\text{Volume of urine/unit time})}{(\text{Concentration of drug in plasma})} \tag{6-2}$$

Since, the term (concentration of drug in urine) × (volume of urine) in the numerator is equal to the amount of drug in urine, equation (6-2) may be written as:

$$\text{ERPF} = \frac{(\text{Amount of drug in urine/unit time})}{(\text{Concentration of drug in plasma})} \tag{6-3}$$

Therefore, ERPF is a measure of amount of drug excreted in urine as a function of concentration of drug in the plasma, i.e. clearance of the drug. The clearance of p-aminohippuric acid (PAH) is estimated at 625 mL/min and is a measure of renal plasma flow. Excretion ratio and ERPF serve two important functions in pharmacokinetic studies. They can be used to determine the rate of excretion of drug and clearance by the kidneys and monitor the changes in kidney function.

Mechanisms of Renal Excretion

There are two mechanisms by which a drug is passed from the blood into glomerular filtrate:

i. Filtration through glomeruli (glomerular filtration)
ii. Active secretion into kidney tubule (tubular secretion).

A third process, which has significant influence on overall drug removal is reabsorption. Drugs may pass from glomerular filtrate into blood by active and passive reabsorption (tubular reabsorption). The net effect of these processes is that a constant fraction of drug present in renal arterial blood is removed and appears in urine.

GLOMERULAR FILTRATION

The kidneys represent about 0.5% of the total body weight and receive a large blood supply via the renal artery. The blood supply received by the kidneys is approximately 20% to 25% of the cardiac output. It is not surprising that the kidneys have a very rich blood supply since they continuously cleanse the blood and adjust its composition. Each kidney contains over 1 million tiny blood-processing units called nephrons, which carry out the processes that form urine. Each nephron consists of a glomerulus, a tuft of capillaries, associated with a renal tubule. The end of the renal tubule is called the glomerular capsule. The glomerular capsule is blind, enlarged and cup-shaped and completely surrounds the glomerulus. The glomerular endothelium is penetrated by many small pores, which makes these capillaries exceptionally porous. They allow large amounts of solute-rich fluid to pass from the blood into the glomerular capsule. This plasma-derived fluid is called the filtrate and it is the raw material that is processed by the renal tubules to form the urine.

Glomerular Filtration Rate: Under resting conditions, blood is constantly circulated through the kidneys at the rate of about 1700 L/day. The rate of plasma flow through the kidneys is about 850 L to 1,000 L per day and about 20 percent of this volume is filtered. Therefore, the amount of fluid filtered from the blood into the glomerular capsule each minute is:

$$\text{GFR} = 20\% \text{ of } (850 \text{ L/day to } 1000 \text{ L/day})$$

$$\text{GFR} = 170 \text{ to } 200 \text{ L/day}$$

$$\text{GFR} = 7 \text{ to } 8 \text{ L/hour}$$

$$\text{GFR} = 118 \text{ to } 140 \text{ mL/min.}$$

The amount of fluid filtered from blood into glomerular capsule per unit time is known as glomerular filtration rate (GFR). A glomerular filtration rate of 130 mL/min is considered normal in healthy state, although 131 ± 22 mL/min is the normal range.

The blood in the kidney passes through many subunits known as glomeruli, which serve as filters. The filtration process is passive in nature and glomerular filtration of solutes is limited by their molecular size and shape. Any drug in plasma, provided its molecular dimensions are small (generally below the colloidal range), will be filtered in the glomeruli. Molecules which are small in size (low-molecular weight) and spherical in shape are filtered easily and long-chain molecules and/or high-molecular weight compounds are not freely filtered.

The glomerular capillaries filter plasma in such a way that any molecule can pass through the capillaries irrespective of its charge, provided its molecular weight is under about 20,000. When the molecular weight exceeds 20,000, the shape of the molecule then becomes the determining factor for filtration. For example, globular hemoglobin molecule (molecular weight = 64,500) readily filters through glomerular capillary wall, but serum albumin (molecular weight = 68,000), which is an elongated molecule, either filters much less readily or is almost completely held back. The upper limit of filterable molecular weight appears to be in the vicinity of about 50,000. This explains why the filtrate in normal kidney is practically free of proteins having a molecular weight of 70,000 or more. So far as drugs are concerned, with the exception of a few macromolecular substances, e.g. dextrans and heparin, all drugs pass the glomerulus as readily as water.

Filtration does not occur if the drug is associated with formed elements of blood or is bound to plasma protein or other tissues in the body. This is because association or binding of drug increases not only the size, but also the molecular weight of the compound. Also, glomerular filtration of drugs is directly related to the free or non-protein bound concentration of drug in the plasma. As the concentration of free drug increases in the plasma, glomerular filtration of the drug will increase proportionally. A drug that is excreted exclusively by glomerular filtration and associated with or bound extensively to the non-filterable components of the blood has an extremely long half-life, unless it undergoes relatively extensive biotransformation.

Factors Influencing Glomerular Filtration: The factors influencing glomerular filtration are those factors, which govern the rate of filtration at the capillary beds. These are:

a. Total surface area available for filtration
b. Permeability of the filtration membrane
c. Net filtration pressure.

The first two factors (total surface area available for filtration and permeability of the filtration membrane) do not pose a problem as far as glomerular filtration is concerned. This is because the glomerular capillaries are exceptionally permeable and have a huge surface area available for filtration. Therefore, GFR is essentially directly proportional to the net filtration pressure. The net filtration pressure is the glomerular hydrostatic pressure minus the sum of glomerular osmotic pressure and capsular hydrostatic pressure. Under normal conditions, the glomerular hydrostatic pressure is about 55 mm of mercury, the glomerular osmotic pressure is about 30 mm of mercury and the capsular hydrostatic pressure is about 15 mm of mercury. Therefore, the net filtration pressure is:

$$55 \text{ mm of mercury} - 30 \text{ mm of mercury} - 15 \text{ mm of mercury} = 10 \text{ mm of mercury}$$

The surface area available for filtration has been estimated to be equal to the surface area of the skin, thus allowing remarkably large amounts of filtrate to be produced even with the modest net filtration pressure of about 10 mm of mercury. On the other hand, a drop in glomerular pressure of only about 15% (which is less than 1 mm of mercury) stops filtration altogether. In other words, a change in the net filtration pressure can change the rate of glomerular filtration significantly. Therefore, an increase in the arterial blood pressure in the kidneys will cause an increase in the glomerular blood pressure, which will result in an increase in the GFR. On the other hand, dehydration, which causes an increase in the glomerular osmotic pressure, will inhibit formation of the filtrate. Although certain disease states may modify any of these pressures, changes in the GFR normally result from changes in the glomerular blood pressure, which is subject to both intrinsic and extrinsic controls.

Determination of Glomerular Filtration Rate: Glomerular filtration rate can be determined by measuring the extent of excretion and the plasma level of a test substance. The substance used to measure filtration rate should have the following properties:

1. It should be removed from plasma by glomerular filtration.
2. It should not be (actively) secreted or reabsorbed by the tubules.
3. It should not be metabolized, stored or protein-bound.
4. It should not affect the filtration rate.

Substances commonly used to measure glomerular filtration rate in humans include mannitol, sodium thiosulfate and inulin (a polymeric carbohydrate). Exogenous administration of creatinine is used to measure GFR in dogs.

GFR can be calculated as follows:

$$\text{GFR} = \frac{(\text{Concentration of drug in urine}) \times (\text{Urine flow/unit time})}{(\text{Concentration of drug in the artery})} \tag{6-4}$$

Since,

$$\text{Concentration} = \frac{\text{Amount}}{\text{Volume}}$$

Therefore,

$$GFR = \frac{(\text{Amount of drug excreted in urine/unit time})}{(\text{Concentration of drug in plasma})} \quad (6\text{-}5)$$

Since amount of drug excreted in urine per unit time is excretion rate, therefore equation (6-5) may be written as follows:

$$GFR = \frac{(\text{Excretion rate})}{(\text{Concentration of drug in plasma})} \quad (6\text{-}6)$$

Since excretion rate is expressed as amount per unit time (amount/min) and concentration is expressed as amount per unit volume (amount/mL), equation (6-6) becomes:

$$GFR = \frac{(\text{amount/min})}{(\text{amount/mL})} = \text{mL/min} \quad (6\text{-}7)$$

$$GFR = \frac{(\text{amount/h})}{(\text{amount/L})} = \text{L/h} \quad (6\text{-}7)$$

GFR is usually expressed as mL/min, although it is not uncommon to express it as L/hour. If a drug is not bound to plasma proteins, it is filtered in the amount equal to:

$$Q = (C_p)(GFR) \quad (6\text{-}8)$$

In equation (6-8), Q = amount of drug filtered through glomeruli (mg/min), Cp = concentration of drug in the plasma (mg/mL) and GFR = glomerular filtration rate (mL/min).

Tubular Secretion

The second mechanism by which a drug is passed from blood into the glomerular filtrate is tubular secretion. Tubular secretion is an active transport process, whereby the drug may is able to be transported against a concentration gradient from the blood capillaries across the tubular membrane into the renal tubule. This active process accounts for the fact that certain drugs, although extensively bound to plasma protein, are rapidly eliminated from the body essentially by renal excretion. The kidney appears to be capable of dissociating the drug-protein complex. The penicillins are an example of drugs that are rapidly eliminated by renal excretion, because the kidney dissociates the drug-protein complex. Two active renal secretion systems have been identified: one for weak acids and another for weak bases. Tubular secretion is important for a variety of functions, for example:

a. To dispose substances not already in the filtrate, e.g. penicillin and phenobarbital.
b. To eliminate undesirable substances that have been reabsorbed by passive diffusion, e.g. urea and uric acid.
c. To control blood pH. When the pH of blood begins to drop, the renal tubule cells actively secrete hydrogen ions into the filtrate and retain more bicarbonate and potassium ions. As a result, the pH of blood rises and urine drains off the excess acid.
d. To remove excessive potassium ions from the body. Nearly all potassium ions in urine are derived from active tubular secretion, because virtually all potassium ions present in the filtrate are reabsorbed in the proximal convoluted tubule.

The secretion process in renal elimination of drugs shares many characteristics of active transport systems of the intestine. It will be recalled that the characteristics of secretory active transport process are:

1. Specificity for chemical structure.
2. Transport against concentration gradient. The drug can be transported (carried) from a region of low concentration to a region of high concentration.

3. Upper rate limit of transport. The system can be saturated, i.e., above a certain blood concentration of drug, the system becomes saturated and reaches a maximum rate of transport.
4. Process can be blocked by metabolic inhibitors.
5. Expenditure of metabolic activity.
6. Functioning of a carrier mechanism.
7. Competitive secretory transport mechanism.

The principle of competition has been employed to provide a longer biological half-life of some drugs. For example, ordinarily, the biological half-life of penicillin is very short because penicillin is eliminated very rapidly. Probenecid is a weak organic acid, which competitively inhibits tubular secretion of benzyl penicillin, thereby decreasing elimination of penicillin. Probenecid has been used clinically to increase biological half-life and therefore the duration of effect of penicillin. The increased duration of effect prolongs therapeutic concentration of penicillin in plasma and this strategy has been found very useful in the treatment of infections, such as meningitis. Similarly, small quantities of salicylic acid competitively inhibit excretion of uric acid, when the concentration of uric acid in urine is high (e.g. in gout). Examples of other commonly used drugs which are eliminated by tubular secretion include the following:

Acids (Anions): Amino acids, acetazolamide, p-aminohippuric acid (PAH), benzyl penicillin, chlorothiazide, furosemide, indomethacin, penicillin, phenylbutazone, probenecid, salicylic acid and thiazide.

Bases (Cations): Cholines, dopamine, histamine, N-methylnicotinamide, dihydro-morphine, quinine, quaternary ammonium compounds and tolazoline.

Determination of Secretion Rate: Active tubular secretion rate of the drug is dependant on renal plasma flow. Therefore, any substance that is actively secreted by the renal tubules can be used to estimate tubular secretion rate, as long as it is not metabolized, stored or protein-bound and it does not affect the tubular secretion rate. Drugs commonly used to measure active tubular secretion include PAH and iodopyracet (diodrast). These substances are not only filtered through the glomerulus but are also vigorously secreted in the kidney tubules. The removal of PAH from arterial blood is 90 percent complete in a single passage through the kidney.

The amount of a drug or a substance secreted by active transport in the tubules is calculated as follows:

$$\text{Amount secreted} = (\text{Amount excreted}) - (\text{Amount filtered}) \tag{6-9}$$

$$\text{Amount secreted} = (C_u)(V) - (C_p)(GFR)(t) \tag{6-10}$$

In equation (6-10), C_u = concentration of drug in urine (in mg/mL), V = volume of urine excreted (in mL), C_p = concentration of drug in plasma (in mg/mL), GFR = glomerular filtration rate (in mL/min) and t = time (in min).

Tubular Reabsorption: Tubular reabsorption may be considered as a reclamation process that begins as soon as the filtrate enters the proximal tubules. Because the total blood volume filters into the renal tubules approximately every 45 minutes, all of the plasma would be drained away as urine within an hour were it not for the fact that most of the tubule contents are quickly reabsorbed (reclaimed) and returned to the blood. The filtered plasma passes through the glomeruli into the renal tubule.

The renal tubule is one of the most energetic sites of transport in the body. Water as well as many other physiologic solutes are reabsorbed from the tubule into the blood capillaries in large amounts. For example, although the glomeruli filter about 7 to 8 L of plasma per hour, the amount of urine formed per hour is only about 60 mL, which represents less than 1 percent of the volume of plasma, filtered by the glomeruli. The balance of the filtered water is reabsorbed. Similarly, glucose (which is a normal component of plasma) is rarely found in the urine of healthy individuals because of its quantitative reabsorption into the tubule. Examples of substances actively reabsorbed from the renal tubule include glucose, various amino acids, lactate, vitamins and most ions.

Drugs that are filtered with plasma are also subject to tubular reabsorption. The mechanism of drug transport from the renal tubule appears to be very similar to passive diffusion of drugs through the gastrointestinal barrier, i.e. the tubule membrane is permeable only to lipid-soluble, non-ionized form of the drug. Consequently, compounds that are charged or possess poor lipid solubility are poorly reabsorbed. Accordingly, tubular reabsorption of drugs that are weak organic acids or weak organic bases is dependent on pH of the fluids in the renal tubule.

URINE pH AND REABSORPTION

To appreciate the effect of urinary pH on the reabsorption of drugs, one needs to know the pH of the fluid in the renal tubule. Although it is very difficult to assess the pH of fluid in the renal tubule, the pH at the beginning and at the terminal processes can be determined fairly easily. The pH of fluid at the beginning of renal tubule is equal to the pH of plasma and the pH of fluid at the terminal process is equal to the pH of urine. Therefore, by measuring the pH of plasma and pH of urine, one can estimate the pH of the fluid at the beginning of the renal tubule and at the terminal processes in the renal tubule. The pH of plasma in human is quite constant at about 7.4, but the normal pH of urine may exhibit large differences. It has been shown that the pH of urine may vary from about 4.5 to about 8 depending on a variety of factors, such as pathophysiology, diet and ingestion of acidic or basic substances. Thus, elimination of certain drugs may be influenced significantly by administration of substances that affect the pH of urine. For example, ingestion of foods rich in proteins has a tendency to lower the pH of urine, making urine more acidic. On the other hand, diets rich in vegetables and carbohydrates result in higher urinary pH, making urine relatively more alkaline. Similarly, some acidic drugs and antacids administered in large quantities may affect the pH of urine.

Based on the pH-partition theory, renal tubular reabsorption of weakly acidic drugs would be expected to be depressed under alkaline (basic) conditions of urinary pH. This is because weakly acidic drugs are more ionized in the alkaline environment; therefore, a lesser fraction of drug is available for diffusion through the renal tubular membrane. However, renal tubular reabsorption of weakly basic drugs would be expected to be increased under alkaline (basic) conditions of urinary pH, because weakly basic drugs are less ionized (more non-ionized) in alkaline environment, therefore, a larger fraction of the drug is available for diffusion through the renal tubular membrane.

Similarly, reabsorption of weakly basic drugs would be expected to be depressed under acidic conditions of urinary pH, because weakly basic drugs are more ionized in the acidic environment and therefore, a lesser fraction of drug is available for diffusion through the tubular membrane. Conversely, renal tubular reabsorption of weakly acidic drugs would be expected to increase under acidic conditions of urinary pH, because weakly basic drugs are less ionized (more non-ionized) in the acidic environment, therefore, a larger fraction of the drug is available for diffusion through the renal tubular membrane.

Acidic Drugs

The influence of urine pH on tubular reabsorption is illustrated by the results of studies with sulfaethidole ($pK_a = 5.6$), a weakly acidic sulfonamide, under conditions of alkalinized and acidified urine. Urine pH was maintained either at pH 5 by continual administration of ammonium chloride or at pH 8 by continual administration of sodium bicarbonate. The average biological half-life of the drug was determined in both cases. The average half-life of sulfaethidole was found to be 11.4 hours, when the urine pH was maintained at pH 5. When the pH of urine was maintained at pH 8, the average biological half-life of sulfaethidole reduced to 4.2 hours.

Using the Henderson-Hasselbalch equation for acidic drugs, the fraction of sulfaethidole unionized at pH 5 can be calculated as follows: The Henderson-Hasselbalch equation for acidic drugs is:

$$pH = pK_a + \log \frac{[\text{Ionized}]}{[\text{Unionized}]} \tag{6-11}$$

Substituting the values of pH of urine (pH = 5.0) and pK_a of sulfaethidole (pK_a = 5.6) into equation (6-11) yields:

$$5.0 = 5.6 + \log \frac{[\text{Ionized}]}{[\text{Unionized}]}$$

which, upon rearrangement gives

$$\log \frac{[\text{Ionized}]}{[\text{Unionized}]} = 5.0 - 5.6 = -0.6$$

Taking inverse logarithms on both side gives:

$$\frac{[\text{Ionized}]}{[\text{Unionized}]} = 0.2512 = \frac{0.2512}{1}$$

$$\%\ \text{Ionized} = \frac{0.2512}{0.2512 + 1} \times 100\% = 20\% \text{ and}$$

$$\%\ \text{Unionized} = \frac{1}{0.2512 + 1} \times 100\% = 80\%$$

Thus, at pH 5, 80% of the administered sulfaethidole is in the unionized form. Similarly, at pH 8, percent sulfaethidole unionized can also be calculated using equation (6-11) as follows:

$$pH = pK_a + \log \frac{[\text{Ionized}]}{[\text{Unionized}]}$$

Substituting the values of pH (= 8.0) and pK_a (= 5.6) into equation (6-11) yields:

$$8.0 = 5.6 + \log \frac{[\text{Ionized}]}{[\text{Unionized}]}$$

$$\log \frac{[\text{Ionized}]}{[\text{Unionized}]} = 8.0 - 5.6 = 2.4$$

Taking inverse logarithms on both sides,

$$\frac{[\text{Ionized}]}{[\text{Unionized}]} = 251.19 = \frac{251.19}{1}, \text{ therefore}$$

$$\%\text{Unionized} = \frac{1}{2510.19 + 1} \times 100 = 0.4\%$$

Thus, only 0.4% of administered sulfaethidole dose is in the unionized form at pH 8. The fraction of sulfaethidole unionized at pH 5 (80%) and at pH 8 (0.4%) correlates with the change in biological half-life of the drug due to change in urinary pH. That is, higher concentration of undissociated drug favors reabsorption from renal tubular fluid, which results in longer biological half-life for the drug. Similar findings have been reported for other acidic drugs. For example, in the case of probenecid,

pH of urine	Ratio of probenecid excreted/filtered
5	0.2
7	1
8	6

Examples of other acidic drugs, which are eliminated faster in alkalinized (basic) urine include amino acids, barbiturates, nitrofurantoin, phenylbutazone, salicylic acid and sulfonamides. Table 6-4 lists the pK_a values of some acidic drugs.

In general, reabsorption of acidic drugs which undergo passive diffusion and have pK_a values between 5 and 8 are most likely to be affected by changes in urinary pH and less likely if pK_a value is less than 5 or greater than 8. This is because, when the difference between the pK_a of drug and the pH of fluid containing the drug becomes large, the ratio of the logarithm of the ionized and non-ionized species of the drug also becomes large and the extent of ionization of the compound at these large differences is not affected to a significant extent.

Table 6-5 shows the effect of difference between pH and pK_a on the degree (extent) of ionization of weakly acidic drugs.

For example, when the difference between the pH of the solution and the pK_a of the drug = 2, then 99% of the drug is in the ionized form and when the difference between the pH of the solution and the pK_a of the drug is equal to 3, then also 99% of the drug is in the ionized form and when the difference between the pH of the solution and the pK_a of the drug = 4, then also 99% of the drug is in the ionized form. This means that when the difference between the pH of the solution and the pK_a of the drug is equal to 2 or more than 2, then 99% of the drug will be in the ionized form. Similarly, when difference between the pH of the solution and the pK_a of the drug = –2, less than 1% of the drug is in the ionized form and when the difference between

Table 6-4 pK_a values of some acidic drugs

Drug	*pK_a*	*Drug*	*pK_a*
Acetaminophen	9.51	Hydrochlorothiazide	$K_1 = 7.9$
Acetazolamide	7.2		$K_2 = 8.6$
Acetylsalicylic acid	3.49	Ibuprofen	4.8
Amobarbital	7.7	Indomethacin	4.5
Ascorbic acid	$K_1 = 4.3$	Lactic acid	3.86
	$K_2 = 11.8$	Levodopa	2.3
Amoxicillin	$K_1 = 2.4$	Naproxen	5.0
	$K_2 = 7.4$	Penicillin V	2.73
Ampicillin	$K_1 = 2.54$	Pentobarbital	8.0
	$K_2 = 7.2$	Phenobarbital	7.41
Barbital	7.91	Phenytoin	8.1
Barbituric acid	3.98	Salicylic acid	2.97
Benzoic acid	4.20	Sulfadiazine	6.48
Benzyl penicillin	2.76	Sulfamerazine	7.06
Boric acid	9.24	Sulfapyridine	8.44
Caffeine	14.0	Sulfathiazole	7.12
Carbenicillin	2.6	Sulfisoxazole	5.0
Cefazolin	2.3	Tetracycline	$K_1 = 3.30$
Cefotaxime	3.4		$K_2 = 7.68$
Chlorpropamide	4.8		$K_3 = 9.69$
Citric acid	$K_1 = 3.15$	Theophylline	9.0
	$K_2 = 4.78$	Thiopental	7.6
	$K_3 = 6.40$	Tolbutamide	5.5
Clofibrate	2.95	Warfarin	4.8

Table 6-5 Effect of pH and pK_a on the extent of ionization of weak acids

$pH - pK_a$	% Ionized	% Unionized
4	99.99	0.01
3	99.90	0.09
2	99.01	0.99
1	90.90	9.09
0	50.00	50.00
–1	9.09	90.90
–2	0.99	99.01
–3	0.09	99.90
–4	0.01	99.99

the pH of the solution and the pK_a of the drug is equal to –3, then also less than 1% of the drug is in the ionized form and when the difference between the pH of the solution and pK_a of the drug = –4, then also less than 1% of the drug is in the ionized form. This means that when the difference between the pH of the solution and the pKa of the drug is equal to –2 or more than –2, then less than 1% of the drug will be in the ionized form.

Basic Drugs

The influence of urinary pH on the elimination of weakly basic drugs which, undergo passive diffusion is very similar to that of acidic drugs, because acidic conditions favor dissociation of basic drugs due to salt formation (e.g. chloride or hydrochloride salt) and the drug tends to be more ionized in acidic environment. Since salt is more water-soluble ionized species than the less water-soluble non-ionized species, salt form of drug is less likely to be reabsorbed and has a tendency to be excreted into the urine more rapidly. Alkaline conditions, on the other hand, favor formation of less water-soluble (and more lipid-soluble) non-ionized species of drug in the basic environment, which favors reabsorption of weakly basic drugs. Thus, half-life of basic drugs will be expected to be greater in patients with alkaline urine than in acidic urine. Table 6-6 lists pK_b values of some basic drugs.

For example, the effect of pH of urine on the elimination of amphetamine (a basic drug) was studied by first increasing the pH of urine by administration of high doses of sodium bicarbonate and then decreasing the pH of urine by administering large doses of ammonium chloride. The following results were obtained:

Urine pH	% of dose excreted unchanged in urine
4.5 – 5.6	57
7.1 – 8.0	7

Only 7 percent of the administered dose was excreted unchanged in the urine, when the pH of urine was in the basic region (pH between 7.1 and 8.0). However, under acidic conditions (pH between 4.5 and 5.6), excretion of the unchanged drug increased eight-fold due to decreased reabsorption of the drug. This is because although the percentage of drug ionized in the acidic environment when pH was 5.0 (about 9%) is not very large, the fraction of drug ionized in the acidic environment is greater than the fraction of drug ionized in the basic environment (less than 1% at pH 7.0) as predicted by the Henderson-Hasselbalch equation for basic drugs:

$$pH = pK_w - pK_b + \log \frac{[\text{Unionized}]}{[\text{Ionized}]} \tag{6-12}$$

In general, reabsorption of basic drugs, which undergo passive diffusion and have pK_b values between 6 and 9 are most likely to be affected by changes in the urinary pH. The effect of urinary pH on the elimination of basic drugs having pK_b values lower than 6 or greater than 9 is not as dramatic as drugs having pK_b values between 6 and 9. As the pK_b value becomes smaller than 6 or greater than 9, the significance of urinary pH on drug elimination starts becoming less important. This is because when the difference between pH and $(pK_w - pK_b)$ of the fluid containing the drug becomes large, the ratio of the logarithm of the unionized form to the ionized form of the basic compound also becomes large. At large ratios of the logarithm of unionized form to the ionized form, the extent of ionization of the compound is not affected to a significant extent. The following example illustrates this concept:

The Henderson-Hasselbalch equation for basic drugs is

$$pH = pK_w - pK_b + \log\frac{[\text{Unionized}]}{[\text{Ionized}]}$$

This upon rearrangement gives

$$\log\frac{[\text{Unionized}]}{[\text{Ionized}]} = pH - (pK_w - pK_b)$$

$$\log\frac{[\text{Unionized}]}{[\text{Ionized}]} = pH + PK_b - pK_w \tag{6-13}$$

Table 6-6 pK_b values of some basic drugs

Drug	pK_b	*Drug*	pK_b
Acebutolol	9.4	Epinephrine	$K_1 = 4.1$
Acetohexamide	6.8		$K_2 = 5.5$
Alprenolol	9.6	Erythromycin	5.2
Amitriptyline	2.2	Hydroquinone	5.33
Amphetamine	10.00	Morphine	6.13
Antipyrine	2.2	Nalorphine	6.2
Apomorphine	7.00	Papaverine	8.1
Atropine	4.35	Physostigmine	$K_1 = 6.12$
Benzocaine	11.22		$K_2 = 12.24$
Brompheniramine	$K_1 = 3.59$	Pilocarpine	$K_1 = 7.2$
	$K_2 = 9.12$		$K_2 = 12.7$
Caffeine	$K_1 = 10.4$	Procaine	5.2
	$K_2 = 13.4$	Quinine	$K_1 = 6.00$
Chloroquine	8.1		$K_2 = 9.89$
Chlorothiazide	$K_1 = 6.8$	Reserpine	7.4
	$K_2 = 9.4$	Scopolamine	5.8
Chlorpheniramine	9.16	Strychnine	$K_1 = 6.0$
Chlortetracycline	$K_1 = 3.3$		$K_2 = 11.7$
	$K_2 = 9.3$	Theobromine	$K_1 = 6.11$
Cimetidine	7.11		$K_2 = 13.3$
Clonidine	8.3	Theophylline	8.80
Cocaine	5.59	Thiourea	11.90
Codeine	5.8	Tolbutamide	8.7
Diazepam	3.4	Urea	13.82

Since, pK_w at room temperature and body temperature is approximately 14, equation (6-13) becomes

$$\log \frac{[\text{Unionized}]}{[\text{Ionized}]} = pH + pK_b - 14 \tag{6-14}$$

If the pH of fluid containing the drug is 6 and pK_b of the drug is 6, then according to equation (6-14),

$$\log \frac{[\text{Unionized}]}{[\text{Ionized}]} = 6 + 6 - 14 = -2$$

$$\frac{[\text{Unionized}]}{[\text{Ionized}]} = \frac{0.01}{1}$$

$$\%\ \text{Unionized} = \frac{0.01}{0.01+1} \times 100 = 0.99\%$$

This means that less than 1% of the drug is unionized, when pH of the fluid containing the drug is 6. Now, if pH of the fluid is still 6, but the pK_b of the drug is 5, then according to equation (6-14),

$$\log \frac{[\text{Unionized}]}{[\text{Ionized}]} = 6 + 5 - 14 = -3$$

And the ratio

$$\frac{[\text{Unionized}]}{[\text{Ionized}]} = \frac{0.001}{1}$$

$$\%\ \text{Unionized} = \frac{0.001}{0.01+1} \times 100 = 0.099\%$$

That is, the percentage of drug unionized is still less than 1%

Similar findings have been reported for other basic drugs, which undergo passive diffusion. Examples of basic drugs eliminated faster in acidic urine include such drugs as amphetamines, chloroquine, codeine, morphine, quinine, quinidine, nicotine, phencyclidine and procaine. As mentioned earlier, in general, reabsorption of basic drugs which undergo passive diffusion and have pK_b values between 6 and 9 are most likely to be affected by changes in the urinary pH.

Table 6-7 shows the effect of difference between pH and pK_b on the degree (extent) of ionization of weakly basic drugs.

Table 6-7 Effect of pH and pK_b on the extent of ionization of weak bases

pH + pK$_b$	*% Ionized*	*% Unionized*
10	99.99	0.01
11	99.90	0.10
12	99.01	0.99
13	90.90	9.10
14	50.00	50.00
15	9.10	90.90
16	0.99	99.01
17	0.10	99.90
18	0.01	99.99

Practicality of Adjustment of Urine pH

In order to increase the duration of therapeutic activity of a drug, the practicality of adjustment of urinary pH to prolong biological half-life of the drug is very questionable. This is in view of the fact that the pH of the urinary tract under normal conditions ranges between 4.5 to about 8; any drastic change in the urinary pH has the potential to cause great discomfort, especially due to the large doses of ammonium chloride or sodium bicarbonate that may be required to achieve the desired urinary pH. However, the technique may be very valuable in the case of drug intoxication or drug overdose situations in which rapid elimination of drug from systemic circulation may be lifesaving. The effect of urine pH on excretion must also be borne in mind in the design of dosage regimen. A large variation in the rate constant of elimination as observed with sulfaethiodole or amphetamine could be significant in determining the success of a course of therapy.

It should be emphasized that administration of certain drugs can change the pH of urine and may cause acidosis or alkalosis because of their acidic or basic nature. Examples of drugs which may cause acidosis include acetylsalicylic acid (Aspirin), ascorbic acid (vitamin C), dimercaprol, lysine hydrochloride and salicylates. Similarly, administration of drugs which may cause alkalosis include antacids and mercurial and thiazide diuretics.

PHARMACOKINETICS AND RENAL EXCRETION

Published literature cites examples of some drugs, which are excreted through the kidneys largely in the unchanged form. There are also other drugs that are excreted partly in the unchanged form and partly in the form of one or more metabolite. However, many drugs are excreted almost completely in the form of one or more metabolite. Determination of the various pharmacokinetic parameters of the parent drug from urinary excretion studies is generally limited to only those drugs, where at least 10 percent of the drug is excreted in the urine in the unchanged form.

Examples of drugs excreted in the unchanged form include barbital, digoxin, gentamicin, streptomycin and vancomycin. Table 6-8 is a partial listing of drugs, which are largely excreted in the unchanged form.

Table 6-8 Examples of drugs excreted largely unchanged

Drug	*% Excreted*	*Drug*	*% Excreted*
Acetazolamide	90	Ethambutol	85
Amoxicillin	70	Furosemide	75
Amphetamine	65	Gentamicin	90
Ampicillin	90	Hetacillin	90
Carbenicillin	90	Hydrochlorothiazide	95
Cefaclor	60	Kanamycin	80
Cefadroxil	95	Methotrexate	95
Cefazoline	85	Oxytetracycline	70
Cephaloridine	70	Penicillin G	80
Cephalothin	60	Pseudoephedrine	95
Chlorothiazide	95	Sulfamethizole	75
Cimetidine	70	Tobramycin	90
Dexamethasone	80	Vancomycin	95
Digoxin	75	Viomycin	80

Some examples of drugs which are excreted in the form of inactive metabolites include Chloramphenicol, isoniazid, morphine and phenacetin.

SUGGESTED READING

1. Delgado J, Remers W, (eds). Wilson and Gisvold's Text Book of Organic Medicinal and Pharmaceutical Chemistry, 9th edition. Lippincott; 1990.
2. Goodman, Gilman's. The Pharmacological Basis of Therapeutics, 9th edition. McGraw Hill; 1996.
3. Guyton AC. Text Book of Medical Physiology, 8th edition. Philadelphia: W. B. Saunders; 1991.
4. Marieb E. Human Anatomy and Physiology, 2nd edition. Benjamin: Cummings Publishing Company; 1991.
5. Mungal D, (ed). Applied Clinical Pharmacokinetics. Raven Press; 1983.
6. Remington. The Science and Practice of Pharmacy, 21st edition. Mack Publishing; 2005.
7. Theoharides T, (ed). Pharmacology. Little Brown and Company; 1992.
8. Wagner J. Fundamentals of Clinical Pharmacokinetics. Drug Intelligence Publications; 1979.

PRACTICE PROBLEMS

6-1. The pK_b of codeine is 5.8. Calculate the percentage of drug in the unionized form in (a) plasma at pH 7.4 and (b) in urine at pH 6.

6-2. The pK_a of phenobarbital is 7.4. Calculate the percentage of drug that will be in the ionized form in urine at (a) pH = 5.0 and (b) pH = 7.5.

6-3. The arterial concentration of a drug is 12 μg/mL. Calculate excretion ratio, if the renal concentration of the drug is 9 μg/mL.

6-4. A 35-year male patient was admitted into a hospital and drug therapy was initiated. According to the laboratory report, the arterial concentration of the drug was 32 μg/mL and the renal concentration of the drug was 24 μg/mL. Calculate the excretion ratio.

6-5. A 50-year female patient was admitted into a hospital and drug therapy was initiated. According to the laboratory report, the arterial concentration of the drug was 20 μg/mL and the renal concentration of the drug was 16 μg/mL. Calculate the excretion ratio.

CHAPTER 7

CLEARANCE

Clearance is a theoretical concept for describing elimination of drug from the body without identifying specific mechanism of the process. The total body clearance (Cl_t, more commonly, Cl) is the sum of clearance of drug by all clearance pathways. Total body clearance considers the entire body as a single drug eliminating system from which all eliminating processes may occur. Instead of describing rate of elimination in terms of a certain quantity or amount of drug eliminated per unit time, clearance describes rate of elimination in terms of volume of fluid that is cleared of drug per unit time. For example, if the apparent volume of distribution of a drug is known to be 41 L and the total body clearance of the drug is 30 mL/min, then by definition, 30 mL of the 41 L body fluid would be cleared of drug per minute, or 1.8 liters of the 41 L would be cleared of drug per hour. Thus, clearance may be defined as "*the volume of plasma from which a measured amount of the substance (drug) can be completely eliminated (or cleared) per unit time*". Clearance is expressed in the units of mL/min or L/hr. The volume concept is not only simple, but it is also convenient because all drugs are dissolved and distributed in the fluids of the body.

There are two major pathways of drug elimination. They are—the kidneys and the liver. Elimination through the kidneys is known as renal clearance and elimination through the liver is called hepatic clearance. Since kidneys and liver play the most prominent role in drug elimination, therefore, only these two organs are usually considered in the clearance of drug. In this regard, since kidney is the major organ of elimination for most drugs, the total body clearance (Cl) is therefore considered as being the result of two clearance processes: renal clearance (kidney) and non-renal clearance (all other pathways).

Total body clearance is defined as:

$$Cl = Cl_r + Cl_{nr} \tag{7-1}$$

where,

Cl = total body clearance

Cl_r = renal body clearance

Cl_{nr} = non-renal body clearance.

Hepatic clearance (Cl_h) is included in non-renal clearance. Other non-hepatic and non-renal pathways of drug elimination, which include lung, saliva, milk and skin are not considered in clearance, because clearance of most drugs from these pathways is negligible.

FACTORS AFFECTING CLEARANCE

Clearance is affected by a number of physiological factors in both healthy subjects as well as in patients suffering from various ailments and conditions. Some of the important factors that affect clearance include the following: age, sex, kidney diseases and cardiac diseases.

1. **Age:** Clearance decreases after the age of 70
2. **Gender**: Clearance is approximately 10% lower in females than in males.

3. **Kidney diseases**: Clearance is reduced in the presence of kidney diseases such as nephritis, pyelonephritis, nephrosclerosis and renal failure. Reduction in clearance during these disease states is somewhat proportional to the reduction in renal function. For example, in slightly reduced renal function, clearance is reduced 20–50% and in mild renal failure, clearance is reduced 50–70%. In moderate renal failure, clearance is reduced 70–90% and in severe renal failure, clearance is reduced more than 90%.
4. **Cardiac diseases**: Cardiac diseases have been shown to affect clearance to varying degrees.

RENAL CLEARANCE

Renal clearance is defined as the volume of drug-containing plasma that is cleared of the drug (removal of the drug) by the kidney per unit time. The volume of plasma cleared of the drug is generally measured in milliliters and time is usually expressed in minutes, therefore, renal clearance, Cl_r, is expressed as mL/min. If the volume of plasma cleared of the drug is expressed in liters, then time would be expressed in hours and renal clearance will be expressed as liters per hour (L/h).

The rate of removal of a drug from the renal arterial blood depends on the mechanisms of renal excretion operating for that drug. Therefore, the values of renal clearance are often employed as an approximation of how the kidney eliminates a drug and these values can hence be used to estimate the glomerular function.

Methods of Measuring Renal Clearance

A number of methods have been used to measure renal clearance. The two more popular methods of measuring renal clearance are:

i. From elimination rate constant
ii. From urinary excretion rate.

From Elimination Rate Constant

The measurement of renal clearance from the rate constant of elimination is a very simple method of determining renal clearance. This method involves the use of two parameters: (i) The rate constant of elimination (K) of drug from the body and; (ii) The apparent volume of distribution (V_d) of the drug. The relationship describing renal clearance (Cl_r) with the rate constant of elimination of drug from the body (K) and the apparent volume of distribution of drug is given by the following equation:

$$\text{Clearance} = (K)(V_d) \quad (7\text{-}2)$$

The two parameters, rate constant of elimination of drug from the body and apparent volume of distribution of drug in the body are determined as follows:

A rapid intravenous bolus dose of the drug is administered and blood samples are collected at predetermined time intervals. The concentration of drug in each blood sample is determined and then plotted as a function of time of withdrawal of the blood sample. From this plasma profile, the rate constant of elimination of drug from the body and the apparent volume of distribution of drug in the body can be determined.

Example 7-1 A 50 mg intravenous bolus dose of a drug, which upon administration, confers upon the body the characteristics of one-compartment pharmacokinetic model, gave the following data: C_0 = 1 mcg/mL and $t_{1/2}$ = 6 hours. Calculate renal clearance of the drug.

Solution

From the data provided,

$$V_d = \frac{\text{Dose}}{C_0} = \frac{50 \text{ mg}}{1 \text{ µg/mL}} = 50 \text{ L},$$

and

$$K = \frac{0.693}{t_{1/2}} = \frac{0.693}{6 \text{ h}} = 0.1155/\text{h}$$

Substituting the values of rate constant of elimination and the apparent volume of distribution of the drug into equation (7-2), one gets:

$$\text{Clearance} = (K)(V_d)$$

$$\text{Clearance} = (0.1155/\text{h})(50 \text{ L}) = 5.775 \text{ L/h}$$

$$\text{Clearance} = 5{,}775 \text{ mL}/60 \text{ min} = 96.25 \text{ mL/min}$$

Example 7-2 Calculate clearance from the following data obtained after 200 mg bolus IV injection.

Time (h):	1	2	3	4	5	6	7
Concentration (µg/mL):	6.5	5.0	4.0	3.2	2.5	2.0	1.6

Solution

A plot of the data on a semilogarithmic graph paper is shown in Figure 7-1. This plot indicates that upon intravenous administration, the drug confers upon the body the characteristics of one-compartment open model.

From Figure 7-1,

$$C_0 = 8 \text{ µg/mL}$$

$$K = \frac{\ln 8 - \ln 1.6}{(0-7)\text{h}} = \frac{1.609}{7 \text{ h}} = 0.23/\text{h}$$

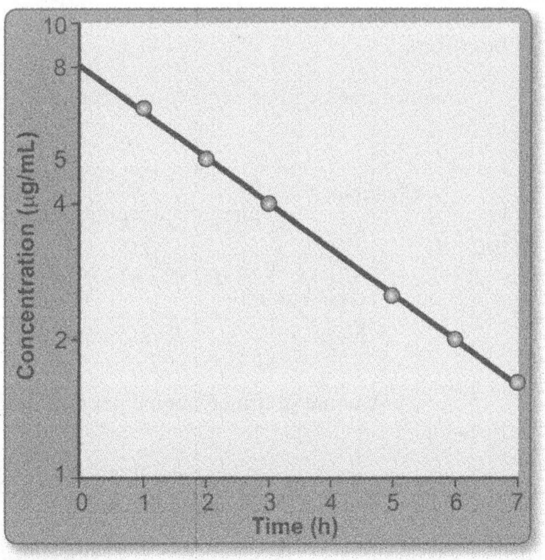

Fig. 7-1 Semilogarithmic plot of data in Example 7-2

Since the drug confers the characteristics of one-compartment model on the body, therefore,

$$V_d = \frac{\text{Dose}}{C_0} = \frac{200\ \text{mg}}{8\ \mu\text{g/mL}} = 25\ \text{L}$$

Substituting the values of K and V_d into equation (7-2):

$$Cl_r = (K)(V_d)$$

$$Cl_r = (0.23/\text{h}) \times (25\ \text{L})$$

$$Cl_r = 5.75\ \text{L/h} = 95.83\ \text{mL/min}$$

From Urinary Excretion Rate

The second method for measurement of renal clearance is based on the concept, as described in Chapter 6, that the amount of drug excreted in urine per unit time (rate of excretion of drug in the urine) is proportional to the concentration of drug in plasma. In other words, this method is based on the concept that clearance may be imagined as the volume of plasma that is "cleaned" of drug per unit time or in technical terms, the volume of plasma that is "cleared" of drug per unit time, i.e.

$$\text{Clearance} = \frac{\text{Volume of plasma cleared of drug}}{\text{Time}} \tag{7-3}$$

Or,

$$\text{Clearance} = \frac{\text{mL of plasma cleared of drug}}{\text{Minutes}} \tag{7-4}$$

The volume of plasma "cleared" of drug is essentially the volume of plasma from which a given amount of drug is excreted through the kidneys. Since,

$$\text{Volume} = \frac{\text{Amount}}{\text{Concentration}}$$

The term "mL of plasma cleared of drug" in the numerator of equation (7-4) may be written as

$$\text{mL of plasma cleared of drug} = \frac{\text{Amount excreted in urine}}{\text{Concentration in renal arterial}} \tag{7-5}$$

Therefore, equation (7-4) becomes

$$\text{Clearance} = \frac{(\text{Amount excreted in urine})/(\text{Concentration in renal arterial})}{\text{Time}} \tag{7-6}$$

$$\text{Clearance} = \frac{(\text{Amount excreted in urine})}{(\text{Time}) \times (\text{Concentration in renal arterial})} \tag{7-7}$$

Equation (7-7) may be written as

$$\text{Clearance} = \frac{(\text{Amount excreted in urine})}{(\text{Time})} \times \frac{1}{(\text{Concentration in renal arterial plasma})} \tag{7-8}$$

Since, $\frac{(\text{Amount excreted in urine})}{(\text{Time})}$ = Amount of drug excreted per unit time = Excretion rate,

$$\text{Clearance} = \frac{\text{Urinary excretion rate}}{\text{Plasma concentration}}\text{, therefore,} \tag{7-9}$$

$$\text{Urinary excretion rate} = (\text{Clearance}) \times (\text{Plasma concentration}) \tag{7-10}$$

This is an equation of a straight line (y = mx + b). In this equation, y is urinary excretion rate of the drug, x is the plasma concentration of the drug and m = slope = clearance. Therefore, a plot of excretion rate of the drug as a function of plasma concentration should be linear with no y-intercept and slope = clearance.

Measurement of Excretion Rate: Excretion rate is the rate at which drug is removed from the body by excretion into the urine. The usual procedure for the determination of excretion rate is to administer the drug dose and collect urine at pre-determined time intervals. The volume of urine collected during each collection interval and the concentration of drug in each urine sample is determined and from this, the amount of drug excreted during each collection interval is calculated as follows:

$$\text{Amount of drug excreted} = (\text{Volume of urine collected}) \times (\text{Concentration of drug in the urine}) \quad (7\text{-}11)$$

Therefore, excretion rate of drug for each time interval is:

$$\text{Excretion rate} = \frac{\text{Amount of drug excreted}}{\text{Time}} \quad (7\text{-}12)$$

The amount of drug excreted during each interval divided by the time interval between urine collections gives excretion rate for each sample.

Measurement of Plasma Concentration: Since concentration of drug in the plasma decreases according to first order kinetics; it is not constant for any length of time. Therefore, plasma concentration of the drug must be determined at frequent time intervals. The selection of time intervals for the determination of plasma concentration of the drug is dictated by the intervals selected for collection of urine for the measurement of excretion rate. For example, let us suppose that the drug was administered as a single IV bolus dose and the first urinary sample was collected at the end of the first hour post dosing. The concentration of drug in the plasma would be at its maximum soon after administration of the dose and excretion of drug would just be beginning. The plasma concentration of drug soon after administration of the dose would not reflect the urinary excretion rate during the first hour because at this time the urinary excretion of the drug has just started. Determination of plasma concentration of the drug at the end of the first hour would also not reflect the urinary excretion rate because at the end of the first hour the concentration of drug in plasma would be much lower than that during the earlier or the middle portion of the time interval during the first hour. The most logical time to determine the drug plasma concentration, which would approximate the urinary excretion rate during the first hour would be the midpoint of this interval, i.e. at 0.5 hour after administration of the drug.

Similarly, to determine the plasma concentration of drug to represent the excretion rate during the second and the fourth hour, the concentration of drug in plasma should not be determined at the second or the fourth hour post dosing, but at the third hour. Therefore, to represent concentration of drug in the plasma for a given excretion rate, it is imperative that the concentration of drug in plasma is determined at the midpoint of corresponding excretion rate. For example, if excretion of drug was determined during the first hour after administration of the dose, the corresponding drug plasma concentration needed to plot the graph would be at the mid point of the first hour, i.e. at 0.5 hour after administration of the dose. If excretion rate of the drug was determined during the third and the fifth hour, then the corresponding plasma concentration needed to plot the graph would be at the mid point of the third and fifth hour after administration of the dose, i.e. at the fourth hour. Similarly, if excretion of drug was determined during the second and the sixth hour after administration of the dose, the corresponding drug plasma concentration needed to plot the graph would still be at the fourth hour. If excretion of drug was determined during the second and the fourth hour after administration of the dose, then the corresponding drug plasma concentration needed to plot the graph would now be at mid point of the second and the fourth hour, i.e. at the third hour.

Determination of Clearance: To determine clearance, a plot of urinary excretion rate as a function of plasma drug concentration is constructed on a rectangular graph paper according to equation (7-10) by plotting urinary excretion rate on the y-axis and concentration of drug in plasma at the midpoints of urinary excretion rates on x-axis. The slope of the straight line yields clearance of the drug.

Mechanism of Drug Excretion

The mechanism of drug excretion can be estimated from a plot of excretion rate versus plasma concentration of drug. The shape of graph and the value of slope obtained from this graph gives a fairly good indication concerning elimination processes involved in clearance of drug, i.e. whether drug excretion is by filtration, secretion or total excretion (filtration and secretion). Figure 7-2 shows hypothetical plots of excretion by these mechanisms.

When the plot of excretion rate versus plasma concentration of drug is not linear, it indicates that excretion proceeds by glomerular filtration and/or active secretion. Since glomerular filtration is a passive diffusion process, the rate of excretion of drug by this route depends on the concentration of drug in plasma.

When the concentration of drug in plasma is low, the rate of excretion of drug is also small. The rate of excretion of drug increases with increasing concentration of drug in plasma and hence the graph must be linear. Secretion, on the other hand, is a process which involves a transport mechanism where saturation of transport mechanism can occur. With some drugs, saturation may occur at normal plasma levels so that the graph may start out linear or exhibit a curve, indicating increase in excretion rate with increasing concentration of drug in plasma, but then attains a plateau once the system reaches saturation. When the drug is excreted by both filtration and active tubular secretion, the two processes (linear for filtration and linear becoming plateau for tubular secretion) combine and the graph becomes curvilinear.

As mentioned earlier, the shape of the graph (linear, curvilinear or linear becoming plateau) and the value of slope obtained from this graph gives a fairly good indication concerning the elimination processes involved in the clearance of drug. As a general rule, if the clearance value exceeds glomerular filtration rate, the drug is filtered as well as secreted by the tubules. If the clearance value is less than glomerular filtration rate, the drug is reabsorbed. The normal value for glomerular filtration rate is taken as 130 mL/min, hence a clearance value of less than 130 mL/min is a good indication of reabsorption. Smaller the value of clearance, larger will be the extent of reabsorption. If clearance is equal to glomerular filtration rate, the drug is possibly filtered only, although it is conceivable that the drug may be filtered, secreted, as well as reabsorbed. Similarly, the normal value for total clearance (glomerular filtration plus active secretion) is considered to be 650 mL/min, therefore, a clearance value of more than 130 mL/min is a good indication of involvement of secretion process in the elimination of the drug.

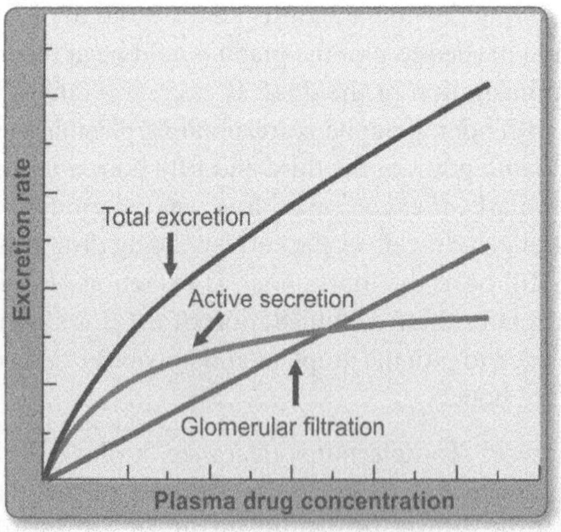

Fig. 7-2 Excretion rate versus plasma concentration

Mechanism of Renal Clearance

The value of renal clearance obtained from the slope of a plot of excretion rate as a function of plasma concentration may be used to extrapolate the actual physiologic clearance process for the renal clearance of a given drug. This is accomplished by comparing renal clearance of the drug to renal clearance of a standard reference.

For example, if inulin (which is cleared through the kidney by the process of glomerular filtration only) is used as the standard, then the ratio of clearance of drug (Cl_{drug}) to inulin clearance (Cl_{inulin}) may be used as an indicator to know whether the drug is only filtered or actively secreted or partially reabsorbed. For instance, if the ratio Cl_{drug}/Cl_{inulin} is more than 1, it means that the clearance of drug is greater than the clearance of inulin. Therefore, the drug is perhaps actively secreted. Similarly, if the ratio Cl_{drug}/Cl_{inulin} is less than 1, it means that the clearance of drug is less than the clearance of inulin. This would be indicative of renal reabsorption of the drug. The degree of renal reabsorption would be indicated by the value of clearance. The larger the value of clearance, the smaller the degree of reabsorption and the smaller the value of clearance, the more extensive is the degree of reabsorption.

When the ratio Cl_{drug}/Cl_{inulin} is equal to 1 (clearance of the drug is equal to the inulin clearance), then the drug is most probably filtered only. It should be borne in mind that a drug which is filtered, secreted, as well as reabsorbed may also have the ratio $Cl_{drug}/Cl_{inulin} = 1$.

The following example illustrates the graphical approach to determine clearance and the mechanism of drug excretion.

Example 7-3 The following data were obtained in 5 human subjects after administration of a single 500 mg oral dose of an antibiotic. Calculate renal clearance of the drug.

Amount of Drug Excreted:

Time (h):	0	2	4	6	8	12	16	20
Amount (mg):	0	80	64	50	46	76	52	4

Plasma Concentration:

Time (h):	0	3	5	7	10	14	18
Concentration (mg/L):	0	6.0	5.0	4.5	3.6	2.5	0.2

Solution

To plot rate of excretion of the drug versus concentration of drug in plasma, the data provided in Example 7-3 should be evaluated in order to develop information, which would be useful to plot excretion rate as a function of plasma concentration. That is, the data should be tabulated to calculate each excretion rate, which would correspond to its respective concentration of drug in the plasma.

The first step is to determine excretion rates during each time interval. This is because the corresponding plasma-drug concentrations depend upon the time interval during which drug excretion was determined. In this case, if excretion of drug was determined during the zero and the second hour after administration of the dose, the corresponding drug plasma concentration needed to plot the graph would be at the midpoint of the zero and the second hour, i.e. at the first hour after administration of the dose. If the excretion of drug was determined during the second and the fourth hour after administration of the dose, then the corresponding drug-plasma concentration needed to plot the graph would be at the midpoint of the second and fourth hour after administration of the dose, i.e. at the third hour. Similarly, if excretion of drug was determined during the fourth and the sixth hour after administration of the dose, the corresponding drug-plasma concentration needed to plot the graph would still be at the fifth hour and so on.

Excretion rates are rates of excretion of the drug. Excretion rates are determined by dividing the amount of drug excreted from the body with the time interval during which that amount of drug was excreted. For example, the excretion rate of drug during the first two hours (between time 0 and 2 hours) is determined by dividing the amount of drug excreted between time 0 and 2 hours (i.e. 80 mg) with the time interval during which this 80 mg of the drug was excreted (i.e. 2 hours):

$$\text{Excretion rate during the first two hours} = \frac{80 \text{ mg}}{2 \text{ h}} = 40 \text{ mg/h}$$

Similarly, excretion rate during the last four hours is determined by dividing amount of drug excreted between 16 and 20 hours (i.e. 4 mg) with time interval during which this 4 mg of drug was excreted (i.e. 4 hours):

$$\text{Excretion rate during the last four hours} = \frac{4 \text{ mg}}{4 \text{ h}} = 1 \text{ mg/h}$$

To obtain the corresponding plasma concentration for each excretion rate, the data given in Example 7-3 are examined. To plot excretion rate of drug during the first two hours (from 0 hour to 2 hours), the corresponding plasma concentration would be at the midpoint of this time interval, i.e. at the first hour. Similarly, to plot excretion rate of the drug during the last 4 hours (from 16 to 20 hours), the corresponding plasma concentration would be at the midpoint of the 16 to 20 hours, i.e. at 18 hours.

Table 7-1 is a retabulation of data given in Example 7-3 and shows the excretion rates of the drug (Column 3) and the plasma concentrations corresponding to each excretion rate (Column 5). In this Table, the first column (Column 1) indicates the time intervals between urinary excretion of the drug given in the data. Column 2 shows the amount of drug excreted during these time intervals and Column 3 is the excretion rate during each time interval which is obtained by dividing the value in Column 2 (amount excreted) by the time interval shown in Column 1. Column 4 indicates the midpoint for each time interval shown in Column 1 and Column 5 lists the plasma concentration of drug (given in the data in Example 7-3) for each of these mid-points. If the plasma concentration of drug for any of the midpoints (Column 3) is not available (e.g. plasma concentration at 1 hour in the data provided here), then the corresponding excretion rate is not used in the plot.

Figure 7-3 is a plot of excretion rate (Column 3 in Table 7-1) as a function of plasma concentration (Column 5 in Table 7-1). It will be noticed that excretion rate during the first two hours (0 to 2 hours) is not plotted because the data do not provide the corresponding plasma concentration of drug at 1 hour. The plot of the data in Fig. 7-3 exhibit a linear relationship, which indicates that elimination of the drug appears to be through glomerular filtration.

Table 7-1 Tabulation of data to obtain excretion rate and plasma concentration

1 *Interval (h)*	2 *Amount excreted (mg)*	3 *Excretion rate (mg/h)*	4 *Midpoint (h)*	5 *Drug-plasma concentration (mg/L)*
0–2	80	80/2 = 40	1	N/A
2–4	64	64/2 = 32	3	6.0
4–6	50	50/2 = 25	5	5.0
6–8	46	46/2 = 23	7	4.5
8–12	76	76/4 = 19	10	3.6
12–16	52	52/4 = 13	14	2.5
16–20	4	4/4 = 1	18	0.2

Determination of Clearance

Clearance, by definition, is the slope of the straight line in Figure 7-3. To calculate the slope, suppose the following two points are chosen: $x_1 = 0$ mg/L, $y_1 = 0$ mg/h and $x_2 = 6.0$ mg/L, $y_2 = 31.0$ mg/h. The excretion rate provided in the data ($y_2 = 32$ mg/h) cannot be chosen as one of the points, because this point is not on the straight line.

$$\text{Slope} = \frac{y_2 - y_1}{x_2 - x_1} = \frac{(31.0 - 0)\,\text{mg/h}}{(6.0 - 0)\,\text{mg/L}} = \frac{31.0\ \text{mg/h}}{6.0\ \text{mg/L}} = 5.1667\ \text{L/h}$$

$$Cl_r = \text{slope} = 5.1667\ \text{L/h} = \frac{0.51667\ \text{L}}{\text{h}} \times \frac{1{,}000\ \text{mL}}{\text{L}} \times \frac{\text{h}}{60\ \text{min}} = 86.1\ \text{mL/min}$$

A linear relationship between excretion rate and plasma concentration obtained in Figure 7-3 indicates that clearance is due to glomerular filtration, because excretion rate of the drug was dependant on the concentration of drug in plasma. A clearance value of 86.1 mL/min indicates the possibility of reabsorption because normal renal clearance value due to glomerular filtration in healthy subjects ranges between 109 and 156 mL/min. If the glomerular filtration rate of 109 mL/min is taken as a normal value in healthy subjects, then a clearance value of 86.1 mL/min indicates about 21% reabsorption. If the glomerular filtration rate of 156 mL/min is taken as a normal value in healthy subjects, then a clearance value of 86.1 mL/min indicates about 44% reabsorption.

It should be mentioned that if the subjects participating in this study were not healthy and had a renal impairment or elimination of the drug was altered due to physiological or medical problems, then the clearance value obtained in this study may not necessarily reflect reabsorption of the drug.

Example 7-4 The following data were obtained in 5 human subjects after administration of a single 200 mg oral dose of an antibiotic. Calculate renal clearance of drug.

Amount of Drug Excreted:

Time (h):	0	1	2	4	8	12	20	24
Amount (mg):	0	25.5	54.5	98.5	142.5	162.5	170.5	171.5

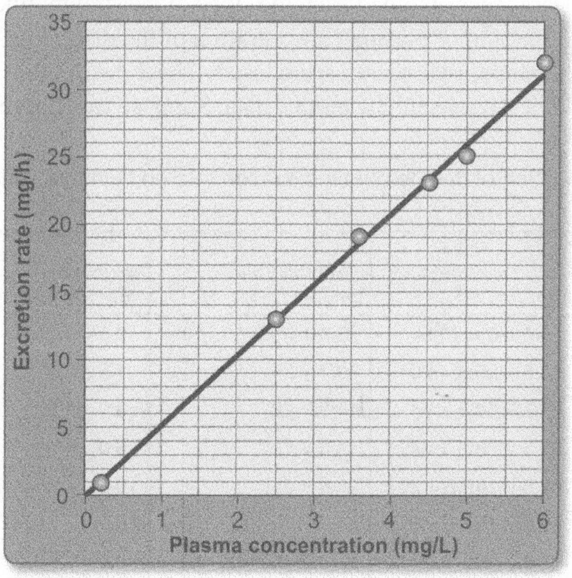

Fig. 7-3 Plot of excretion rate versus plasma concentration

Plasma Concentration:

Time (h):	0	0.5	1.5	3.0	6.0	10	16
Concentration (mg/L):	0	7.0	9.6	7.4	3.8	1.6	0.4

Solution

The data show that the amount of drug excreted in the urine increases with each time interval indicating that the amount excreted given in the data is cumulative amount excreted. Therefore, the amount of drug excreted during each time interval should be determined first. The amount of drug excreted during each time interval is obtained by subtracting the total amount of drug excreted during the preceding interval from the total amount of drug excreted during the time interval in question. In the data provided, the amount of drug excreted in urine at time 0 is 0 mg, at the end of 1 hour, a total amount of 21.5 mg is excreted and at the end of 2 hours a total of 54.5 mg is excreted. This means that:

The amount of drug excreted from 0 to 1 hour = 25.5 mg – 0 mg = 25.5 mg
The amount of drug excreted from 1 to 2 hour = 54.5 mg – 25.5 mg = 29 mg
The amount of drug excreted from 2 to 4 hour = 98.5 mg – 54.5 mg = 44 mg.

Since the midpoint of excretion rate for the first hour (time 0 to 1 hour) is 0.5 hour, therefore plasma concentration at 0.5 hour will be plotted for the excretion rate from 0 to 1 hour. Similarly, the mid-point of excretion rate for amount of drug excreted between 1 hour and 2 hours is 1.5 hours, therefore plasma concentration at 1.5 hour will be plotted for the excretion rate from 1 to 2 hours. And because the mid-point of excretion rate for the amount of drug excreted between 2 hours and 4 hours is 3 hours, therefore plasma concentration at 3 hours will be plotted for the excretion rate from 2 to 4 hours. The plasma concentration for each excretion rate will be at the midpoint of excretion rate in question.

Table 7-2 lists excretion rates (Column 3) and the corresponding plasma concentrations (Column 5).

Figure 7-4 shows the plot of excretion rate (Column 3 in Table 7-2) as a function of plasma concentration (Column 5 in Table 7-2) on a regular coordinate graph paper. Each excretion rate is plotted against its corresponding plasma concentration. It will be noticed that excretion rate during the last 4 hours (from 20 to 24 hours) is not plotted because the data do not provide the corresponding plasma concentration (at 22 hours).

The value of clearance is obtained from the slope of the straight line obtained when excretion rate is plotted as a function of plasma concentration of the drug (Fig. 7-4).

To calculate the slope, two points are chosen. These two points should be as far apart as possible and should best represent the plotted data. Suppose we choose the following two points:

Table 7-2 Tabulation of data to obtain excretion rate and plasma concentration

1 *Interval (h)*	2 *Amount excreted (mg)*	3 *Excretion rate (mg/h)*	4 *Midpoint (h)*	5 *Drug plasma concentration (mg/L)*
0–1	25.5 – 0 = 25.5	25.5/1 = 25.5	0.5	7.0
1–2	54.5 – 25.5 = 29	29/1 = 29	1.5	9.6
2–4	98.5 – 54.5 = 44	44/2 = 22	3.0	7.4
4–8	142.5 – 98.5 = 44	44/4 = 11	6.0	3.8
8–12	162.5 – 142.5 = 20	20/4 = 5	10.0	1.6
12–20	170.5 – 162.5 = 8	8/8 = 1	16.0	0.4
20–24	171.5 – 170.5 = 1	1/4 = 0.25	22.0	N/A

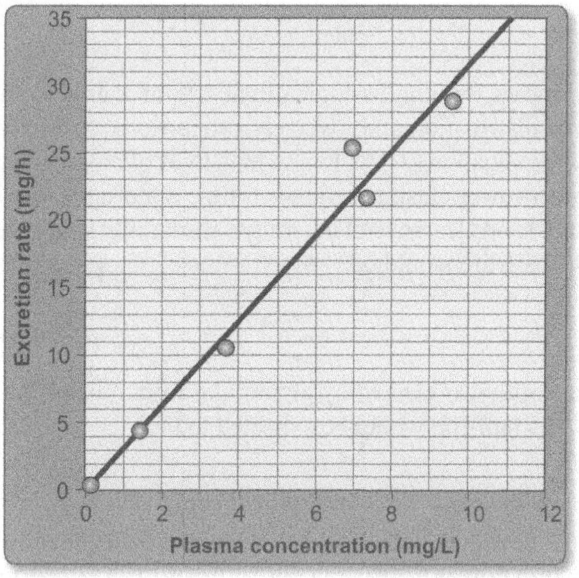

Fig. 7-4 Plot of excretion rate versus plasma concentration

$x_1 = 0$ mg/L, $y_1 = 0$ mg/h; and $x_2 = 11.0$ mg/L, $y_2 = 35.0$ mg/h.

It will be noticed that the data point, $x_2 = 9.6$ mg/h is not chosen to calculate the slope because this point is not on the straight line.

$$\text{Slope} = \frac{y_2 - y_1}{x_2 - x_1} = \frac{(35-0)\text{ mg/h}}{(11-0)\text{ mg/h}}$$

$$\text{Slope} = \frac{35\text{ mg/h}}{11\text{ mg/L}} = 3.18\text{ L/h}$$

$$Cl_r = \frac{3.18\text{ L}}{\text{h}} \times \frac{1{,}000\text{ mL}}{\text{L}} \times \frac{\text{h}}{60\text{ min}} = 53\text{ mL/min}$$

A linear relationship between excretion rate and plasma concentration in Fig. 7-4 indicates clearance by glomerular filtration. The clearance value of 53 mL/min indicates the possibility of reabsorption.

DRUGS ELIMINATED SOLELY BY RENAL EXCRETION

The main route of removal of many drugs is via renal excretion. The half-life of drugs principally eliminated through the kidneys can be determined if clearance and apparent volume of distribution are known. For a large number of drugs, such as penicillin, tetracycline, streptomycin, sulfonamides, hydrochlorothiazide, gentamicin, lithium, etc. the main route of removal of drug from the body is via renal excretion. In these cases the half-life of drug in the body can be determined if clearance and apparent volume of distribution of the drug are known.

$$\text{Since } Cl = (K)(V_d) \text{ and } K = \frac{0.693}{t_{1/2}}$$

$$\text{Therefore, } Cl = \frac{(0.693)\times(V_d)}{t_{1/2}} \tag{7-13}$$

$$\text{and } t_{1/2} = \frac{(0.693)\times(V_d)}{Cl} \tag{7-14}$$

This equation shows that the biological half-life of a drug is directly proportional to its apparent volume of distribution and inversely proportional to its clearance. According to the relationship shown in equation (7-14), longer half-lives of most drugs are due to larger volumes of distribution and/or lower clearance values. Thus, if a drug is distributed only in the plasma fluid (V_d = 3,000 mL) and clearance of the drug is essentially by glomerular filtration (clearance = 130 mL/min), its half-life would be:

$$t_{1/2} = \frac{(0.693)\times(3{,}000\text{ mL})}{130\text{ mL/min}} = 16\text{ min}$$

But, if the same drug was cleared by glomerular filtration and was distributed in total body fluids (V_d = 41 L), its half-life would be expected to be:

$$t_{1/2} = \frac{(0.693)\times(41{,}000\text{ mL})}{130\text{ mL/min}} = 219\text{ min}$$

This is about 14 times the half-life when drug was distributed in plasma only, because the volume of distribution now is approximately 14 times (41 L/3 L = 13.7). Similarly, if the drug was distributed in plasma fluid only and was cleared by total excretion, its half-life would be expected to be:

$$t_{1/2} = \frac{(0.693)\times(3{,}000\text{ mL})}{650\text{ mL/min}} = 3\text{ min}$$

This is one-fifth the value obtained when clearance was due to glomerular filtration only, because

$$\frac{\text{Clearance by filtration}}{\text{Clearance by total excretion}} = \frac{130\,\text{mL/min}}{650\,\text{mL/min}} = \frac{1}{5}$$

Similarly, if one calculated the half-life of a drug, which was distributed in total body fluids and the drug was cleared by glomerular filtration as well as by tubular secretion, then the half-life of the drug will be found to be:

$$t_{1/2} = \frac{(0.693)\times(41000\text{ mL})}{650\text{ mL/min}} = 44\text{ min}$$

This is approximately one-fifth of the half-life found when clearance was by filtration only:

$$\frac{\text{Clearance by total excretion}}{\text{Clearance by filtration}} = \frac{44\text{ min}}{219\text{ min}} = \frac{1}{5}$$

Clearly, there is no upper limit on elimination half-life, because: (a) renal clearance may be as low as 0 mL/min (e.g. extensive renal insufficiency or complete reabsorption and (b) the apparent volume of distribution can (and does in many cases) exceed the volume of total body fluids (e.g. extensive tissue binding).

Example 7-5 A drug is eliminated solely by glomerular filtration (GFR = 130 mL/min) and is 70% reabsorbed. If the apparent volume of distribution of this drug is known to be 12 L, calculate half-life of the drug.

Solution

There are two ways to handle this question:

a. Since reabsorption is 70%, therefore clearance = 100 – 70 = 30% of glomerular filtration. Clearance = 30% of 130 mL/min = (0.3)(130 mL/min) = 39 mL/min. Substituting the values of clearance and apparent volume of distribution into equation (7-14),

$$t_{1/2} = \frac{(0.693)\times(1,2000\text{ mL})}{39\text{ mL/min}} = \frac{8316\text{ mL}}{39\text{ mL/min}} = 213\text{ min}$$

b. Alternatively, if there was no reabsorption, half-life of the drug would be:

$$t_{1/2} = \frac{(0.693)\times(V_d)}{Cl} = \frac{(0.693)\times(1,2000\text{ mL})}{130\text{ mL/min}} = \frac{8316\text{ mL}}{130\text{ mL/min}} = 64\text{ min}$$

But, in this case, since reabsorption is 70%, therefore, filtration is only 30%.

therefore, $t_{1/2} = \frac{64\text{ min}}{30\%} = 213\text{ min}$

CREATININE CLEARANCE

Creatinine clearance represents the rate at which creatinine is removed from the blood by the kidneys. Creatinine is a metabolic breakdown product of the muscle creatinine phosphate and has a relatively constant level of daily production. However, creatinine production in an individual varies with the age, weight and sex of the individual. Under normal circumstances creatinine production is roughly equal to creatinine excretion; therefore, concentration of creatinine in the serum is more or less constant in a given individual. The normal serum creatinine values range between 0.6 mg/dL and 1.2 mg/dL, but the normal values vary with the amount of muscle mass. For example, serum creatinine levels are high in a muscular athlete and creatinine values are low in a person with fewer muscles. That is to say that while a value of 1.2 mg/dL is considered normal in the case of a muscular athlete, the same value is considered too high in a person who is small, sedentary and has little muscle mass.

Creatinine is excreted by glomerular filtration. Although it is not reabsorbed, a small amount of creatinine may be actively secreted by the renal tubules. Therefore, the values for glomerular filtration rate obtained by creatinine clearance tend to be slightly higher than the glomerular filtration rate measured by inulin clearance. For all practical purposes excretion of creatinine closely parallels glomerular filtration rate within a relatively narrow range (± 10%). The normal creatinine clearance for average healthy adult males is approximately 100 mL/min (± 25 mL/min).

Elevation of serum creatinine concentration is a good indicator of renal damage. This is because renal impairment is almost always the only cause of elevated serum creatinine levels. In a patient with reduced glomerular filtration, accumulation of serum creatinine will be usually in accordance with the degree of loss of glomerular filtration in the kidney. As a general rule, the value of serum creatinine doubles with each 50% decrease in glomerular filtration rate. For example, if the normal serum creatinine level in a patient is 1 mg/dL, then a serum creatinine concentration of 2 mg/dL will represent 50% renal function. In other words, if 1 mg/dL serum creatinine concentration represents 100% renal function in this particular patient, then a serum creatinine concentration of 2 mg/dL in this patient would represent 50% renal function. Similarly, a serum creatinine concentration of 4 mg/dL in this patient would represent 25% renal function. As an approximation, the degree of loss of glomerular filtration in the kidney can be estimated by dividing 100 with the patient's serum creatinine concentration (in mg/dL). Mathematically, this concept may be expressed by the following relationship:

$$\frac{100\%}{\text{Serum creatinine concentration}} = \%\text{ Renal function}$$

For example, if 1 mg/dL serum creatinine concentration represents 100% renal function in a particular patient, then a serum creatinine concentration of 2 mg/dL in this patient would represent

$$\frac{100\%}{2} = 50\%\text{ Renal function}$$

Similarly, if 1 mg/dL serum creatinine concentration represents 100% renal function in a particular patient, then a serum creatinine concentration of 4 mg/dL in this patient would represent

$$\frac{100\%}{4} = 25\% \text{ Renal function}$$

Calculation of Creatinine Clearance

Creatinine clearance (Cl_{cr}) is calculated using the relationship between the rate of excretion of creatinine by the kidneys and the concentration of creatinine in the serum. To obtain a reliable rate of urinary excretion of creatinine, the excretion rate of creatinine is measured over a relatively long period of time, e.g. over a 24 hour period.

In actual practice, the amount of creatinine excreted by the kidneys is determined from a 24 hour pooled urine sample by determining the concentration of creatinine in the pooled sample. If C_u is the concentration of creatinine in urine (in mg/mL) and V is the volume (in mL) of urine voided (total volume of urine collected in 24 hours), then the amount of creatinine excreted in 24 hours is calculated as follows:

Since,

$$\text{Amount} = (\text{Concentration}) \times (\text{Volume}), \quad (7\text{-}15)$$

$$\text{Therefore, amount of creatinine excreted} = (C_u \text{ in mg/mL})(V \text{ in mL}) \quad (7\text{-}16)$$

$$\text{or, amount of creatinine excreted} = (C_u)(V) \text{ mg} \quad (7\text{-}17)$$

The rate of urinary excretion of creatinine is calculated as follows:

$$\text{Since, rate} = \frac{\text{Amount}}{\text{Time}} \quad (7\text{-}18)$$

$$\text{Creatinine excretion rate} = \frac{(C_u)\times(V)}{t} \text{ mg/h} \quad (7\text{-}19)$$

The serum creatinine concentration is determined at the midpoint of the urinary collection period to reflect serum creatinine concentration during the period of urinary excretion. Thus, if urine is collected over a 24 hour period, then the serum creatinine concentration is determined at the 12th hour of the urine collection period.

If C_{cr} is serum creatinine concentration (in mg/mL) during this period, then

$$Cl_{cr} = \frac{\text{Excretion rate}}{\text{Serum creatinine concentration}}$$

$$Cl_{cr} = \frac{\{(C_u)\times(V)/t\} \text{ in mg/h}}{C_{Cr}\text{, in mg/mL}}$$

$$Cl_{cr} = \frac{(C_u)\times(V)}{(t)\times(C_{Cr})} \text{ mL/h} \quad (7\text{-}20)$$

Creatinine clearance is clinically expressed in mL/min. Since clinical laboratories express serum creatinine concentration in mg% (mg/dL or mg/100 mL) and if the volume of urine collected in 24 hours is expressed in mL, then equation (7-20) may be written as:

$$Cl_{cr} = \frac{(C_u)\times(V)\times(100)}{(1{,}440)\times(C_{Cr})} \text{ mL/min} \quad (7\text{-}21)$$

Example 7-6 The serum creatinine concentration in a hospital patient was found to be 1.1 mg/dL. Over a 24 hour period, 1.73 L of urine was collected and the concentration of creatinine in the urine was found to be 0.98 mg/mL. Calculate creatinine clearance in this patient.

Solution

Substituting $C_u = 0.98$ mg/mL, V = 1.73 L = 1730 mL and $C_{cr} = 1.1$ mg/dL into equation (7-21):

$$Cl_{cr} = \frac{(C_u) \times (V) \times (100)}{(1,440 \text{ min}) \times (C_{cr})} \text{ mL/min}$$

$$Cl_{cr} = \frac{(0.98 \text{ mg/mL}) \times (1,730 \text{ mL}) \times (100)}{(1,440 \text{ min}) \times (1.1 \text{ mg})} = \frac{169,540 \text{ mL}}{1,584 \text{ min}}$$

$$Cl_{cr} = 107 \text{ mL/min}$$

RENAL FUNCTION IN ADULTS

As mentioned earlier, clearance is affected by a variety of factors, including age, sex and kidney and cardiac diseases. Since renal clearance depends on renal function, it follows that any change in renal clearance will reflect a corresponding change in renal function. Studies have shown that renal function normally declines with increasing age. Therefore therapeutic monitoring may be required in middle-age and older patients and also in patients with nephrotoxicity or acute or chronic renal failure. This is especially important if a large amount of the administered drug dose is excreted unchanged in the urine.

Determination of creatinine clearance using the relationship between rate of creatinine excretion in urine and concentration of creatinine in the serum poses a few problems. Specifically, determination of urinary excretion rate of creatinine is the most time-consuming element. This is because determination of excretion rate of creatinine in the urine involves the time necessary for complete 24 hour urine collection from the patient and time necessary for the analysis of urine sample. These problems preclude direct estimation of creatinine clearance. Since serum creatinine concentration is related to creatinine clearance, therefore, in practice, creatinine clearance is most often estimated from the concentration of creatinine in the plasma (serum) of the patient. The advantage of estimating creatinine clearance from serum creatinine concentration is that serum creatinine is measured routinely in the clinical laboratory.

Creatinine Clearance from Serum Creatinine Concentration

Various methods have been proposed to estimate creatinine clearance based on concentration of creatinine in the plasma. The concentration of creatinine in the plasma is also referred to as the serum creatinine concentration of the patient. Most of the methods proposed to estimate creatinine clearance are essentially based on the age and/or the weight of the patient and the concentration of creatinine in the serum of the patient. These methods make two important assumptions:

a. The first assumption is stable creatinine clearance during renal insufficiency, i.e. stable renal function. It is assumed that renal function in the patient does not change during renal insufficiency
b. It is assumed that no abnormal muscle disease (e.g. muscular dystrophy or hypertrophy) occurs during renal insufficiency.

These two assumptions are important because if renal function undergoes further changes during renal insufficiency, it is conceivable that a change may also occur in serum creatinine concentration of the patient. If, during renal insufficiency, a change occurs in the serum creatinine concentration of the patient, then it may be essential to monitor the serum creatinine concentration of patient during the course of therapy. And, if the serum creatinine concentration of the patient does change during the course of therapy, then it may be necessary to reevaluate creatinine clearance as needed. Creatinine clearance in obese patients may be based on lean body weight or on actual body weight, whichever is lower.

Of the various methods available for the estimatation of renal function, three methods are frequently used. They are:

1. Jelliffe method
2. Cockcroft and Gault method
3. Siersback-Nielsen method.

Cockcroft and Gault method and Siersback-Nielsen method are based upon similar parameters. Therefore, creatinine clearance values obtained using these two methods are generally found comparable.

Jelliffe Method

Jelliffe method of determining creatinine clearance is based on age and serum creatinine concentration of the patient. This method is not intended for patients under 20 years of age and should be used to calculate creatinine clearance in mature adults only. This method is generally applicable for adult patients up to the age of 80 years.

Jelliffe method uses the following two equations for the determination of creatinine clearance in males and in females:

a. Creatinine clearance in males,

$$Cl_{cr} \text{ in males} = \frac{98 - 0.8 \times (y - 20)}{(C_{cr})} \quad (7\text{-}22)$$

In this equation,
y is age in years and
C_{cr} is serum creatinine concentration in mg/dL.

b. Creatinine clearance in females:
According to Jelliffe method, creatinine clearance in females is 90% that in males. Therefore, in the case of females, equation (7-22) is multiplied by 90% or 0.9, i.e.

$$Cl_{cr} \text{ in females} = (0.9) \times \frac{98 - 0.8 \times (y - 20)}{(C_{cr})} \quad (7\text{-}23)$$

Example 7-7 Calculate creatinine clearance in a 75-year-old female having a serum creatinine concentration value of 0.8 mg/dL.

Solution

Creatinine clearance in an adult female is given by equation (7-23):

$$Cl_{cr} \text{ in females} = (0.9) \times \frac{98 - 0.8 \times (y - 20)}{(C_{cr})}$$

$$= (0.9) \times \frac{98 - 0.8 \times (75 - 20)}{0.8}$$

$$= (0.9) \times \frac{98 - 44}{0.8} = (0.9) \times (67.5)$$

$$= 60.75 \text{ mL/min}$$

Example 7-8 Calculate creatinine clearance in a 95-year-old female having a serum creatinine concentration of 0.8 mg/dL.

Solution

Creatinine clearance in an adult female is given by equation (7-23) is:

$$Cl_{cr} \text{ in females} = (0.9) \times \frac{98 - 0.8 \times (95 - 20)}{(C_{cr})}$$

$$= (0.9) \times \frac{98 - 0.8 \times (95 - 20)}{0.8}$$

$$= (0.9) \times \frac{98 - 60}{0.8}$$

$$= (0.9) \times (47.5)$$

$$= 42.75 \text{ mL/min}$$

From Examples (7-7) and (7-8) it is seen that according to Jelliffe method, creatinine clearance is smaller for the older patient even though both patients had the same serum creatinine concentration.

Cockcroft and Gault Method

Cockcroft and Gault method differs from Jelliffe method in that it takes into account the weight of the patient also, i.e. this method is based upon age, weight and serum creatinine concentration of the patient. Cockcroft and Gault method uses the following equations to estimate creatinine clearance.

a. Creatinine clearance in males

$$Cl_{cr} \text{ in males} = \frac{(140 - y) \times (w)}{(72) \times (C_{cr})} \tag{7-24}$$

where,
y is age of patient in years,
C_{cr} is serum creatinine concentration in mg/dL and
w is weight of the patient in kilograms.

The lean body weight of patient may be used in this method. The lean body weight is determined using the following equation:

$$\text{Lean body weight in males} = 0.3281\ W + 0.3393\ H - 29.5336 \tag{7-25}$$

where,
W is weight in kilograms and
H is height in centimeters.

b. Creatinine clearance in females

According to the method of Cockcroft and Gault, creatinine clearance in females is about 85% of creatinine clearance in males. Therefore, in the case of females, the value obtained in equation (7-24) is multiplied by 0.85, i.e.

$$Cl_{cr} \text{ in females} = (0.85) \times \frac{(140 - y) \times (w)}{(72) \times (C_{cr})} \tag{7-26}$$

where,
y is age of the patient in years,
C_{cr} is serum creatinine concentration in mg/dL and
w is weight of the patient in kilograms.

The lean body weight of patient may be used in this method. The lean body weight is determined using the following equation:

$$\text{Lean body weight in females} = 0.2967\ W + 0.4181\ H - 43.2933 \tag{7-27}$$

where,
W is weight of the patient in kilograms and
H is height of the patient in centimeters.

Example 7-9 Calculate creatinine clearance in a 75-year-old female, weighing 110 lb, having a serum creatinine concentration of 0.8 mg/dL.

Solution

The creatinine clearance in an adult female is given by equation (7-26):

$$Cl_{cr} \text{ in females} = (0.85) \times \frac{(140 - y) \times (w)}{(72) \times (C_{cr})}$$

The weight of the patient in kg is:

$$w = \frac{110 \text{ lbs}}{2.2 \text{ lbs/kg}} = 50 \text{ kg}$$

Substituting the values, y = 75, w = 50 and C_{cr} = 0.8 into equation (7-26), one obtains

$$Cl = (0.85) \times \frac{(140 - 75) \times (50)}{(72) \times (0.8)}$$

$$= (0.85) \times \frac{(65) \times (50)}{57.6}$$

$$= 48 \text{ mL/min}$$

It will be noticed that creatinine clearance obtained by this method is different from that obtained in Example 7-7 using Jelliffe method although age, gender and serum creatinine concentrations were same in both cases. This is because Jelliffe method does not take into account the weight of the patient, while the method of Cockcroft and Gault does. Thus, for patients with same age, gender and serum creatinine concentration, creatinine clearance values obtained by the method of Cockcroft and Gault will vary depending upon the weight of the patient, while those obtained by Jelliffe method will not.

Siersback-Nielsen Method

The Siersback-Nielsen method of determining creatinine clearance is similar to the method of Cockcroft and Gault. This method also makes use of serum creatinine concentration, weight, age and gender of the patient. The difference in the two methods is that instead of an equation, this method uses a nomogram (Fig. 7-5). Although use of a nomogram is relatively easier than using an equation, use of an equation generally provides a more accurate answer.

The nomogram shown in Figure 7-5 consists of five vertical lines, drawn parallel to and at suitable distances from each other. These lines are labeled (from left to right) in the following order:

Clearance (in mL/min)
Weight (in Kg)
R (no units, because this line represents the point of reference)
Age (in years)
Serum Creatinine Concentration (in mg/dL).

The vertical line labeled "Age" is marked separately for males and females, the markings on the right-hand side of this line are for females and markings on the left hand-side are for males. The nomogram is used as follows:

a. Draw a straight line to connect patient's weight (on the second line from left) to the patient's age (on the second line from right). This gives a point of intersection on the middle line R.
b. Draw a straight line to connect the patient's serum creatinine value (in mg/dL) on the first line on right to the point of intersection on line R and extrapolate this straight line to the first line on left to read creatinine clearance.

Example 7-10 Using the Siersback-Nielsen method, calculate the creatinine clearance in a 75-year-old male, weighing 170 lbs. The serum creatinine concentration in this patient is 0.95 mg/dL.

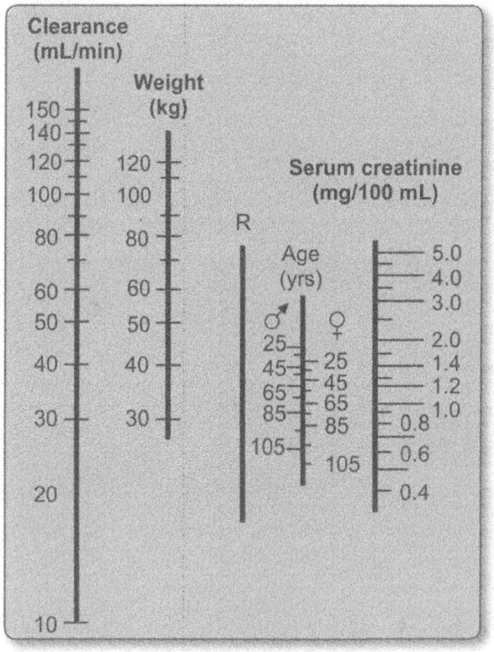

Fig. 7-5 Siersback-Nielsen nomogram for determination of creatinine clearance. *Courtesy:* K Siersback-Nielsen, JM Hansen, J Kampmann and M Kristensen "Rapid Evaluation of Creatinine Clearance," Lancet. 1971;1:1133-34

Solution

In the Siersback-Nielsen nomogram (Fig. 7-6), mark the patient's age (75 years, on the left-hand side of the second line from right) with the patient's weight (170 lbs, which is 77.3 kg, on the second line from left). Now connect these two points (patient's age and patient's weight) with a straight line.

This will give a point of intersection on the line labeled "*R*". This is the reference point. Now, draw a straight line to connect the patient's serum creatinine concentration (0.95 mg/dL, on the first line on right) with the intersection point on the line labeled "*R*" and extrapolate this straight line to the first line on left. It reads creatinine clearance of approximately 70 mL/min.

From the Siersback-Nielsen nomogram, the patient's creatinine clearance is determined to be approximately 70 mL/min.

Example 7-11 Using the data given in Example 7-10, calculate the creatinine clearance by the method of Cockcroft and Gault and Jelliffe method, and compare the results with the answer obtained by the Siersback-Nielsen method.

Solution

a. Cockcroft and Gault method

Creatinine clearance in males by Cockcroft and Gault method is given by equation (7-24):

$$\text{Cl}_{\text{cr}} \text{ in males} = \frac{(140 - y) \times (w)}{(72) \times (C_{cr})}$$

$$= \frac{(140 - 75) \times (170/2.2)}{(72) \times (0.95)}$$

$$= \frac{(65) \times (77.3)}{68.4}$$

$$= 73.46 \text{ mL/min}$$

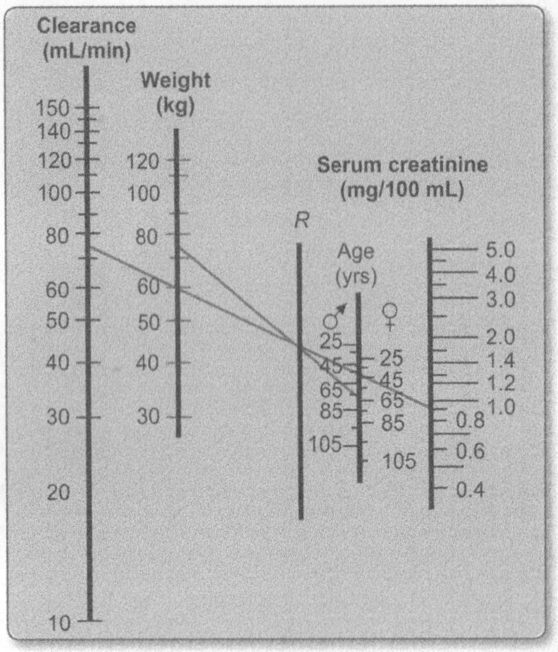

Fig. 7-6 Determination of creatinine clearance in Example 7-10 with Siersback-Nielsen nomogram

b. Jelliffe method

Creatinine clearance in males by Jelliffe method is given by equation (7-22):

$$Cl_{cr} \text{ in males} = \frac{98 - 0.8 \times (y - 20)}{(C_{cr})}$$

$$= \frac{98 - 0.8 \times (75 - 20)}{0.95}$$

$$= \frac{54}{0.95} = 56.84 \text{ mL/min}$$

c. Siersback-Nielsen Method

The value of creatinine clearance obtained in Example 7-10 using the nomogram of Siersback-Nielsen was approximately 70 mL/min. Although this value is very similar to the value obtained by the method of Cockcroft and Gault, it is very different from the value obtained by the Jelliffe method.

RENAL FUNCTION IN INFANTS

Incomplete development of renal function at birth is a potential source of differences in pharmacokinetics and pharmacology of some drugs in premature newborns, infants and children under the age of 2 years. These differences are due to two reasons: (i) variation in body composition and (ii) lack of maturity of kidney function. The lack of maturity of kidney function in infants and young children affects both modes of renal elimination—tubular secretion as well as glomerular filtration.

Tubular Secretion: There are two tubular functions—secretory mechanism and reabsorption. The primary reason for reduced renal tubular function in infants (secretory mechanism and absorptive capacity) is that the enzyme systems involved in the secretory mechanisms are not completely developed in infants. Some of the drugs that are affected by this immaturity are salicylic acid, penicillins and phenylbutazone.

Glomerular filtration: The reduced renal excretion by glomerular filtration in infants and young children is due to two reasons:

a. Poor permeability of glomerular membrane
b. Reduced renal blood flow relative to the volume of body water.

Because of these two reasons, reduction in renal clearance in the premature newborns and in infants is about 30% to 50% per unit of body weight. For example, inulin clearance (glomerular filtration) in an average adult is 1.86 mL per min per kg of body weight, whereas in the newborns inulin clearance is only 0.86 mL per min per kg of body weight.

Similarly, the clearance of p-aminohippuric acid (PAH) in average adults is 9.29 mL per min per kg of body weight, but in the newborns the clearance of PAH is only 3.43 mL per min per kg body of weight. Therefore, drugs that depend heavily on renal excretion will exhibit significantly reduced elimination and consequently a sharp increase in their biological half-lives. For example, since penicillins are predominantly excreted through the kidneys, the elimination half-lives of these drugs are sharply increased in infants and newborn babies. In addition to the lack of maturity of kidney function, the pH of the newborn's urine is more acidic, which allows the reabsorption of slightly acidic drugs. Some examples of these drugs include chlorates, ethacrynic acid, furosemide, indomethacin, penicillins, phenobarbital and phenytoin.

The renal function in newborns quickly improves by about 4 weeks of age, therefore the excretion rate is sufficient to follow most of the standard dosage schedule. Full adult capacity, however, may not be achieved until the end of the first year of life. A comparison of renal clearance (glomerular filtration as well as tubular secretion) in adults and newborn babies is shown in Table 7-3.

The significant effect of renal immaturity on drug treatment is the potential of drug toxicity. Although drug toxicity in the newborn and young children has been commonly attributed to incomplete or slow metabolism of drug, inefficient renal function should not be overlooked as a potential contributory factor. If a drug is administered as a single dose treatment for an acute condition (e.g. a single dose analgesic), it does not matter if the biological half-life is increased significantly. In some cases it may be desirable if the half-life of the drug is increased because then the duration of action of the drug is prolonged. But, in the case of chronic diseases and in those conditions when the drug is administered for longer periods (e.g. multiple dose administration of analgesics or treatment of infection with antibiotics), the increase in the biological half-life of drug poses a potential danger of drug accumulation. It is important that the pharmacist alert and counsel parents concerning long-term administration of over-the-counter medications to newborns and premature infants.

Table 7-3 Comparison of renal clearance in adults and newborns

Parameter	*Average Adult*	*Average Newborn*	*% of Adult*
Body Weight (kg)	70	3.5	5
Body Water (L)	41	2.7	6.6
(L per kg body weight)	0.59	0.77	130
Inulin Clearance			
(mL/min)	130	3	2.3
(per kg body weight)	1.86	0.86	46
(half-life, min)	219	630	287
PAH* Clearance			
(mL/min)	650	12	1.8
(per kg body weight)	9.3	3.4	37
(half-life, min)	43	160	372

*PAH = P-aminohippuric acid.

Calculation of Creatinine Clearance

In pediatric practice, determination of creatinine clearance using the relationship between urinary creatinine excretion rate and creatinine concentration in the serum is not used, because collection of a 24 hour pooled sample of urine for determination of creatinine excretion rate in urine is just not feasible in infants and children. Among the methods available for calculating creatinine clearance in children, the two more popular methods are the method of Schwartz and associates and the method of Traub and Johnson. Both methods use body length (height) and serum creatinine concentration of the child. However, the method of Schwartz and associates uses an equation and the method of Traub and Johnson makes use of a nomogram.

Method of Schwartz and Associates

The method of Schwartz and Associates uses the following equation for calculating creatinine clearance in children. Creatinine clearance obtained is expressed in mL/min/1.73 m^2.

$$Cl_{cr} = \frac{(0.55) \times (\text{height in cm})}{(C_{cr})} \text{ mL/min/1.73 m}^2 \quad (7\text{-}28)$$

According to equation (7-28), creatinine clearance is directly proportion to the height of those children who have similar serum creatinine concentration.

Example 7-12 What is the creatinine clearance for a 120 cm tall 9-year old child, having a serum creatinine concentration of 1 mg/dL?

Solution

According to the method of Schwartz and Associates, creatinine clearance for a child is

$$Cl_{cr} = \frac{(0.55) \times (\text{height, in cm})}{(C_{cr})} \text{ mL/min/1.73 m}^2$$

$$= \frac{(0.55) \times (120)}{1} = 66 \text{ mL/min/1.73 m}^2$$

Since the equation of Schwartz and Associates used for the calculation of creatinine clearance is based only on the height of the child and does not take into consideration either the age or the weight of the child, it follows that this equation will give identical creatinine clearance values for two children with differing age and weight, but having the same height.

Method of Traub and Johnson

This method uses a nomogram, which requires the height of the patient and serum creatinine concentration of the patient. According to the authors of this method, the development of this nomogram was based upon the observations of 81 children between the ages of 6 and 12 years.

The nomogram, shown in Fig. 7-7, consists of three vertical straight lines, drawn parallel to each other and at suitable distances from each other. These straight lines are:

a. The vertical straight line on the left represents serum creatinine concentration of the patient. This straight line can be used for serum creatinine concentration ranging between 0.4 mg/dL to 6 mg/dL. This straight line is subdivided into units expressing serum creatinine concentration in mg/dL.
b. The vertical straight line on the right represents height. This straight line is subdivided into units expressing height of the child in centimeters. This straight line can be used for height ranging between 30 cm and 200 cm.

c. The vertical straight line in the middle of these two parallel lines represents creatinine clearance. This straight line is subdivided into units and expresses creatinine clearance in terms of mL/min/1.73 m^2. This straight line can be used to "read" creatinine clearance values ranging between 2 mL/min/1.73 m^2 and 160 mL/min/1.73 m^2.

To use this nomogram, a straight line is drawn to connect the value of patient's serum creatinine concentration (in mg/dL) to the patient's height (in cm). The point of intersection of this straight line on the vertical straight line in the middle of nomogram gives creatinine clearance in mL/min/1.73 m^2.

As can be seen from the nomogram shown in Figure 7-7, the method of Traub and Johnson for the determination of creatinine clearance of a child does not take into consideration the age of the child or the weight of the patient. It means that the method of Traub and Johnson will yield the same value of creatinine clearance for all children regardless of their age or weight, as long as these children have the same height and the same serum creatinine concentration.

Example 7-13 Using the method of Traub and Johnson, determine the creatinine clearance for a 9-year-old child who stands 120 cm tall and having a serum creatinine concentration of 1 mg/dL.

Solution

To determine creatinine clearance of the child using the method of Traub and Johnson, the nomogram shown in Figure 7-8 is used.

i. Draw a straight line to connect patient's height (120 cm) with patient's serum creatinine concentration (1 mg/dL).
ii. The point of intersection of this straight line on the middle straight line reads creatinine clearance = 57 mL/min/1.73 m^2.

It will be noticed that this value is much different from the value obtained by the method of Schwartz and associates.

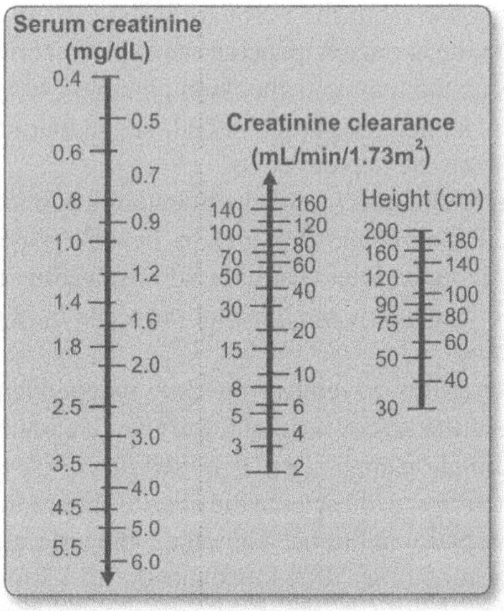

Fig. 7-7 Traub and Johnson nomogram for determination of creatinine clearance. *Courtesy:* SL Traub and CE Johnson. "Comparison methods of estimating creatinine clearance in children." Am J Hosp Pharm. 1980;37:195-201

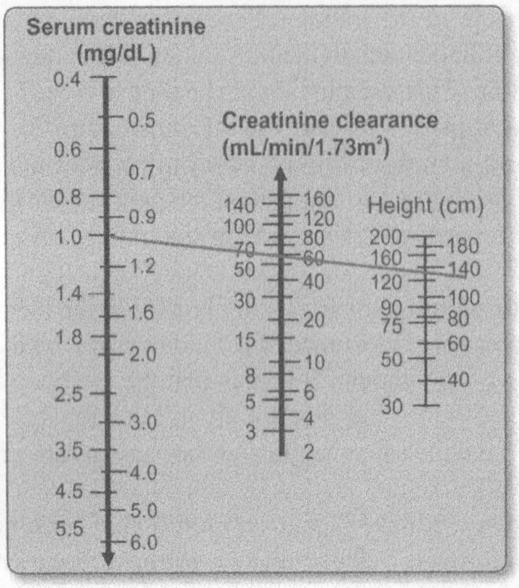

Fig. 7-8 Determination of creatinine clearance in Example 7-13 using the nomogram of Traub and Johnson

HEPATIC CLEARANCE

The liver is the largest gland in the body and performs an astonishingly large number of tasks that impact all body systems. One consequence of this complexity is that hepatic disease has widespread effect on virtually all organ systems in the body.

The hepatic vascular system has several unique characteristics relative to other organs. The circulatory system of the liver is unlike that seen in any other organ. Of great importance is the fact that a majority of the liver's blood supply is venous blood. Roughly 75% of the blood entering the liver is venous blood from the portal vein. Importantly, all of the venous blood returning from the small intestine, stomach, pancreas and spleen converges into the portal vein. One consequence of this is that the liver gets the "first pickings" of everything absorbed in the small intestine, which is where all nutrients are absorbed. The remaining 25% of the blood supply to the liver is arterial blood from the hepatic artery.

Hepatic clearance refers to the volume of drug-containing plasma that is cleared of the drug by liver per unit time. Blood enters the liver by hepatic portal vein and hepatic artery and leaves the liver by hepatic vein. After oral drug administration, the drug is absorbed from gastrointestinal tract into the mesenteric vessels and proceeds to hepatic portal vein, to liver, and then to systemic circulation.

The liver has the intrinsic ability to remove the drug independently of blood flow. This is called *intrinsic clearance*. As the name suggests, intrinsic clearance is primarily due to the inherent ability of biotransformation enzymes (e.g. mixed function oxidase) to biotransform the drug as it enters liver. The activity of these enzymes varies due to the presence of other drugs or the presence of environmental conditions. Therefore, intrinsic clearance varies depending on concomitant administration of other drugs or exposure to various environmental factors. Some drugs and environmental factors increase activity of these enzymes and some drugs and environmental factors do just the opposite. For example, phenobarbital (or drugs which produce phenobarbital as biotransformation product) or exposure to tobacco smoke increases the level of these enzymes, while administration of drugs such as cimetidine or exposure to acute lead poisoning has an inhibitory effect on these enzymes.

Hepatic clearance also includes excretion of drug into the bile. Biliary drug excretion is an active transport process and involves excretion of the following:

a. Drugs with a relatively high molecular weight (generally, a molecular weight greater than 500)
b. Polar drugs
c. Glucuronide conjugates of various drugs.

Some drugs are absorbed from the gastrointestinal tract by the mesenteric and hepatic portal vein into the liver. The liver may secrete some of the drug (either unchanged or as a glucuronide metabolite) into the bile. From the bile the drug may empty back (through bile duct) into the gastrointestinal tract for absorption once again. Glucuronide metabolite of the drug may also empty from the bile into gastrointestinal tract where bacteria may hydrolyze the glucuronide conjugate allowing the released drug to be reabsorbed.

Reabsorption of the drug after hepatic pass is known as *enterohepatic circulation* and is responsible for the drug being recycled.

Calculation of Hepatic Clearance

Hepatic clearance is usually not measured directly. Hepatic clearance is most often estimated indirectly either from total body clearance and renal body clearance or from hepatic extraction ratio. The following two methods are used for estimating hepatic clearance:

From Renal and Total Clearance: In this method, hepatic clearance is determined as the difference between total body clearance and renal clearance. The following equation describes this method:

$$Cl_h = Cl - Cl_r \quad (7\text{-}29)$$

where,
Cl_h = hepatic clearance,
Cl = total body clearance
Cl_r = renal clearance.

Since the total body clearance, by definition, is the sum total of renal clearance (Cl_r) and non-renal clearance (Cl_{nr}), it follows that hepatic clearance is equivalent to non-renal clearance (Cl_{nr}).

From Hepatic Extraction Ratio: Hepatic clearance may also be calculated by using the following relationship between hepatic blood flow and hepatic extraction ratio:

$$Cl_h = (Q_H) \times (HER) \quad (7\text{-}30)$$

where,
Q_H = hepatic blood flow
HER = extraction ratio.

Hepatic Extraction Ratio

Hepatic extraction ratio is the fraction of drug removed from plasma by the liver. The fraction of drug removed by the liver is expressed as a ratio and this fraction is obtained as a fractional difference between the arterial concentration of drug in plasma entering the liver, the venous concentration of drug in plasma exiting the liver. This fractional difference is determined by dividing the amount of drug removed from plasma by the amount of drug contained in the plasma as it enters liver. Thus, if

C_A = the arterial concentration of drug in plasma entering the liver
C_V = the venous concentration of drug in plasma exiting the liver, then

the amount of drug removed from plasma by the liver is represented by the difference between the arterial and the venous concentrations of drug in the plasma, i.e. ($C_A - C_V$).

Therefore, the fraction of drug removed by the liver, i.e. hepatic extraction ratio is given by the relationship:

$$\text{Hepatic extraction ratio} = \frac{C_A - C_V}{C_A} \tag{7-31}$$

The concept of extraction ratio used in the removal of drug by the liver is similar to the concept of excretion ratio used in the removal of drug by the kidneys (renal excretion). Similar to the renal excretion ratio, the value of hepatic extraction ratio may range from 0 to 1. When extraction ratio is 0, it indicates that no drug is removed by the liver and when extraction ratio is 1.0, it means that the entire quantity of drug is removed as the drug-containing plasma perfuses through the liver. For example, hepatic extraction ratio of 0.25 indicates that 25% of the drug was removed by liver as the drug-containing plasma perfused through the liver.

Generally speaking, hepatic extraction ratio of less than 0.2 indicates a low extraction ratio and hepatic extraction ratio higher than 0.7 indicates a high extraction ratio. For some drugs, such as, isoproterenol, lidocaine and nitroglycerin, the hepatic extraction ratio is high (greater than 0.7) and the drug is removed by liver as rapidly as the drug-containing blood perfuses through the organ. Examples of drugs having an extraction ratio less than 0.5 include acetaminophen, diazepam, digoxin, phenytoin, theophylline tolbutamide and warfarin.

Table 7-4 lists some examples of drugs and their hepatic extraction ratios.

Hepatic Blood Flow

Hepatic blood flow plays an important role in hepatic clearance, because hepatic clearance is affected by blood flow to the liver. An increase in hepatic blood flow is likely to increase the rate of removal of drug by the liver and a decrease in hepatic blood flow is likely to decrease the rate of removal of drug by the liver. Under normal conditions, the rate of blood flow to the liver is approximately 1.5 liters per minute. However, this value changes due to changes in the environment and/or physical activity of the individual patient. Various conditions have been reported to alter the flow of blood to the liver. The more important factors include the following:

i. Presence of drugs
ii. Presence of disease state
iii. Exercise.

For example, propranolol, a beta-adrenergic blocking agent, has been shown to decrease hepatic blood flow by decreasing cardiac output. Therefore, this drug decreases its own hepatic clearance when it is administered orally.

Table 7-4 Hepatic extraction ratios of some drugs

Drugs with extraction ratio greater than 0.5	
Labetalol	Pentazocine
Lidocaine	Pethidine
Metoprolol	Propoxyphene
Morphine	Propranolol
Nortriptyline	Verapamil
Drugs with extraction ratio less than 0.5	
Binding Sensitive	**Binding Insensitive**
Chlorpromazine	Acetaminophen
Diazepam	Chloramphenicol
Digitoxin	Hexobarbital
Phenytoin	Theophylline
Tolbutamide	Quinidine
Warfarin	

Example 7-14 Calculate the fraction of drug removed by liver if arterial plasma concentration of a drug entering the liver is 1.85 mg/L and venous plasma concentration of the drug is 1.12 mg/L.

Solution

Here, C_A = 1.85 mg/L and C_V = 1.12 mg/L, therefore, hepatic extraction ratio is

$$\text{Hepatic extraction ratio} = \frac{C_A - C_V}{C_A}$$

$$= \frac{1.85 \text{ mg/L} - 1.12 \text{ mg/L}}{1.85 \text{ mg/L}}$$

$$= 0.395$$

FIRST-PASS EFFECT

First-pass effect is a phenomenon, which usually occurs with an orally administered drug. In this phenomenon, a portion of the orally administered drug undergoes elimination before it has a chance to be absorbed into systemic circulation. It is for this reason that this phenomenon is also known as *presystemic elimination.*

Determination of First-Pass Effect

First-pass effect is usually determined and measured by comparing the extent of absorption of orally administered drug with that of an intravenously administered rapid bolus dose. Since, area under the plasma concentration versus time curve is an indicator of extent of absorption, the area under the curve obtained from an orally administered dose is compared with that obtained from an intravenous rapid bolus dose of an aqueous solution of identical dose of the drug. If area under the curve obtained from oral dose is less than that obtained from intravenous dose, then it is suspected that the drug undergoes first-pass effect. In order for a drug to undergo first-pass effect, the following conditions must be met:

a. The entire drug dose administered orally is released from dosage form and is made available for absorption,
b. The drug is not acid-labile,
c. The drug is not destroyed in the gastrointestinal tract by the gastrointestinal enzymes
d. The area under the plasma concentration versus time curve from the orally administered dose is less than area under the plasma concentration versus time curve from the intravenously administered dose.

The extent to which an orally administered dose undergoes first pass effect is determined by the fractional difference between area under the plasma concentration versus time curve obtained from intravenous dose and area under the plasma concentration versus time curve obtained from the oral dose. The fractional difference between the two areas is determined using the equation:

$$\text{Fractional difference} = \frac{AUC_{IV} - AUC_{oral}}{AUC_{IV}} \qquad (7\text{-}32)$$

where,

AUC_{IV} = area under the plasma concentration versus time curve obtained from the intravenous dose, and

AUC_{oral} = area under the plasma concentration versus time curve obtained from the oral dose.

The fractional difference represents the fraction of orally administered dose that was removed before the drug was absorbed into systemic circulation. For example, if fractional difference = 0.27, it indicates that 27% of the administered dose was not able to be absorbed into systemic circulation.

Drugs that demonstrate high hepatic extraction ratio exhibit first-pass effect. Drugs which exhibit high first pass effect (greater than 0.9) are best administered by routes other than those involving the gastrointestinal tract. Insulin and nitroglycerin are examples of popular drugs, which exhibit high first pass effect. Examples of other drugs that exhibit first-pass effect include dopamine, imipramine, lidocaine, morphine, propoxyphene and salicylamide. Box 7-1 lists examples of some drugs that exhibit first-pass effect.

Example 7-15 The area under plasma concentration versus time curve from an aqueous solution of a drug administered intravenously is 237 μg × h/mL and area under the plasma concentration versus time curve from an identical dose of the same drug administered orally is 190 μg × h/mL. What is fractional difference between the two areas?

Solution

$$\text{Fractional difference} = \frac{AUC_{IV} - AUC_{oral}}{AUC_{IV}}$$

$$= \frac{237\ \mu g \times h/mL - 190\ \mu g \times h/mL}{237\ \mu g \times h/mL}$$

$$= \frac{47\ \mu g \times h/mL}{237\ \mu g \times h/mL} = 0.2$$

This fractional difference, 0.2, represents the fraction of the administered dose that was removed before the drug was absorbed into the systemic circulation. In other words, 20% of the administered dose was not able to be absorbed.

DOSAGE IN CHILDREN

One of the most difficult tasks in pediatric therapy is the calculation of dosage in children, particularly in newborn babies, premature babies, infants and very young children. Various methods have been reported for calculating the dosage for children and infants, all of which calculate the child's dose as a fraction of the adult dose. For many years, the pharmacist relied on four popular and traditional methods of computing the child's dose based upon one of the following criteria:

(i) Age in months, (ii) Age in years, (iii) Age next birthday, and (iv) Weight in pounds.

The first three methods use age of the child. Depending upon whether the dose was calculated for an infant or a child, the method used age in years for the child and age in months for the infant. None of these four methods considered body surface area or kidney function in children and newborn babies in calculating the dose. These four methods were:

i. Fried's Rule

$$\text{Dose for infant} = \left(\frac{\text{Age in months}}{150}\right)(\text{Adult dose}) \qquad (7\text{-}33)$$

Box 7-1 Examples of drugs that exhibit first-pass effect

Acetylsalicylic acid	Isoproterenol	Nortriptyline
Alprenolol	Lidocaine	Pentazocine
Amitriptyline	Meperidine	Prozacin
Desipramine	Metoprolol	Propoxyphene
Dopamine	Morphine	Propranolol
Imipramine	Nitroglycerin	Salicylamide

ii. Young's Rule

$$\text{Dose for child} = \left(\frac{\text{Age in years}}{\text{Age} + 12}\right)(\text{Adult dose}) \qquad (7\text{-}34)$$

iii. Cowling's Rule

$$\text{Dose for child} = \left(\frac{\text{Age next birthday}}{24}\right)(\text{Adult dose}) \qquad (7\text{-}35)$$

iv. Clark's Rule

$$\text{Dose for infant} = \left(\frac{\text{Weight in pounds}}{150}\right)(\text{Adult dose}) \qquad (7\text{-}36)$$

Although these methods are still used by many pharmacists, newer methods for the determination of dose for children started appearing in the literature in recent years. Some of these methods depend upon the weight and/or age of the child; others consider body surface area as the determining factor in calculating the dose for the child. Some of these methods, classified into six major categories are described here:

Methods Based on the Weight of Child: In these methods the calculation of the child's dose (CD) is based upon the child's weight (CW) in kg, the adult dose (AD) and adult's weight (AW).

a. Augsberger method : $CD = \frac{(1.5)(CW + 10)}{100}(AD)$ (7-37)

b. Clark method : $CD = \frac{(CW)}{(AW)}(AD)$ (7-38)

Methods Based on the Age of Child: In these methods the child's dose is calculated as a fraction of the adult dose based upon the age of the child next birthday in years and a correction factor. The correction factor depends on the method developed by the innovator.

a. Augsberger method : $CD = \frac{4(CA + 20)}{100}(AD)$ (7-39)

b. Bastedo method : $CD = \frac{CA + 3}{30}(AD)$ (7-40)

c. Brunton method : $CD = (0.4)(CA)(AD)$ (7-41)

d. Fried' s method : $CD = (0.08)(CA)(AD)$ (7-42)

e. Gaubius method :

 i. Up to the age of 1 year: $CD = \frac{(AD)}{12}$ (7-43)

 ii. Between the ages of 1 and 2 years: $CD = (0.125)(AD)$ (7-44)

f. Martinet method : $CD = (0.05)(AD)$ (7-45)

g. Sagel method :

 i. Up to the age of 4 months: $CD = \frac{5 + 13(CA)}{100}(AD)$ (7-46)

 ii. Between the ages of 4 and 12 monthrs: $CD = \frac{7 + 8(CA)}{100}(AD)$ (7-47)

Method Based on the Age and Weight of Child: In this method, the child's dose is calculated as a fraction of the adult dose based on a factor (which relates the age of the child), the weight of the child and the weight of the adult.

a. Von Harnack method:

i. Up to the age of 1 year: $CD = \frac{(1.8)(CW)}{(AW)}(AD)$ (7-48)

ii. Between the ages of 1 and 6 years: $CD = \frac{(1.6)(CW)}{(AW)}(AD)$ (7-49)

Method Based on Body Surface Area: In this method of calculating the child's dose, the body surface area of the child (BSA) is compared to the body surface of the adult (1.73 m^2).

$$\text{Crawford-Terry-Rourke method: } CD = \frac{\text{Body surface area of child}}{1.73 \text{ m}^3}(AD) \quad (7\text{-}50)$$

The value of the body surface area of the child/infant at certain ages is taken as follows: newborn = 0.21 m^2, 3 months = 0.29 m^2, 6 months = 0.36 m^2, 1 year = 0.45 m^2, 2 years = 0.54 m^2 and 3 years = 0.6 m^2.

The body surface area of an in between age child may be extrapolated, e.g. body surface area of a 2.5 year child = 0.5 (0.54 + 0.6) = 0.57 m^2. The following equations may be used to calculate the body surface area:

$$BSA\ (m^2) = \sqrt{\frac{(\text{Height in inches})(\text{Weight in pounds})}{3131}}; \quad (7\text{-}51)$$

$$BSA\ (m^2) = \sqrt{\frac{(\text{Height in centimeters})(\text{Weight in kilograms})}{3600}}; \quad (7\text{-}52)$$

These two equations can also be used to determine the body surface area of an adult, as long as the adult is of normal height, weight and built.

Methods Based on Body Surface Area and Age: In these methods a factor is used in calculating the child's dose. This factor takes into account the body surface area and the age of the child.

a. Denekamp method: $CD = \frac{13 + (12)(CA)}{100}(AD)$ (7-53)

b. Sagal method:

   i. Up to the age of 4 months: $CD = \frac{12 + (19)(CA)}{100}(AD)$ (7-54)

   ii. Between the ages of 4 and 12 months: $CD = \frac{15 + (11)(CA)}{100}(AD)$ (7-55)

c. Von Harnack method

   i. Up to the age of 3 months: $CD = \frac{(AD)}{6}$ (7-56)

   ii. Between the ages of 3 and 6 months: CD = (0.2)(AD) (7-57)

   iii. Between the ages of 6 months and 1 year: CD = (0.25)(AD) (7-58)

Method Based on Body Surface Area and Weight: In this method, body surface area (assessed on body weight) is used to calculate the child's dose.

$$\text{Wagner method: } CD = \frac{(4.7)(CW)^{0.73}}{100}(AD) \quad (7\text{-}59)$$

SUGGESTED READING

1. Delgado J, Remers W (eds). Wilson and Gisvold's Text Book of Organic Medicinal and Pharmaceutical Chemistry, 9th edition. Lippincott; 1990.
2. Goodman and Gilman's: The Pharmacological Basis of Therapeutics, 9th edition. McGraw Hill; 1996.
3. Guyton AC. Text Book of Medical Physiology, 8th edition. WB Saunders: Philadelphia; 1991.

4. Marieb E. Human Anatomy and Physiology, 2nd edition. The Benjamin/Cummings Publishing Company; 1991.
5. Mungal D (ed). Applied Clinical Pharmacokinetics. Raven Press; 1983.
6. Remington: The Science and Practice of Pharmacy, 21st edition. Mack Publishing; 2005.
7. Theoharides T (ed). Pharmacology. Little Brown and Company; 1992.
8. Wagner J. Fundamentals of Clinical Pharmacokinetics. Drug Intelligence Publications; 1979.

PRACTICE PROBLEMS

7-1. The following data were obtained in human subjects after oral administration of a single 500 mg dose of an experimental antibiotic. Plot the data on a suitable graph paper and (a) calculate clearance, and (b) determine the mechanism of renal excretion.

Amount Excreted in Urine:

Time (h):	1	3	5	7	9	11	13	15
Amount (mg):	35	129	105	82	38	30	19	8

Plasma Concentration:

Time(h):	2	4	6	8	10	12	14
Concentration (mg/dL)	13.2	10.9	7.8	3.9	3.1	2.1	1.05

7-2. The following data were obtained following intramuscular injection of a single 1 g dose of an experimental antibiotic. Plot the data and (a) calculate clearance, (b) determine mechanism of excretion, and (c) calculate biological half-life if apparent volume of distribution is 12 L.

Plasma concentration	
Time (h)	Concentration (mg/dL)
1.5	0.6
2.5	0.5
3.5	0.44
5.0	0.36
7.0	0.25
8.5	0.20
9.5	0.16
10.5	0.14
11.5	0.11

Urinary excretion	
Time (h)	Amount (mg)
1.0	0.8
2.0	6.4
3.0	5.1
4.0	4.5
6.0	7.6
8.0	5.2
9.0	2.0
10.0	1.7
11.0	1.4
12.0	1.0

7-3. A drug is eliminated solely by glomerular filtration (GFR = 130 mL/min). If the volume of distribution of this drug is 12 L, calculate half-life of the drug.

7-4. A drug is eliminated solely by glomerular filtration (GFR = 130 mL/min). If the volume of distribution of this drug is 60 L, calculate half-life of the drug.

7-5. A drug is eliminated solely by glomerular filtration (GFR = 130 mL/min) and is 40% reabsorbed. If the volume of distribution of this drug is 41 L, calculate half-life of the drug.

7-6. A drug is eliminated solely by glomerular filtration (GFR = 130 mL/min) and is 85% reabsorbed. If the volume of distribution of this drug is 20 L, calculate half-life of the drug.

7-7. A drug is eliminated by glomerular filtration as well as by tubular secretion. If the volume of distribution of this drug is 20 L, calculate half-life of the drug.

7-8. A drug is eliminated by glomerular filtration as well as by tubular secretion and is 30% reabsorbed. If the volume of distribution of this drug is 41 L, calculate half-life of the drug.

7-9. Using the method of Schwartz and associates, calculate the creatinine clearance for a 150 cm tall 10-year-old child having a serum creatinine concentration of 1 mg/dL.

7-10. The serum creatinine concentration in a patient is 1.2 mg/dL and the concentration of creatinine in a 24 hour pooled sample of urine (volume of urine collected in the 24 hour pooled sample = 1.5 L) was found to be 0.92 mg/mL. Calculate creatinine clearance in this patient.

7-11. Using Jelliffe method, calculate creatinine clearance in a 75-year-old female having a serum creatinine concentration of 0.9 mg/dL.

7-12. Using Jelliffe method, calculate creatinine clearance in a 65-year-old male having a serum creatinine concentration of 0.85 mg/dL.

7-13. Calculate the fraction of drug removed by liver if the arterial plasma concentration of a drug is 1.65 mg/L and the venous plasma concentration of the drug is 1.32 mg/L.

7-14. The area under the plasma concentration versus time curve from a single 300 mg bolus dose of a drug administered intravenously as an aqueous solution is 356 μg × h/mL and area under the plasma concentration versus time curve from an identical dose of the same drug administered orally as an aqueous solution is 200 μg × h/mL. Calculate the percent administered dose that was removed before systemic absorption of the drug.

CHAPTER 8

BIOAVAILABILITY

During the early 1960's, drug product development was at its peak, propelled by the early 1940's and late 1950's discovery of a significant number of very important antibiotics such as chlortetracycline, oxytetracycline and chloramphenicol. Competing drug companies claimed superiority for their antibiotic on the basis of attaining higher plasma levels of the antibiotic following oral administration of their product. The significance of adding an extra ingredient (adjuvant) on enhancing oral absorption of the drug was heavily promoted by the pharmaceutical companies. For example, Bristol Laboratories added the adjunct sodium hexametaphosphate to their tetracycline capsules, Pfizer Laboratories added glucosamine hydrochloride and Lederle Laboratories added citric acid. Soon afterwards, the pharmaceutical industry introduced many new products.

Some of the new products introduced were chemical compounds that exhibited variations in their pharmacologic and therapeutic activity when slight modification was made in their chemical structure. In some cases, a small modification in the chemical structure of the compound led to a slight change in biological activity, whereas in some other compounds, even a minor modification led to extreme variations. For example, phenoxymethylpenicillin (penicillin V) was marketed as penicillin, which produced higher plasma levels than benzylpenicillin (penicillin G) after oral administration. It was shown that the greater acid-stability of the antibiotic penicillin V accounted for the higher plasma concentration of this penicillin. This led to recognition of the fact that a great deal of knowledge is required for studying the many factors that affect biological and therapeutic activity of the administered drug.

In recent years, however, the number of new products introduced by the pharmaceutical companies has declined substantially, partly because of the stringent regulations imposed by the Food and Drug Administration and partly because pharmaceutical companies believe that there are not too many new products left to be discovered. Therefore, a large number of manufacturers shifted, in part, their attention to marketing old products either in new dosage forms (marketed as new drug delivery systems) or in the same dosage form as generic products. It is for this reason, that many multinational companies are involved in the manufacture of generic products at the present time, although, in the past, generic products were mainly the domain of generic companies. Therefore, the availability of a large number of generic products has given further impetus to research in assessing biological availability of the drug from the administered dosage form. With a large number of generic, as well as multinational companies competing for a larger share of the generic products business, it is no wonder that such terms as bioavailability, drug product selection, generic equivalency, therapeutic efficacy and drug substitution have become common household words.

The term bioavailability may be translated to mean availability of drug or the active ingredient(s) to the biological system. The extent to which the active ingredient in a dosage form intended for extravascular administration becomes available for absorption is dependent on a variety of factors. Some of the factor which are known to affect drug absorption are:

1. Physicochemical properties of the drug substance (e.g. aqueous solubility, lipid solubility, partition coefficient, extent of ionization, etc.).
2. Method of manufacture of the dosage form (e.g. wet granulation, direct compression, dry granulation and tablet hardness, etc.).
3. Manufacturing aides used in the fabrication of the dosage form (e.g. bulking agents, binders, lubricants, dyes, disintegrants, coating materials, etc.).

Hence, these factors may require special consideration in determining bioavailability of the active ingredient from the dosage form.

Bioavailability, as the name implies, refers to availability of the administered drug dose to the biological system. An intravenously administered dose of a drug in an aqueous solution is considered to be completely available to the biological system, because the entire drug dose is placed directly into the bloodstream. The drug from an extravascularly administered dose, on the other hand, may or may not be completely available. A number of factors may be responsible for the lack of complete availability of drug from an extravascularly administered dosage form. These include: incomplete absorption of the drug dose, inactivation of part of the administered dose in the biological environment, metabolism of part of the drug dose at the absorption site or other similar reasons. Since biologic response is a result of an interaction between the drug substance and the functionally important molecules (receptors) in the living system, unavailability of a portion of the administered drug from the dosage form may result in variation in the expected therapeutic response.

Bioavailability is loosely defined as the rate at which and extent to which the active drug ingredient is absorbed from a drug product (dosage form) and becomes available at the site of drug action. In actual practice it is difficult, if not impossible, to measure the actual concentration of drug at the site of action. Therefore, one usually measures concentration of drug in the blood or plasma as an indicator of the rate and extent of availability of drug at the site of action. This concept is based on the premise that most drugs reach the site of action or the biophase, through systemic circulation and therefore, the concentration of drug in blood or plasma reflects the concentration of drug at the site of action. Another approach to correlate concentration of drug at the site of action is to use urinary excretion of unchanged drug as an index of concentration of drug in the plasma. Since the rate of excretion of drug in the urine is a function of concentration of drug in the blood, it follows that the rate of urinary excretion of drug is representative of the rate of absorption of the drug. Similarly, the extent of urinary excretion of the drug is representative of the extent of drug absorption.

As can be seen from this definition, the term bioavailability is defined as a measure, relative to some standard of the rate and amount of drug which reaches systemic circulation unchanged after administration of the drug dose. This definition includes two parameters:

1. Rate of drug absorption
2. Extent of drug absorption.

The definition of bioavailability precludes dosage forms administered intravenously, because in these dosage forms there is no rate of absorption.

The data generated during bioavailability studies can be used to obtain a variety of information. This is because bioavailability studies are concerned most with the fraction of the dose that is released *in vivo* and is capable of reaching systemic circulation intact, rather than the 'label dose' stated on the packaged form of the drug. Some examples, where bioavailability data provide useful information concerning efficacy of the drug include the following:

1. Determine the extent of absorption, i.e. the amount or fraction of the administered drug dose absorbed from a dosage form.
2. Determine rate of absorption of the drug.
3. Determine the length (duration) of the presence of drug in the biological fluids or tissues.
4. Correlate relationship between concentration of drug in the plasma and clinical response.

5. Compare systemic availability of drug from different production batches of the dosage form.
6. Determine duration of activity of the drug.
7. Compare systemic availability of drug from different dosage forms of the same drug manufactured by the same manufacturer.
8. Compare systemic availability of drug from the same dosage form produced by different manufacturers.
9. Determine plasma concentration of drug at which toxicity occurs.
10. Determine the design of the proper dosage regimen for the patient.

DETERMINATION OF BIOAVAILABILITY

The ideal method of determining bioavailability is clinical evaluation of therapeutic effectiveness of the drug or drug product. In some instances, it is relatively easy to evaluate the effectiveness of the drug, e.g. effect of the drug in lowering blood pressure or the effect of the drug in reducing the blood glucose level. Unfortunately, in many cases, therapeutic efficacy of the drug or the drug product is very difficult to quantify, especially where evaluation of the effectiveness of drug is more subjective than objective in nature (e.g. the perception of effectiveness of an analgesic drug in an individual patient). Also, because of inter- and intra-subject variability, sound clinical studies call for a large number of subjects to participate in the study and this requirement adds more ethical and economic restrictions on the successful execution of the clinical study.

As mentioned earlier, one usually measures concentration of drug in an easily accessible biological fluid as long as the concentration of drug in this fluid correlates with the concentration of drug at the receptor site. Two fluids are commonly employed for this purpose:

1. Blood or plasma
2. Urine.

This is because bioavailability studies based on plasma levels or urinary excretion data are relatively less costly and tend to be more time-saving procedures. Also, if the study is well designed and executed properly, it can provide a quantifiable and highly reliable evaluation of the pharmacokinetic parameters of the new drug product.

Blood or Plasma

Blood or plasma is the most commonly used body fluid to correlate concentration of drug at the receptor site or the site of action due to the fact that most drugs reach the site of action or biophase, through systemic circulation, hence, concentration of drug in blood or plasma reflects concentration of drug at the site of action. Therefore, bioavailability is sometimes referred to as biological availability or systemic availability. The venous and arterial blood is considered systemic circulation during absorptive phase after oral administration and blood in the portal vein is excluded. In this method, blood samples are collected at predetermined time intervals after extravascular administration of the drug dose. Concentration of drug in each blood sample is determined using a suitable assay method and these concentrations are plotted as a function of time on a suitable graph paper. The plasma profile thus obtained is used to estimate rate and extent of drug absorbed into systemic circulation. It is important to collect blood samples at reasonable time intervals in order to obtain a comprehensive plasma profile.

The major drawback of using plasma concentration as an indicator of systemic availability of the drug is that the subjects participating in the study have to be under medical supervision and blood samples must be withdrawn by qualified individuals. The advantage of using plasma concentration is that if the study is well designed and executed properly, it can provide a quantifiable and highly reliable evaluation of pharmacokinetic parameters of the drug product.

Urine

Another approach to correlate concentration of drug at the site of action is to use urinary excretion of unchanged drug. Since the rate of excretion of drug in the urine depends on the concentration of drug in blood (or plasma), it follows that the rate of urinary excretion of drug is representative of the rate of absorption of drug and cumulative amount of drug excreted in the urine is representative of the extent of drug absorption.

In this method, the drug dose is administered by an extravascular route and the patient is asked to void their bladder at frequent time intervals. The volume of urine voided at each interval is determined and concentration of drug in each urine sample is calculated. The amount of drug excreted during each time interval is determined by multiplying the volume of urine voided with the concentration of drug in each sample of urine. Urinary excretion rate during each interval is then determined by calculating the amount of drug excreted per unit time.

One major advantage of using urinary excretion to correlate systemic absorption of drug is that collection of urine is much simpler, least troublesome and least painful to the subjects participating in the bioavailability study than the collection of blood samples of the subjects.

There are several problems with using urinary excretion data to correlate systemic absorption of the drug. The two main problems, however, are as follows:

1. Collection of urine samples is limited due to an individual's ability to void bladder at frequent time intervals. During the earlier part of the bioavailability study, one is able to void bladder more frequently than during the later part of the study. This limits the number of data points that can be obtained for the study.
2. Determination of various pharmacokinetic parameters of the parent drug from urinary excretion studies is generally limited to only those drugs, where at least 10% of the drug is excreted in urine in the unchanged form. Literature cites examples of some drugs, which are excreted largely in the unchanged form, while others are excreted partly in the unchanged form and partly in the form of one or more metabolite and yet many drugs are excreted almost completely in the form of one or more metabolite. Examples of drugs excreted in the unchanged form include the following drugs: barbital, digoxin, gentamicin, streptomycin and vancomycin.

Bioavailability Studies

As mentioned earlier, the most reliable and sensitive method of determining bioavailability is an analysis of plasma concentrations of drug at various time intervals after administration of the drug dose. The data are then plotted on a rectilinear graph paper and this plot provides important and useful information concerning the rate and extent of availability of drug from the dosage form.

A typical plot of concentration of drug in plasma as a function of time after extravascular administration of a single dose of a drug is shown in Figure 8-1. In this profile, MEC is minimum effective concentration and MTC is minimum toxic concentration. The peak drug plasma concentration, C_{max} (also known as peak concentration, peak height or intensity of action) is 24 mcg/mL. The time at which the peak plasma concentration (C_{max}) occurs is T_{max} (time of peak concentration or time of maximum concentration). In Figure 8-1, T_{max} is 2 hours. In plasma profiles obtained after intravenous administration of a bolus dose of a drug, the intensity of action (or C_{max}) would be plasma drug concentration immediately after administration of the dose (C_0) and time of peak concentration or T_{max} would be at time 0 (immediately after administration of the dose).

The drug starts exhibiting its therapeutic effect when its concentration in plasma achieves minimum therapeutic (effective) concentration (MEC). The time at which the minimum therapeutic concentration is achieved is when the drug starts exhibiting its therapeutic effect.

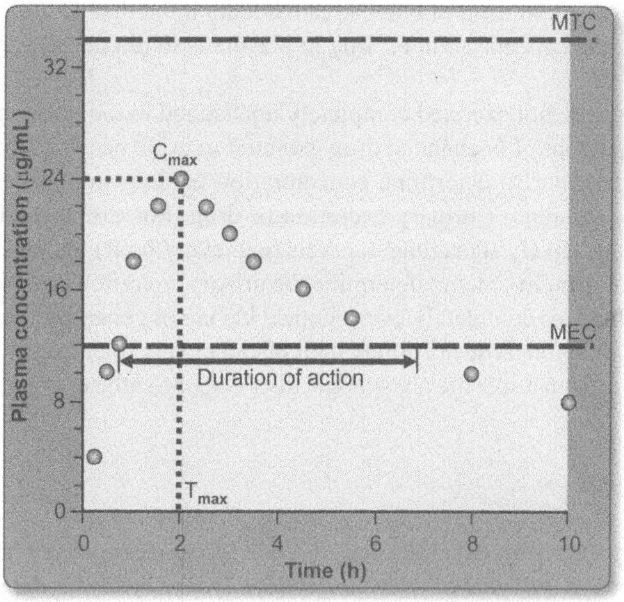

Fig. 8-1 Typical plot of plasma concentration versus time

This is known as onset of action. The drug continues to exert its therapeutic effect, as long as plasma levels of the drug remain above the MEC. The activity of the drug ceases when the concentration of drug in plasma falls below the MEC. The time interval between the onset of action and cessation of activity is known as duration of action.

In the typical plasma profile shown in Figure. 8-1, the drug starts exhibiting its therapeutic effect at about 0.5 hours after administration of the dose and the activity of the drug ceases at about 7.0 hours. Therefore, the onset of action of drug from this dosage form is about 0.5 hours and the duration of action is 7.0 hours – 0.5 hour = 6.5 hours.

Parameters of Bioavailability

Any number of parameters may be used in conducting bioavailability studies, as long as the parameters used reflect the rate of drug absorption and the extent of drug absorption. In estimating bioavailability of a drug or the bioavailability of a drug from a dosage form, it is customary to use data derived from either concentration of drug in plasma (blood or serum) or excretion of the unchanged drug in urine.

Plasma Concentration Data

When drug plasma concentration data are used to estimate bioavailability, the following three parameters estimate the extent of absorption and rate of absorption of the drug:

1. Peak plasma concentration (C_{max})
2. Time of peak plasma concentration (T_{max})
3. Area under the plasma concentration versus time curve (AUC).

The area under the plasma concentration versus time curve (AUC) is an estimate of the extent of absorption of the drug. The peak plasma concentration (C_{max}) and the time of peak plasma concentration (T_{max}) are indicative of rate of absorption of the drug.

Most bioavailability studies use the drug plasma concentration data rather than the urinary excretion data. This is because:

1. The appearance of drug in bloodstream occurs immediately after the drug is absorbed and therefore, the concentration of drug in plasma is in direct relation to the rate of absorption of drug.
2. Most drugs are not excreted completely unchanged in the urine. In such cases, determining the total amount of unchanged drug excreted in urine becomes difficult.
3. It is much easier to determine concentration of drug in plasma at any time than it is to determine the rate of urinary excretion of drug. For example, if plasma concentration is needed at relatively short time intervals (e.g. every hour), blood samples can be withdrawn every hour. But, in order to determine the urinary excretion rate every hour, the patient must void the bladder completely every hour. This is not generally feasible at all times, because normally individuals do not empty their bladder every hour except, perhaps, when the patient is suffering from a specific physiologic disorder, or a catheter is placed in the patient to collect urine.

Urinary Excretion Data

When urinary excretion data are used, the rate of excretion of unchanged drug in the urine is used as an indicator of rate of drug absorption. This is based on the premise that as the rate of absorption of drug increases, so does the rate of excretion of drug in the urine. Similarly, the cumulative amount of unchanged drug excreted in the urine indicates extent of absorption of the drug, because greater the extent of absorption, greater the amount of drug excreted in the urine.

Rate of Absorption

In practice, the actual rate of drug absorption is rarely determined to estimate the bioavailability of drug from its dosage form, because indirect methods are available to indicate relative rates of drug absorption from a dosage form.

Consider the three plasma profiles shown in Figure 8-2. In these three profiles, the curves A, B and C represent the plasma profile of identical doses of three different formulations of the same drug administered by the same extravascular route. Evidently, faster rate of absorption of drug should reach higher peak concentration of drug in plasma and slower rate of drug absorption will exhibit a much lower peak plasma concentration. Therefore, one may use peak concentration

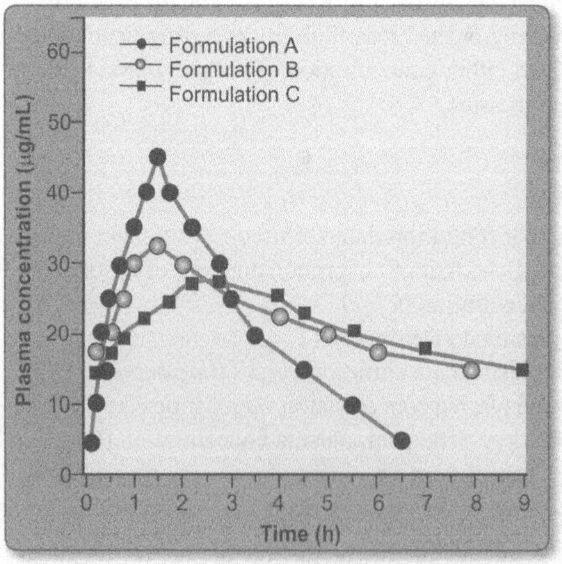

Fig. 8-2 Plasma concentration of three different formulations

of drug in plasma (C_{max}) as an indicator of rate of absorption of drug, i.e. higher the peak concentration, faster the rate of absorption of the drug. According to the three plasma profiles shown in Figure 8-2, the peak concentration of drug in the plasma follows the rank order: A > B > C. This indicates that the rates of absorption of drug from these three formulations follow the rank order A > B > C. Therefore, C_{max}, the peak plasma concentration of drug is used as one of the indicators of rate of absorption of the drug.

Similarly, faster rate of absorption of the drug should exhibit the time of attaining peak plasma concentration of drug a lot sooner than the relatively slower rate of absorption of the drug. Thus, the sooner the drug attains T_{max}, the faster the rate of drug absorption and longer the time of attaining T_{max}, the slower the rate of drug absorption. Therefore, the time of peak plasma drug concentration (T_{max}) may also be used as another indicator of rate of absorption of the drug.

It is seen in Figure 8-2 that the time of peak concentration occurs most rapidly in plasma profile A, which also exhibits the highest peak plasma concentration of the drug. The time of maximum concentration of the drug occurs less rapidly in plasma profile B and this profile also exhibits a lower peak plasma concentration of drug than that exhibited in profile A. The time of peak plasma dug concentration occurs after a long time in profile C and this profile also exhibits the lowest peak plasma concentration of the drug.

Hence, the two parameters C_{max} and T_{max} reflect the rate of absorption of the drug.

Thus, during bioavailability studies based on the data derived from the plasma concentration of the drug, the following are the two indicators traditionally used for the rate of absorption of the drug from an extravascularly administered dosage form are:

1. Peak concentration of drug in plasma, C_{max}. This is read directly from the concentration of drug in plasma versus time graph (Figure 8-3). The peak concentration of drug in plasma, according to Figure 8-3 is 45 μg/mL.
2. Time of peak concentration of drug in plasma, T_{max}. This is also read directly from the concentration of drug in plasma versus time graph (Figure 8-3). The time of peak concentration of drug in plasma, according to Figure 8-3 occurs at 1.5 hour.

Extent of Drug Absorption

The extent of drug absorption signifies the fraction of administered dose that is actually absorbed and appears in the systemic circulation. The concept of extent of drug absorption applies only

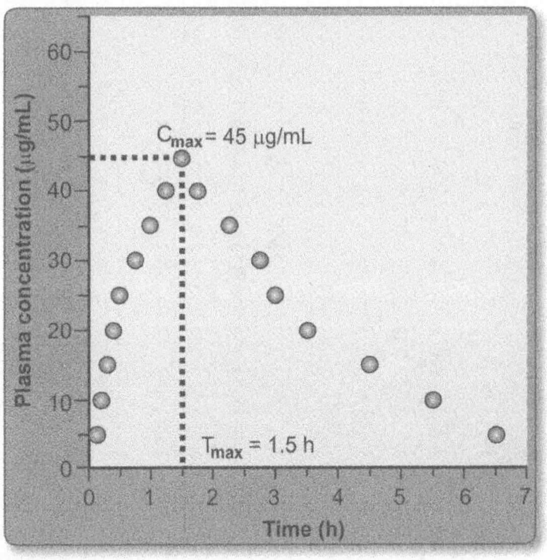

Fig. 8-3 Plasma concentration versus time profile after oral administration

to the extravascular drug administration, because one does not know, whether the entire dose administered reaches systemic circulation or some portion of the administered dose was not absorbed (e.g. due to incomplete release of drug from the dosage form, or incomplete absorption of the drug, or degradation of the drug in the environment at the site of administration, or inactivation of drug at the site of administration). If the drug is administered intravenously, it is assumed that the extent of absorption is 100%, because the entire drug dose is placed in the systemic circulation.

Since it is not possible to directly determine the fraction of dose that is actually absorbed, indirect methods must be used to estimate extent of absorption. The most popular method of estimating extent of absorption is to use area under the plasma concentration versus time curve as an indicator of extent of absorption.

The technique used in the determination of area under the plasma concentration versus time curve is as follows.

Following administration of a given dose, blood samples are collected at predetermined time intervals. These samples are analyzed to determine the concentration of drug in plasma and the data thus obtained (concentration of drug in the plasma as a function of time) are plotted on a rectilinear coordinate graph paper. A smooth curve is then drawn to represent the concentration data points and the area bounded by the concentration-time curve is determined. For example, let us suppose that a 325 mg dose of drug was administered orally and a plot of the concentration of drug in the plasma as a function of time was obtained as shown in Figure 8-4. The area covered by this plasma concentration versus time plot (generally referred to as the area under the curve, or AUC) thus represents the quantity of drug, which appears in the bloodstream (i.e. the extent of absorption from the administered dose). It should be mentioned that area under the curve (AUC) thus determined has the units of (drug plasma concentration) (time) and not the amount of drug in the plasma.

The AUC obtained following administration of an extravascular dose only represents the extent of absorption. It does not indicate the exact amount of drug absorbed from the administered dose. In order to determine the amount of drug actually absorbed or the percent of administered dose reaching systemic circulation, the following method is used.

A similar dose of the drug is administered intravenously as an aqueous solution containing no additives (e.g. colorants or flavoring agents) or formulation aides (e.g. buffering agents, antioxidants, cosolvents, etc.). The area under the plasma concentration versus time curve of the

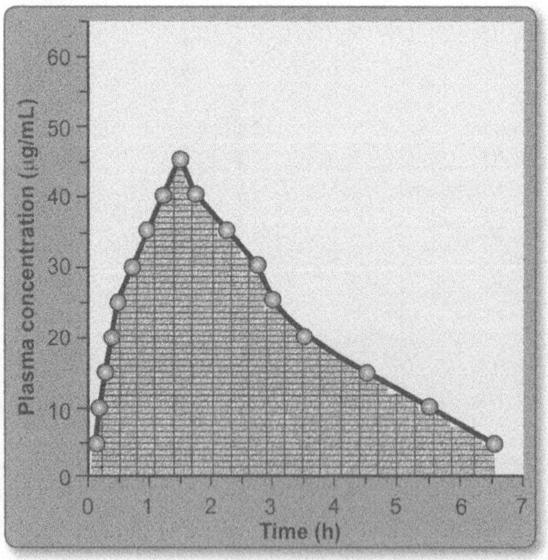

Fig. 8-4 Plasma concentration versus time plot (shaded area is AUC)

intravenously administered dose is then determined. Since it can be assumed that availability of drug from the intravenous administration of the aqueous solution is 100%, a comparison of AUC from the intravenously administered dose with the AUC from the extravascularly administered dose, therefore, provides an indication of the fraction of dose absorbed into the bloodstream from the extravascularly administered dosage form.

RELATIVE BIOAVAILABILITY

Relative bioavailability, as the name implies, is bioavailability in relation to a given standard. Relative bioavailability is defined as the extent of drug absorption from the test preparation (or product) relative to the extent of drug absorption from the reference (or standard) preparation (or product). The test preparation is the product being evaluated and reference preparation is the preparation (or product), which is used to compare the test product with. The test preparation may be a new dosage form being introduced by the manufacturer of an existing drug product or a new strength in the same dosage form being introduced by the same manufacturer. The test preparation may also be a generic product being introduced by a competitive company. For a generic product the reference preparation used for comparison is generally the innovator's product already existing in the same dosage form.

If a commercial reference preparation does not exist, e.g. when a new product is marketed by a manufacturer, the reference product used is an aqueous intravenous solution without any formulation additives (e.g. buffers, preservatives, etc.).

The following relationship is used to estimate relative bioavailability:

$$\text{Relative bioavailability} = \frac{AUC_{test}}{AUC_{ref}} \tag{8-1}$$

In this equation,

AUC_{test} = area under the curve from test preparation (preparation under investigation)

AUC_{ref} = area under the curve from the reference preparation (preparation against which the test preparation is being compared).

The use of relative bioavailability is not limited to the comparison of two different dosage forms of the same product. It is also used when one wishes to compare two products of the same drug made by different manufacturers or two different strengths of the same drug manufactured by the same company. For example, if a manufacturer markets a 100 mg tablet and then decides to market the same drug as a 100 mg capsule or as a 50 mg tablet, the extent of absorption from the new dosage forms (100 mg capsule or 50 mg tablet) can be estimated by administering separately a single 100 mg dose of the drug in various dosage forms and calculating the areas under the curve from each of these dosage forms. The relative bioavailability is then determined by comparing the areas under the curve from these dosage forms with the AUC from the 100 mg tablet. In these cases, the 100 mg tablet is used as the reference preparation, because the manufacturer simply wishes to compare the extent of absorption from the new products relative to the already existing dosage form.

Example 8-1 The area under the plasma concentration versus time curve from a 325 mg dose of a drug administered as an oral suspension was found to be 105 μg × h/mL and area under the plasma concentration versus time curve from a similar dose administered orally, as a tablet dosage form was found to be 130 μg × h/mL. Calculate relative bioavailability of the drug from the suspension formulation.

Solution

The test product here is the suspension formulation and the reference product is the tablet formulation. Using equation (8-1), we have

$$\text{Relative bioavailability} = \frac{150\ \mu g \times h/mL}{130\ \mu g \times h/mL}$$

$$\text{Relative bioavailability} = 0.808$$

$$\text{Relative bioavailability} = 80.8\%$$

If the entire 325 mg of drug is absorbed from the tablet dosage form, then the amount of drug absorbed from the suspension formulation is 80.8% of 325 mg = 262.6 mg.

Example 8-2 The area under the curve following administration of a single dose of each of the following dosage forms was determined to be as follows:

$$\text{One 100 mg tablet} = 120\ mg \times h/L$$

$$\text{One 100 mg capsule} = 126\ mg \times h/L$$

$$\text{Two 50 mg tablets} = 110\ mg \times h/L$$

Calculate the extent of absorption of drug from the 100 mg capsule and the 50 mg tablet dosage forms (relative to the 100 mg tablet dosage form).

Solution

Here, the reference product is 100 mg tablet and test products are 100 mg capsule and 50 mg tablet.

The extent of absorption of drug from the 100 mg capsule and the 50 mg tablet is as follows:

$$\text{100 mg capsules} = \frac{126\ mg \times h/mL}{120\ mg \times h/mL} = 1.05 = 105\%$$

$$\text{50 mg tablets} = \frac{110\ mg \times h/L}{120\ mg \times h/L} = 0.917 = 91.78\%$$

As can be seen from these examples, the extent of absorption from the test preparation is not necessarily identical to the extent of absorption from the reference product. Depending on the formulation factors used in the fabrication of the dosage form, the extent of absorption from the test product may be greater than the extent of absorption from the reference product (as in the case of the capsule dosage form in Example 8-2) or it may be less than the extent of the absorption from the reference product (as in the case of the 50 mg tablet formulation in Example 8-2).

DETERMINATION OF AREA UNDER THE CURVE

Various methods are available for determination of area under the plasma concentration versus time curve. Four methods are recognized in bioavailability studies—use of planimeter, counting squares, trapezoidal rule, and cutting and weighing. These methods can only provide AUC from time 0 to the time of last plasma concentration point, i.e. AUC_{0-t}.

All of these methods can be used either for the determination of AUC of a drug product, or for comparing the areas under the curve of two or more different products (or dosage forms of the same drug). The method involving the use of the planimeter somehow never gained popularity, perhaps due to the lack of availability of the instrument. The second method, the method of counting squares, gained initial popularity, but is falling out of use now, because this method is somewhat eye-straining. The most popular method of determining AUC is the method of trapezoidal rule, because this method is relatively simple, least time consuming and most reproducible. The cutting and weighing method is more commonly used when one wishes to compare bioavailability of drug from two preparations.

Planimeter

Planimeter is an instrument, which mechanically measures area of plane figures. It consists of an arm attached to a rotating wheel, which moves a dial with the movement of the arm. To measure area under the plasma concentration versus time curve, plasma concentration of drug as a function of time is plotted on a rectilinear graph paper and a smooth curve is drawn to best represent the data. The arm of the planimeter is traced over the concentration versus time curve to obtain the dial reading. The dial is equipped with vernier calipers to ensure accurate reading on the dial. The reading on the dial is then converted into AUC by using a factor obtained by tracing the arm over a square or a circle of known area. Although this method was considered to be the simplest and most reliable method of determining AUC, it is not in common use. It never gained popularity and most research facilities never acquired this instrument.

Counting Squares

In counting squares method, as the name suggests, the total number of squares enclosed by the plasma concentration versus time curve are counted. The methodology for this technique is as follows.

The plasma concentration as a function of time is plotted on a regular rectilinear graph paper and instead of joining the points with straight lines, a smooth curve is drawn to best represent the data points. No attempt is made to extrapolate the curve beyond the last concentration-time point. Instead, a straight line is drawn to connect the last concentration data point with the corresponding time point on the time-axis. The squares enclosed within this bounded plasma concentration versus time curve are now counted. The area of each square is determined using the relationship:

$$\text{Area} = (\text{height})(\text{width})$$

It should be pointed out that the height and width of the squares is not measured in inches, centimeters or any other conventional linear unit of measurement. The height is measured in the units of concentration on y-axis and the width is measured in the units of time on the x-axis. For example, if 70 divisions on the x-axis were used to represent 14 hours, then each division on x-axis equals 0.2 hours. Similarly, if 100 divisions on the y-axis were used to represent 25 mg/mL, then each division on y-axis equals 0.25 mg/mL. Thus, the area of a square composed of each division on the two axes is:

$$(0.25 \text{ mg/mL})(0.2 \text{ h}) = 0.05 \text{ mg} \times \text{h/mL}$$

Alternatively, the area of each square may be determined as follows:

Since, there are 70 divisions on the x-axis and 100 divisions on the y-axis, therefore,

$$\text{Total number of squares on the graph} = (70)(100) = 7{,}000.$$

The 70 divisions on the x-axis represent 14 hours and the 100 divisions on the y-axis represent 25 mg/mL, therefore, the 7,000 squares represent:

$$(25 \text{ mg/mL})(14 \text{ h}) = 350 \text{ mg} \times \text{h/mL}$$

This means that the area of each square is:

$$50 \text{ mg tablets} = \frac{350 \text{ mg} \times \text{h/mL}}{7{,}000}$$

$$50 \text{ mg tablets} = 0.05 \text{ mg} \times \text{h/mL}$$

The area thus obtained has the units of (concentration)(time). Knowing the area of one square, it is then possible to calculate area under the curve using the following relationship:

$$\text{AUC} = (\text{\# of squares})(\text{area of one square})$$

It should be mentioned that when counting squares, it is customary to count only the complete squares bounded by the plasma concentration versus time curve. To accomplish this, one counts only the whole squares and squares that are covered 50% or more than 50%. This means that all those squares that are covered less than 50% are not counted, which negates the effect of counting partial squares as full squares.

Obviously, the accuracy of determining the area under the curve depends on:

i. The number of squares per linear inch on the graph paper
ii. The investigator counting the squares.

A graph paper with a large number of small squares will provide an answer that is closer to the actual AUC than a graph consisting of a small number of relatively large-sized squares. It is therefore suggested that a graph paper containing 20 squares per linear inch should be used for the determination of AUC by the method of counting squares.

The disparity in the final count of squares due to counting by different investigators arises, because when counting squares that are not completely covered, each individual uses their judgment in deciding whether a given square is covered 50% or more than 50% and therefore, should be counted as a full square, or the square is covered less than 50% and should not be counted.

Counting a large number of small squares can be very tedious and eye-straining. To make it less stressful and somewhat easier on the eye, it is suggested that one should use a graph paper, where a group of small squares can be grouped together into a few large squares. This not only makes the counting of squares less strenuous but also minimizes errors because when counting a large number of small squares, one may count some squares more than once and neglect to count some squares all together. Counting squares to determine the AUC is a simple technique and is illustrated in the following example.

Example 8-3 Plasma concentration (mg/mL) as a function of time (hr) following oral administration of a single 500 mg dose of a drug is shown below. Calculate area under the curve from 0 to 5 hours.

Time (h)	0.5	1.0	1.5	2.0	2.5	3.0	3.5	4.0	4.5	5.0
Concentration (mg/mL)	1.5	16.0	35.0	45.0	32.0	20.0	14.0	10.0	8.0	5.0

Solution

The plot of data is shown in Figure 8-5. A smooth curve is drawn to represent these points. The data points are not joined with straight lines, but a smooth curve is drawn to best represent the data points.

As can be seen from Figure 8-5, the area bounded by the plasma concentration versus time curve consists of 26 large squares (like the square shown as A outside the graph), 21 medium squares (like the square shown as B outside the graph) and 555 small squares (like the square shown as C outside the graph). Since the area of a square is length times its width, therefore,

Area of one large square (area A of inset in Figure 8-5) = (5.0 μg/mL)(0.50 h)
= 2.500 μg × h/mL,

Area of one medium square (area B of inset in Figure 8-5) = (2.5 μg/mL)(0.25 h)
= 0.625 μg × h/mL, and

Area of one small square (area C of inset in Figure 8-5) = (0.5 μg/mL)(0.05 h)
= 0.025 μg × h/mL

The total areas of these large, medium and small squares are:

Area of 26 large squares = (26)(2.500 μg × h/mL) = 65.000 μg × h/mL
Area of 21 medium squares = (21)(0.625 μg × h/mL) = 13.125 μg × h/mL
Area of 555 small squares = (555)(0.025 μg × h/mL) = 13.875 μg × h/mL
Area under the curve from 0 to 5 hours = (65.000 + 13.125 + 13.875) μg × h/mL
Area under the curve from 0 to 5 hours = 92 μg × h/mL.

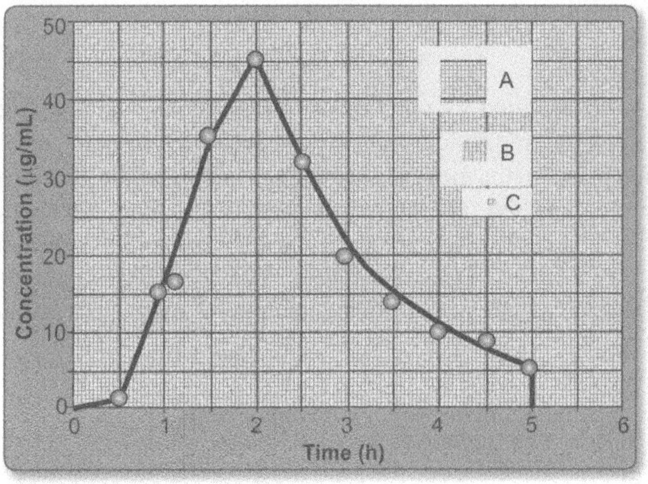

Fig. 8-5 Area under the curve by counting squares

Trapezoidal Rule

In trapezoidal method, plasma concentration as a function of time is plotted on a rectilinear graph paper. The plot is divided into geometric figures whose area can be determined individually using an appropriate geometric formula for each figure. Therefore, the concentration versus time plot is not drawn as a smooth curve, but adjacent concentration points are joined with straight lines. A perpendicular on x-axis is drawn from each concentration point to obtain a geometric figure. All but one or two segments in this plot tend to be trapezoids, hence the name trapezoidal rule.

Most plasma concentration versus time data do not provide concentration of drug in plasma immediately after administration of the dose (concentration at time 0). If concentration at time 0 is not provided, the following rules apply:

1. In extravascular administration, concentration at time 0 is taken as 0, if the drug is delivered using an immediate-release dosage form.
2. In intravascular administration, concentration at time 0 is the maximum concentration of drug in the plasma. Concentration at time 0 is generally not available, because a blood sample is not drawn at time 0. Therefore, the concentration of drug at time 0 must be determined using an appropriate method. The best method of determining plasma concentration at time 0 is to plot plasma concentration as a function of time on a semi-logarithmic graph paper and back-extrapolate the straight line to time 0. This is the concentration at time 0 and this concentration is plotted on the rectilinear graph paper to draw the first segment.

In intravascular administration, the first segment will be a trapezoid and in extravascular administration, the first segment will be a triangle. The following relationships are used to calculate the area of each geometric figure:

Area of a triangle:

$$\text{Area of a triangle} = (0.5)(\text{Height})(\text{Base}) \quad (8\text{-}2)$$

Area of a trapezoid:

Two formulas can be used to calculate the area of a trapezoid:

$$\text{Area of a trapezoid} = (0.5)(\text{Base})(\text{Sum of the two parallel sides}) \quad (8\text{-}3)$$

Since a trapezoid is a triangle attached to a rectangle with a common base, its area can also be determined by adding together the areas of the triangle and the rectangle:

$$\text{Area of a trapezoid} = \text{Area of triangle} + \text{Area of rectangle} \quad (8\text{-}4)$$

It will be recalled that the area of a rectangle is:

$$\text{Area of a rectangle} = (\text{Length})(\text{Width})$$

The AUC determined by counting squares usually yields a slightly different value than that obtained by the trapezoidal rule. This is because a smooth curve is drawn to represent the concentration points in the method of counting squares, while the concentration points are joined in the trapezoidal method. The smooth curve drawn to represent the data points tends to cover a slightly different area than that obtained when the data points are connected with straight lines.

Example 8-4 Using the data given in Example 8-3, calculate area under the curve by trapezoidal rule.

Solution

Figure 8-6 shows a plot of the data given in Example 8-3. Since concentration of drug in plasma at time 0 is given in the data, one does not need to determine plasma drug concentration at time 0 using a semi-logarithmic graph paper. The adjacent concentration points are joined with straight lines and a perpendicular is drawn on x-axis from each concentration point to obtain the various geometric figures (segments) that comprise the curve from time 0 to 5 hours.

The AUC from time 0 to 5 hours calculated by the trapezoidal rule depends on the number of concentration points obtained from time 0 to 5 hours. Greater the number of concentration points, the more accurate the AUC. As can be seen in Figure 8-6, this plot consists of 10 segments, marked A through J. Only the first segment, segment A is a triangle, whereas all other segments (segments B through J) are trapezoids, i.e. this plot contains 1 triangle and 9 trapezoids. The area of each segment is calculated using the formula of the geometric figure of the segment (triangle for segment A and trapezoid for segments B through J). The sum of areas of all these 10 segments yields AUC from time 0 to the time of last data point plotted in the graph.

The calculations used for the determination of area of each geometric figure (segment) in this graph are shown in Table 8-1. The area of each segment is then added to obtain area under the plasma concentration versus time curve from time 0 to 5 hours.

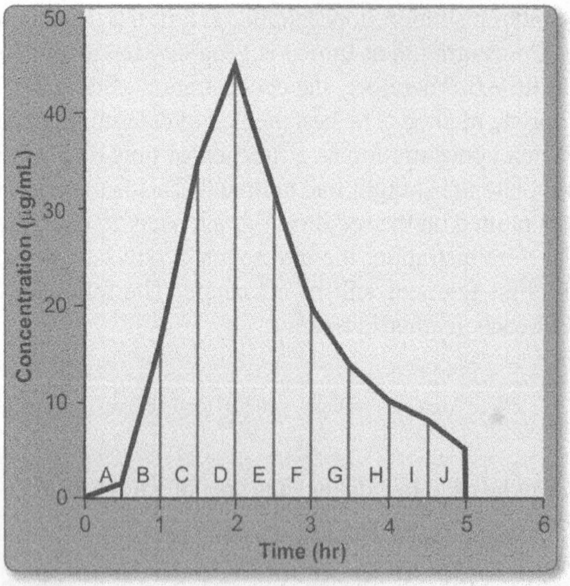

Fig. 8-6 Area under the curve by trapezoidal rule

Table 8-1 Area under the curve by trapezoidal rule for data in Fig. 8-6

Segment	*Geometric Figure*	*Area (µg × h/mL)*
A	triangle	(0.5)(1.5)(0.5) = 0.375
B	trapezoid	(0.5)(0.5)(1.5 + 16) = 4.375
C	trapezoid	(0.5)(0.5)(16 + 35) = 12.750
D	trapezoid	(0.5)(0.5)(35 + 45) = 20.00
E	trapezoid	(0.5)(0.5)(45 + 32) = 19.250
F	trapezoid	(0.5)(0.5)(32 + 20) = 13.000
G	trapezoid	(0.5)(0.5)(20 + 14) = 8.500
H	trapezoid	(0.5)(0.5)(14 + 10) = 6.000
I	trapezoid	(0.5)(0.5)(10 + 8) = 4.500
J	trapezoid	(0.5)(0.5)(8 + 5) = 3.250
	Area under the curve from 0 to 5 hours = 92.000	

Cutting and Weighing

Cutting and weighing method involves plotting the plasma profile on a graph paper and then, as the name of this method implies, cutting and weighing the plasma profile. The plasma concentration as a function of time is plotted on a rectilinear graph paper and instead of joining the points with a straight line (as was done in the trapezoidal method), a smooth curve is drawn to represent the data points. The curve thus obtained is cut from the graph paper and its weight is determined. The weight of the curve is then converted into the area bounded by the curve as follows.

Briefly, the method involves using two graphs: one graph paper is used to plot the data and another graph paper is used as a reference graph paper. The only requirements are:

a. The graph papers used must be identical in all respects (e.g. size and dimensions of the graph paper, weight of the graph paper, markings on the graph paper, etc.)
b. The scales used for x-axis and the y-axis in each case must also be identical.

The first requirement is easily met if:

i. One uses two graph papers from the same batch
ii. One graph paper is divided into two equal parts and these two equal parts are used as two graph papers.

The second requirement is easily met by using identical scales for x-axis on the two graphs and identical scales for y-axis on each graph paper.

The plasma concentration of drug as a function of time is plotted on one of the graph papers and a smooth curve is drawn to best represent the concentration points. The curve is then carefully cut with a pair of sharp scissors and weighed accurately on an analytical balance. Let us suppose that the weight of the curve is w_1. It does not matter what units are used for the weight. The weight may be in grams, or milligrams, or grains, or any other scientific units. This means that area under the plasma concentration versus time curve (AUC_1) is proportional to the weight of graph paper (w_1) of this curve, i.e.

$$AUC_1 \propto w_1 \tag{8-5}$$

To determine the relationship between the AUC and weight of the curve, the second identical graph paper is used. The x-axis and the y-axis are marked on this paper using the same scale that was used to plot the plasma concentration versus time curve. The area of this graph paper is calculated using the relationship:

$$\text{Area} = (\text{Length})(\text{Height}) \tag{8-6}$$

For example, if the y-axis (concentration of drug in the plasma) on this graph paper was plotted from 0 μg/mL to 100 μg/mL and the x-axis (time) was from 0 to 14 hours, then the area of this graph paper is:

$$(100\ \mu g/mL)(14\ h) = 1{,}400\ \mu g \times h/mL$$

Let us call this AUC_2. The margins of this graph paper are now removed with a pair of sharp scissors and the graph paper is weighed accurately on an analytical balance. The units of weight used for this graph paper must be same as were used for the weight of the plasma concentration versus time curve. Let us suppose that the weight of this graph paper is found to be w_2 g. This means that the weight w_2 g of this graph paper is equivalent to an area of AUC_2 (1,400 μg × h/mL in this case), i.e.,

$$AUC_2 \propto w_2 \quad (8\text{-}7)$$

Knowing the relationship between weight and area of the paper, the area of concentration of drug in plasma versus time curve can be calculated from the weight of the plasma concentration curve by combining equations (8-5) and (8-7):

$$\frac{AUC_1}{w_1} = \frac{AUC_2}{w_2} \quad (8\text{-}8)$$

The following relationship is used to determine AUC represented by the plasma concentration versus time data:

$$AUC_1 = \frac{(AUC_2)(w_1)}{w_2} \quad (8\text{-}9)$$

where,
AUC_1 = area under the plasma concentration versus time curve
AUC_2 = area of reference graph paper
w_1 = weight of curve
w_2 = weight of the reference graph paper.

This method is frequently used to compare AUC of two or more formulations, e.g. determination of relative bioavailability from two different dosage forms, or from products in the same dosage form manufactured by different manufacturers, or from similar dosage forms made by the same manufacturer, but containing different strengths of active ingredient. The following example illustrates the use of cutting and weighing technique for determination of AUC.

Example 8-5 The data given in Example 8-3 were plotted on a graph paper. The entire length of y-axis represented 50 μg/mL and the entire length of the x-axis represented 7 hours. The curve was cut and its weight was 1.1507 g. An identical graph paper, with margins removed and representing 50 μg/mL on the y-axis and 7 hours on the x-axis weighed 4.3775 g. Calculate area under the curve.

Solution

The graph paper weighing 4.3775 g is the reference graph paper and the graph paper weighing 1.1507 g is the test graph paper.

The area of reference graph paper = (50 μg/mL)(7 hours) = 350 μg × h/mL, therefore,

$$AUC_{ref} = 350\ \mu g \times h/mL,$$
$$w_{ref} = 4.3775, \text{ and}$$
$$w_{test} = 1.1507g$$

Substituting the relevant values into equation (8-9):

$$\text{Area of graph weighing } 1.1507\ g = \frac{(350\ \mu g \times h/mL)(1.1507\ g)}{4.3775\ g} = 92\ \mu g \times h/mL$$

Example 8-6 Formulation A is a generic product and formulation B is innovator's formulation. The data from the two formulations are plotted on separate graph papers using identical x- and y-axis. The plasma profiles are cut and accurately weighed. If the weight of curve A is 0.6198 g and the weight of curve B is 0.6887 g, what is the extent of absorption of drug from formulation A relative to formulation B?

Solution

From the data provided, the relative extent of absorption from formulation A is

$$\frac{\text{AUC of A}}{\text{AUC of B}} = \frac{\text{weight of curve A}}{\text{weight of curve B}}$$

$$\frac{\text{AUC of A}}{\text{AUC of B}} = \frac{0.6198}{0.6887} = 0.9 = 90\%$$

Since AUC from formulation A is 90% that of formulation B, it means that extent of absorption from formulation A is 90% compared to extent of absorption from formulation B.

INTRAVENOUS ADMINISTRATION

The discussion and examples pertaining to the determination of AUC has so far been limited to situations, where the drug dose is administered extravascularly as a single bolus dose. It has been seen that when a drug is administered extravascularly, the concentration of drug in plasma at time 0 is 0 and hence, plasma profile can be obtained by drawing a smooth curve starting at time 0. However, when the drug is administered intravenously as a single bolus dose, the concentration of drug in plasma is at time 0 is not 0. Therefore, in order to obtain the plasma profile starting at time 0, the plasma concentration of drug at time 0 must first be determined. It is customary to obtain this concentration of drug at time 0 from a linear plot of plasma concentration versus time (e.g. by plotting the data according to first order kinetics on a semi-logarithmic graph paper and back-extrapolating the straight line to time 0). This concentration (at time 0) is then plotted on the graph being prepared for the determination of AUC to obtain the plasma profile starting from time 0. The area under the plasma concentration versus time curve is the determined either by drawing a smooth curve (and counting squares, or cutting and weighing technique), or geometrical figures are drawn to calculate area of these geometrical figures and thus obtain area under the plasma concentration-time curve.

The following example illustrates the methodology used for the determination of AUC after intravenous administration of a single bolus dose of a drug.

Example 8-7 The plasma concentration as a function of time following a single bolus intravenous 10 mg dose of a drug is shown below. Calculate area under the curve from 0 to 7 hours.

Time (h)	1	2	3	4	6	7
Concentration (μg/L):	16	13	10	8	5	4

Solution

A plot of plasma concentration versus time on a rectilinear graph paper is shown in Figure 8-7.

Although any one of the four methods discussed earlier may be used to calculate area under the plasma concentration versus time curve, it will be necessary to determine the concentration of drug at time 0 in order to determine AUC for the first hour (the first segment of the plasma profile).

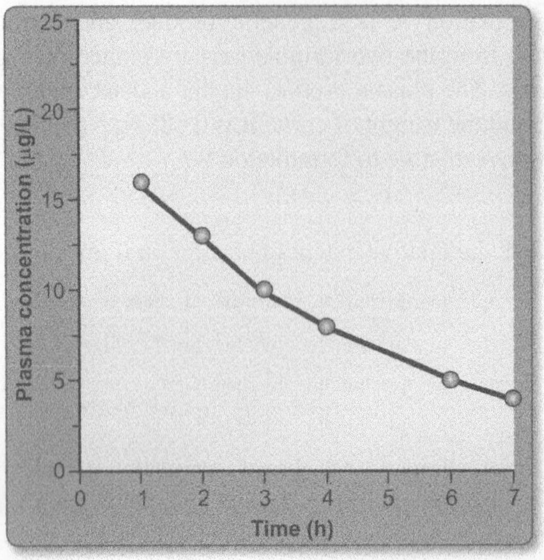

Fig. 8-7 Plot of the data in Example 8-7 on a rectangular graph paper

The plasma profile shown in Figire 8-7 does not show a linear relationship between the concentration of drug in plasma versus time. This indicates that elimination of drug from the plasma does not follow zero-order kinetics.

The graph shown in Figure 8-7 should not be used to determine concentration of drug at time zero, because the curve cannot be back-extrapolated to time zero (with a reasonable degree of accuracy) to determine concentration of drug in plasma at time zero (concentration of drug in the plasma immediately after administration of the dose). The data are therefore, plotted on a semi-logarithmic graph paper to determine if the plasma profile follows first-order kinetics. If a linear relationship is found between the concentration of drug in plasma and time according to first-order kinetics, then one can determine concentration at time 0 by simply back-extrapolating the straight line to time 0.

A plot of the data on a semi-logarithmic graph paper is shown in Figure 8-8. This plot indicates elimination of drug according to first-order kinetics. The linear relationship between concentration of drug in the plasma and time is back-extrapolated to time zero to determine concentration of drug in plasma at time 0. The y-intercept in this graph reads 20 μg/L, meaning that concentration of drug in the plasma at time zero (immediately after the administration of the dose) = 20 μg/L.

As mentioned earlier, to determine the area under the plasma concentration versus time curve from time zero to 7 hours, one may use any of the four methods for estimating AUC described earlier (the use of planimeter, the method of counting squares, the trapezoidal method, or the method of cutting and weighing the curve). For the sake of simplicity and convenience, the trapezoidal method is used here to calculate AUC from time 0 to 7 hours.

The data plotted on a rectilinear graph paper (shown in Figure 8-7) are used, except that a new concentration point at time 0 is added. This concentration point was determined from the graph (shown in Figure 8-7) by back-extrapolation of the straight line to time zero. Instead of drawing a smooth curve to best represent the concentration data points, the adjacent concentration points are joined together with straight lines and a perpendicular is drawn from each of these concentration points on the x-axis, resulting into geometric figures. Thus, one develops geometric figures for the entire plasma profile from zero to 7 hours.

Figure 8-9 shows the geometric figures developed by this method. As can be seen from Figure 8-9, the plasma profile from time zero to 7 hours is divided into six trapezoidal segments, because there only six plasma concentration points were provided in the data (the data did not provide a concentration point at 5 hours). These trapezoids are identified in Figure 8-9 as segments A through F.

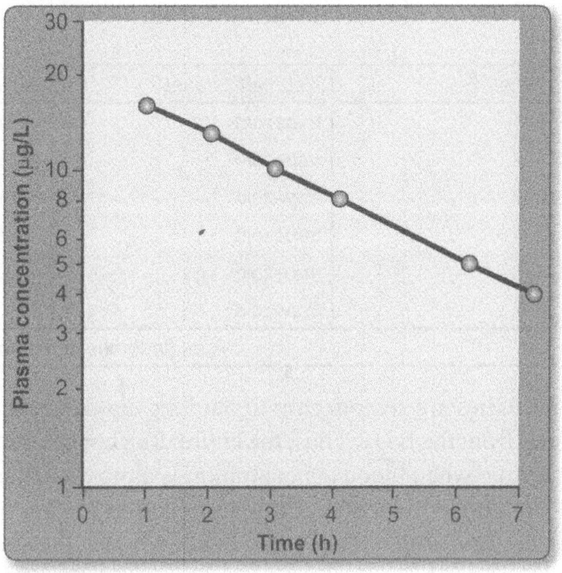

Fig. 8-8 Semi-logarithmic Plot of Data in Example 8-7

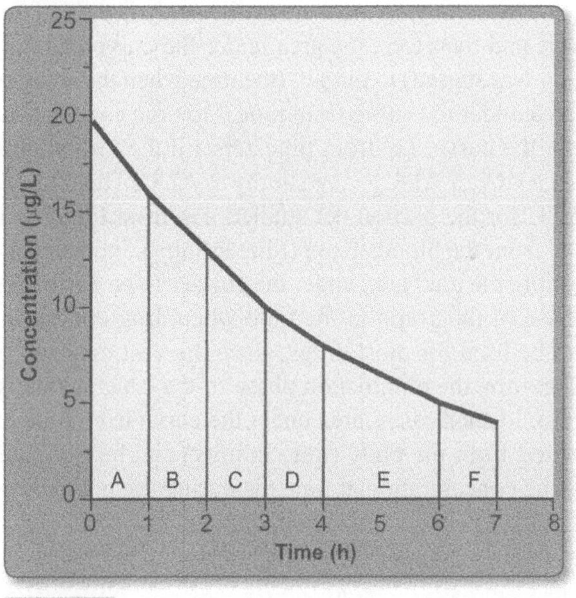

Fig. 8-9 Estimation of area under the curve (AUC) by trapezoidal rule

The area of each segment (trapezoid) is calculated using the formula given in equation (8-7) for the area of a trapezoid. Table 8-2 shows calculations used for determining area of the six trapezoids shown in Figure 8-9 and determination of AUC from 0 to 7 hours using trapezoidal method.

Total Area Under the Curve

Total area under the curve is area under the plasma concentration versus time curve from the time the drug appears in systemic circulation to the time that the drug is virtually eliminated from the systemic circulation. Since most drugs are absorbed almost immediately after administration of the drug dose, the appearance of drug in plasma is considered to have taken place at time zero. Therefore, total area under the curve is also referred to as AUC from time zero to infinity.

Table 8-2 Determination of AUC using trapezoidal rule for the data shown in Fig. 8-9

Segment	*Time (h)*	*Geometric figure*	*Area (μg × h/L)*
A	0–1	trapezoid	(0.5)(1.0)(20 + 16) = 18.0
B	1–2	trapezoid	(0.5)(1.0)(16 + 13) = 14.5
C	2–3	trapezoid	(0.5)(1.0)(13 + 10) = 11.5
D	3–4	trapezoid	(0.5)(1.0)(10 + 8) = 9.0
E	4–6	trapezoid	(0.5)(2.0)(8 + 5) = 13.0
F	6–7	trapezoid	(0.5)(1.0)(5 + 4) = 4.5
			Area under the curve from 0–7 h = 70.5

Pharmacokinetic studies are seldom carried out long enough to allow the drug to be almost completely eliminated from the body. Thus, the entire drug concentration versus time curve (i.e. from time zero to the time when blood concentration is almost zero) is usually not available for estimating the total area under the curve. Early termination of pharmacokinetic study is partly due to time constraints (for a drug having a half-life of 6 hours, the study may have to be carried for more than 2 days) and partly because very low concentrations of drug in the plasma samples (when the drug is almost virtually eliminated from the body) are very difficult to determine with a reasonable degree of accuracy. In most cases, the study is carried out only sufficiently beyond the absorptive phase and therefore, the area under the curve can only be estimated from time zero (when the study was started) to time 't' (the time when the study was terminated). The AUC thus estimated is area under the curve from time 0 to time t and is usually indicated as AUC_{0-t}.

Total area under the curve, i.e. from time zero till the virtual elimination of drug from the body is indicated as AUC_{total}, $AUC_{0-\infty}$ or simply as AUC. The total area under the curve (AUC) is AUC_{0-t} plus AUC for the portion not studied, i.e. from time t to the time when the drug is virtually eliminated from the bloodstream (time infinity), indicated as $AUC_{t-\infty}$. If drug follows zero-order elimination, the total area under the curve can be easily determined by extrapolating the elimination phase of the graph to the time when drug concentration reaches 0. However, this method cannot be used for most drugs, since the vast majority of drugs follow first-order elimination and therefore, the elimination phase of the drug profile is neither linear nor attains a value equal to zero. In such cases, area under the curve from time t to the time when the drug is virtually eliminated from the body (time infinity) can be estimated by using the following equation provided the concentration at time t is during the post-absorptive phase:

$$AUC_{t-\infty} = \frac{C_t}{K} \tag{8-10}$$

where,

C_t = concentration of drug in the plasma at time t (this is the last concentration point in the plasma profile shown in, Figure 8-6)

K = apparent first order elimination rate constant.

This area, added to the area calculated from time 0 to time t gives the total area under the plasma concentration-time curve. As mentioned above, equation (8-10) is applicable only if:

i. The concentration at time t (C_t) is during the post-absorptive phase (i.e. there is no input of drug in the systemic circulation).
ii. Elimination follows first-order kinetics.

The use of equation (8-10) is not limited to the last concentration data point. This equation can be used for concentration at any data point as long as there is no more drug input after this concentration point, i.e. the absorption phase is virtually complete. Thus, for drugs administered by intravenous bolus injection and eliminated by first-order kinetics, equation (8-10) can be modified to calculate total area under the curve. In this case, since the drug does not undergo absorption, the concentration of drug in plasma immediately after the administration of the dose (C_0) is concentration of drug in the post-absorptive phase. Therefore, in equation (8-10) if the term t (for time t) is changed to zero, then the concentration at time t, C_t, should also be changed to C_0.

Equation (8-10) now becomes:

$$AUC_{0-\infty} = \frac{C_0}{K} \quad (8\text{-}11)$$

Equation (8-11) describes the total area under the curve (AUC_{total}) following the administration of a single intravenous bolus dose.

Example 8-8 Using the data given in Example 8-7, calculate total area under the curve (AUC from time 0 to infinity).

Solution

Two methods can be used to calculate total area under the plasma concentration versus time curve:

A. Using the trapezoidal rule: Determine area under the curve from 7 hours to infinity using equation (8-10) and add this area to area under the curve from 0–7 hours calculated in Example 8-7. The sum of these two would be the total area under the curve.
B. Using the relationship between C_0 and K
   Equation (8-11) is used to calculate total area under the curve following intravenous administration of the drug.

A. Using the trapezoidal rule:

1. The trapezoidal rule is used to calculate area under the curve from 0 to 7 hours. This was calculated in Example 8-7 and was found to be 70.5 μg × h/L
2. The area under the curve from 7 hours to infinity is calculated using equation (8-10). To use this equation we need the values of C_0 and K. From the plot of concentration of drug in plasma versus time shown in Figure 8-8, C_0 = 20 μg/L. Also from Figure 8-8,

$$K = -\text{slope}\ \frac{\ln 20\ \mu g/L - \ln 4\ \mu g/L}{0\ h - 7\ h} = \frac{1.6094}{-7\ h} = 0.23/h$$

Therefore, using equation (8-10) and substituting the values of C_t = 4 μg/L at t = 7 hours,

$$AUC_{t-\infty} = \frac{C_t}{K} = \frac{4\ \mu g/L}{0.23/h} = 17\ \mu g \times h/L$$

Thus,

$$AUC_{0-7} = 70.5\ \mu g \times h/L, \text{ and}$$

$$AUC_{7-\infty} = 17\ \mu g \times h/L. \text{ Therefore,}$$

$$AUC_{0-\infty} = AUC_{0-7} + AUC_{7-\infty}$$

$$AUC_{0-\infty} = 17\ \mu g \times h/L + 70.5\ \mu g \times h/L$$

$$AUC_{0-\infty} = 87.5\ \mu g \times h/mL$$

B. Using the relationship between C_0 and K

Equation (8-11) is used to calculate total area under the curve following intravenous administration of the drug. C_0 = 20 μg/L

$$AUC_{0-\infty} = \frac{C_0}{K} = \frac{20\ \mu g/L}{0.23/h} = 87\ \mu g \times h/L$$

Example 8-9 A patient was administered a 325 mg oral dose of a drug. The concentration of drug in plasma after 8 hour was 5 mg/L. If biological half-life of the drug is 4 hour, calculate area under the plasma concentration versus time curve from 8 hours till the virtually complete elimination of drug from the body.

Solution

Since, $t_{1/2}$ = 4 h, therefore, the rate constant of elimination, K is

$$K = \frac{0.693}{t_{1/2}} = \frac{0.693}{4\ h} = 0.17325/h$$

$$AUC_{8-\infty} = \frac{C_8}{K} = \frac{5\ mg/L}{0.17325/h} = 28.86\ \mu g \times h/L$$

Example 8-10 A patient was administered a 500 mg oral dose of a drug. The concentration of drug in plasma after 10 hour was 3 mg/L. If biological half-life of the drug is 8 hour, calculate area under the plasma concentration versus time curve from 10 h till the virtually complete elimination of drug from the body.

Solution

Since, $t_{1/2}$ = 8 h, therefore, the elimination rate constant, K is

$$K = \frac{0.693}{t_{1/2}} = \frac{0.693}{8\ h} = 0.086625/h$$

$$AUC_{10-\infty} = \frac{C_{10}}{K} = \frac{3\ mg/L}{0.086625/h} = 34.632\ mg \times h/L$$

Amount of Drug Absorbed

When a drug is administered intravenously, the entire drug dose is placed into the systemic circulation. Therefore, the amount of drug 'absorbed' from an intravenous dose is considered to be equal to the amount of drug administered. However, when the drug is administered extravascularly, the amount of drug absorbed from the administered dose may vary considerably. For some drugs, the amount of drug absorbed from an extravascularly administered dose is equal to the amount of drug dose administered. But, for many drugs the amount of drug aborbed is not necessarily equal to the amount of dose administered. Some orally administered drugs are acid-labile and unless administered as an enteric-coated product, a portion of the administered dose may be destroyed before it can be absorbed. Some drugs are inactivated in the presence of enzymes and the entire administered dose may not be available for absorption, because a portion of the drug dose administered may undergo degradation in the gastrointestinal environment. Similarly, a portion of the intramuscularly administered dose may be bound to the skin before it is absorbed.

To determine the amount of drug absorbed from an extravascularly administered dose, a similar dose is administered intravenously as an aqueous solution. The drug solution should not contain additives or formulation aides in order to be sure that the drug is not bound to or complexed with the additives or formulation aides.

The area under the plasma concentration versus time curve of the intravenously administered dose is determined. As mentioned previously, since the availability of drug from intravenous solution is 100%, a comparison of area under the curve from the extravascularly administered dose relative to the area under the curve from the intravenous dose provides the fraction of dose absorbed from the extravascular dosage form.

Example 8-11 The area under the plasma concentration versus time curve from a 325 mg bolus dose of a drug administered intravenously as an aqueous solution was found to be 185 μg × h/mL and the area under plasma concentration versus time curve from a similar dose administered orally as a tablet was found to be 153 μg × h/mL. What is the extent of absorption from the tablet formulation?

Solution

Compared to the intravenous dose, the extent of absorption from the oral tablet is 153 μg × h/mL

$$\text{Extent of absorption from the tablet} = \frac{153\ \mu g \times h/mL}{185\ \mu g \times h/mL}$$

$$\text{Extent of absorption from the tablet} = 0.827$$

For the sake of convenience, the extent of absorption of drug is usually expressed as a percent, rather than a fraction. Therefore,
Extent of absorption of the from the tablet = (0.827)(100) = 82.7%, and
The amount of drug absorbed from the 325 mg dose = 82.7% of 325 mg = 268.775 mg.

Example 8-12 The areas under the plasma concentration versus time curve obtained after administration of identical doses of a drug from five dosage forms are shown in the following table:

Dosage Form	*AUC (μg x h/mL)*
Intravenous solution	1,900
Capsule	1,700
Tablet	1,520
Oral solution	1,830
Suspension	1,600

Calculate the extent of absorption of the drug from the following dosage forms:
1. Capsule relative to the tablet dosage form
2. Oral solution relative to the intravenous injection
3. Suspension relative to the oral solution dosage form
4. Tablet relative to the suspension dosage form
5. Capsule relative to the intravenous solution.

Solution

1. Extent of absorption from capsule relative to the tablet dosage form is:

$$\frac{1,700\ \mu g \times h/mL}{1,520\ \mu g \times h/mL} = 1.118$$

2. Extent of absorption from oral solution relative to the intravenous dosage form is:

$$\frac{1,830\ \mu g \times h/mL}{1,900\ \mu g \times h/mL} = 0.9632$$

3. Extent of absorption from suspension relative to oral solution dosage form is:

$$\frac{1,600\ \mu g \times h/mL}{1,830\ \mu g \times h/mL} = 0.8743$$

4. Extent of absorption from tablet relative to the suspension dosage form is:

$$\frac{1,520\ \mu g \times h/mL}{1,600\ \mu g \times h/mL} = 0.95$$

5. Extent of absorption from capsule relative to the intravenous injection is:

$$\frac{1,700\ \mu g \times h/mL}{1,900\ \mu g \times h/mL} = 0.8947$$

SUGGESTED READING

1. American Pharmaceutical Association. Guidelines for biopharmaceutical studies in man. Acad Pharm Aci, Washington DC. 1972.
2. Madan PL. Bioavailability and bioequivalence: The underlying concepts. US Pharmacist. 1992;17(11):H10-H30.
3. Madan PL. Bioavailability and patient variances. US Pharmacist. 1996;21(5):3-14.

PRACTICE PROBLEMS

8-1. The area under plasma concentration versus time curve after a 500 mg IV bolus dose of a drug was 285 μg × h/mL and AUC from a similar dose given orally as a tablet was 265 μg × h/mL. What is the extent of absorption from the tablet formulation?

8-2. Calculate the relative bioavailability of a drug from a suspension formulation if the area under the curve from a 325 mg dose was 135 μg × h/mL and area under the curve from a similar tablet dose was 170 μg × h/mL.

8-3. The plasma concentration versus time data obtained after oral dose of a drug were plotted on a rectilinear graph paper representing 100 μg/mL on the y-axis and 14 hours on the x-axis. The curve was cut and it weighed 2.1515 g. An identical graph paper representing 14 hours on the x-axis and 100 μg/mL on the y-axis weighed 4.7705 g. Calculate the area under the curve.

8-4. From the following data obtained after administration of a single 1,000 mg dose, calculate: (a) onset of action, (b) intensity of action, (c) duration of action and (d) area under the plasma concentration versus time curve from the time of drug administration to 14 hours. The minimum effective concentration of drug is 12 mg/L.

Time (h)	*Concentration (mg/L)*	*Time (h)*	*Concentration (mg/L)*
1	26.0	8	22.8
2	36.0	10	17.4
4	35.4	12	13.2
6	29.0	14	10.0

8-5. Calculate the area under the plasma concentration versus time curve from the time of drug administration to14 hours from the following data obtained after the administration of a 500 mg dose of an antibiotic. If MEC is 7.2 μg/mL, calculate: (a) onset of action, (b) intensity of action and (c) duration of action.

Time (h)	*Concentration (mg/L)*	*Time (h)*	*Concentration (mg/L)*
1	5.8	8	10.0
2	9.2	10	8.5
4	12.0	12	7.1
6	11.5	14	6.0

8-6. Calculate the total area under the curve (AUC_{total}) from the following data obtained after the administration of a single 1 g dose of a drug. The rate constant of elimination of the drug is known to be 0.036/h.

Time (h)	*Concentration (mg/L)*	*Time (h)*	*Concentration (mg/L)*
1	6.0	8	12.5
2	9.6	10	11.5
4	12.8	12	10.7
6	13.2	14	10.0

8-7. Calculate the total area under the curve from the following data obtained after administration of a single 0.5 g dose of a drug. The rate constant of elimination of the drug is 0.124/h and the minimum effective concentration of this drug has been reported to be 1.5 mg/mL.

Time (h)	Concentration (mg/L)	Time (h)	Concentration (mg/L)
1	4.9	8	7.4
2	7.6	10	5.8
4	8.9	12	4.5
6	9.4	14	3.5

8-8. The following data were obtained after administration of a single 200 mg dose of the drug. If the minimum effective concentration of the drug is 1.5 mg/mL, calculate: (a) onset of action, (b) the intensity of action, (c) duration of action and (d) total area under the plasma concentration versus time curve. The rate constant of elimination of the drug is 0.238/h.

Time (h)	Concentration (mg/mL)	Time (h)	Concentration (mg/mL)	Time (h)	Concentration (mg/mL)
0.5	2.40	2.0	4.25	5.0	2.54
1.0	3.70	3.0	3.80	6.0	1.95
1.5	4.15	4.0	3.10	7.0	1.50

8-9. The plasma concentration versus time data obtained after oral dose of a drug were plotted on a rectilinear graph paper representing 100 mcg/mL on y-axis and 14 hours on x-axis. The curve was cut and it weighed 3.515 g. An identical graph paper, with margins removed and representing similar x- and y-axis weighed 4.275 g. Calculate area under the curve from the oral dose.

8-10. The area under plasma concentration versus time curve from a 325 mg dose of an oral suspension was 185 μg × h/mL and area under the curve from a similar 325 mg single dose from a tablet was 170 μg × h/mL. Calculate the relative bioavailability of drug from the suspension formulation.

8-11. If minimum effective concentration of a drug is 6 mg/L, calculate onset of action, intensity of action, duration of action and total area under the curve from the following data obtained after administration of a single 200 mg dose of the drug. The rate constant of elimination is 0.215/h.

Time (h)	Concentration (mg/L)	Time (h)	Concentration (mg/L)
1	12.0	8	9.1
2	17.5	10	6.6
4	17.3	12	4.3
6	12.9	14	2.8

8-12. Administration of a single 300 mg dose of an antibiotic by intravenous injection, oral tablet, or oral capsule gave the following data. If minimum effective concentration is 3 μg/mL, calculate:

a. Absolute bioavailability
b. Relative bioavailability from tablet and capsule dosage forms and
c. Onset, intensity and duration of action from each dosage form.

Time (h)	Plasma concentration (mg/L)		
	IV Injection	Tablet	Capsule
0.5	9.0	2.4	3.0
1.0	8.0	3.0	3.3
2.0	6.2	3.7	4.1
3.0	5.0	3.9	4.0
4.0	4.0	3.6	3.9
5.0	3.2	2.8	3.1
6.0	2.5	2.2	2.4
7.0	2.0	1.8	1.9

8-13. The plasma concentration as a function of time following a single bolus intravenous 10 mg dose of a drug is shown below. Calculate total area under the curve.

Time (h)	1	2	3	4	6	7
Concentration (μg/L)	16	13	10	8	5	4

CHAPTER 9

BIOEQUIVALENCE

The term bioequivalence indicates biological equivalence. Bioequivalence has also been referred to as comparative bioavailability. The concept of bioequivalence started to gain increasing attention during the last forty years or so, after it became evident that some marketed products containing the same amount of drug marketed in the same dosage form exhibited marked differences between their therapeutic responses. In many instances different therapeutic responses observed with these products were correlated successfully to dissimilar levels of drug concentration in the plasma, which was caused mainly because of differences in the rate of absorption of drug from these products.

It is now very well established that the rate at which and the extent to which an administered drug dose reaches systemic circulation for systemic effect and therefore the bioavailability of the drug depends on a number of very important factors. From a pharmaceutical standpoint, there are three inherent factors that are known to affect drug absorption and therefore systemic availability of a drug after administration of the drug dose. These are:

a. Formulation technique used in the development of the dosage form
b. Method and equipment used in the manufacture of dosage form
c. Materials used in the formulation of dosage form even though these materials are considered inert. These include: the particle size and crystal form or polymorphic form of the drug substance, diluents and excipients used in the dosage form including binders, disintegrating agents, fillers, lubricants, coating materials, solvents, suspending agents and dyes. Lubricants and coating materials are foremost among the materials that are suspect in the bioavailability problems.

The formulation of the same drug by different manufacturers in similar dosage forms or the formulation of the same drug by the same manufacture in different dosage forms or the formulation of a drug by the same manufacturer in different countries may exhibit different bioavailability characteristics and therefore potentially different clinical effectiveness. For example, two or more products may appear identical or equivalent because they contain the same drug, in same dosage strength, and in the same dosage form. But, if some formulation materials (e.g. diluents, binders, disintegrants, lubricants, etc.) used in their manufacture were different, then it is possible that these products may exhibit differences in bioavailability of the drug and thus in clinical effectiveness of the drug. The classic case of Dilantin is an example of this situation. A few years ago, a number of Dilantin toxicity cases were reported in Australia. The patients reporting toxicity had been taking Dilantin for some time not only in the same dosage form, but also in the same strength of the dosage form. Later, it was discovered that the company had started manufacturing Dilantin locally using the same formula, but because of availability problems, a different diluent was used in the domestic product. The change in diluent was identified to be responsible for the differing availability of drug from the locally manufactured dosage form. It was found that the diluent previously used in the imported product was binding a fraction of drug in the dosage form, whereas the binder used in the domestic product did not bind to the drug at all. Thus, due to no binding of drug to the new diluent, larger amount of the drug was released from the new formulation. Thus, the bioavailability of drug from the domestic product had increased and a larger amount of the drug was reaching systemic circulation, thereby exhibiting toxic effects.

In another widely publicized study, digoxin was shown to exhibit varying availability from different manufacturers although each dosage form contained the same drug in the same strength. Also, differences in the availability of digoxin from different batches of the same dosage form made by the same manufacturer were reported in several studies published in scientific journals. Many researchers have shown that a variety of factors in the preparation of a formulation of a dosage form can result in differing bioavailability of drug from the dosage form and possibly clinical effectiveness. These factors include the following:

a. Use of different formulation materials
b. Use of similar material obtained from different suppliers
c. Validity of process variables
d. Method of manufacture
e. Equipment used in the manufacturing process.

It is therefore clear that equivalency of drug products, which may appear identical in many respects becomes questionable.

EQUIVALENCE

Equivalence is a comparative term and is used to indicate that two or more substances labeled as equivalent are presumed to be similar to one another with respect to a specific characteristic or function. The term bioequivalence is used in pharmaceutical industry to indicate that when different products or dosage forms are labeled as equivalent products, there are certain similarities in these products with respect to a defined set of standards. The following terms are used to define the type or level of 'equivalency' between such drug products.

Pharmaceutical Equivalents

The Food and Drug Administration (FDA) defines the term 'pharmaceutical equivalent' products as follows:

> *Drug products are considered to be pharmaceutical equivalents if they contain the same active ingredient(s) and are identical in strength or concentration, dosage form and route of administration.*

According to this definition, pharmaceutically equivalent drug products must contain the same amount or concentration of active ingredient in the same dosage form and must be administered by the same route of administration. This means that these products may or may not contain the same inert ingredients, both qualitatively as well as quantitatively. Thus, all brands of diazepam 5 mg oral tablets manufactured by various manufacturers are pharmaceutically equivalent as long as each brand of tablets contains 5 mg of diazepam, regardless of the type and amount of inert ingredient or ingredients used in the formulation of the tablet dosage form. For example, one manufacturer may use lactose as the diluent, another manufacturer may use dicalcium phosphate as the diluent and another manufacturer may use starch as the diluent in the production of their tablet dosage forms. Similarly, different manufacturers may use different amounts and different types of other excipients (for example, binder, disintegrant, lubricant, etc.) in the fabrication of their tablet dosage forms.

All pharmaceutically equivalent products are formulated to meet the same standards that have been established for that particular product. These standards may be standards established by the compendial requirements or they may be established by other applicable standards (i.e. standards concerning strength, quality, purity and identity of the product). However, pharmaceutically equivalent products may differ from each other in a variety of physical characteristics, e.g. shape and size of the dosage form, scoring and/or embossing configuration on the product, packaging of the finished product, expiration time of the product and within certain limits, labeling on the finished product. In addition, they may not necessarily contain the same formulation excipients (e.g. binders, lubricants, disintegrating agents, etc.), including colors, preservatives, flavors, etc.

Pharmaceutical equivalents have sometimes been referred to as chemical equivalents, because the only requirement of pharmaceutically equivalent products is that they must contain the same chemical entity (drug) in the same strength. Since pharmaceutical equivalents are not required to contain identical amounts of same formulation excipients, it is conceivable that differing amounts and/or types of inert ingredient used in the manufacture of pharmaceutically equivalent products may not necessarily provide similar availability of active ingredient for systemic effect.

Example 9-1 Which of the following three tablet formulations are pharmaceutically equivalent?

Ingredient	*Function*	*Tablet A*	*Tablet B*	*Tablet C*
Acetaminophen	Drug	300 mg	–	300 mg
Aspirin	Drug	–	300 mg	–
Lactose	Filler	100 mg	100 mg	-
Avicel	Filler	–	–	100 mg
Starch	Disintegrant	50 mg	50 mg	–
Avicel	Disintegrant	–	–	50 mg
Magnesium stearate	Lubricant	2 mg	2 mg	2 mg
Gelatin	Binder	10 mg	10 mg	10 mg

Solution

All three formulations are tablet formulations and are formulated to provide analgesic effect. Also, all three formulations contain the same amount of active ingredient and all three tablets are intended to be administered by the same route of administration. However, the type and quantities of inert ingredients in the three formulations are not similar.

Although formulations A and B contain identical quantities of the same inert ingredients, their active ingredient (drug entity) is not the same. Therefore, tablets A and B are not pharmaceutically equivalent.

A comparison of tablet formulation B with the tablet formulation C shows that these two formulations contain different inert ingredients, as well as different active ingredient. Therefore, tablets B and C are not pharmaceutical equivalents because they do not contain the same active ingredient.

Formulations A and C contain different inert ingredients, but they contain the same active ingredient in the same amount. By definition, products are pharmaceutical equivalents if they contain the same active ingredients and are identical in strength, dosage form and route of administration. Therefore, according to this definition, tablets A and C are pharmaceutical equivalents.

Pharmaceutical Alternatives

The FDA defines pharmaceutical alternatives as follows:

> *Pharmaceutical alternatives are those drug products that contain the same therapeutic moiety, but are different salts, esters or complexes of that moiety or are different dosage forms or strengths.*

According to this definition, different dosage forms of the same drug product (e.g. tablets versus capsules, tablets versus suspension, capsules versus suspension, syrup versus suspension, etc.) are pharmaceutical alternatives. Similarly, different dosage strengths manufactured within a product line (e.g. 250 mg tablets versus 500 mg tablets, 500 mg tablets versus 250 mg capsules, or 125 mg tablet versus a suspension containing 125 mg per teaspoonful) manufactured by a single manufacturer are considered pharmaceutical alternatives.

Since, the definition of pharmaceutical alternatives does not specify that these products must also be pharmaceutical equivalents, therefore, pharmaceutical alternatives also include extended release products when compared with immediate-release formulations (or standard-release formulations) of the same active ingredient (e.g. phenytoin 100 mg immediate release oral capsules versus phenytoin 100 mg extended release oral capsules).

Since, by definition, products are considered pharmaceutical alternatives as long as they contain the same therapeutic moiety, not necessarily the same drug entity, a variety of dosage forms of the given drug product may fall in this category. Examples of pharmaceutical alternatives include such products as similar strengths of the antibiotic tetracycline hydrochloride capsules versus tetracycline phosphate complex capsules and similar strengths of quinidine sulfate tablets versus quinidine sulfate capsules.

Example 9-2 Five formulations of drug products are shown below. The amount of active ingredient listed for these products is per tablet, per capsule or per teaspoonful. Which of the following five formulations are pharmaceutical alternatives?

Ingredient	*Tablet A*	*Tablet B*	*Capsule C*	*Syrup D*	*Suspension E*
Ibuprofen	200 mg	–	–	–	200 mg
Aspirin	–	–	300 mg	–	–
Acetaminophen	–	250 mg	–	250 mg	–

Solution

The active ingredient in all five products provides analgesic effect. However, these products are formulated using different analgesics. The following products contain different drug entities: Products A, B and C; Products A, C and D; Products B, C and E; and products C, D and E, Therefore, these products are neither pharmaceutical equivalents nor pharmaceutical alternatives. Products A and E contain the same active ingredient in the same amount, therefore, these two products are pharmaceutical alternatives, but they are not pharmaceutical equivalents because the dosage form is different (one is a tablet and the other is a suspension). Similarly products B and D contain the same active ingredient in the same amount, therefore these two products are pharmaceutical alternatives, but they are not pharmaceutical equivalents because the dosage forms are different (one is a tablet and the other is a syrup).

Biological Equivalents

The FDA defines biological equivalents or bioequivalents as follows:

> *Biological equivalents or bioequivalents are pharmaceutical equivalents that exhibit comparable bioavailability when studied under similar experimental conditions.*

According to this definition, biological equivalent or bioequivalent drug products are those pharmaceutical equivalents that display similar rate of absorption and similar extent of absorption of therapeutic drug moiety when studied under similar experimental conditions. Although the definition specifies comparison of pharmaceutical equivalents, it is obvious that pharmaceutical alternatives are also included in this definition, because the comparison being made here is between therapeutic drug ingredient (drug moiety) and not between identical chemical compound. It is important to note that the comparison of rate and extent of absorption is made when the study is conducted under similar experimental conditions.

The FDA defines and describes conditions under which a test and reference drug must be bioequivalent. These conditions include (but are not limited to) the following:

a. The rate and extent of absorption of the test drug do not show a significant difference from the rate and extent of absorption from the reference drug when the therapeutic moiety (drug) is administered at the same molar dose under similar experimental conditions, either as a single dose or in multiple dose regimen. The similarity in the rate and extent of absorption is established by comparing the parameters of bioavailability (rate and extent of absorption or peak concentration, time of peak concentration and area under the curve) of the therapeutic moiety from the test product with those of the reference product.
b. Similarity in the extent of absorption when the difference in the rate of absorption from reference drug is intentional and is reflected in the proposed labeling of the test drug. This is acceptable only if difference in the rate of absorption is not essential to attainment of the effective concentration of drug in the body when administered for chronic use and is considered medically insignificant for the drug.
c. For topically applied products intended for local rather than systemic effect, other *in vivo* tests of bioequivalence may be appropriate.
d. Bioequivalence may sometimes be demonstrated using a suitable *in vitro* bioequivalence standard, especially when such an *in vitro* test has been correlated with human *in vivo* bioavailability data.

Therapeutic Equivalents

The FDA defines therapeutic equivalents as follows:

> *Therapeutic equivalents are those pharmaceutical equivalents that can be expected to have the same clinical effect when administered to patients under the conditions specified in the labeling.*

According to the FDA, the concept of therapeutic equivalence as used here applies only to those products that contain the same active ingredients, e.g. tetracycline hydrochloride tablets manufactured by different manufacturers or different strengths of tetracycline hydrochloride tablets made by the same manufacturer. The concept of therapeutic equivalence does not include a comparison of different therapeutic agents used for the same condition, i.e. different chemical compounds used for a therapeutic effect, e.g. aspirin versus acetaminophen or aspirin versus ibuprofen or ibuprofen versus acetaminophen for pain relief or propoxyphene hydrochloride versus pentazocine hydrochloride for the treatment of pain.

The FDA classifies only those products as therapeutically equivalent, that meet specified general criteria. Some of these criteria are:

1. They are approved as safe and effective, or approved under section 505(j) of the Federal Food, Drug and Cosmetic Act.
2. They are pharmaceutical equivalents in that:
   a. They contain identical amounts of the same active drug ingredient in the same dosage form, and
   b. Meet compendial or other applicable standards of identity, strength, purity and quality.
3. They are bioequivalent in that:
   a. They do not present a known or potential bioequivalence problem and they meet an acceptable *in vitro* standard, or

   b. If they do present such a known or potential problem, they are shown to meet an appropriate bioequivalence standard demonstrating comparable rate and extent of absorption.
4. They are adequately labeled.
5. They are manufactured in compliance with current good manufacturing practice (CGMP) regulations.

The FDA generally considers drug products to be therapeutically equivalent if they meet the criteria outlined above, even though they may differ in certain other characteristics. These characteristics include: shape and size of the dosage form, scoring and/or embossing configuration on the product, packaging of the finished product, expiration time of the product, certain minor aspects of labeling on the finished product (for example, presence of specific pharmacokinetic data and/or information). In addition, therapeutic equivalent products may not necessarily contain the same formulation excipients (e.g. fillers or diluents, disintegrating agents, binders, lubricants, etc.), including colors, flavors, preservatives, etc. The FDA concedes that when such differences are important in the care and treatment of a patient, it may be appropriate for the prescriber to require that a particular brand be dispensed as a medical necessity. The FDA also believes that with this limitation, products classified as therapeutically equivalent can be substituted with the full expectation that the substituted product will produce the same clinical effect as the originally prescribed product.

Many clinicians tend to believe that just because two or more drug products are bioequivalent, it does not necessarily mean that these products are also therapeutically equivalent. However, based on the findings of the FDA, this does not appear to be the case. According to the FDA, it is not aware of one single clinical study that compared two drug products evaluated by the FDA as bioequivalent or therapeutic equivalent that demonstrates therapeutic inequivalence.

Bioinequivalency

While the above defined terms explain the level of equivalency, they do not necessarily imply that all bioequivalent products must contain the same inert ingredients. Despite this, however, in most cases pharmaceutical equivalent products are also bioequivalent as well as therapeutically equivalent. The differences arise only when the active ingredient in two or more products is 'incompatible' with one or more inert ingredient. For example, if the diluent used in a tablet or capsule formulation binds or forms a complex with the active ingredient, then this formulation is not likely to be bioequivalent to a formulation prepared using a diluent, which does not interact with the active ingredient. Similarly, a tetracycline dosage form prepared using no calcium containing ingredient will be pharmaceutically equivalent to calcium-containing ingredients (e.g. dicalcium phosphate as on of the excipients), but in all probability will be neither bioequivalent nor therapeutically equivalent.

Until the late 1960's, disintegration time of tablets was considered an adequate test to ensure the availability of drug from the dosage form. However, in the case of some drugs, serious deficiency in bioavailability was noted to exist even if the dosage form disintegrated fully *in vivo*. The following discussion highlights some examples of wide variation in the bioavailability of some critical drugs. This discussion demonstrates serious consequences on the safety and therapeutic efficacy of some important drug products.

Aspirin

A study dealing with three commercial aspirin tablet products (Comparison of dissolution and absorption rates of different commercial aspirin tablets) was published in *J. Pharm. Sci.* **50**, 388, 1961. In this study it was reported that absorption rates, as well as the incidence and severity of localized gastric irritation (and possibly bleeding) following administration of aspirin tablets were interrelated. Both were a function of dissolution rate of aspirin from its particular dosage form. The rank order of the *in vivo* results showed excellent correlation to the *in vitro* dissolution rates of the three aspirin products. The study pointed out that disintegration time (which was the major test for *in vitro* bioequivalence at the time of publication of this study) had no bearing on the rate of absorption of aspirin from the tablets studied.

A comparison of disintegration times and dissolution rates (or initial absorption rates) of the three products tested indicated that the product with a longer disintegration time was actually most rapidly absorbed. The authors concluded that while delayed disintegration can interfere with absorption, it does so only by its effect on dissolution. Interestingly, the rank order of absorption of the three brands of aspirin tablets (and hence the side-effects) reported in this study coincided with an earlier study, which determined gastrointestinal blood loss in 120 subjects taking various forms of salicylates. According to the earlier report, fecal blood loss increased in the order: salicylate solution < product A < product B = product C. According to this study, it appears that the longer the aspirin tablet stayed in the stomach, the lower the absorption, the greater the irritation and the more chance that severe side effects such as gastric bleeding can take place.

Later, another study was conducted by Levy and his co-workers. In this study (G Levy, J Leonards, and J Procknal, 'Development of *in vitro* dissolution tests, which correlate quantitatively with dissolution rate-limited drug absorption in man', published in 1965 in the *J. Pharm. Sci.*, **54**, 1719, 1965), the authors investigated bioavailability of the following four dosage forms of aspirin: a solution, plain tablet, plain tablet containing alkaline additive as a buffer to enhance dissolution and aspirin in the form of microencapsulated aspirin particles. The study found that absorption of aspirin from the four dosage forms occurred at widely different rates. The shortest absorption half-life of aspirin (time required for 50% of the dose to be absorbed) was 5 minutes and was observed when aspirin was administered as a solution dosage form. On the other end of the scale, the longest absorption half-life of aspirin was 80 minutes and was found with microencapsulated aspirin particles.

Seventeen commercial of enteric-coated sodium salicylate tablets were evaluated for their ability to resist release of their active ingredient in the acidic gastric environment. The coating on at least ten brands failed to provide the necessary protection (PL Madan and M Minisci, "*In-Vitro* determination of the resistance of commercial enteric-coating to acidic conditions," *Drug Intell. Clin. Pharm.*, **10**, 588 1976).

Chloramphenicol

In the early 1960's, chloramphenicol was promoted by the manufacturer (Parke-Davis) as a safe and effective broad spectrum antibiotic. At the time when the product was facing competition from various generic manufacturers of chloramphenicol, a major finding regarding bioequivalence of chloramphenicol products was reported in the literature in the late 1960's in a study conducted by A Glazko, A Kinkel, W Alegnani and E Holmes. This study, titled "An evaluation of the absorption characteristics of different chloramphenicol preparations in normal human subjects," was published in *Clin. Pharmacol. Ther.*, **9**, 472, 1968. In this study, the authors compared bioequivalence of the marketed chloramphenicol products by comparing absorption of the antibiotic chloramphenicol. The authors used blood levels of chloramphenicol and urinary excretion of the chloramphenicol and its metabolites to show that after oral administration, absorption of chloramphenicol from a generic product was only one-third as compared to the absorption of chloramphenicol from the innovator chloromycetin capsules (Parke-Davis). Two other generic products used in this study exhibited intermediate absorption characteristics, but absorption from the generic products was still significantly less than absorption from the innovator's capsules. Later, the differences in the absorption of the drug were attributed to the fact that chloramphenicol exists in four different polymorphic forms, only one of which was the active drug.

Digoxin

Digoxin is one of the most widely used cardiac glycosides. It exhibits a steep dose/response curve, meaning that a small increase in the dose exhibits a steep increase in the response. Also, there is a very small margin between therapeutic and toxic levels of the drug (narrow therapeutic margin). This becomes a critical issue from a clinical stand-point, because a narrow margin between therapeutic and toxic levels can cause significant fluctuations in blood levels, which can result either in subclinical response or in toxic side effects. For digoxin, the problem is exacerbated by its poor aqueous solubility and incomplete absorption from the gastrointestinal tract. Some reports indicating frequent occurrence of serious intoxication of patients under treatment with digitalis glycosides were published in the literature in the early 1970's (G Beller, T Smith, W Abelmann, E Haber and W Hood, "Digitalis intoxication: A prospective clinical study with serum level correlations," *New Engl. J. Med.*, **284**, 989, 1971). Since digoxin is a life-saving drug, bioinequivalence of digoxin tablets became a major concern.

An awareness of bioinequivalence of digoxin preparations was prompted by a report published in the early 1970's (J Lindenbaum, M Mellow, M Blackstone and V Butler, "Variations in the biologic availability of digoxin from four preparations," *New Engl. J. Med.*, **285**, 1344, 1971). The authors reported that substantial differences in dosage regimens were required to stabilize patients on digoxin tablets. Subsequent bioavailability studies showed that there were four-to seven-fold differences in serum levels of the glycoside in the same patient not only between products of different manufacturers, but also between products from the same lots of the same manufacturer. The existence of a serious bioinequivalence problem with digoxin preparations was later confirmed by other authors (B Whitting, J Rodger and D Summer, "New formulation of digoxin," *Lancet*, **2**, 922, 1972).

Marked differences in the bioavailability of digoxin are attributed largely to changes in the formulation of the product and/or in the manufacturing process used in the fabrication of the dosage form. These changes can lead to significant modifications in the dissolution rate of the tablet and hence in the bioavailability of the drug. This fact was highlighted by several reports that were published in Great Britain. These reports indicated that a change in the manufacturing process of Lanoxin, the most widely used brand of digoxin in Great Britain, had resulted in the production and distribution of Lanoxin tablets that possessed almost double the effective potency of batches of Lanoxin tablets that were marketed before the manufacturing process was changed (M Stewart and E Simpson, "New formulation of Lanoxin: expected plasma levels of digoxin," *Lancet*, **2**, 541, 1972). Another study reported that the particle size of digoxin used in the manufacture of digoxin tablets played an important role in the bioavailability of the drug (A Jounela, P Pantikainen and A Sothmann, "Effect of particle size on the bioavailability of digoxin," *Eur. J. Clin. Pharmacol.*, **8**, 365, 1975). According to this report, reduction of particle size of digoxin from 102 μm to about 10 μm resulted in doubling its bioavailability.

Nitrofurantoin

Nitrofurantoin had been the subject of various studies dealing with the biological availability of the drug. In a study published by H Paul, J Kenyon, M Paul and A Borgmann, the particle size of nitrofurantoin used in the formulation of the tablet dosage form was shown to have a very large influence on the bioavailability of the drug (H Paul, J Kenyon, M Paul and A Borgmann, "Laboratory studies with nitrofurantoin: relationship between crystal size, urinary excretion in the rat and man, and emesis in dogs," *J. Pharm. Sci.*, **56**, 882, 1967). Many other reports pointing to bioequivalence of several nitrofurantoin products have appeared in the literature, one of which compared fourteen commercially available nitrofurantoin products (M Meyer, G Slywka, R Dann and P Wyatt, "Bioavailability of fourteen nitrofurantoin products," *J. Pharm. Sci.*, **63**, 1693, 1974).

It appears that the bioequivalence problem of nitrofurantoin may have been augmented by the early United States Pharmacopeia (USP) dissolution time specification for the tablet dosage forms. Since rapid dissolution and absorption of nitrofurantoin can cause gastrointestinal upset and nausea, the early USP dissolution time specification of nitrofurantoin was designed to minimize these side effects. In order to prevent acceptance of drug products with extremely low bioavailability, the USP XX modified the dissolution limit from '60 percent must dissolve in not less than 1 hour' to 'not less than 25 percent must dissolve in 1 hour.' This means that the dissolution requirement was changed from a minimum of 60 percent of the drug to dissolve within 1 hour, to a minimum of 25 percent of the drug to dissolve in 1 hour. A minimum of 25 percent means that as much as 100% of the drug could dissolve in 1 hour and meet the USP dissolution specification.

Phenytoin

Phenytoin is an extensively used antiepileptic drug. The therapeutic serum level of phenytoin should be maintained within a narrow range (10-20 mg/L) in order to assure efficacy, while avoiding intoxication. In 1968, several toxic episodes attributed to overdosage were reported in Australia ("Diphenylhydantoin overdosage," *Clin. Alert* **287**, Dec. 31, 1968). The manufacturer confirmed that a change had been made in one of the excipients used in the manufacture of phenytoin tablets. It was discovered that the change in the excipient caused a significant increase in bioavailability of the product, which led to the overdose side effect (intoxication).

In the middle 1970's, many investigators reported significantly wide variations in plasma levels of phenytoin marketed products (K Albert, E Sakmar, M Hallmark, D Weidler and J Wagner, "Bioavailability of diphenylhydantoin," *Clin. Pharmacol. Ther.*, **16**, 727, 1974). It was also reported that phenytoin preparations containing the sodium salt of the drug exhibited greater bioavailability than phenytoin products containing phenytoin as the free acid (L Lund, "Clinical significance of generic inequivalence of three different pharmaceutical preparations of phenytoin," *Eur. J. Clin. Pharmacol.*, **7**, 119, 1974).

In a study dealing with the evaluation of relative bioavailability of eleven batches of phenytoin sodium capsules representing eight different manufacturers (A Melikian, A Straughn, G Slywka, P Whyatt and M Meyer, "Bioavailability of eleven phenytoin products," *J Pharmacokinet. Biopharm.*, **5**, 133, 1977), the mean peak concentration of phenytoin in plasma of one product was found to be consistently lower than other products at each sampling time. Also, certain products exhibited significantly higher area under the plasma concentration versus time curve and significantly higher concentration of drug in plasma at certain sampling points than the reference product. Based upon various published reports citing serious bioavailability-bioequivalence problems and because of physicochemical properties of phenytoin, its narrow therapeutic range and dose-dependent kinetics, phenytoin has been identified as a critical drug, which exhibits potential bioavailability-bioequivalence problems. Therefore, because of wide divergence in dissolution rate of its marketed products and because of the slow dissolution characteristics of the most commonly prescribed reference product, the FDA and the USP were prompted to designate phenytoin capsules as either extended-release product or prompt-release product (USP XX, p.621, 1980). The monographs included in USP 23 - NF 18 on phenytoin are: phenytoin tablets (chewable), extended phenytoin sodium capsules, prompt phenytoin sodium capsules and phenytoin sodium injection.

Prednisone

The discovery of bioequivalence problems associated with prednisone tablets has a very interesting historical background. In 1963, prednisone tablets were used successfully to control a familial Mediterranean fever in a patient. The patient was responding favorably to the treatment. For some reason, the brand of prednisone was switched during the treatment. Immediately after switching the brand, the new prednisone tablets failed to produce any relief, but when the patient was put back on the original brand, full clinical response was observed in the patient. Upon *in vitro* dissolution testing of the two products, it was found that the dissolution rate of the biologically inactive prednisone tablets was significantly slower than that of the original brand. In the following year, a similar case was also reported with an arthritic patient receiving prednisone tablets (G Levy, N Hall and E Nelson, "Studies on inactive prednisone tablets, USP XVI," *Am. J. Hosp. Pharm.*, **21**, 402, 1964).

Several other bioavailability and dissolution studies on commercially available prednisone tablets from different manufacturers showed that prednisone tablets were prone to bioavailability problems. The tablets differed in the rate of appearance of prednisone in plasma (an indication of differing absorption rates of prednisone from the tablets), but not in the amount of prednisone that reached the general circulation (extent of absorption). It is interesting to note that although in some of these cases, clinical effectiveness of such tablets was correlated positively to the *in vitro* dissolution rate of prednisone (T Sullivan, E Sakmar, K Albert, D Blair and J Wagner, "*In vitro* and *in vivo* availability of commercial prednisone tablets," *J. Pharm. Sci.*, **64**, 1723, 1975), in some other cases, wide differences in the rate of dissolution of prednisone from the tablets did not result in significant differences in the bioavailability of prednisone (A DiSanto and K. DeSante, "Bioavailability and pharmacokinetics of prednisone in humans," *J. Pharm. Sci.*, **54**, 109, 1975).

Oxytetracycline

In the late 1960's, serious bioequivalence problems were reported for the broad spectrum antibiotic, oxytetracycline. A bioavailability study was conducted by G Brice and H Hammer on products from 16 different lots of the antibiotic manufactured by 13 different manufacturers. This study (G Brice and H Hammer, "Therapeutic non-equivalence of oxytetracycline capsules," *J. Am. Med. Assoc.*, **208**, 1189, 1969) revealed that Terramycin, the innovator's product, had superior average serum levels than all other generic products, in spite of the fact that all of these lots had received approval from the FDA for the marketing of these products. Concerned about these results, the FDA commissioned another scientific group to investigate the bioavailability of all oxytetracycline products marketed in the USA. This study was conducted by Blaire and co-workers on all manufacturing sources that were supplying oxytetracycline. Interestingly, this study (D Blair, R Barnes, E Wildner and W Murray, "Biological availability of oxytetracycline hydrochloride capsules. A comparison of all manufacturing sources supplying the United States market," *J. Am. Med. Assoc.*, **215**, 251, 1971) simply confirmed the earlier report that there was a serious bioequivalence problem with the marketed products of this antibiotic. Consequently, several lots of the antibiotic oxytetracycline capsules were recalled as a result of these reports.

Tetracycline

Parallel to the episode of oxytetracycline products, serious bioequivalence problems were reported with the products of another important antibiotic, tetracycline. A comparative bioavailability study of 12 batches of tetracycline representing nine different manufacturers reported that the average drug serum peak levels of certain products were only one-half the concentration of others. The bioequivalence problem with tetracycline was confirmed from the data of another separate study by H MacDonald, F Pisano, J Berger, A Dornbush and E Palcak, which compared blood levels of tetracycline after oral ingestion of three generic tetracycline capsules. This study found that concentration of tetracycline in the plasma was significantly lower from the generic products than that obtained from the innovators' product (H MacDonald, F Pisano, J Berger, A Dornbush and E Palcak, "Physiological availability of various tetracyclines," *Drug Inf. Bull.*, **3**, 76, 1969).

Thyroid

One of the earlier reports on the clinical ineffectiveness of a USP thyroid product appeared in the literature in the early 1960's (B Catz, E Ginsburg and S Salenger, "Clinically inactive Thyroid USP, A preliminary report," *New Eng. J. Med.*, **266**, 136, 1962). This publication reported that a generic product containing thyroid USP was clinically ineffective in treating hypothyroidism. But, substitution of the generic brand by levothyroxine USP in the same patients suffering from hypothyroidism produced satisfactory clinical efficacy. These findings were later confirmed in another independently published study, which evaluated the bioavailability of two prominent brands of the drug in 34 patients (A. Ramos-Gabatin, J. Jacobson, and R. Young, "*In vivo* comparison of levothyroxin preparations," *J. Am. Med. Assoc.*, **247**, 203, 1982). Based on their findings, the authors recommended that patients receiving thyroid preparations for the treatment of hypothyroidism should be treated consistently with a single brand. The reason given for this recommendation was based on the fact that adjustment of dose may be necessary if brands of the drug are switched.

Tolbutamide

The clinical failure of some generic tolbutamide tablets was reported in the Canadian literature by Carminetsky in the early 1960's (S. Carminetsky, "Substitution for brand name drugs," *Can. Med. Assoc. J.*, **88**, 950, 1963). In the following year, the bioinequivalence problem with tolbutamide tablets was confirmed by other published studies. Later, another Canadian study was conducted on a much larger scale by F. Lu, W. Rice, C. Mainville. This study reported that the time for the *in vitro* dissolution of 50 percent of drug for 26 batches of tolbutamide tablets representing 21 manufacturers varied from as little as 3 minutes to as much as 2 hours (F. Lu, W. Rice, C. Mainville, "A comparative study of some brands of tolbutamide in Canada: II. Pharmaceutical aspects," *Can. Med. Assoc. J.*, **92**, 1166, 1965). The implication of such a wide range in tolbutamide dissolution on the clinical effectiveness of the drug upon switching from one brand to another was evident.

Even a minor change in the amount of an exipient in the formulation of the product can have a significant effect on the bioavailability and clinical efficacy of the drug product. A well controlled clinical study compared the brand name product, Orinase and an experimental tablet formulation containing half the amount of the disintegrant, *Vee Gum*. Ten healthy nondiabetic subjects participated in this study (A. Varley, "The generic inequivalence of drugs," *J. Am. Med. Assoc.*, **206**, 1745, 1968). Bioavailability was measured by concentration of the drug in serum and therapeutic efficacy was measured by the ability of the drug to lower serum glucose levels. The area under the curve over an 8 hour period was 3.5 times greater with Orinase than with the experimental tablet (the tablet fabricated with half the amount of the disintegrant in the Orinase tablet) and the difference between average glucose levels for the two formulations differed markedly at the 1.5 hours and 3 hours sampling intervals. This study showed that slight and/or minor changes in the formulation of a product can produce considerable differences in the bioavailability of the drug and its eventual therapeutic efficacy. Therefore, the FDA recognized that tolbutamide products were prone to bioavailability problems and compiled a list of 12 manufacturers' products as therapeutically inequivalent to each other.

Another study, published in 1964, compared the dissolution profiles of tolbutamide for 62 lots of tolbutamide tablets from 6 manufacturers. This study (J. Ayers, H. Huang, and K. Albert, "Generic tolbutamide tablet dissolution: Intralot and interlot variation," *J. Pharm. Sci.*, **73**, 1629,

1964) found that the interlot and intralot variation was highly dependent on the manufacturer. The interlot range for mean dissolution of drug for a generic brand ranged between 58 % and 104% and one lot failed to meet the USP rotating-basket dissolution specifications as well as the paddle-stirrer dissolution specifications. In addition, tablet response to aging (storage of tablets after manufacture) at various relative humidity conditions exhibited large differences between manufacturers. While the innovator's product showed no significant change on storage, the dissolution of some generic tablets decreased dramatically on aging under high humidity conditions. These studies indicated that if variations of such magnitude can occur between different formulations of the same drug, then the specifications regulating the bioavailability of these products needed reevaluation.

Concern for Bioinequivalency

In response to concerns for bioavailability, the USP added dissolution requirements to tablet and capsule dosage forms starting in the 1970s. In 1976, the USP adopted a policy favoring a dissolution test for essentially all tablet and capsule dosage forms. By 1990, about 400 monographs in the USP contained dissolution testing requirement and in 1995, the USP 23 contained *Dissolution* or *Drug release* requirements in 532 monographs. This trend continues to grow and with each USP revision more monographs will have a *Dissolution Test* requirement. According to the USP, whenever a medically significant difference in bioavailability has been found among supposedly identical articles, a dissolution test has discriminated among these articles. The USP considers dissolution test discriminating and satisfactory, because, according to studies conducted by the USP, dissolution requirements can exclude definitively any unacceptable article. Therefore, the USP feels that there is no need for compendial requirements for *in vivo* bioavailability. Based upon its studies, the USP feels that dissolution tests are so discriminating of even those formulation factors that may only sometimes affect bioavailability of immediate-release products that it is not uncommon for a clinically acceptable article to perform poorly in a typical dissolution test. In such cases, the USP has been mindful of including as many acceptable articles as possible, without setting forth dissolution specifications so generous as to raise reasonable scientific concern for bioequivalence.

In the case of immediate-release articles, the USP is of the opinion that there is no medically significant bioequivalence problem with those articles where 75 percent of an article is dissolved in water or 0.1 N Hydrochloric Acid at 37°C in 45 minutes in the official basket or paddle apparatus operated at the usual speed. In the case of modified-release articles, USP 23 contains monographs for delayed-release and extended-release articles.

Bioavailability is particularly important for drugs, which have a narrow therapeutic index and/or exhibit a steep dose/response curve. Marked differences in the bioavailability of such drugs as digoxin, phenytoin, tolbutamide, thyroid and many other critical drugs and the demonstration of serious consequences on the safety as well as therapeutic efficacy of the drug, propelled the issue of bioequivalence from being an academic topic to a major concern among physicians, pharmacists, pharmaceutical manufacturers, as well as compendial and governmental agencies.

Recognizing the importance of these issues, two relevant new chapters appear in USP 23: *In Vitro and In Vivo Evaluation of Dosage Forms* and *In Vivo Bioequivalence Guidelines*. The publication of five specific and two general bioavailability-bioequivalence guidelines in USP 23 provides practitioners and pharmaceutical scientists the assurance that a number of substantive issues of bioavailability and bioequivalence have been addressed.

According to the USP, medically significant cases of bioinequivalence in drug products containing the same active ingredient and marketed by different manufacturers are mainly due to four reasons (see USP 23, p. lvi, 1995 or the latest USP). These four reasons, not necessarily in the order in which they are listed, are as follows:

a. Particle size of active ingredient
b. Excessive amount of magnesium stearate as lubricant
c. The polymer used in coating dosage form (especially shellac)
d. Insufficient quantity of disintegrant.

These four reasons are self-explanatory. For example, particle size of the active ingredient translates into the surface area of the drug particles exposed to the dissolution medium. Larger the particle size, smaller the surface area and hence, slower the rate of dissolution of drug in the dissolving fluid. Similarly, the use of excessive amount of magnesium stearate (or other hydrophobic materials) as the lubricant in a formulation tends to create a water-proofing effect on the tablet granules; thereby causing water-repelling property on the drug particles. If the tablet granules become water-repelling, then the dissolution medium cannot wet the drug particles, and therefore, the drug particles cannot undergo dissolution.

Various polymers are used in the coating of tablet formulations. Each polymer exhibits different affinity for the dissolution medium. Some polymers dissolve in the aqueous medium rather quickly, but many polymers are slow dissolving and hence retard drug dissolution in the gastrointestinal tract. Similarly, use of insufficient quantity of disintegrant in the formulation of a solid dosage form may retard disintegration and consequently result in slow dissolution of the active ingredient.

Several drugs have been identified as particularly prone to bioavailability problems. Box 9-1 is a partial listing of drugs for which bioequivalence has been suspected.

Box 9-1 Drugs for which bioinequivalence has been suspected

Acetazolamide	Methaqualone
Acetohexamide	Nalidixic Acid
Acetaminophen	Nitrofurantoin
Aminophylline	Oxytetracycline
d-Amphetamine	Paraminosalicylate Sodium
p-Aminosalicylic Acid	Papaverine
Ampicillin trihydrate	Pentaerythritol tetranitrate
Ascorbic Acid	Penicillin G Potassium
Aspirin	Penicillin V
Bishydroxycoumarin	Pentobarbital
Chloramphenicol	Phenobarbital Sodium
Chlortetracycline	Phenacetin
Chlordiazepoxide	Phenylbutazone
Chlorpropamide	Phenytoin
Diazoxide	Prednisone
Diethylstilbestrol	Propantheline
Digitoxin	Quinidine
Digoxin	Reserpine
Erythromycin	Riboflavin
Furosemide	Salicylamide
Ferrous Sulfate	Secobarbital Sodium
Griseofulvin	Spironolactone
Hydrochlorothiazide	Sulfadiazine
Hydrocortisone	Sulfisoxazole
Ibuprofen	Sulfamethoxazole
Indomethacin	Tetracycline hydrochloride
Isoniazid	Theophylline
Levodopa	Thyroid
Meprobamate	Tolbutamide
Methandrostenolone	Triamterene

As mentioned earlier, bioinequivalency has been shown to exist not only in products manufactured by different manufacturers and different dosage strengths of the dosage form manufactured by the same manufacturer, but also in different batches of the same drug product manufactured by the same manufacturer. This bioinequivalency can cause variations in the bioavailability of the drug, which may cause potential therapeutic problems. When a patient takes two bioinequivalent drug products during the course of a therapy, variations in the bioavailability can lead to complications in the treatment and can potentially cause therapeutic failures. This raises an important question:

Is bioavailability testing necessary for all drug products?

The answer is:

In principle, yes!

It is a very well known fact that bioavailability studies are very time-consuming and very expensive to conduct. Understandably, bioavailability testing for all products is economically difficult, and for some drugs such studies may not necessarily be essential. The question of determining bioavailability, however, is of particular interest for drug products, which fall into one or more of the following categories:

a. Where it is necessary to maintain a defined minimum effective concentration of drug in the biological fluids during the course of therapy,
b. Potent drugs, and
c. Drugs, which are poorly soluble in the gastrointestinal fluids (for the orally administered drugs) or in the body fluids (for drugs, which are administered rectally and by extravascular parenteral route).

Thus, candidates for the potential of reduced bioavailability are those drugs, which exhibit the following characteristics:

a. All drugs, which have a low solubility at the site of administration or absorption (< 0.3% solubility)
b. All drug products from which the active ingredient is too slowly or incompletely released
c. All drugs with a narrow therapeutic index.

BIOEQUIVALENCY OF GENERIC DRUGS

As indicated earlier, according to the FDA, a generic drug product is considered bioequivalent if bioavailability from the generic product is not significantly different from that of the innovator product. That is, the rate and extent of absorption from the two products do not exhibit significant differences when both products are administered in the same dosage form, by the same route of administration, at the same dose of the therapeutic ingredients and under the same experimental conditions. Under the Federal Food, Drug and Cosmetic Act of 1984, to gain approval from the FDA, a generic drug product must meet certain specific requirements. Some of these requirements are as follows:

1. Contain the same active ingredient(s) as the innovator drug. The inert ingredients may vary.
2. Be identical in strength, dosage form and route of administration.
3. Have the same indications and precautions for use.
4. Meet the same batch-to-batch requirements for identitying strength, purity and quality.
5. Have the same labeling instructions.
6. Be bioequivalent.
7. Be manufactured under the same strict standards of FDA's Good Manufacturing Practice regulations as required for the innovator products.

Generic Substitution

The FDA recommends generic substitution only among products that it has evaluated to be therapeutically equivalent. Through its publication *Approved Drug Products with Therapeutic Equivalence Evaluations* (referred to by the FDA as *the List*), the FDA provides information on multiple source drugs that are deemed therapeutically equivalent or inequivalent. *The List* identifies currently marketed drug products approved on the basis of safety and effectiveness by the FDA. This publication is available to the pharmacists and is commonly referred to as the *FDA Orange Book*, because the color of its cover is orange colored. This publication is not an official national compendium. Its purpose is to merely display the FDA's therapeutic equivalence recommendations on approved multiple source drug products. The FDA does not mandate or enforce substitution based on its Orange Book. Substitution programs are administered by each state because generic substitution is a policy administered at the state level intended to minimize the cost of drug to the consumers and the practices of pharmacy and medicine are state functions.

The FDA has published the Orange Book, since 1980 and this publication is updated monthly. The Orange Book identifies currently marketed prescription and non-prescription drug products approved by the FDA on the basis of safety and effectiveness under the Federal Food Drug and Cosmetic (FD and C) Act. The non-prescription drug products included in the Orange Book are those that require approved applications for marketing. This Book contains information on about 10,000 approved prescription drug products, about 7,500 of which are available from more than a single manufacturer, with only approximately 10 percent considered therapeutically inequivalent to the innovator products. For example, the FDA rates all conjugated estrogens and esterified estrogen products as being not therapeutically equivalent, because no manufacturer has as yet has submitted an acceptable *in vivo* bioequivalence study. Therefore, the FDA does not recommend substitution of these products for each other. Several categories of products are excluded from this publication even though many may be marketed legally. These include:

a. Unapproved drugs legally on the market. These are drugs on the market that are approved only on the basis of safety covered by the ongoing drug efficacy study implementation (DESI) review (e.g. Donnatal Tablets and Librax Capsules).
b. Products not subject to enforcement action.
c. Products not recognized by the FDA as new drugs.
d. Over the counter (OTC) drug products that do not require approved applications for marketing.
e. Products that are known to be no longer marketed. This knowledge is based on information furnished in the approved new drug application.
f. Approved drug products solely marketed abroad.
g. Drug products marketed prior to 1938 that are not subject to the pre-market clearance procedure of the law are also excluded from this publication (e.g. Synthroid Tablets). There are three drugs, which were marketed prior to 1938 and therefore are not included in either category.
h. Products approved as drugs, but now regarded as medical devices, biologics, or foods.

THERAPEUTIC EQUIVALENCE EVALUATIONS

A coding system is used for therapeutic equivalence evaluations, which allows the users to determine whether an approved product is therapeutically equivalent to other pharmaceutically equivalent products.

In this coding system, multisource drugs are classified by placing them into two major classification categories. These are Category A and Category B. For these two categories, a two-letter coding system is used. The first letter is the basic classification (either 'A' or 'B') to which an individual drug product has been assigned. Thus, the first letter of products included in Category A will be A; and the first letter of all products included in Category B will be B. The change in first letter of the code changes the status of the product. For example, if the first letter of the code is changed from A to B, it changes the status of the product from category A to category B. Similarly, if the first letter of the code is changed from B to A, it changes the status of the product from category B to category A. The second letter in each category designates a more specific reason for placing the individual product in that category, i.e. it provides additional information on the basis of the FDA's evaluation of the particular dosage form. In some instances, however, the second letter is also an indication of the type of dosage form. For example, if the second letter is a P, it indicates a parenteral product and if the second letter is a T, it indicates a topical product.

Category A

Drug products designated with an **A** code contain only those drug products that the FDA considers to be therapeutically equivalent to other pharmaceutically equivalent products. Only those drug products are listed in category **A** that have no known or suspected bio-equivalency problems or if they have had any actual or potential bioequivalence problems these problems have been resolved with adequate *in vivo* and/or *in vitro* evidence supporting bioequivalence. Drug products designated with an **A** code fall under one of the following two main policies. These policies are:

1. The first main policy for drug products, which are designated with an **A** code is designed for active ingredients or dosage forms for which no *in vivo* bioequivalence issue is known or suspected. For these active ingredients or dosage forms, the information necessary to show bioequivalence between pharmaceutically equivalent products is presumed and considered self-evident based on other data in the application of some dosage forms, e.g. solution dosage forms. For solid oral dosage forms, bioequivalence may be satisfied by a showing that an acceptable *in vitro* standard is met. Such products are assigned a therapeutically equivalent rating so long as they are manufactured in accordance with current goods manufacturing practice (CGMP) regulations and meet the other requirements of their approved applications. Active ingredients or dosage forms that fall under this main policy are designated **AA, AN, AO, AP or AT**, depending on the dosage form.
2. The second main policy for drug products, which are designated with an **A** code is designed for
   i. (DESI) products containing active ingredients on dosage forms that have been identified by the FDA as having actual or potential bioequivalence problems, and
   ii. Drug products that were marketed after 1962 in a dosage form, which presents a potential bioequivalence problem.

These pharmaceutical equivalents are assigned a therapeutic equivalence evaluation only if the approved application of the product contains adequate scientific evidence, which establishes through adequate *in vivo* and/or *in vitro* studies, the bioequivalence of the product to a selected reference product. These products are designated as AB.

There are some general principles that may affect the substitution of pharmaceutically equivalent products in specific cases. One should be alert to these principles so as to deal appropriately with situations that will require professional judgement and discretion. The specific sub-codes are defined here briefly. The detailed description of these codes is given in the Orange Book.

AA: These are *products in conventional dosage forms that do not present bioequivalence problems*. Products coded AA contain products and active ingredients and dosage forms that are not regarded as presenting either actual or potential bioequivalence problems or drug qualities or standard issues. Nonetheless, in order to be approved, all oral dosage forms must meet an appropriate *in vitro* bioequivalence standard that is acceptable to the FDA.

AB: The AB evaluation denotes *products that meet the necessary bioequivalence requirements.* The **AB** evaluation denotes those products that contain an active ingredient in a dosage form that is subject to a bioequivalence requirement or for which the submission of bioavailability or clinical data are required for approval or to permit therapeutic equivalence evaluations. Products generally will be coded **AB** if a study is submitted demonstrating bioequivalence, even if the study currently is not required for approval. This category also includes those few drugs for which there is more than one approved application, but only one manufacturer. The only instance in which a multisource product will be rated AB on the basis of bioavailability rather than bioequivalence is where the innovator product is the only one listed under that ingredient heading and has completed an acceptable bioavailability study. It does not signify that this product is therapeutically equivalent to the other drugs under the same heading. Drugs coded **AB** under an ingredient heading are considered therapeutically equivalent only to other drugs coded AB under that heading.

AN: The **AN** code denotes *solution and powders for aerosolization.* Solution and powders for aerosolization that are marketed for use in any of the several delivery systems are considered to be pharmaceutically and therapeutically equivalent. Uncertainty regarding therapeutic equivalence of aerosolized products arises primarily because of differences in the drug delivery system used for the product. Therefore, those products that are compatible only with a specific delivery system or those products that are packaged in and with a specific delivery system are not coded AN, but are coded **BN**, unless they have met an appropriate bioequivalence standard. The change in first letter of the code (from **A** to **B**) changes the status of the product from category **A** to category **B**. This is because drug products in their respective delivery systems are not necessarily pharmaceutically equivalent to each other and therefore, are not therapeutically equivalent.

AO: The **AO** code denotes *injectable oil solutions.* Injectable oil solutions are considered pharmaceutically and therapeutically equivalent only when the active ingredient, its concentration and type of oil used as a vehicle are identical, because absorption of drugs in injectable oil solutions may vary substantially with the type of oil used as a vehicle and the concentration of the active ingredient used in the product.

AP: This code denotes *aqueous injectable (parenteral) solutions.* It should be noted, however, that even though injectable (parenteral) products under a specific listing may be evaluated as therapeutically equivalent, there may be important differences among the products in the general category, *Injectable; Injection.* For example, some injectable products that are rated therapeutically equivalent are labeled for different routes of administration. In addition, some products evaluated as therapeutically equivalent may have different preservatives or no preservatives at all. Also, such products as injectable products available as dry powders for reconstitution, concentrated sterile solutions for dilution and sterile solutions ready for injection, are all considered to be pharmaceutically and therapeutically equivalent provided they are designed to produce the same concentration of the active ingredient prior to injection and are similarly labeled. It should be remembered, however, that consistent with accepted professional practice, it is the responsibility of the prescriber, dispenser or the individual administering the product, to be familiar with a product's labeling to assure that it is given only by the route(s) of administration stated in the labeling.

Certain commonly used large volume intravenous products in glass containers are not included on the list (e.g. dextrose injection 5%, dextrose injection 10% and sodium chloride injection 0.9%) because these products are on the market without FDA approval and the FDA has not published conditions for marketing such parenteral products under approved new drug applications (NDAs). When packaged in plastic containers, FDA regulations require approved applications prior to marketing. All large volume parenteral products are manufactured under similar standards, regardless of whether they are packaged in glass or plastic, therefore, the FDA has no reason to believe that the packaging container of large volume parenteral drug products that are pharmaceutically equivalent would have any effect on their therapeutic equivalence.

AT: The **AT** code represents Topical Products. All solutions and DESI drug products containing the same active ingredient in the same topical dosage form for which a waiver of *in vivo* bioequivalence has been granted and for which chemistry and manufacturing processes are adequate are considered therapeutically equivalent and coded **AT**. There are a variety of topical dosage forms available for dermatologic, ophthalmic, otic, rectal, and vaginal administration. These are available in solution, cream, ointment, gel, lotion, paste, spray and suppository dosage forms. These dosage forms are not considered pharmaceutically equivalent, even though different topical dosage forms may contain the same active ingredient and potency. Therefore, these dosage forms are not considered therapeutically equivalent. Pharmaceutically equivalent topical products that raise questions of bioequivalence, including all post-1962 topical drug products, are coded **AB** when supported by adequate bioequivalence data and **BT** in the absence of such data.

Category B

This category includes drug products that the FDA does not at this time consider to be therapeutically equivalent to other pharmaceutically equivalent products. This category includes only those drug products for which actual or potential bioequivalence problems have not been resolved by adequate evidence of bioequivalence. Often the problem with products listed under this category is with specific dosage forms rather than with the active ingredients. Drug products designated with a **B** code fall under one or more of the following three main policies:

1. The drug products either contain active ingredients or the drug products are manufactured in dosage forms that have been identified by the FDA as either having documented bioequivalence problems or a significant potential for such problems and for which no adequate studies have been submitted to the FDA demonstrating bioequivalence.
2. The quality standards of the products are either inadequate or the FDA has an insufficient basis to determine therapeutic equivalence.
3. The drug products are under regulatory review.

Products included in this category are designated with a **B** code, i.e. the first letter used in identifying this category is **B**. Depending on the dosage form, the drug products in this category are designated as **B*, BC, BD, BE, BN, BP, BR, BS, BT or BX**.

B*: Drug products included in the **B*** code are those *drug products that require further FDA investigation and review to determine therapeutic equivalence*. This code is assigned to products that were previously assigned an **A** or **B** code and if the FDA receives new information that raises a significant question regarding therapeutic equivalence that can be resolved only through further FDA investigation and/or review of data and information submitted by the applicant. The **B*** code signifies that the FDA will take no position regarding the therapeutic equivalence of the product until the FDA completes its investigation and review.

BC: The **BC** code includes *extended-release dosage forms (capsules, injectables and tablets)*. The official compendia define an extended-release dosage form as one that allows at least a two-fold reduction in dosing frequency as compared to that drug marketed as a conventional dosage form (e.g. as a solution or a prompt drug-releasing conventional solid dosage form). Although bioavailability studies have been conducted on these dosage forms, they may be potentially subject to bioavailability differences, primarily because different manufacturers developing extended-release products for the same active ingredient rarely employ similar formulation approaches in the fabrication of their extended-release products. Therefore, the FDA does not consider different extended-release dosage forms containing the same active ingredient in identical strength to be therapeutically equivalent unless equivalence (in both rate and extent) between individual products has been specifically demonstrated through appropriate bioequivalence studies. Extended-release products for which such bioequivalence data have been submitted are coded **BC,** while those for which such data are available are coded **AB.**

BD: This code is used for *active ingredients and dosage forms with documented bioequivalence problems*. The **BD** code denotes products containing active ingredients with known bioequivalence problems and for which adequate studies have not been submitted to the FDA demonstrating bioequivalence. The FDA assigns **AB** code to those products where studies demonstrating bioequivalence have been submitted.

BE: The code **BE** denotes *delayed-release oral dosage forms*. The official compendia define delayed-release dosage forms as those products that release their active ingredient(s) at a time other than promptly after administration. Enteric-coated articles are delayed-release dosage forms. Delayed-release dosage forms containing the same ingredients marketed by different manufacturers as are subject to significant differences in the absorption of the drug. Therefore, unless otherwise specifically noted, the FDA considers different delayed-release products containing the same active ingredients as presenting a potential bioequivalence problem. The FDA, therefore, codes these products **BE** in the absence of *in vivo* studies showing bioequivalence. If adequate *in vivo* studies have demonstrated the bioequivalence of specific delayed-release products, such products are then coded **AB.**

BN: Drug products included in the code **BN** are *products in aerosol-nebulizer drug delivery systems*. This code applies to drug solution or powders that are marketed only as a component of or as compatible with, a specific drug delivery system. The FDA feels that there may, for example, be significant differences in the dose of drug and particle size delivered by different products of this type. Therefore, the FDA does not consider different metered aerosol dosage forms containing the same active ingredient(s) in equal strengths to be therapeutically equivalent unless the drug products meet an appropriate bioequivalence standard.

BP: This code includes *active ingredients and dosage forms with potential bioequivalence problems*. FDA's bioequivalence regulations contain criteria and procedures for determining whether a specific active ingredient in a specific dosage form has a potential for causing a bioequivalence problem. It is FDA's policy to consider an ingredient meeting these criteria as having potential bioequivalence problem even in the absence of positive data demonstrating inequivalence. Therefore, pharmaceutically equivalent products containing these ingredients in oral dosage forms are coded **BP,** until adequate *in vivo* bioequivalence data are submitted to the FDA. Injectable suspensions containing an active ingredient suspended in either an aqueous or an oleaginous vehicle have also been coded **BP** by the FDA. Injectable suspensions are subject to bioequivalence problems because differences in particle size, polymorphic structure of the suspended active ingredient or the suspension formulation can significantly affect the rate of release and absorption of drug. Therefore, the FDA does not consider pharmaceutical equivalents of these products bioequivalent without adequate evidence of bioequivalence.

BR: Drug products included in code **BR** are *suppositories or enemas that deliver drugs for systemic absorption*. The absorption of active ingredients from suppositories or enemas that are intended to have a systemic effect (as distinct from suppositories administered for local effect of the active ingredient) can vary significantly from product to product.

Therefore, the FDA considers pharmaceutically equivalent systemic suppositories or enemas bioequivalent only if *in vivo* evidence of bioequivalence is available. In those cases where *in vivo* evidence is available, the product is coded **AB.** If such evidence is not available, the products are coded **BR.**

BS: This code is used for *products having drug standard deficiencies*. If the drug standards for an active ingredient in a particular dosage form are found by the FDA to be deficient so as to prevent an FDA evaluation of either pharmaceutical or therapeutic equivalence, then all drug products containing that active ingredient in that dosage form are coded **BS**. For example, if the standards permit a wide variation in pharmacologically active components of the product such that pharmaceutical equivalence is in question, then all products containing that active ingredient in that dosage form are coded **BS.**

BT: The **BT** code is assigned to *topical products with bioequivalence issues*. This code applies mainly to the post-1962 dermatologic, ophthalmic, otic, rectal and vaginal products for topical administration, including creams, ointments, gels, lotions, pastes and sprays, as well as suppositories not intended for systemic absorption of the drug. Topical products evaluated as having acceptable clinical performance, but that are not bioequivalent to other pharmaceutically equivalent products or that lack sufficient evidence of bioequivalence are coded **BT**.

BX: This code includes *drug products for which the data are insufficient to determine therapeutic equivalence*. The code **BX** is assigned to specific drug products for which the data that have been reviewed by FDA are insufficient to determine therapeutic equivalence under the policies, which are used to define equivalence. In these situations, the drug products are presumed to be therapeutically inequivalent until the FDA determines that there is adequate information to make a full evaluation of therapeutic equivalence.

Substitution Laws

In order to contain costs of drugs to the patient, almost every state in USA has adopted laws that encourage the substitution of less expensive therapeutically equivalent drug products, commonly referred to as the generic products. A universal formulary applicable to all states in the USA is not available because FDA cannot serve the needs of each state on individual basis. Each state publishes its own formulary, which enables the pharmacist to determine whether or not a drug product may be substituted. The FDA, however, does provide in its Orange Book, a list of all prescription drug products approved by the FDA for safety and effectiveness, with therapeutic recommendations being made on all multiple source drug products in the list. This list can be used by each state in implementing its own law so as to relieve the FDA of expending an enormous amount of resources to provide individualized service to all states. It must be remembered that the

FDA does not mandate, which drug products may or may not be substituted. The therapeutic equivalence evaluations in the Orange Book are recommendations only.

Some states publish a formulary that lists products, which are considered bioequivalent and therefore can be substituted for other products. This type of formulary is called the positive formulary. Other states publish a formulary that lists products, which are considered bio-inequivalent and should not be substituted for other products. This type of formulary is known as the negative formulary. In the positive formulary approach, the state law requires that the substitution be limited to drugs listed in the formulary and in the negative formulary approach, the state law requires that substitution is permitted for all drugs except those prohibited by the formulary.

The New York state publishes a positive formulary of *Approved Drug Products with Therapeutic Equivalence Evaluations*. Although it carries the same title as that used by the FDA for its Orange Book, the book published by the New York state is popularly known as the *Green Book*, because of color of its cover when the book was first published. The cover of the current edition of the book is white and green, but it is still called the Green Book. The state of New Jersey also publishes a positive formulary, known as *New Jersey Generic Formulary*.

BIOEQUIVALENCE STUDIES

The simplest and the most common experimental design for the comparison of bioavailability of two drug products is the 'crossover design study'. In this method, an adequate number of human subjects are divided into two groups and each group receives both products at two different occasions. The number of subjects constituting an adequate size is determined by the drug being evaluated and the therapeutic effect being monitored. In most cases, a small number of healthy subjects (generally 24) between 18 and 40 years of age and preferably of similar height and weight are selected. The individuals are divided equally into two carefully matched groups. Each test subject is randomly assigned one of the two products. In the first segment of the study all subjects are administered the assigned product and in the second segment of the study the subjects are assigned another product. This procedure avoids bias of the test results. Depending on the nature of drug and the therapeutic effect for which the drug is indicated, some bioequivalence studies may require a relatively larger population of subjects (up to 100) to evaluate the bioavailability of the product being studied.

In the first segment of study, the first assigned product is administered. The blood samples are drawn from the subjects at predetermined time intervals and analyzed for drug concentration. For the second segment of study, an appropriate time interval is allowed for the drug to be virtually eliminated. This is known as 'wash-out period' and ensures that there is no residual drug or metabolite from the first administered product. After the wash-out period, the procedure used in the first segment is repeated with the second product. This technique is called crossover technique because each subject is now receiving another product. The advantage of crossover design experiment is that each individual serves his/her own control by taking each of the two products. Thus, inherent differences between individuals, which may exhibit different patterns of drug absorption, metabolism and excretion are minimized. After the second segment of study, the data are analyzed to determine the parameters used to assess and compare bioavailability (i.e. peak concentration [C_{max}], time to peak concentration [T_{max}] *and area under the plasma concentration versus time curve*). These parameters are analyzed using the principle of superimposition or statistical procedures are used in order to determine whether or not differences in bioavailability parameters are significant. In the principle of superimposition, the data from both products are plotted on the same graph paper. If the two products exhibit similar bioavailability, the curve from the test product should superimpose the curve from the reference product. The statistical procedures used to determine bioequivalency of the products being compared are discussed in the next section. It should be mentioned here that statistical differences in the bioavailability parameters are not necessarily clinically significant in therapeutic outcome of the drug.

In most bioequivalence studies, researchers conducting the study as well as patients receiving the treatment are not informed as to which subject is receiving what product. Both products are made to look exactly alike so that physical appearance or other characteristics (e.g. smell, taste, size and shape of the tablet or capsule, etc.) cannot identify the product. This is known as a double-blind study (blind, because everybody involved in the bioequivalence study is 'blind' to the product and double, because the patient as well as the researcher is unaware of the product being administered).

In the design and evaluation of bioequivalence studies, the FDA requires that the study should be large enough to provide a good probability to detect reasonable differences in average bioavailability. The FDA uses hypothesis testing and confidence intervals to determine the probability that the parameters fall within acceptable limits. The standards vary among drugs and drug classes, e.g. antiarrhythmic agents may be allowed a 25 percent variation and antipsychotic agents may fall within a 30 percent variation. In the past, the FDA required the bioavailability of the drug measured in 75 percent of the subjects to fall within 25 percent of the mean bioavailability of the population test, i.e. within the range of 75% and 125%. This means that two products could be considered bioequivalent even if the variation between these two products ranged between 75% and 125%, i.e. almost a two-fold difference. This was popularly known as the 75/75 rule (75% subjects, 75% bioavailability). However, this test was determined not to be scientifically valid. Current criteria have allowed up to a 20 percent variation between the bioavailability parameters, i.e. the FDA considers an 80 percent probability to be a good probability and a 20 percent difference as a reasonable difference. This has come to be known as the '80/20 rule', meaning that the study should be large enough to provide an 80 percent probability to detect a 20 percent difference in average bioavailability. This bioequivalence rule applies to both the innovator reformulated products and generic products. It should be mentioned, however, that consultants to the FDA have suggested applying more stringent statistical testing. The current thinking is to reduce the acceptable difference to within 10 percent of the mean area under the curve (AUC) of the reference product, and increase the probability level to 90 percent. If accepted, this will likely be known as the '90/10' requirement. The industry, on the other hand, considers that this is too harsh a requirement and that such stringent criteria would increase the difficulty of approval of a generic product within these limits.

Guidance for Bioequivalence

At the request of the manufacturer, the Division of Bioequivalence of the FDA may provide guidance for *in vivo* bioequivalence and *in vitro* dissolution studies for the specific dosage form of the drug. These documents may be obtained by writing to the FDA. Given below is guidance for *in vivo* bioequivalence and *in vitro* dissolution studies for indomethacin capsules. This guidance was issued by the Division of Bioequivalence on January 25, 1988. This guidance document carries the following foot-note:

> *"This statement is an informal communication under 21 CFR 10.90 (b) (9) that represents the best judgement of the Division of Bioequivalence at this time. This statement, however, does not necessarily represent the formal position of the Center for Drug Evaluation and Research, Food and Drug Administration and does not bind or otherwise obligate the Center for Drug Evaluation and Research, Food and Drug Administration to the views expressed."*

Division of Bioequivalence
Guidance for In Vivo Bioequivalence
and In Vitro Dissolution
Studies for Indomethacin Capsules

I. Introduction: Indomethacin is a potent non-steroidal anti-inflammatory and analgesic agent. Due to the potential side effects, it is frequently reserved for use when other anti-inflammatory agents are ineffective.

The drug is almost completely absorbed (98%) following oral administration of the capsule. Peak plasma levels are achieved within 3 hours under fasting conditions and elimination half-life of the parent drug estimated from plasma data is about 2 to 3 hours. Indomethacin is 90 percent bound to plasma proteins and is largely converted to O-demethylates and conjugates. Enterohepatic recycling of the conjugates occurs. About 10 to 20% of the parent drug is excreted unchanged in the urine and 2 to 5% of the dose is recovered as demethylindomethocin and dechlorobenzoylindomethacin metabolites in urine.

Because indomethacin exhibits extensive enterohepatic recycling, which may affect the serum drug levels, the Division of Bioequivalence requires that the bioequivalence of the test and the reference products be demonstrated in urine, when the serum data are inconclusive.

II. Guidance for In Vivo Bioequivalence: The bioequivalence study for indomethacin should be conducted with 16 or more subjects in a randomized 2-way crossover design. All subjects should be given physical examinations and appropriate clinical laboratory tests to ensure that they are healthy. Subjects with a history of serious gastrointestinal, hepatic, renal or hematological diseases are to be excluded from the study.

The test product should be from production lot or from a lot produced under production conditions. The bioequivalence study should compare the test capsule against reference capsule. A single oral dose of 50 mg of the test product or the reference product (Indocin, 50 mg by Merck, Sharpe and Dohme) should be given to the subjects after an overnight fast. Water may be taken *ad lib*, but food should be limited to standard meals and should not be given within 4 hours after the dose.

Blood samples should be collected at 0 (pre-dose), 0.33, 1, 1.5, 2, 3, 4, 5, 6, 8, 10, 12 and 24 hours post dose. Urine should be collected during the first 48 hours after dosing. Blood samples should be assayed for the serum levels of indomethacin at each sampling time by a sensitive, indomethacin-specific method. Urine should be assayed only when blood data are inadequate for demonstrating bioequivalence. Urine samples should be assayed for total indomethacin (free and conjugates) over the entire collection period.

The serum and urine data should be analyzed statistically by suitable method such as t-test and (ANOVA) analysis of variance. Bioavailability parameters, such as AUC, C_{max} (peak serum level), T_{max} (time to peak) and percent total recovery of indomethacin and its conjugates should all be evaluated. In addition, the 90 percent shortest confidence interval of the estimated difference in sample means should be reported for AUC, C_{max} and T_{max}.

Bioequivalence requirements for 25 mg capsules of indomethacin will be deemed to have been met under the following conditions:

1. The 25 mg capsules are proportionally similar in their active and inactive ingredients to the 50 mg capsule.
2. The 25 mg capsules have satisfactory dissolution performance compared to that of the 50 mg capsules.
3. An acceptable *in vivo* bioequivalence study has been conducted for the 50 mg capsules.

III. In Vitro Studies:

a. *Dissolution Guidance:* Dissolution testing of indomethacin capsules should be conducted on 12 dosage units of the same lots of the test and reference products as used in the *in vivo* bioequivalence study. The dissolution testing should be conducted using the following conditions (Table 9-1):

Table 9-1: The dissolution testing requirements

Requirements	*Particulars*
a. Apparatus	USP I (basket)
b. RPM	100
c. Medium	Phosphate buffer pH 7.2, diluted 1:4 with water
d. Volume of medium	750 mL
e. Temperature	37°C
f. Sampling times	5, 10 and 20 minutes
g. Specifications	NLT 80% (not less than 80% dissolved in 20 minutes

b. *Content Uniformity Guidance:* Content uniformity for 10 test capsules from the lots used in the *in vitro* and *in vivo* testings should be submitted along with the dissolution testing data. The content uniformity test should be conducted using the guidelines specified in the USP.

IV. Potency: Prior to initiation of the bioequivalence study the applicant should determine the potency of the lot of the test drug to be used in the study. It is recommended that the applicant should ensure that the potency of the lot of the listed product to be used as a reference in the bioequivalence study is within 5 percent of that for the test drug product. The data on potency should be submitted along with the dissolution data.

Statistical Criteria for Bioequivalence

Under the Drug Price Competition and Patent Term Restoration Act of 1984 (the Waxman-Hatch Amendments of 1984), manufacturers seeking approval to market generic product of a drug must submit data to the FDA demonstrating that the generic drug product is bioequivalent to the pioneer (innovator) drug product. A major premise underlying the Act of 1984 is that bioequivalent products are therapeutically equivalent and therefore, these products are interchangeable.

The Division of Bioequivalence of the FDA in the Office of Generic Drugs usually evaluates bioequivalence by comparing the *in vivo* rate and extent of drug absorption of a test product and reference formulation in healthy subjects. In a standard *in vivo* bioequivalence study design, study participants receive test and reference products on separate occasions with random assignment to the two possible sequences of product administration. The bioequivalence study may be conducted either as a single dose or in multiple doses. The study involves collection of samples of an accessible biologic fluid such as blood or urine and analysis of each sample for concentrations of drug and the metabolites. The pharmacokinetic parameters (area under the curve, maximum concentration of drug in plasma and time of maximum concentration) are obtained from the resulting concentration versus time curves. These pharmacokinetic parameters are then analyzed statistically to determine if the test and reference products yield comparable values.

The Division of Bioequivalence of the FDA employs a testing procedure termed the two one-sided tests procedure to determine whether average values for the pharmacokinetic parameters measured after administration of the test and reference products are comparable. This procedure involves the calculation of a confidence interval for the ratio (or difference) between the test and reference product pharmacokinetic variable averages. The limits of observed confidence interval must fall within a predetermined range for the ratio (or difference) of the product averages. The determination of confidence interval range and statistical level of significance are judgments made by the Division of Bioequivalence of the FDA. The primary comparison of interest in a bioequivalence study is the ratio of the average parameter data from the test and reference formulations rather than the difference between them. Using log transformation (i.e. converting the data into logarithm of the data), the general linear statistical model employed in the analysis of bioequivalence data allows inferences about the difference between the two means on the log scale, which can then be retransformed into inferences about the ratio of the two averages (means or medians) on the original scale. Logarithmic transformations achieve the general comparison based on the ratio rather than the difference.

To facilitate bioequivalence comparisons, pharmacokinetic parameters for each individual subject are displayed in parallel for the formulations tested. For example, the comparison between test (T) and reference (R) product is listed as follows:

$$\text{Difference between test and reference product} = \text{T} - \text{R}$$

$$\text{Ratio between test and reference product} = \frac{\text{T}}{\text{R}}$$

$$\text{Logarithm of ratio between test and reference product} = \log \frac{T}{R} \text{ or } \ln \frac{T}{R}$$

In addition to the arithmetic mean for the test and reference products, the geometric means (antilog of the means of logs), means of the logs and standard deviations and coefficients of variation, are included in the report. For a broad range of drugs, the FDA Division of Bioequivalence used a range of 80 to 120% for the ratio of the product averages as the standard equivalence criterion. This corresponds to a range of ± 20% for the relative difference between the product averages. When log-transformed data are used in the analysis of area under the curve and C_{max}, the FDA uses the 80/125 rule. According to this rule, two formulations are generally considered bioequivalent if their rate and extent of absorption differ by – 20% to + 25% or less (i.e. the ratio of their averages are within a range of 80 to 125%). The advantage of using a range of 80 to 125% for the ratio of averages over the 80 to 120% criterion is that for the analysis of log-transformed data, the probability of concluding equivalence is at a maximum if the ratio of averages is in fact 1.0 (i.e. the two averages are exactly equal). For the analysis of log-transformed data with a criterion of within 80 to 120%, the maximum probability of concluding equivalence occurs when the ratio of averages of the two products equals approximately 0.98. Thus, an equivalence criterion of within 80 to 125% (80/125 rule) is used for the ratio of the product averages.

The use of the 80/125 rule is based on a medical decision that, for most drugs, a difference in concentration of the active ingredient in blood within the limits of – 20% to + 25% will not be clinically significant.

Comparing Arithmetic Averages: The statistical analysis on both the ratios and the difference of the logarithms (the difference of the logarithms is actually the logarithm of the ratio) is performed using a paired t-test. This test is a statistical test, which is used for comparing arithmetic averages. This test was developed by Gosset who was writing under the pseudonym of 'Student' (hence the name *Student's t-test,* usually shortened to *t-test*), because Gosset's employer did not want any employee of the company to publish their scientific work.

The *t*-distribution has the following properties:

a. It has a mean (arithmetic average) of 0.
b. It is symmetrical about the mean.
c. The *t*-distribution approaches normal distribution as (n – 1) approaches infinity.
d. Compared to the normal distribution, the *t*-distribution is less peaked in the center and has higher tails.
e. The variable t ranges from – ∞ to + ∞.

Although a requirement for the valid use of the t-distribution is that the sample must be drawn from a normal distribution, experience has shown that moderate departures from this requirement can be tolerated. As a consequence, the t-distribution is used even when it is known that the parent population deviates from normality. The t-distribution is used when the sample size is small (less than 30).

The t-test is applied:

i. When the ratio of the parameters is used for comparison or
ii. When the differences of the logarithms of the parameters are used for comparison.

The use of *t-test* in both of these situations is described below:

i. **When the ratio of the parameters is used for comparison:** When the ratio of the parameters is used for comparison, the *t*-statistic is calculated using the following equation:

$$t = \frac{|\bar{X} - 1|}{(sd)/(N)^{0.5}} = \frac{|\bar{X} - 1|(N)^{0.5}}{sd} \quad (9\text{-}1)$$

where,

t = the t-statistic,

$\bar{X}$ = the arithmetic average of the pharmacokinetic parameter being compared,

1 = the number 1 in the numerator indicates the probability of concluding equivalence is at a maximum, if the ratio of averages is in fact exactly equal to 1.0 (i.e. the two averages are exactly equal)

sd = standard deviation of the sample, and

N = the number of subjects participating in the study.

The term $|\bar{X} - 1|$ in the numerator of equation (9-1) is the absolute difference between 1 and the arithmetic average.

The value of the *t*-statistic calculated using equation (9-1) is compared with the published value of t-statistic (Table 9-2) at the chosen confidence level for (N – 1) degrees of freedom. The two products are considered equivalent only if the calculated value of *t*-statistic is less than the published value of t-statistic.

The values of t-distribution for (N – 1) degrees of freedom at various levels of confidence for the one-sided as well as two-sided tests are listed in Table 9-2.

ii. **When differences of the logarithms of the parameters are used for comparison:** The difference of the logarithms is actually the logarithm of the ratio). When this ratio is used for comparison, the following equation is used:

Table 9-2 t-Distributions

Two-sided	*40%*	*20%*	*10%*	*5%*	*1%*
One-sided	*20%*	*10%*	*5%*	*2.5%*	*0.5%*
Degrees of Freedom	$t_{0.80}$	$t_{0.90}$	$t_{0.95}$	$t_{0.975}$	$t_{0.99}$
1	1.38	3.08	6.31	12.71	63.66
2	1.06	1.89	2.92	4.30	9.92
3	0.98	1.64	2.35	3.18	5.84
4	0.94	1.53	2.13	2.78	4.60
5	0.92	1.48	2.02	2.57	4.03
6	0.91	1.44	1.94	2.45	3.71
7	0.90	1.42	1.89	2.36	3.50
8	0.89	1.40	1.86	2.31	3.36
9	0.88	1.38	1.83	2.26	3.25
10	0.88	1.37	1.81	2.23	3.17
11	0.88	1.36	1.80	2.20	3.11
12	0.87	1.36	1.78	2.18	3.05
13	0.87	1.35	1.77	2.16	3.01
14	0.87	1.35	1.76	2.14	2.98
15	0.87	1.34	1.75	2.13	2.95
16	0.86	1.34	1.75	2.12	2.92
17	0.86	1.33	1.74	2.11	2.90
18	0.86	1.33	1.73	2.10	2.88
19	0.86	1.33	1.73	2.09	2.86
20	0.86	1.33	1.72	2.09	2.85
25	0.86	1.32	1.71	2.06	2.79
30	0.85	1.31	1.70	2.04	2.75
40	0.85	1.30	1.68	2.02	2.70
60	0.85	1.30	1.67	2.00	2.66
120	0.85	1.29	1.66	1.98	2.62
Infinity	0.84	1.282	1.645	1.96	2.576

$$t = \frac{\left|\bar{X} - 0\right|}{(sd)/(N)^{0.5}} = \frac{\left|\bar{X} - 0\right|(N)^{0.5}}{sd} \tag{9-2}$$

In this equation,

t = the t-statistic,

$\bar{X}$ = the arithmetic average (mean) of the difference of the logarithms of the pharmacokinetic parameter being compared,

0 = the number 0 in the numerator of equation (9-2) indicates the probability of concluding equivalence is at a maximum if the difference of the logarithms of the parameter is in fact 0 (i.e. the two averages are exactly equal), sd is standard deviation of the sample, and

N = the number of subjects in the study. The term $\left|\bar{X} - 0\right|$ in the numerator of equation (9-2) is absolute difference between 0 and the arithmetic average. This term is similar to the term $\left|\bar{X} - 1\right|$ in equation (9-1), because logarithm of 1 = 0.

The value of the t-statistic calculated using equation (9-2) is compared with the published value of the t-statistic at the chosen confidence level for (N – 1) degrees of freedom. The two products are considered equivalent only if the calculated value of t-statistic is less than the published value of t-statistic.

Constructing Confidence Intervals

The purpose of constructing confidence intervals for the population mean is to define an interval that, with a specified degree of confidence, includes the parameter being estimated. In bioequivalence studies, the parameter being estimated is the arithmetic average (mean) of the pharmacokinetic parameter of interest. The usual pharmacokinetic parameters of interest in bioequivalence studies include the following: area under the plasma concentration versus time (AUC), time of maximum concentration of drug in the plasma (T_{max}) and maximum concentration of drug in the plasma (C_{max}). The general procedure for constructing confidence interval for population mean (arithmetic average) is to use the following relationship:

$$\text{Population mean} = \text{Estimator} \pm (\text{Reliability Coefficient}) \times (\text{Standard Error})$$

In this relationship:

Estimator is the arithmetic average (mean) of the sample,

Reliability coefficient is the value of the t-statistic at the chosen confidence level, and

Standard Error (also known as standard error of the mean) is computed using the following relationship:

$$\text{Standard error} = \frac{\text{Sample stan dard deviation}}{(\text{Number of subjects in the sample})^{0.5}}$$

For example, to calculate 95% confidence interval for the one-sided t-test, the reliability coefficient is the value of the t-statistic at $t_{1-0.05} = t_{0.95}$. When a two-sided t-test is used, the reliability coefficient is the value of the t-statistic at $t_{1-(0.05/2)} = t_{1-0.025} = t_{0.975}$

Hence, the 95% confidence interval is calculated using the following relationship:

$$\text{The 95\% confidence interval is} = \bar{X} \pm \frac{(t_{0.975})(sd)}{(N)^{0.5}} \tag{9-3}$$

where,

$\bar{X}$ = arithmetic average of the pharmacokinetic parameter under comparison,

N = number of subjects participating in the study,

Sd = standard deviation, and

$t_{0.975}$ = the value of the t-statistic obtained from t-distribution table for (N – 1) degrees of freedom for the one-sided test.

To verify, for a particular pharmacokinetic parameter, that 80/125 rule (– 20 to + 25%) is satisfied, two one-sided statistical tests are carried out using the log transformed data from the bioequivalence study. One test is used to verify that the average response for generic product is no more than 20 percent below that for the innovator product, and the other test is used to verify that the average response for the generic product is no more than 25 percent above that for the innovator product. The current practice is to carry out two one-sided tests at the 0.05 level of significance.

The two one-sided tests are carried out by computing a 90 percent confidence interval. For the approval of ANDA's (abbreviated new drug applications), in most cases, the generic manufacturer must show that a 90 percent confidence interval for the ratio of mean response (usually area under the curve and maximum concentration of drug in the plasma) of its product to that of the innovator product is within the limits of 0.8 and 1.25, using the log transformed data. If the true average response of the generic product in the population is near 20 percent below or 25 percent above the innovator average, then one or both of confidence limits is likely to fall outside the acceptable range and the product will fail bioequivalence test. Thus an approved product is likely to differ from that of the innovator by far less than this quantity.

The current practice of carrying out two one-sided tests at the 0.05 level of significance ensures that if the two products truly differ by as much or more than is allowed by the equivalence criteria (usually within – 20 to + 25% of the innovator product average for the bioequivalence parameter, such as area under the curve or Cmax) there is no more than a 5 percent chance that they will be approved as an equivalent. This reflects the fact that the primary concern (from the regulatory point of view) is the protection of the patient against acceptance of bioequivalence if it does not hold true. The results of a bioequivalence study must usually be acceptable for more than one pharmacokinetic parameter. As such, a generic product that truly differs by – 20 to + 25% or more from the innovator product with respect to one or more pharmacokinetic parameters would actually have less than 5 percent chance of being approved.

A detailed analysis of a typical data (generated during equivalence studies of a product) illustrating the application of the FDA requirement for bioequivalency goes in great depth and therefore, it is beyond the scope of discussion in this Chapter. The compilation and analysis of data are not only time-consuming, but these compilations also involve statistical analysis using such statistical tests as ANOVA. However, in order to provide some degree of understanding of statistical analysis used in these studies, Example 9-3 illustrates the application of the *t*-statistic for comparison of means of two products for their equivalency.

Example 9-3 The area under the plasma concentration versus time curve for 12 healthy subjects who participated in a bioavailability study comparing two formulations (A and B) of the same drug (administered in the same dosage form and in the same dosage strength) is shown below.

Perform a two-sided paired *t*-test on the average of the ratios and the difference of the logarithms of the average, comparing the average ratio to 1.

Subject	A	B	Subject	A	B
1	95	125	7	100	125
2	105	95	8	135	95
3	90	135	9	100	120
4	98	138	10	95	135
5	100	120	11	100	120
6	130	138	12	98	120

Solution

In order to perform the t-tests on the ratios and the difference of the logarithms, the data given above are tabulated as follows:

Subject	*Product A*		*Product B*		*A/B*	*Ratio*
	AUC	*log AUC*	*AUC*	*log AUC*		*log A – log B*
1	95	1.9777	125	2.0969	0.76	-0.1192
2	105	2.0212	95	1.9777	1.11	0.0453
3	90	1.8542	135	2.1303	0.67	-0.1739
4	98	1.9913	138	2.1399	0.71	-0.1487
5	100	2.0000	120	2.0792	0.83	-0.0809
6	130	2.1139	138	2.1399	0.94	-0.0269
7	100	2.0000	125	2.0969	0.80	-0.0969
8	135	2.1303	95	1.9777	1.42	0.1522
9	100	2.0000	120	2.0792	0.83	-0.0809
10	95	1.9777	135	2.1303	0.70	-0.1549
11	100	2.0000	120	2.0792	0.83	-0.0809
12	98	1.9913	120	2.0792	0.82	-0.0862
			Average		0.87	-0.0710
			standard deviation		0.21	0.0917

t Test on the Ratios: From equation (9-1), the value of the t-statistic is:

$$t = \frac{|\bar{X} - 1|(N)^{0.5}}{sd}$$

$$t = \frac{|0.87 - 1|(12)^{0.5}}{0.21} = \frac{(0.13)(3.464)}{0.21}$$

$$t = \frac{0.45}{0.21} = 2.142$$

According to the *t* distribution table (shown in Table 9-2), at p = 0.5 and 11 degrees of freedom (N – 1 = 12 – 1 = 11), the value of *t* statistic is 2.20 and the calculated value of t statistic in this Example is 2.825. Since the calculated value of *t* statistic in this Example (2.825) is greater than the published value of *t* statistic (2.20), it is concluded that the parameter being compared (area under the curve) is not similar, i.e. the two products are not bioequivalent.

t Test on the Difference of the Logarithms: From equation (9-2), the value of the t-statistic is:

$$t = \frac{|\bar{X} - 0|(N)^{0.5}}{sd}$$

$$t = \frac{|-0.071 - 0|(12)^{0.5}}{0.0917} = \frac{(0.071)(3.464)}{0.917} = \frac{0.2459}{0.0917} = 2.682$$

According to the *t* distribution table (shown in Table 9-2), at p = 0.5 and 11 degrees of freedom (i.e. N – 1 = 12 – 1 = 11), the value of t statistic is 2.20.

Since the calculated value of t (2.682) is greater than the published value of t (2.20), it is concluded that the parameter being compared (area under the curve) is not similar, i.e. the two products are not bioequivalent.

95% Confidence Interval: From equation (9-3), the 95% confidence interval is:

$$\text{The 95\% confidence interval} = \bar{X} \pm \frac{(t_{0.975})(sd)}{(N)^{0.5}}$$

$$\text{The 95\% confidence interval} = 0.87 \pm \frac{(2.2)(0.21)}{3.464} = 0.87 \pm \frac{0.462}{3.464} = 0.87 \pm 0.1334$$

Therefore, the range is from (0.87 – 0,1334) to (0.87 + 0.1334)

Therefore, the range is from 0.7366 to 1.0035.

ORAL DOSAGE FORMS THAT SHOULD NOT BE CRUSHED

There are many instances when the contents of a solid dosage form are removed from the dosage form and crushed or divided into smaller doses for administration to children or to patients who have difficulty in swallowing the intact dosage form. For example, a dosage form contained in a hard gelatin capsule may be removed from its shell or a tablet may be crushed prior to administration to a patient in a suitable liquid as a suspension. Some may feel that in order to give one-half or one-quarter of the adult dose to a child, the adult dose may be divided into two or four equal parts, e.g. the tablet can be cut into two or four equal parts or the contents of a capsule may be divided into two or four equal parts and administered in a suitable medium.

There are many examples of situations, which may prompt this decision. Some of these include:

a. The patient is unable to take the solid dosage form, but can take a liquid dosage form, or
b. The patient may have difficulty swallowing the tablet or the capsule, or
c. Mixing of powdered medication with food or drink may make the drug more palatable, or
d. The patient may have nasogastric tubes, which do not permit administration of tablets or capsules, or
e. The patient does not like to take the medication. In such cases mixing the drug with food or a beverage may be the only way of making the patient take the drug.
f. An oral solution for a particular medication may not be available from the manufacturer or readily prepared by pharmacy.

While it may not affect the absorption characteristics of many drugs administered from a divided or crushed tablet or administration of the powder obtained from emptying the contents of a hard gelatin capsule, there are instances where absorption characteristics of some drugs may be affected. Therefore, some tablet and capsule dosage forms should be administered intact without destroying the integrity of the dosage form. It is therefore recommended that individual drug monograph, Physician's Drug Reference or manufacturer's literature should be consulted prior to emptying the capsule or crushing the tablet. Dosage forms, which should not be crushed or divided by the pharmacist or by the patient fall into one of the following categories.

Enteric-coated Products

The purpose of enteric coating on a dosage form is to resist the release of drug from the dosage form in the gastric environment. Tablet and capsule dosage forms are usually protected with a coating of a polymer that is insoluble (or resists dissolution) in the acidic environment of the stomach. Therefore, crushing the tablet or removing contents from the capsule breaks this protective coating thus allowing drug release in the acidic environment of the stomach. In some capsule formulations, however, the capsule shell is not coated with an enteric polymer, but drug particles are individually coated with the protective coating. In such cases, removal of the contents from a capsule shell does not necessarily destroy the integrity of the dosage form and it may be safe to assume that the granules will resist drug dissolution in the acidic environment of the stomach.

Extended-release Products

The term extended release as used here also includes such designations as long-acting, slow-release, controlled release, etc. Many specialized techniques have been used in the formulation of these products, which allows the medication within it to be slowly released into the body fluids. Crushing or dividing the tablet or crushing the capsule contents may therefore destroy the mechanism used for modifying drug release from the intact dosage form. For example, the drug may be centered within the core of the tablet and coated with alternating layers of a polymer and drug. The drug is released with a subsequent shedding of multiple layers around the core. Some tablets are formulated with a low melting wax or wax-like material that surrounds the drug particles. Wax melts in the gastrointestinal tract releasing drug particles for dissolution.

Slow-K is an example of this. Similarly, capsules may contain multiple types of beads, each type coated with layers of polymers that dissolve at different rates providing a continuous release of drug. This technique was pioneered by Smith Kline and French. Tampering the dosage form or its contents may destroyed any of these mechanisms, thereby converting the extended-release dosage form into conventional-release dosage form.

Unpleasant Tasting Medication

Some drugs are very unpleasant to taste. In order to improve their palatability and facilitate acceptance by the patient, the manufacturers coat the tablet dosage forms of these drugs with a polymer film or with sugar. By crushing the tablet, this coating is lost and the patient tastes the unpleasant tasting drug, thus defeating the purpose of coating the tablet. If the unpleasant tasting drug is marketed in a capsule formulation, the manufacturer feels that there is no need to coat the dosage form, because the capsule shell provides adequate barrier to the unpleasant taste of the drug. Thus, removing the contents of a capsule from its shell no longer provides this barrier to the unpleasant taste of the drug.

Sublingual Tablets

Sublingual tablets usually contain drugs that are not administered via the gastrointestinal tract. These tablets are not swallowed and are intended to be placed under the tongue because this dosage form allows rapid absorption of the drug and/or prevent degradation of drug in the gastric environment. Crushing a sublingual tablet means that the patient will be administered a powder. Since the patient will not be able to keep the powder under the tongue, the powder will be swallowed by the patient, hence defeating the purpose of the dosage form. Also, it may substantially alter the pharmacokinetics of the dosage form. Dosage forms intended for sublingual use should not be crushed. Some products may not state on the label that the dosage form is for sublingual administration. Thus, it may not be easy to determine if a medication is to be used sublingually. Sublingual medications should indicate on the package that they are intended for sublingual use.

Effervescent Tablets

Effervescent tablets are formulated to contain an acid and a base (both in the solid state) in the tablet formulation. The base is usually a bicarbonate so that when the acid and the base neutralize each other, the resulting reaction produces carbon dioxide. This evolution of gas produces effervescence. Since the acid and the base in the tablet formulation are in solid state, they cannot interact with each unless they come into contact with water. Hence, these tablets effervesce when they come into contact with an aqueous solution. Thus, when dropped into a liquid, the tablet dissolves quickly to yield a solution. Many effervescent tablets, when crushed, lose their ability to effervesce and quick dissolution. Also, when the powder from the crushed tablets is placed in the mouth, the powder may produce effervescence when it comes into contact with saliva and the liquid used to wash down the powder. The effervescence thus produced either in the mouth or in the stomach may be very uncomfortable to the patient.

Miscellaneous

Miscellaneous is evident that several dosage forms do not lend themselves to crushing or dividing even when the dosage form is a scored (or quadri-scored) tablet. Crushing or chewing may substantially alter the dosage form's pharmacokinetics, exhibit poor taste, irritant properties or carcinogenic potential. Table 9-3 is an alphabetical listing of drug products and their dosage forms that should not be crushed. It should be noted that some listed products may have been discontinued, reformulated or have availability in limited areas.

Table 9-3 Oral dosage forms that should not be crushed

Product Name	*Dosage form*	*Reason (S)*
	A	
Aciphex	Tablet	Extended release/slow release
Accutane	Capsule	Liquid-filled capsule
Actifed 12-hour	Capsule	Extended release/slow release
Acutrim	Tablet	Extended release/slow release
Adalat CC	Tablet	Extended release/slow release
Aerolate SR	Capsule	Extended release/slow release
Aerolate JR	Capsule	Extended release/slow release
Afrinol Repetabs	Tablet	Extended release/slow release
Allegra-D	Tablet	Extended release/slow release
Allerest 12-hour	Capsule	Extended release/slow release
Ammonium Chloride Extended Release	Tablet	Enteric-coated
Artane Sequels	Capsule	Extended release/slow release
Arthritis Bayer (Time Release)	Capsule	Extended release/slow release
Arthrotec	Tablet	Enteric-coated
ASA Enseals	Tablet	Enteric-coated
Asacol	Tablet	Extended release/slow release
Ascriptin A/D	Tablet	Enteric-coated
Ascriptin ES	Tablet	Enteric-coated
Atrohist LA	Tablet	Extended release/slow release
Atrohist Plus	Tablet	Extended release/slow release
Atrohist Sprinkle	Capsule	Extended release/slow release
Azulfidine EN-tabs	Tablet	Enteric-coated
	B	
Baros	Tablet	Effervescent product
Bayer Low Adult 81 mg	Tablet	Enteric-coated
Bayer Regular strength 325 mg	Tablet	Enteric-coated
Bayer enteric-coated	Tablet	Enteric-coated
Betachron E-R	Capsule	Extended release/slow release
Betapen-VK	Tablet	Bitter/unacceptable taste
Biaxin-XL	Tablet	Extended release/slow release
Biohist-LA	Tablet	Extended release/slow release
Bisacodyl	Tablet	Enteric-coated
Bontril SR	Capsule	Extended release/slow release
Breonesin	Capsule	Extended release/slow release
Brexin LA	Capsule	Extended release/slow release
Bromfed	Capsule	Extended release/slow release
Bromfed PD	Capsule	Extended release/slow release
	C	
Calan SR	Tablet	Scored tablet, may be broken in half
Cama Arthritis Pain Reliever	Tablet	Enteric-coated
Carbatrol	Capsule	Extended release/slow release
Carbiset-TR	Tablet	Extended release/slow release
Cardizem	Tablet	Extended release/slow release
Cardizem CD	Capsule	Extended release/slow release

Contd...

Contd...

Cardizem SR	Capsule	Extended release/slow release
Carter's Little Pills	Tablet	Enteric-coated
Ceclor CD	Tablet	Extended release/slow release
Ceftin	Tablet	Bitter/unacceptable taste
CellCept Roche	Capsule	Potentially carcinogenic, handle with adequate protection
Charcoal Plus	Tablet	Enteric-coated
Chloral Hydrate	Capsule	Liquid-filled capsule
Chlorpheniramine Maleate time release	Capsule	Extended release/slow release
Chlor-Trimeton 8-Hour	Tablet	Extended release/slow release
Chlor-Trimeton 12-Hour	Tablet	Extended release/slow release
Choledyl SA	Tablet	Extended release/slow release
Cipro	Tablet	Bitter/unacceptable taste
Claritin-D	Tablet	Extended release/slow release
Claritin-D 24 Hour	Tablet	Extended release/slow release
Codimal-LA	Capsule	Extended release/slow release
Codimal-LA Half	Capsule	Extended release/slow release
Colace	Capsule	Bitter/unacceptable taste
Comhist LA	Capsule	Extended release/slow release
Compazine Spansule	Capsule	Extended release/slow release
Congress JR	Capsule	Extended release/slow release
Congress SR	Capsule	Extended release/slow release
Contac 12-Hour	Capsule	Extended release/slow release
Contac Maximum Strength	Capsule	Extended release/slow release
Cotazym S	Capsule	Enteric-coated
Covera-HS	Tablet	Extended release/slow release
Creon 5	Capsule	Enteric-coated
Creon 10	Capsule	Enteric-coated
Creon 20	Capsule	Enteric-coated
Cystospaz-M	Capsule	Extended release/slow release
Cytovene	Capsule	Potentially carcinogenic, handle With adequate protection
Cytoxan	Tablet	Potentially carcinogenic, handle with adequate protection
Cordilox	Tablet	Scored tablet, may be broken in half
	D	
D.A. II	Tablet	Extended release/slow release
Dairycare	Tablet	Extended release/slow release
Dallergy	Tablet	Extended release/slow release
Dallergy-D, JR	Tablet	Extended release/slow release
D-amine SR	Tablet	Extended release/slow release
Deconamine Sr	Tablet	Extended release/slow release
Decongest II	Tablet	Extended release/slow release
Decongestine	Tablet	Extended release/slow release
Deconhist LA	Tablet	Extended release/slow release
Deconomed SR	Tablet	Extended release/slow release
Deconsal II, Sprinkle	Capsule	Extended release/slow release
Defen-LA	Tablet	Extended release/slow release
Demazin Repetab	Tablet	Enteric-coated

Contd...

Contd...

Depakene	Capsule	Slow release, mucous membrane irritant
Depakote	Tablet	Extended release/slow release
Depakote ER, Sprinkles	Capsule	Enteric-coated
Desal II	Tablet	Extended release/slow release
Desoxyn Gradumets	Tablet	Extended release/slow release
Desyrel	Tablet	Enteric-coated
Despec SR	Caplets	Extended release/slow release
Detrol LA	Capsule	Extended release/slow release
Dexaphen SA	Tablet	Extended release/slow release
Dexatrim Ext Duration	Capsule	Extended release/slow release
Dexadrine Spansule	Capsule	Extended release/slow release
D-Feda II	Tablet	Extended release/slow release
Diamox Sequels	Capsule	Extended release/slow release
Dilacor XR	Capsule	Extended release/slow release
Dilantin Kapseals	Capsule	Extended release/slow release
Dilatrate SR	Capsule	Extended release/slow release
Diltia XT	Capsule	Extended release/slow release
Dimetane Extentabs	Tablet	Extended release/slow release
Dimetapp Extentabs	Tablet	Extended release/slow release
Disobrom	Tablet	Extended release/slow release
Disophrol Chronotab	Tablet	Extended release/slow release
Dital	Capsule	Extended release/slow release
Ditropan XL	Tablet	Extended release/slow release
Docusate w/ Casanthrol	Capsule (soft)	Bitter/unacceptable taste
Docusate	Capsule (soft)	Bitter/unacceptable taste
Dolobid	Tablet	Enteric-coated, bitter/unacceptable taste
Donnatal Extentab	Tablet	Extended release/slow release
Donnazyme	Tablet	Enteric-coated
Doryx	Capsule	Extended release/slow release
Doxidan Liquigels	Capsule (soft)	Liquid-filled capsule
Drexophed	Tablet	Extended release/slow release
Drisdol	Tablet	Extended release/slow release
Dristan 12-Hour	Nasal Spray	Bitter/unacceptable taste
Drituss GP	Tablet	Extended release/slow release
Drixomed	Tablet Extended	Release/slow release
Drixoral	Tablet	Extended release/slow release
Drixoral Plus, Sinus	Tablet	Extended release/slow release
Drize-R	Tablet	Extended release/slow release
Drysec	Tablet	Extended release/slow release
Duagen	Capsule (soft)	Liquid-filled capsule
Dulcolax	Tablet	Enteric-coated
Duotrate	Capsule	Extended release/slow release
Duradryl JR	Capsule	Extended release/slow release
Duralex	Capsule	Extended release/slow release
Duraquin	Tablet	Extended release/slow release
Durasal II	Tablet	Extended release/slow release
Dura-Tap PD	Tablet	Extended release/slow release
Duratuss	Tablet	Extended release/slow release
DuratussG, GP	Tablet	Extended release/slow release

Contd...

Contd...

Dura-Vent A	Tablet	Extended release/slow release
Dura-Vent/DA	Tablet	Extended release/slow release
Dylaxol	Tablet	Enteric-coated
Dynabac	Tablet	Enteric-coated
Dynabac D5-Pak	Tablet	Enteric-coated
Dynacirc CR	Capsule	Extended release/slow release
Dynahist-ER Pediatric	Capsule	Extended release/slow release
Dynex	Tablet	Extended release/slow release
	E	
Easpirin	Tablet	Enteric-coated
EC Naprosyn	Tablet	Enteric-coated
Ecotrin	Tablet	Enteric-coated
Ecotrin Adult low Strength	Tablet	Enteric-coated
Ecotrin Maximum Strength	Tablet	Enteric-coated
E.E.S. 400	Tablet	Enteric-coated
Effexor XR	Capsule	Extended release/slow release
Efidac 24 Chlorpheniramine	Tablet	Extended release/slow release
Efidac 24 Pseudoephedrine	Tablet	Extended release/slow release
Elixophyllin SR	Capsule	Extended release/slow release
E- Mycin	Tablet	Enteric-coated
Entex LA	Tablet	Extended release/slow release
Entex PSE	Tablet	Extended release/slow release
Entocort EC	Capsule	Enteric-coated
Equanil	Tablet	Bitter/unacceptable taste
Ergostat	Tablet	Sublingual tablet
Eryc	Capsule	Enteric-coated
Ery- Tab	Tablet	Enteric-coated
Erythromycin Stearate	Tablet	Enteric-coated
Erythromycin Base	Tablet	Enteric-coated
Eskalith- CR	Tablet	Extended release/slow release
Eudal SR	Tablet	Extended release/slow release
Extendryl JR	Capsule	Extended release/slow release
Extendryl SR	Capsule	Extended release/slow release
Extress	Tablet	Enteric-coated
	F	
Fedahist Timecaps	Capsule	Extended release/slow release
Feen- A- Mint	Tablet	Enteric-coated
Femilax	Tablet	Enteric-coated
Fenesin	Capsule	Extended release/slow release
Fenisin DM	Capsule	Extended release/slow release
Feosol	Tablet	Enteric-coated
Feratab	Tablet	Enteric-coated
Fergon	Capsule	Extended release/slow release
Fero-Grad 500	Tablet	Extended release/slow release
Ferro-Sequels	Tablet	Extended release/slow release
Ferro-Time	Capsule	Extended release/slow release
Ferrous Fumarate DS	Tablet	Extended release/slow release
Feverall Sprinkle	Capsule	Capsule content intended to be Placed in a teaspoonful of water or soft food

Contd...

Contd...

Flagyl ER	Tablet	Extended release/slow release
Fleets bisacodyl	Tablet	Enteric-coated
Flomax	Capsule	Extended release/slow release
Fumatinic	Capsule	Extended release/slow release
	G	
Gastrocrom	Capsule	Effervescent product (contents may be dissolved in water for administration)
Gaviscon	Tablet	Effervescent product
Geocillin	Caplets	Bitter/unacceptable taste
Glucotrol XL	Tablet	Extended release/slow release
GrisPEG	Tablet	Crushing may result in precipitation of larger particles
Guaifed PD	Capsule	Extended release/slow release
Guaifenex LA	Tablet	Extended release/slow release
Guaifenex PPA	Tablet	Extended release/slow release
Guaifenex PSE	Tablet	Extended release/slow release
Guaimax-D	Tablet	Extended release/slow release
	H	
Halfprin	Tablet	Enteric-coated
Humibid DM	Tablet	Bitter/unacceptable taste
Humibid DM sprinkle	Capsule	Extended release/slow release
Humibid LA	Tablet	Extended release/slow release
Humibid sprinkle	Capsule	Extended release/slow release
Hydergine LC	Tablet	Extended release/slow release (product is in liquid form within a special capsule)
Hydergine sublingual	Tablet	Sublingual tablet
Hytakerol	Capsule	Liquid-filled capsule
	I	
Iberet	Tablet	Enteric-coated
Iberet Folic 500	Tablet	Enteric-coated
Icaps Plus	Tablet	Extended release/slow release
Icaps Time Release	Tablet	Extended release/slow release
Ilotycin	Tablet	Enteric-coated
Imdur	Tablet	Extended release/slow release
Inderal LA	Capsule	Extended release/slow release
Inderide LA	Capsule	Extended release/slow release
Indocin SR	Capsule	Extended release/slow release
Ionamin	Tablet	Enteric-coated
Isoptin SR	Tablet	Extended release/slow release
Isordil Sublingual	Tablet	Sublingual tablet
Isordil Tembids	Tablet	Extended release/slow release
	K	
K + 8	Tablet	Extended release/slow release
K + 10	Tablet	Extended release/slow release
Kadian	Capsule	Extended release/slow release

Contd...

Contd...

Kaon Cl	Tablet	Extended release/slow release
K-Dur	Tablet	Extended release/slow release
K-Lease	Capsule	Extended release/slow release
Klor-Con	Tablet	Extended release/slow release
Klotrix	Tablet	Extended release/slow release
K-lyte	Tablet	Effervescent product
K-lyte Cl	Tablet	Effervescent product
K-lyte DS	Tablet	Effervescent product
K-Norm	Capsule	Extended release/slow release
K-tab	Tablet	Extended release/slow release
	L	
Levbid	Tablet	Extended release/slow release
Levsinex Timecap	Capsule	Extended release/slow release
Lexxel	Tablet	Extended release/slow release
Lithobid	Tablet	Extended release/slow release
Lodine XL	Tablet	Extended release/slow release
Lodrane LD	Capsule	Extended release/slow release
	M	
Mag-Tab SR	Tablet	Extended release/slow release
Mestinon Timespan	Tablet	Extended release/slow release
Mi-Cebrin	Tablet	Enteric-coated
Mi-Cebrin T	Tablet	Enteric-coated
Micro-K	Capsule	Extended release/slow release
Monafed	Tablet	Extended release/slow release
Monafed DM	Tablet	Extended release/slow release
Motrin	Tablet	Bitter/unacceptable taste
MS Contin	Tablet	Extended release/slow release
Muco-Fen-DM	Tablet	Extended release/slow release
Muco-Fen-LA	Tablet	Extended release/slow release
	N	
Naldecon	Tablet	Extended release/slow release
Nalex A	Tablet	Extended release/slow release
Naprelan	Tablet	Extended release/slow release
Nasabid SR	Capsule	Extended release/slow release
Nasahist Capsule	Capsule	Extended release/slow release
Nasatab LA	Tablet	Scored tablet, may be broken in half
Nd Clear	Capsule	Extended release/slow release
Nexium	Capsule	Extended release/slow release
Nia-Bid	Capsule	Extended release/slow release
Niacin time release (Generic)	Tablet	Extended release/slow release
Niaspan	Tablet	Extended release/slow release
Nico 400	Tablet	Extended release/slow release
Nicotinic acid (Generic)	Tablet	Extended release/slow release
Nifedical XL	Tablet	Extended release/slow release
Nifedipine ER (Generic)	Tablet	Extended release/slow release
Nitrobon	Capsule	Extended release/slow release
Nitrocine Timecaps	Capsule	Extended release/slow release
Nitrocot	Capsule	Extended release/slow release

Contd...

Contd...

Nitrogard	Tablet	Extended release/slow release
Nitroglyn	Capsule	Extended release/slow release
Nitrong	Tablet	Sublingual tablet
Nitroquick	Tablet	Sublingual tablet
Nitrostat	Tablet	Sublingual tablet
Nitro Tab	Tablet	Sublingual tablet
Nitrotime	Capsule	Extended release/slow release
Noctec	Capsule	Extended release/slow release
Nolamine	Tablet	Extended release/slow release
Nolex LA	Tablet	Extended release/slow release
Norflex	Tablet	Extended release/slow release
Norpace CR	Capsule	Extended release/slow release
Novafed	Capsule	Extended release/slow release
Novafed A	Capsule	Extended release/slow release
	O	
Omeprazole (Generic)	Capsule	Enteric-coated
Omnihist LA	Tablet	Extended release/slow release
Ondrox	Tablet	Extended release/slow release
Optilets-500	Tablet	Enteric-coated
Optilets-M-500	Tablet	Enteric-coated
Ordrine AT ER,SR	Capsule	Extended release/slow release
Oragrafin	Capsule	Liquid-filled capsule
Oramorph SR	Tablet	Extended release/slow release
Ornade Spansule	Capsule	Extended release/slow release
Oruvail	Capsule	Extended release/slow release
Oxycontin	Tablet	Extended release/slow release
	P	
Pabalate	Tablet	Enteric-coated
Pancrease	Capsule	Enteric-coated
Pancrease MT	Capsule	Enteric-coated
Panmist Jr, LA	Tablet	Extended release/slow release
Panmycin	Capsule	Bitter/unacceptable taste
Pennaz	Tablet	Extended release/slow release
Papaverine SA	Capsule	Extended release/slow release
Pathilon Sequels	Capsule	Extended release/slow release
Pavabid Plateau	Capsule	Extended release/slow release
Paxil CR	Tablet	Extended release/slow release
PBZ-SR	Tablet	Extended release/slow release
Pentasa	Tablet	Extended release/slow release
Peritrate SA	Tablet	Extended release/slow release
Permitil Chronotab	Tablet	Extended release/slow release
Phazyme	Tablet	Extended release/slow release
Phenergan	Tablet	Bitter/unacceptable taste, antacids or milk may prematurely dissolve the coating
Phyllocontin	Tablet	Extended release/slow release
Plendil	Tablet	Extended release/slow release
Pneumomist	Tablet	Extended release/slow release
Prevacid	Capsule	Enteric-coated, extended release/slow release

Contd...

Contd...

Prilosec	Capsule	Enteric-coated, extended release/slow release
Pro-Banthine	Tablet	Bitter/unacceptable taste
Procanbid	Tablet	Extended release/slow release
Procainamide SR	Tablet	Extended release/slow release
Procardia	Capsule	Bitter/unacceptable taste
Procardia XL	Tablet	Extended release/slow release
Profen II	Tablet	Extended release/slow release
Profen LA	Tablet	Extended release/slow release
Pronestyl-SR	Tablet	Extended release/slow release
Propecia	Tablet	Potentially carcinogenic, handle with adequate protection
Proscar	Tablet	Potentially carcinogenic, handle with adequate protection
Protonix	Tablet	Enteric-coated, extended release/slow release
Proventil Repetabs	Tablet	Extended release/slow release
Prozac (Weekly)	Capsule	Extended release/slow release
	Q	
Quibron-T SR	Tablet	Extended release/slow release
Quinaglute Dura-Tabs	Tablet	Extended release/slow release
Quinidex Extentabs	Tablet	Extended release/slow release
Quin-Release	Tablet	Extended release/slow release
	R	
Respa-1st	Tablet	Extended release/slow release
Respa-DM	Tablet	Extended release/slow release
Respa-GF	Tablet	Extended release/slow release
Respahist	Capsule	Extended release/slow release
Respaire SR	Capsule	Extended release/slow release
Respbid	Tablet	Extended release/slow release
Ritalin SR	Tablet	Extended release/slow release
Robimycin	Tablet	Enteric-coated
Rondec TR	Tablet	Extended release/slow release
Ru-Tuss DE	Tablet	Extended release/slow release
	S	
Sinemet CR	Tablet	Extended release/slow release
Singlet for Adults	Tablet	Extended release/slow release
Slo-bid Gyrocaps	Capsule	Extended release/slow release
Slo-Niacin	Tablet	Extended release/slow release
Slo-Phyllin GG	Capsule	Extended release/slow release
Slo-Phyllin Gryocaps	Capsule	Extended release/slow release
Slow-FE	Tablet	Extended release/slow release
Slow-FE with Folic Acid	Tablet	Extended release/slow release
Slow-K	Tablet	Extended release/slow release
Slow-Mag	Tablet	Extended release/slow release
Sorbitrate SA	Tablet	Extended release/slow release
Sorbitrate Sublingual	Tablet	Sublingual tablet
Sparine	Tablet	Bitter/unacceptable taste

Contd...

Contd...

S-P-T	Capsule	Liquid-filled capsule
Sudafed 12 hour	Capsule	Extended release/slow release
Sudal 60/500	Tablet	Extended release/slow release
Sudal 120/600	Tablet	Extended release/slow release
Sudex	Tablet	Extended release/slow release
Sular	Tablet	Extended release/slow release
Sustaire	Tablet	Extended release/slow release
Syn-RX	Tablet	Extended release/slow release
Syn-RX DM	Tablet	Extended release/slow release
	T	
Tavist-D	Tablet	Extended release/slow release
Teczem	Tablet	Extended release/slow release
Tedral SA	Tablet	Extended release/slow release
Tegretol-XR	Tablet	Extended release/slow release
Teldrin Maximum Strength	Capsule	Extended release/slow release
Tepanil Ten-Tab	Tablet	Extended release/slow release
Tessalon Perles	Capsule	Extended release/slow release
Theo-24	Tablet	Extended release/slow release
Theobid Duracaps	Capsule	Extended release/slow release
Theoclear LA	Capsule	Extended release/slow release
Theochron	Tablet	Extended release/slow release
Theo-Dur	Tablet	Extended release/slow release
Theo-Dur Sprinkle	Capsule	Extended release/slow release
Theolair SR	Tablet	Extended release/slow release
Theo-Sav	Tablet	Extended release/slow release
Theo-Span-SR	Capsule	Extended release/slow release
Theo-Time SR	Tablet	Extended release/slow release
Theo-X	Tablet	Extended release/slow release
Theovent	Capsule	Extended release/slow release
Thorazine Spansule	Capsule	Extended release/slow release
Toprol XL	Tablet	Extended release/slow release
Touro A&D	Capsule	Extended release/slow release
Touro EX	Tablet	Extended release/slow release
Touro LA	Tablet	Extended release/slow release
T-Phyl	Tablet	Extended release/slow release
Trental	Tablet	Extended release/slow release
Triaminic	Tablet	Enteric-coated
Triaminic 12	Tablet	Extended release/slow release
Triaminic TR	Tablet	Extended release/slow release
Tri-Phen-Chlor Time Released	Tablet	Extended release/slow release
Tri-Phen-Mine SR	Tablet	Extended release/slow release
Triptone Caplets	Tablet	Extended release/slow release
Tuss LA	Tablet	Extended release/slow release
Tuss Ornade Spansule	Capsule	Extended release/slow release
Tylenol Extended Relief	Capsule	Extended release/slow release
	U	
ULR-LA	Tablet	Extended release/slow release
Ultrabrom	Capsule	Extended release/slow release
Ultrabrom PD	Capsule	Extended release/slow release

Contd...

Contd...

Ultrase	Capsule	Enteric-coated
Ultrase MT	Capsule	Enteric-coated
Uni Decon	Tablet	Extended release/slow release
Uni-dur	Tablet	Scored tablet, may be broken in half
Uniphyl	Tablet	Scored tablet, may be broken in half
Urimax	Tablet	Enteric-coated
Uni Multihist D	Capsule	Extended release/slow release
Urocit K	Tablet	Extended release/slow release
	V	
Vanex Forte-D	Tablet	Extended release/slow release
Vanex Forte-R	Capsule	Extended release/slow release
Vantin	Tablet	Bitter/unacceptable taste
V Dec M	Tablet	Extended release/slow release
Verelan	Capsule	Extended release/slow release
Verelan PM	Capsule	Extended release/slow release
Versacaps	Capsule	Extended release/slow release
Videx EC	Capsule	Enteric-coated
Vivotif Berna	Capsule	Enteric-coated
Volmax	Tablet	Extended release/slow release
Voltaren	Tablet	Enteric-coated
Voltaren XR	Tablet	Extended release/slow release
	W	
We Mist LA	Tablet	Extended release/slow release
Wellbutrin SR	Tablet	Extended release/slow release
Wellbutrin XL	Tablet	Extended release/slow release
Westrim LA	Capsule	Extended release/slow release
West-Decon	Tablet	Extended release/slow release
	X	
Xanax XR	Tablet	Extended release/slow release
	Z	
Zephrex LA	Tablet	Extended release/slow release
Zorprin	Tablet	Extended release/slow release
Zyban	Tablet	Extended release/slow release
Zymase	Tablet	Enteric-coated
Zyrtec-D	Tablet	Extended release/slow release

SUGGESTED READING

1. Gibaldi M. Biopharmaceutics and Clinical Pharmacokinetics, 4th edition. Lea and Febiger; 1991.
2. Gosset WS. The Probable Error of a Mean. Biometrika. 1908;6:1-25.
3. Washington DC. Guidelines for biopharmaceutical studies in man. Amer Pharm Assoc. Acad Pharm. Sci., 1972.
4. Madan PL. Are your patients getting the drugs you prescribe? The Medical Society of the State of New York. June; 1994.

5. Madan PL. Bioavailability and Bioequivalence: The Underlying Concepts. US Pharmacist. 1992;17(11):H10-H30.
6. Madan PL. Bioavailability and patient variances. US Pharmacist Suppl. 1996;21(5):3-14.
7. Madan PL. Introduction to bioavailability and pharmacokinetics. In: Lamba and Walker (eds). Antibiotics and Microbial Transformations. CRC Press, Boca Raton, Florida; 1987.
8. Pharmaceutical Manufacturers Association, Bioequivalence of Solid Oral Dosage Forms, US Food and Drug Administration Hearing. Sept 29-Oct 1, 1986.

PRACTICE PROBLEMS

9-1. Which of the following three tablet formulations are pharmaceutically equivalent?

Ingredient	*Function*	*Tablet A*	*Tablet B*	*Tablet C*
Acetaminophen	Drug	300 mg	–	300 mg
Aspirin	Drug	300 mg	300 mg	–
Lactose	Filler	100 mg	100 mg	–
Avicel	Filler	–	–	100 mg
Starch	Disintegrant	50 mg	50 mg	–
Avicel	Disintegrant	–	–	50 mg
Magnesium stearate	Lubricant	2 mg	2 mg	2 mg
Gelatin	Binder	10 mg	10 mg	10 mg

9-2. Which of the following five formulations are pharmaceutical alternatives? The amount of active ingredient listed for these products is per tablet, per capsule or per teaspoonful.

Ingredient	*Tablet A*	*Tablet B*	*Capsule C*	*Syrup D*	*Suspension E*
Ibuprofen	200 mg	–	–	–	200 mg
Aspirin	–	–	300 mg	–	–
Acetaminophen	–	325 mg	–	325 mg	–

9-3. The area under the plasma concentration versus time curve for 12 subjects who participated in a bioavailability study, which compared two products of the same drug in the same strength and same dosage form is shown below. Perform a two-sided paired t-test on both the ratios and the difference of the logarithms, comparing the average ratio to 1.

Subject	*A*	*B*
1	201	200
2	231	236
3	221	216
4	260	233
5	228	224
6	237	216

Subject	*A*	*B*
7	326	296
8	235	195
9	240	207
10	267	247
11	284	210
12	201	209

9-4. The area under the plasma concentration versus time curve for 12 subjects comparing two products of the same drug in the same strength and the same dosage form made by two manufacturers is shown below. Perform a two-sided paired t-test on both the ratios and the difference of the logarithms, comparing the average ratio to 1.

Subject	A	B
1	102	110
2	95	112
3	101	101
4	100	114
5	98	117
6	109	112

Subject	A	B
7	114	108
8	108	116
9	97	109
10	104	109
11	119	125
12	117	121

9-5. Which of the following four formulations are pharmaceutical alternatives? The amount of active ingredient listed for these products is per tablet, per capsule or per teaspoonful.

Ingredient	Tablet A	Tablet B	Capsule C	Syrup D
Ibuprofen	200 mg	–	–	200 mg
Aspirin	–	–	300 mg	–
Acetaminophen	–	250 mg	250 mg	–

9-6. Twenty healthy subjects participated in a bioavailability study undertaken to compare two formulations (A and B) of the same drug (administered in the same dosage form and in the same dosage strength). The t-tests performed on the ratios and the difference of the logarithms gave the following data:

	Ratio A/B	log A – log B
Average	0.5	–0.042
Standard Deviation	0.12	0.061

Perform the t-test on the ratios and the t-test on the difference of the logarithms and determine, if the two products are bioequivalent.

9-7. Twelve healthy subjects participated in a bioavailability study undertaken to compare two formulations (A and B) of the same drug (administered in the same dosage form and in the same dosage strength). The *t*-tests performed on the ratios and the difference of the logarithms gave the following data:

	Ratio A/B	log A – log B
Average	0.7	–0.040
Standard Deviation	0.12	0.059

Perform the t-test on the ratios and the t-test on the difference of the logarithms and determine if the two products are bioequivalent.

9-8. The area under the plasma concentration versus time curve for 12 healthy subjects who participated in a bioavailability study comparing two formulations (C and D) of the same drug (administered in the same dosage form and in the same dosage strength) is shown below. Perform a two-sided paired t-test on the average of the ratios and the difference of the logarithms of the average, comparing the average ratio to 1.

Subject	C	D
1	1235	1625
2	1365	1235
3	1170	1755
4	1274	1794
5	1300	1560
6	1690	1794

Subject	C	D
7	1300	1625
8	1755	1235
9	1300	1560
10	1235	1755
11	1300	1560
12	1274	1560

CHAPTER 10

COMPARTMENT MODELS

Following the administration of a drug dose and the appearance of drug in the plasma, the drug may undergo distribution into other body fluids (e.g. the extracellular fluids or total body fluids) and various body tissues (such as proteins minerals or the adipose tissue). The concentration of drug in the plasma, various other body fluids and tissues undergoes changes as a result of several processes working simultaneously. This is because the drug is always in a dynamic state within the body and in a biologic system, such as human body, drug events often happen simultaneously. Also, the handling of a drug by the body is generally a very complex process, which is usually difficult to understand unless a number of simplifying assumptions are made concerning the movement and transfer of drug into various other body fluids and tissues. Therefore, simplification of body processes is essential to predict the behavior of drug in the body. It is for this reason that pharmacokinetic studies are usually described in terms of pharmacokinetic models and compartments.

A *pharmacokinetic model* is a mathematical description of a biologic system, which can be used to simulate the rate processes describing the movement of drug in the body. Various mathematical models can be devised to simulate these rate processes. In pharmacokinetic studies, a model is often used as a concise way to accomplish the following objectives:

a. Develop equations, which describe drug concentration
b. Express quantitative relationships between various parameters
c. To predict drug concentration in the body as a function of time.

A basic and elementary type of model used in pharmacokinetic studies is the compartment model. The term *compartment* as used here does not necessarily represent a specific tissue, fluid or a particular portion of the body. The term compartment is used to describe a group of tissues, which are similar in certain characteristics (e.g. rate of blood flow to the tissue or partition properties) or specific entities (e.g. drug affinity, fat, plasma proteins), etc. The compartments are considered to be connected to each other by pathways, which may be reversible or irreversible. Examples of reversible pathways include weak binding of a drug to plasma proteins and renal elimination with complete reabsorption. An example of an irreversible pathway is elimination of drug from body through urine or other excretory pathway.

A compartment is not a real physiologic or anatomic region of the body. It may comprise of as little as a few, to as large as many different regions of the body. In pharmacokinetic studies, compartment models have been termed 'deterministic' because the amount and concentration of drug in the plasma can often be used to determine the type of model required to describe pharmacokinetics of the drug.

The most commonly employed approach to pharmacokinetic characterization of a drug is to represent the body as if it consisted of a system of compartments, between which the drug distributes. As a rule, drugs intended for systemic effect distribute rapidly to tissues with high blood flow (e.g. heart, lungs, liver and kidneys) and more slowly to those tissues where blood circulation is poor. If distribution of drug into these groups is rapid and instantaneous, the drug confers the characteristics of one-compartment model on the body, i.e. drug moves freely between these groups as if there were no barriers separating these groups. If the distribution of drug between these groups is not instantaneous but relatively slow, then the distribution of drug in the body may be described as a two-, three-, or more than three-compartment model, i.e. the drug confers upon the body the characteristics of a multi-compartment model. If the distribution of a drug into the tissues is instantaneous, but the drug accumulates in tissues either as a result of the drug's physicochemical characteristics or because of a special affinity of tissue for the drug, the drug then confers upon the body the characteristics of a multiple compartment pharmacokinetic model. For example, lipid-soluble drugs may accumulate in fat (the adipose tissue) and drugs having affinity for proteins may bind to albumin. In most instances binding of drugs to adipose tissue or proteins is reversible and such binding results in a depot action. Also, drugs which have a greater affinity for these tissues may displace other drugs, which are not as strongly bound.

COMPARTMENT MODELING

Compartment models are mathematical models devised to simulate rate processes of drug absorption, distribution metabolism and elimination. These models are used to develop equations, which describe concentration of drug in the body as a function of time. The key to compartment modeling is simplicity. In constructing compartment models, the simplest and most reasonable model is proposed first. The simplest and most reasonable model is one-compartment model. It is tested for its goodness of fit between experimental data and calculated values. If prediction with the proposed model does not appear adequate, then the next complex model is proposed and tested. The next complex model will be two-compartment model. If data prediction with the two-compartment model also proves inadequate, then the next higher model (three-compartment model) is proposed and tested. This procedure continues until a good fit is obtained with physiologically meaningful parameters. Since, the key to compartment modeling is simplicity; one-compartment model is the starting point. If there is an acceptable and reasonable goodness of fit between experimental data and calculated values, one stops here and one-compartment model is developed and proposed. The pharmacokinetics of most drugs is adequately described by one-compartment model.

As mentioned earlier, in pharmacokinetic modeling the body is represented as a series or systems of compartments that communicate reversibly with each other. Within each of these compartments the drug is considered to be mixed rapidly and homogeneously. In addition, the drug is considered to be uniformly distributed in each compartment. Thus, a pharmacokinetic compartmental model provides a simple way of grouping all drug-containing tissues into one-, two-, three-, or more compartments in which the drug moves to and from the central compartment.

Open and Closed Models

Pharmacokinetic models are referred to as open models (as opposed to closed models), e.g. one-compartment open model, two-compartment open model, etc. The term open refers to the fact that the administered drug dose is removed from the body by an excretory mechanism, as the unchanged drug and/or as a metabolite. For most drugs, the organ for excretion is the kidneys, while some drugs may also be removed from the body by other excretory organs. If the drug was not removed from the body by an excretory mechanism, then the proposed model would be referred to as a closed model, e.g. one-compartment closed model or two-compartment closed model, etc meaning that the proposed pharmacokinetic model is 'closed' as far as removal of drug from the body is concerned and the administered drug will persist in the body forever. Since all drugs administered into the body are removed by one or more excretory mechanism, all pharmacokinetic models are essentially 'open' models and for this reason the term 'open' is not used in describing a given model. Unless otherwise stated, it is understood that the model being proposed is an open model and not a closed model.

ONE-COMPARTMENT MODEL

In one-compartment pharmacokinetic model, after the administered drug dose appears in plasma, the drug is either distributed in plasma volume only, or if it distributes between plasma and other fluids and tissues, distribution is almost instantaneous and equilibrium is reached immediately. Blood and all readily accessible fluids and tissues may generally be treated kinetically as a common homogeneous unit, generally referred to as central compartment. One-compartment model assumes that any changes that occur in concentration of drug in the plasma will also be reflected by proportional changes in concentration of drug in the fluids and/or tissues in which the drug is distributed. This model does not assume that concentration of drug in each fluid or tissue is the same at any given time. Elimination of drug takes place from plasma and reduction in concentration of drug in plasma due to elimination is quantitatively reflected in similar reduction of drug concentration in other tissues and/or fluids, which comprise central compartment. It should be pointed out that while reduction of concentration of drug in each tissue of the central compartment is quantitatively proportional, the reduction in the amount of drug may not necessarily be exactly by the same amount. Figure 10-1 is a schematic of one-compartment model. Only one rectangular box in this schematic indicates that upon administration, the drug confers the pharmacokinetic characteristics of one-compartment model on the body.

In compartment modeling, the term 'central compartment' is sometimes used by some to indicate the plasma volume only. This is not always the case. For example, the volume of central compartment of some drugs is much greater than the plasma volume, suggesting that the central compartment consists of plasma and some other body fluids and/or tissues. Therefore, the term central compartment should actually be used to include plasma volume and other highly perfused tissues. This would signify the fact that the distribution of drug between plasma and other highly perfused tissues is instantaneous. Therefore, the volume of the central compartment is not necessarily limited to the plasma volume only and may in fact be much greater than the volume of the plasma fluid. Thus, if the concentration of drug were to decrease in the plasma (due to elimination), then the concentration of drug will also decrease in the other tissues by the same factor.

Multi-compartment Models

Drugs that exhibit multi-compartment pharmacokinetics distribute into different tissues at different rates. In general, highly perfused tissue groups equilibrate with drug more rapidly than poorly perfused tissue groups. Also, a drug will concentrate in a tissue in accordance with affinity of drug for that tissue. For example, highly lipid-soluble drugs accumulate in the adipose tissue more readily than less lipid-soluble drugs. Similarly, drugs that bind proteins may be more concentrated in plasma due to presence of proteins in plasma and because protein-bound drugs do

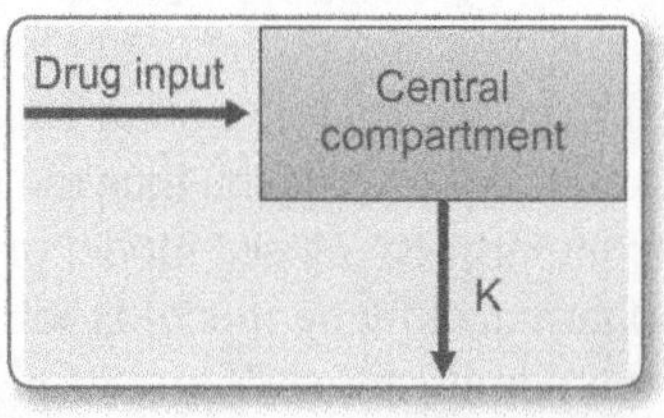

Fig. 10-1 Schematic of one-compartment pharmacokinetic model

not diffuse into the tissues. Thus, concentration as well as amount of drug in various tissues will depend on the nature of tissue and physicochemical characteristics of drug, e.g. lipid solubility, partition coefficient, etc. The accumulation of tetracycline in calcium-containing tissues, such as teeth and bones due to tetracycline-calcium complexation is a well-known example.

Terminology and Rate Constants

The terminology as well as the rate constants associated with multi-compartment models in pharmacokinetics is simple and self-explanatory. For example, the administered drug dose (regardless of the route and method of administration) is drug input and drug elimination from the central compartment is known as drug output. The various compartments into which the drug undergoes distributions are identified by the chronological path of drug transport into these compartments. The compartment of drug input is called the central compartment and the compartments into which the drug distributes (from the central compartment) are referred to as the tissue compartments. The various rate constants of transfer of drug associated with these compartments are identified in the simplest possible manner. The following terminology is used in a multi-compartment model:

Drug Input: The term drug input refers to the dose and/or route of drug administration. If the drug is administered by an extravascular route (e.g. oral, rectal, transdermal route or by intramuscular injection, etc.), then the drug input is associated with a rate constant of absorption (K_a). The rate constant of absorption, almost always, follows first-order kinetics. If the drug is administered by constant intravenous infusion, the rate constant of drug input is K_0 (zero-order rate of administration). If the drug is administered by rapid intravenous bolus injection, then there is no rate constant associated with drug input because the drug is placed into the central compartment all at once.

Drug Output: Drug output indicates the removal of drug from the central compartment. For the purposes of our discussion, this term will be limited to the removal of drug via the kidneys (renal elimination). Since kidneys remove the drug from plasma volume only, drug removal is therefore indicated by the symbol K or K_e, and is referred to as the overall rate constant of renal elimination. The elimination rate constant (K_e) also almost always follows first-order kinetics.

Central Compartment: As indicated earlier in reference to Figure 10-1, the central compartment is the compartment where the drug first appears in systemic circulation after administration of the dose. Therefore, this is compartment #1. Drug elimination from the body takes place from the central compartment.

Peripheral Tissue Compartment: This is the second compartment where the drug appears after the administered dose appears in the central compartment. Therefore, this compartment is compartment #2. In order for the drug to appear in this compartment, the drug must first be present in the central compartment. If the drug distributes into more than one tissue compartment, then the peripheral tissue compartment (compartment #2) is identified as the shallow tissue compartment.

Deep Tissue Compartment: This is the third compartment where drug may appear after the administered dose appears in the central compartment. Therefore, this is compartment #3. The third compartment is distinguished from compartment #2 because the distribution of drug in this compartment is not similar to the distribution of drug in compartment #2.

Transfer Rate Constants: The various rate constants of transfer of drug are indicated by the letter K and a subscript. The subscript identifies the compartments involved in the transfer of the drug. The subscripts used to indicate the various rate constants of transfer of drug are two-digit numbers. The first digit represents the compartment number from where the drug is coming and the second digit represents the compartment number where the drug is going. For example, subscript 12 indicates that the drug is coming from compartment #1 and is going into compartment #2 and the subscript 21 means that the drug transfers from compartment #2 into compartment #1. The subscript 10 is used to indicate "from compartment #1 to out of the body", i.e. elimination via the kidneys. Thus, K_{10} here has the same meaning as K_e in one-compartment model.

Apparent Volume of Distribution: The apparent volume of distribution of drug (generally referred to as the volume of distribution) is the volume of tissues or fluids in which the drug appears to be distributed. In the one-compartment model, the volume of distribution is the volume of the central compartment because this is the only compartment where the drug is distributed. In multi-compartment models, the apparent volume of distribution of drug represents the sum of the apparent volumes of distribution of all compartments into which the drug is distributed. Thus, if the pharmacokinetic model indicates a central compartment, a peripheral (shallow) tissue compartment and a deep tissue compartment, then the apparent volume of distribution of drug is the sum of the apparent volumes of distribution of the central compartment and the two tissue compartments.

Two-compartment Model

In the two-compartment model, immediately after appearance of drug in the plasma, the drug distributes rapidly into the highly perfused tissues. The blood and the readily accessible fluids and tissues may often be kinetically treated as a common homogeneous unit. As mentioned earlier, this is known as the central compartment. After the appearance of drug in the central compartment, the concentration of drug in the plasma exhibits an initial rapid decline because the drug from the central compartment undergoes elimination (removal) by two first-order processes:

i. Loss of drug due to elimination
ii. Loss of drug due to transfer of drug from the central compartment into the components of a second compartment.

This second compartment is generally known as the peripheral compartment or the tissue compartment. Since, the central compartment is reversibly connected to the tissue compartment, a portion of the drug, which had initially transferred into the tissue compartment will start returning to the central compartment according to the first-order rate constant of transfer, K_{21}, the rate constant of transfer of drug from the tissue compartment into the central compartment. After some time, the distribution of drug between these two compartments (central compartment and the tissue compartment) attains an equilibrium, i.e. a portion of the drug is lost from the central compartment into the tissue compartment according to the first-order rate constant of transfer, K_{12} and a portion of the drug returns from the tissue compartment into the central compartment according to the first-order rate constant of transfer K_{21}. At that time the initial rapid decline in concentration of drug in the plasma is followed by a slow decline in the concentration of drug in plasma, because part of the drug which had earlier transferred from the central compartment into the tissue compartment starts returning from the tissue compartment into the central compartment due to the establishment of an equilibrium between these two compartments.

Pharmacokinetically, a two-compartment model is depicted schematically as two rectangular boxes. One box represents the central compartment and the other box represents tissue compartment and both are reversibly connected to each other with first-order rate constants. That is, the drug transfers between these two compartments through reversible first-order processes. The drug input is represented in the central compartment by an irreversible process. This is usually a first-order process, except when the drug is administered by continuous intravenous infusion or by special drug delivery systems capable of zero-order release of drug. The elimination of drug also takes place from the central compartment, but by an irreversible mechanism (e.g. elimination via kidney through the urinary tract). Figure 10-2 shows a schematic of the two-compartment model. In the two-compartment model, the rate constants of transfer of drug between the compartments are:

K_{12} = Apparent first-order rate constant of transfer of drug from the central compartment into the tissue compartment.

K_{21} = Apparent first-order rate constant of transfer of drug from the tissue compartment into the central compartment.

K_{10} = Apparent first-order rate constant of drug elimination from central compartment (= K in one-compartment model).

In the two-compartment pharmacokinetic model, one would expect that K_{12} (the first-order rate constant of transfer of drug from the central compartment into the tissue compartment) would be greater than K_{21} (the first-order rate constant of transfer of drug from the tissue compartment into the central compartment). This expectation is based upon common sense, which dictates that in order for the drug to exhibit concentration in the tissue compartment, the rate of transfer of drug from central compartment into the tissue compartment must be greater than the rate of transfer of drug from the tissue compartment into the central compartment. That is, unless the drug enters the tissue compartment at a faster rate than it leaves the tissue compartment, the drug cannot accumulate in the tissue compartment. This may be true if transfer of drug between these two compartments followed zero-order kinetics. In actual practice, this is not necessarily the case, because in most cases the transfer of drug between these two compartments follows first-order kinetics. Since, in first-order kinetics, the rate of transfer of drug from one compartment to the other is concentration dependent, therefore, it is possible for the rate constant of transfer of drug from central compartment into the tissue compartment to be equal to or even smaller than the rate constant of transfer of drug from tissue compartment into the central compartment. There are numerous examples in the literature where K_{12} is either less than or approximately equal to K_{21}.

Three-compartment Model

The three-compartment pharmacokinetic model is a two-compartment model (one central compartment and one peripheral or shallow tissue compartment), with an additional third compartment (a deep tissue compartment) attached either to the central compartment or to the peripheral (shallow tissue) compartment. This third compartment represents a deep tissue compartment (e.g. such poorly perfused tissue as fat), or it may represent the binding of drug to the tissues, e.g. plasma proteins. In order to differentiate the two tissue compartments, the first tissue compartment is usually labeled as the *peripheral tissue compartment* or *shallow tissue compartment* and the second tissue compartment is usually labeled as the *deep tissue compartment*.

The rate constants of transfer of drug in a three-compartment model are labeled as follows:

K_{12} = Apparent first-order rate constant of transfer of drug from the central compartment into the peripheral tissue compartment.

K_{21} = Apparent first-order rate constant of transfer of drug from the peripheral tissue compartment into the central compartment.

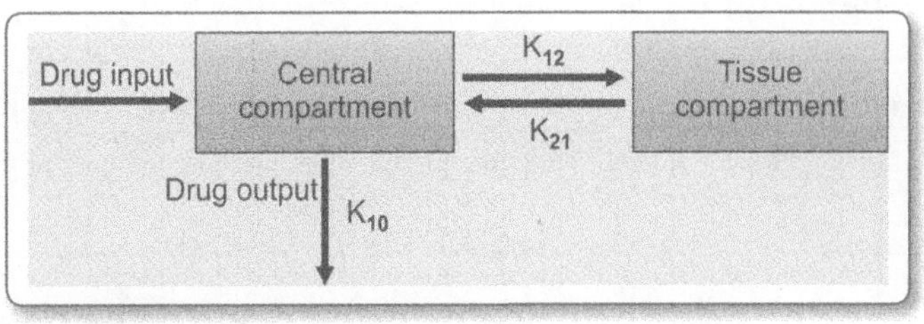

Fig. 10-2 Schematic of two-compartment model

K_{13} = Apparent first-order rate constant of transfer of drug from the central compartment into the deep tissue compartment.

K_{31} = Apparent first-order rate constant of transfer of drug from the deep tissue compartment into the central compartment.

K_{23} = Apparent first-order rate constant of transfer of drug from the peripheral tissue compartment into the deep tissue compartment.

K_{32} = Apparent first-order rate constant of transfer of drug from the deep tissue compartment into the peripheral tissue compartment.

While the pharmacokinetics of most drugs can be easily explained by fitting the experimental data either to the one-compartment pharmacokinetic model or to the two-compartment pharmacokinetic model, some drugs may exhibit the characteristics of a three-or more than three-compartment pharmacokinetic model. Examples of drugs, which exhibit the characteristics of a three-compartment model include diazepam, digoxin and tubocurarine. A drug, which demonstrates the necessity of the three-compartment pharmacokinetic model usually appears to be distributed most rapidly to a highly perfused compartment (this is central compartment), less rapidly to a second compartment (this is the peripheral or shallow tissue compartment) and very slowly to the third compartment (this is the deep tissue compartment). The third compartment may be a poorly perfused tissue (e.g. bone or fat) or may represent tightly bound drug in the tissues.

Types of Multi-compartment Models

The schematic of a two-compartment pharmacokinetic model can be represented in only one fashion: a central compartment reversibly connected to the tissue compartment. On the other hand, a multi-compartment model may be represented in more than one way, because central compartment and the two tissue compartments may be reversibly connected in more than one configuration. Three acceptable models have been proposed to represent a multi-compartment pharmacokinetic model: catenary model, mammillary model and perfusion model.

Catenary Model: The catenary model consists of a series of compartments joined to one another like the compartments of a train. In three-compartment catenary model, the central compartment is connected to the first tissue compartment and first tissue compartment is connected to the second tissue compartment. Central compartment represents plasma and highly perfused tissues which equilibrate with the drug rapidly. Figure 10-3 is a schematic of three-compartment catenary model. The drug transfers from central compartment into the shallow tissue compartment first and from this compartment it then transfers into the deep tissue compartment (second tissue compartment). The drug cannot transfer from central compartment into the deep tissue compartment without first going through shallow tissue compartment, because shallow tissue compartment is 'sandwiched' between the central and deep tissue compartments. Similarly, in a four-compartment catenary

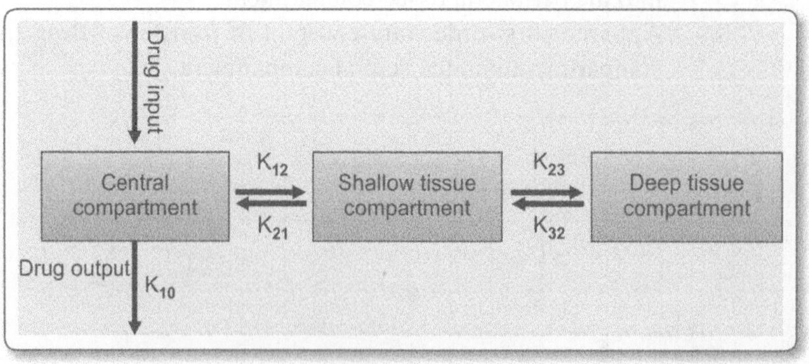

Fig. 10-3 Schematic of three-compartment catenary model

model, a third tissue compartment (very deep tissue compartment) will be reversibly connected to the second tissue compartment. In order for the drug to appear in the third tissue compartment, the drug will have to be present in the first tissue compartment, followed by its appearance in the second tissue compartment before it could appear in the last tissue compartment.

The catenary model has not found universal acceptance due to several reasons. The most important objection to this model is that while most functional organs in the body are directly connected to plasma (central compartment), the catenary model depicts the connections otherwise.

Mammillary Model: The mammillary model depicts every tissue compartment connected directly to the central compartment. This is similar to connections between most functional organs of the body and plasma (hence the name mammilary model).

Figure 10-4 is schematic of a three-compartment mammillary model showing a central compartment with two tissue compartments.

In the mammilary model, all tissue compartments, (e.g. the peripheral shallow tissue compartment, the deep tissue compartment and any other compartment with which the drug undergoes distribution), are connected directly to the central compartment like satellites. Each tissue compartment is independently connected to the central compartment. That is, no tissue compartment is sandwiched between the central compartment and another tissue compartment or between two tissue compartments. In the mammilary model also, the central compartment represents plasma and highly perfused tissues, which rapidly equilibrate with the drug.

One of the advantages of using the mammillary model is that it is possible to estimate the amount of drug in any compartment after the drug is introduced into a given compartment. This is because the mammillary model may be considered as a strongly connected system. As in other models, in this model also, elimination of drug occurs from the central compartment since organs predominantly involved in elimination (kidney and liver) are well-perfused tissues. The mammillary model is preferred in pharmacokinetic studies and is used most commonly because it seems to follow the pattern of drug distribution in the body. The schematic of a four-compartment mammillary pharmacokinetic model will be depicted with a third tissue compartment (very deep tissue compartment) reversibly connected to the central compartment.

Figure 10-5 is a schematic of the four-compartment mammillary model.

Perfusion Model: The perfusion model has been referred to by various other names, such as the physiologic model or the blood flow model. This is because perfusion models are based on known anatomic and physiologic data. The main advantage of perfusion models is that perfusion models kinetically describe data with the consideration that the drug is carried from the site of administration by blood flow to various body organs, where the drug rapidly equilibrates with the interstitial fluid in the organ. Drugs are carried to organs by arterial blood and leave organs

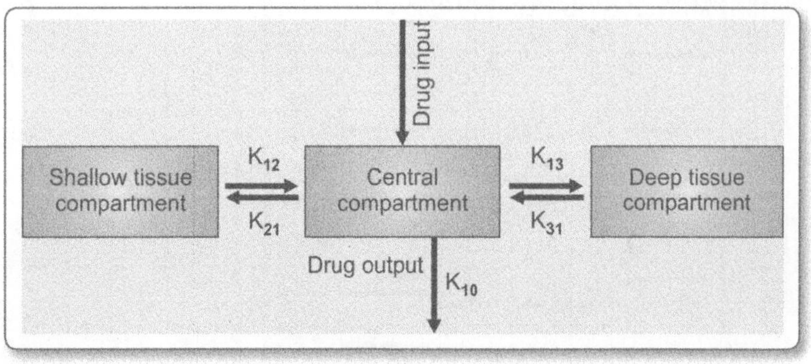

Fig. 10-4 Schematic of three-compartment mammillary model

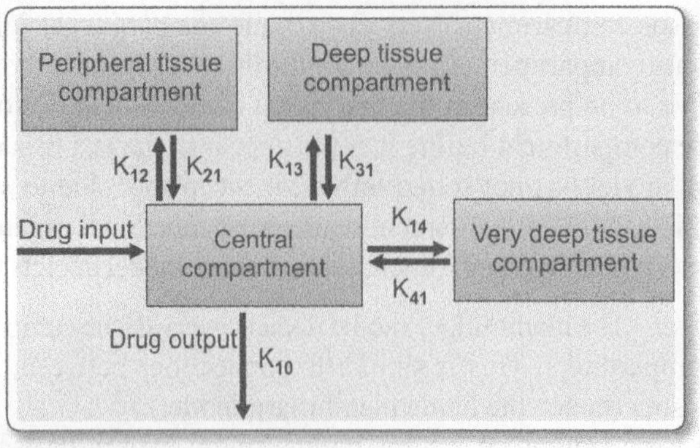

Fig. 10-5 Schematic of four-compartment mammillary model

by venous blood. Therefore, these models have been used in pharmacokinetic studies to describe distribution of drugs in blood and into various other organs. In these models, the concentration of drug in various tissues is predicted by the following three factors:

a. The size of the organ tissue
b. Blood flow to the organ tissue
c. The experimentally determined ratios of drug concentration between the tissue and the blood.

The number of compartments in the perfusion model varies with the drug because only those tissues are included in this model, which exhibit presence or penetration of drug into the tissue. For example, most drugs have little penetration into the brain, into the bones and into other parts of the central nervous system. These organs are therefore generally not included in a perfusion model. It is for this reason that the number of pharmacokinetic compartments in a perfusion model is determined by the number of organ tissues into which the drug penetrates.

Figure 10-6 shows a schematic of an example of a perfusion model.

A perfusion model has been successfully used to describe distribution of lidocaine in blood and various organs. The concentration of lidocaine in such tissues as lung, liver, brain, muscle

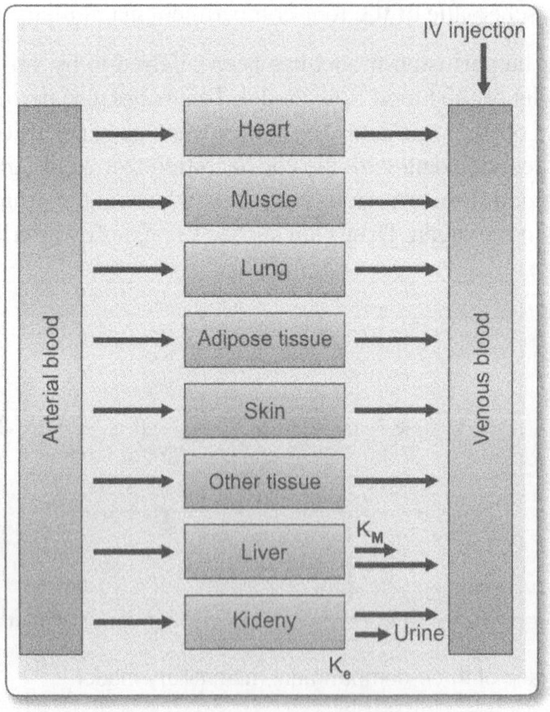

Fig. 10-6 Example of the perfusion model

and adipose tissue showed that adipose tissue accumulates drugs slowly because of low blood supply. Vascular tissues, for example, the lungs, equilibrate rapidly with blood and lidocaine concentration in these tissues starts to decline as soon as the concentration of lidocaine in the blood starts to fall.

Examples of drugs described by perfusion model include biperiden, Cisplatin, Methotrexate and thiopental.

Perfusion models have some advantages and some disadvantages. The major advantage of perfusion models is that the information derived from these models can be applied to several species, e.g. humans and experimental animals. The mammillary model and the catenary model do not offer this advantage because species differences are noticed in these models. Thus, the information derived from studies conducted on animals in a perfusion model may be applied to predict pharmacokinetics in the humans. For example, when human experimentation is restricted or difficult, the physiological and anatomical parameters can be used to predict the side effects of drugs on humans from the effects of drugs on animals. The drawback of perfusion models is that there are fewer data points than parameters that one tries to fit and therefore the projected data are not well constrained.

SUGGESTED READING

1. Gerlowski LE, Jain RK. Physiologically based pharmacokinetic modeling: Principles and applications. J Pharm Sci. 1983;72(10):1103-27.
2. Gibaldi M. Biopharmaceutics and Clinical Pharmacokinetics, 4th edition. Lea and Febiger; 1991.
3. Wagner JG. "Do you need a pharmacokinetic model, and if so, which one? J. Pharmacokinet. Biopharm. 1975;3(6):457-78.
4. Wagner JG. Fundamentals of Clinical Pharmacokinetics. Drug Intelligence Publications; 1979.

CHAPTER 11

INTRAVENOUS BOLUS DOSE

The plasma profile obtained following the administration of a rapid intravenous bolus injection of a drug is less complicated than that obtained after administration of the same dose of the same drug by an extravascular route. This is because intravenous administration does not involve an absorption process and the entire drug dose enters the plasma immediately after administration of the drug dose, i.e. the fraction of administered dose entering the plasma is equal to 1 (F = 1). The process of elimination begins immediately after administration and depending on distribution characteristics of the drug (if drug distributes between plasma and other body fluids and/or tissues), distribution also begins. The concentration of drug in central compartment declines as a function of time due to one or more first-order processes responsible for removal of drug from the plasma.

ONE-COMPARTMENT MODEL

In one-compartment model, after a rapid intravenous bolus injection, the entire drug dose enters plasma all-at-once. If the drug distributes between plasma and other components of the body (e.g. some other body fluids, tissues or tissue organs), then the distribution is considered instantaneous and an equilibrium is reached rapidly. The drug is said to confer upon the body the characteristics of one-compartment model. As soon as drug enters plasma, the process of elimination begins. Since elimination is a first-order kinetic process with an overall rate constant = K, this rate constant is the sum of all rate constants involved in elimination of drug from the body (e.g. rate constant of renal elimination, rate constant of non-renal elimination and rate constant of metabolism or bio-transformation, etc.

One-compartment model can be described by the first-order rate process using equation (3-27) as described in Chapter 3:

$$C_t = C_0(e^{-K(t)}) \qquad (11\text{-}1)$$

which, in the logarithmic form is

$$\ln C_t = \ln C_0 - K(t)$$

This is an equation of a straight line (y = mx + b). A plot of ln C versus t on a coordinate graph paper would yield a straight line, with y-intercept = $\ln C_0$ and slope = – K(K > 0). *If a semi-logarithmic* graph paper is used, a plot of concentration versus time will yield a straight line with y-intercept = C_0 and slope = – K(K > 0).

Pharmacokinetic Parameters

The pharmacokinetics parameters associated with one-compartment model following rapid intravenous bolus dose are as follows:

Elimination Rate Constant, K: It is determined from the slope of the straight line obtained when logarithms of concentrations are plotted as a function of time.

Biological Half-Life, $t_{1/2}$: It can be either read directly from the plasma profile or can be calculated from elimination rate constant using equation (3-32) as described in Chapter 3:

$$t_{1/2} = \frac{0.693}{K} \qquad (11\text{-}2)$$

Apparent Volume of Distribution, V_d: This is also apparent volume of central compartment, V_c, and, is determined using equation (5-8) as described in Chapter 5:

$$V_d = V_c = \frac{Dose}{C_0} \qquad (11\text{-}3)$$

Area Under the Curve, (AUC): Calculation of area under the curve depends on whether one wishes to calculate area under the curve from time 0 to a certain time t or it is desired to know the total area under the curve (from time 0 to infinity).

AUC_{0-t}: Area under the curve from time 0 to a certain time t can be determined using any one of following methods described previously:

a. Counting squares.
b. The trapezoidal rule
c. Cutting and weighing.

$AUC_{0-\infty}$: The total area under the curve is determined using one of the following equations (8-11) as described in Chapter 8:

$$AUC_{0\to\infty} = \frac{C_0}{K} \qquad (11\text{-}4)$$

$$AUC_{0\to\infty} = \frac{Dose}{Clearance} \qquad (11\text{-}5)$$

Example 11-1 The plasma concentration as a function of time after 250 mg intravenous bolus dose of an antibiotic is given below. Plot the data and describe the pharmacokinetics model.

Time (hour):	1.0	2.0	3.0	4.0	5.0	6.0	7.0
Concentration (μg/mL):	8.0	6.3	4.9	4.0	3.2	2.5	1.9

Solution

Since the smallest concentration to be plotted is 1.9 μg/mL (at 7 hours) and the highest concentration (at 1 hour) is 8.0 μg/mL, one-cycle semi-log paper will be needed. But one-cycle graph paper may not suffice if concentration at time 0 is greater than 10 μg/mL, in which case, one would need a two-cycle semi-log graph paper. Figure 11-1 shows the data plotted on one-cycle semi-log paper. A linear relationship indicates one-compartment model according to equation (11-1).

Pharmacokinetic Parameters

Elimination Rate Constant: The straight line in Figure 11-1 represents drug elimination from the central compartment, i.e. from the body. The slope of this straight line is used to calculate the rate constant of elimination, K.

One chooses two points on this straight line to calculate the slope. If the two points are:

$$x_1 = 0 \text{ h},\ y_1 = 10.0\ \mu g/mL \text{ and } x_2 = 7.0 \text{ h},\ y_2 = 2.0\ \mu g/mL,$$

then the rate constant of elimination, K is:

$$K = -\text{slope} = -\frac{\ln y_2 - \ln y_1}{x_2 - x_1}$$

$$K = -\frac{\ln 2.0 - \ln 10.0}{7.0\text{ h} - 0\text{ h}}$$

$$K = -\frac{0.6931 - 2.3026}{7.0\text{ h}} = -\frac{-1.6095}{7.0\text{ h}} = 0.2299/\text{h}$$

Biological Half-Life: There are two methods of determining biological half-life ($t_{1/2}$):

1. *From the graph* Concentration at time 0 is 10.0 μg/mL. Time when concentration becomes one-half of 10 μg/mL (i.e. 5 μg/mL) is read from the graph. Figure 11-1 shows $t_{1/2}$ = approximately 3 hours.
2. *Using equation (11-2)*

$$t_{1/2} = \frac{0.693}{K} = \frac{0.693}{0.2299/\text{h}}$$

$$t_{1/2} = 3.01\text{ h}$$

Volume of Distribution: Apparent volume of distribution (V_d) is calculated using equation (11-3):

$$V_d = \frac{\text{Dose}}{C_0} = \frac{250\text{ mg}}{10\ \mu\text{g/mL}}$$

$$V_d = \frac{250\text{ mg}}{10\text{ mg/L}} = 25\text{ L}$$

Area Under the Curve: Total area under the curve can be determined as follows:

1. *Using equation (11-4):*

$$AUC_{0\to\infty} = \frac{C_0}{K} = \frac{10\ \mu\text{g/mL}}{0.2299/\text{h}}$$

$$AUC_{0\to\infty} = 43.5\ \mu\text{g} \times \text{h/mL}$$

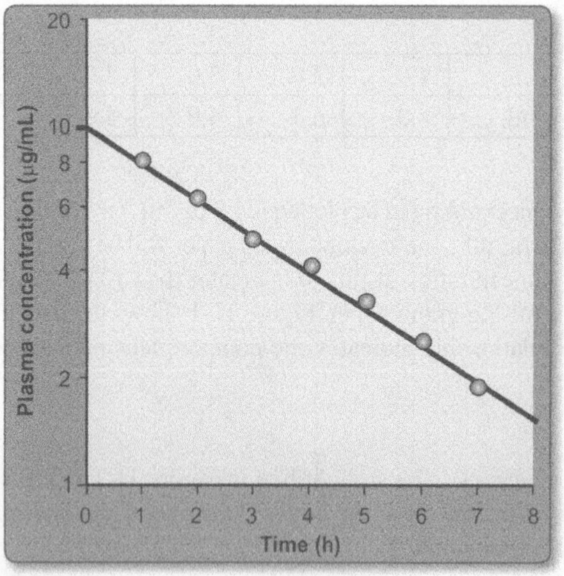

Fig. 11-1 Semi-logarithmic plot of data in Example 11-1

2. Using equation (11-5)
   Since clearance = (K)(V_d) = (0.2299/h)(25 L) = 5.7475 L/h, therefore, AUC according to equation (11-5) is:

$$AUC_{0\to\infty} = \frac{\text{Dose}}{\text{Clearance}} = \frac{250 \text{ mg}}{5.7475 \text{ L/hr}} = 43.5 \text{ mg} \times \text{h/L}$$

Description of the Model

This one-compartment model can be described either schematically or by an equation.

Description by Equation: From the parameters found in Example 11-1, the plasma profile is described by the equation:

$$C_t = (10) \times (e^{-0.2299(t)})$$

In this equation, C_0 = 10 and K = 0.2299. Since the units of time or concentration are not given, only numerical values of C_0 and K can be obtained.

Schematic Representation: A schematic of pharmacokinetic model, which describes the plasma profile is shown in Figure 11-2.

This schematic shows that a 250 mg rapid bolus dose is administered intravenously. The apparent volume of distribution (which is also the apparent volume of central compartment) is 25 L and the rate constant of elimination is 0.2299/h.

MULTI-COMPARTMENT MODEL

The pharmacokinetics of multi-compartment model differs from that of one-compartment model in several respects, but most predominantly in plasma profile. A first-order plot of drug concentration in plasma as a function of time following rapid intravenous bolus dose exhibits an entirely different plasma profile than that seen in one-compartment pharmacokinetic model.

Plasma Concentration Versus Time Plot

The first-order plot of plasma drug concentration versus time in one-compartment model results in a mono-exponential decline. In multi-compartment models the plasma profile exhibits a multi-exponential curve. The nature of the profile depends on the number of compartments exhibited in the model. A two-compartment pharmacokinetic model results in a bi-exponential curve and a three-compartment model yields a tri-exponential curve.

The reason for multi-exponential profile in multi-compartment models is that in one-compartment model, the loss of drug from the central compartment is due to only one first-order process (i.e., elimination of drug from the body). But in a multi-compartment model, the loss of drug from the central compartment is due to more than one first-order processes: (i) the elimination of drug from the body and (ii) the distribution of drug in the body. Also, each distribution process consists of two first-order processes: (a) The transfer of drug from the central

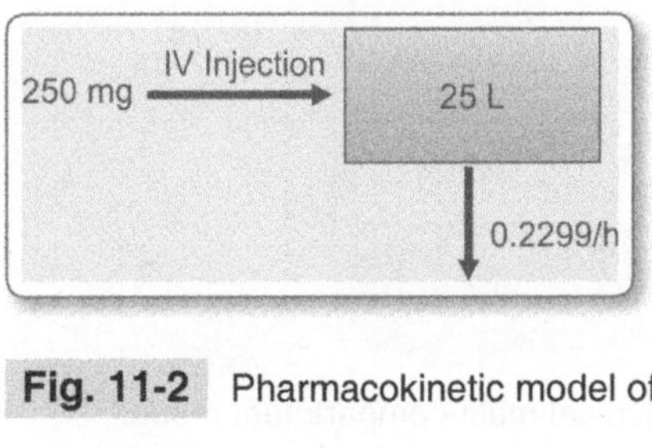

Fig. 11-2 Pharmacokinetic model of data in Example 11-1

compartment into tissue compartment, and (b) The transfer of drug from the tissue compartment into the central compartment. Since the drug is removed from the central compartment by more than one first-order process, the concentration of drug in the central compartment shows an initial decline which is much more rapid than that seen in one-compartment model. This rapid decline gradually tapers to a relatively slow decline because of transfer of drug from the tissue compartment(s) into the central compartment and because the drug starts to establish an equilibrium between the central and the tissue compartment(s). Figure 11-3 is a typical profile of a multi-compartment model.

The initial rapid decline in drug concentration is known as distributive phase and slower rate of decline toward the tail-end is known as elimination phase. Although distribution is predominant process in distributive phase and elimination is the predominant process in elimination phase, both processes are in progress throughout the course of drug kinetics. To determine number of compartments in the model, the multi-exponential profile is resolved. Resolution of plasma profile, called *feathering* the data or *stripping* the curve, is used to determine the number of first-order rate processes that comprise the plasma profile. If the plasma profile is stripped to yield two straight lines then two compartments comprise the plasma profile. If stripping yields three straight lines then it is a three-compartment model, and if stripping yields four straight lines then we have a four-compartment pharmacokinetic model, and so on.

Feathering or Stripping the Curve

Feathering the data or stripping the curve uses the method of residuals. This method is based on the following premise: if the multi-exponential curve consists of n first-order processes, then first develop the simplest first-order process and subtract this process from the multi-exponential curve. The data thus obtained will now represent (n-1) first-order processes. If the original multi-exponential profile represented a two-compartment model, then for this multi-exponential plasma profile, n = 2, meaning that the multi-exponential curve comprised of two first-order processes. Therefore, subtraction of the first first-order process from the plasma profile should yield a linear relationship for the second first-order process. Similarly, if the original curve represented a pharmacokinetic model consisting of more than two compartments, then subtraction of the first first-order process from the plasma profile results in more than one first-order process. Therefore, subtraction will yield a curve (not a straight line) when the first first-order process is subtracted from the original plasma profile.

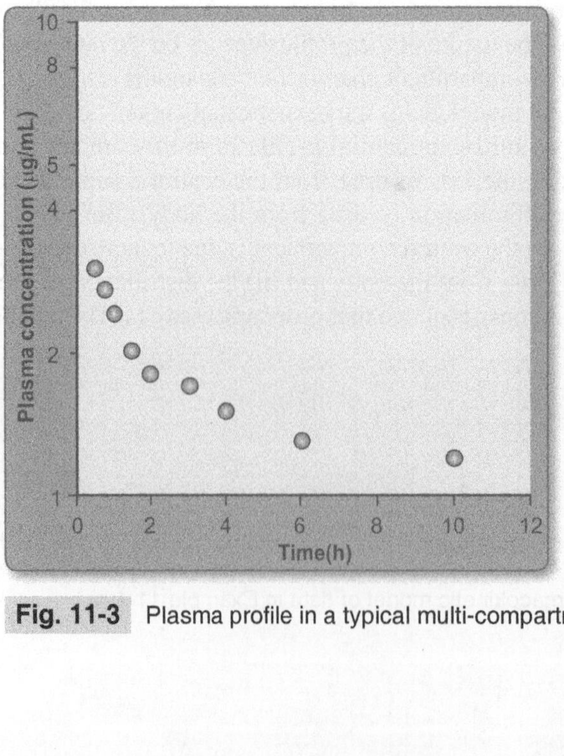

Fig. 11-3 Plasma profile in a typical multi-compartment model

TWO-COMPARTMENT MODEL

The bi-exponential equation describing the plasma profile in a two-compartment model is given by the following equation:

$$C = B(e^{-\beta t}) + A(e^{-\alpha t}) \quad (11\text{-}6)$$

where,
C = plasma concentration at time t
B = y-intercept of first-order rate process of elimination phase
A = y-intercept of first-order rate process of distributive phase rate process
β = hybrid-rate constant for elimination phase
α = hybrid-rate constant for distributive phase
t = time.

The exponents β and α are not simple rate constants but are a complex function of all rate constants associated with two-compartment model. Therefore, the exponents β and α are called hybrid rate constants or micro-rate constants. The complexity of these hybrid constants can be appreciated from the following equations:

$$\alpha = \tfrac{1}{2}\{K_{12} + K_{21} + K_{10} + [(K_{12} + K_{21} + K_{10})^2 - 4K_{21}K_{10}]^{1/2}\} \quad (11\text{-}7)$$

$$\beta = \tfrac{1}{2}\{K_{12} + K_{21} + K_{10} - [(K_{12} + K_{21} + K_{10})^2 - 4K_{21}K_{10}]^{1/2}\} \quad (11\text{-}8)$$

The values of the hybrid rate constants β and α are determined from slopes of the straight lines having y-intercepts B and A, respectively. If natural logarithms are used, then slope of the straight line having B as the y-intercept = $-\beta$ and slope of the straight line having A as the y-intercept = $-\alpha$. Hybrid rate constant α is always greater than hybrid rate constant β.

Since hybrid-rate constant α is always greater than β, it follows that some time after distributive phase, $A(e^{-\alpha t})$ will approach 0 while $B(e^{-\beta t})$ will still have a finite value, indicating end of distributive phase, but continuation of elimination phase. At that time, equation (11-6) becomes

$$C = B(e^{-\beta t}) + 0 = B(e^{-\beta t}) \quad (11\text{-}9)$$

Subtracting equation (11-9) from equation (11-6),

$$C = A(e^{-\alpha t}) \quad (11\text{-}10)$$

where, C' is residual plasma drug concentration obtained after subtraction of elimination phase from the plasma profile. Equation (11-10) is a first-order equation of straight line with a y-intercept of A and first-order rate constant = α.

Pharmacokinetic Parameters

The pharmacokinetic parameters associated with a two-compartment model are: biological half-life ($t_{1/2}$), first-order rate constant of elimination of drug from central compartment (K_{10}), first-order rate constant of transfer of drug from central compartment into tissue compartment (K_{12}), first-order rate constant of transfer of drug from tissue compartment into central compartment (K_{21}), apparent volume of distribution of central compartment (V_c), apparent volume of distribution of tissue compartment (V_t), apparent volume of distribution of drug (V_d) and total area under the curve (AUC).

Biological Half-Life: The rate constant K_{10} is not used to calculate biological half-life, because K_{10} represents elimination of drug from the central compartment. In equation (11-9), β represents the first-order rate constant of elimination from the body; therefore biological half-life is calculated using β.

$$t = \frac{0.693}{\beta} \tag{11-11}$$

Rate Constants: Three rate constants are associated with a two-compartment model: One rate constant is the first order rate constant of removal of drug from the central compartment (K_{10}), and the other two are first order rate constant of transfer of drug between the central and the tissue compartment (K_{12} and K_{21}).

$$K_{21} = \frac{A\beta + B\alpha}{B + A} \tag{11-12}$$

$$K_{10} = \frac{\alpha\beta}{K_{21}} \tag{11-13}$$

$$K_{12} = \alpha + \beta - K_{21} - K_{10} \tag{11-14}$$

Volume of Distribution: The apparent volume of distribution of drug in two-compartment model is the sum of apparent volumes of distribution of central and tissue compartments.

Apparent Volume of Central Compartment (V_c): At time 0, equation (11-6) becomes

$$C_0 = B + A \tag{11-15}$$

Since at time 0 distribution of drug has not yet started, C_0, therefore reflects concentration of drug in the central compartment only. If D is dose administered, then

$$C = \frac{D}{V_c} \tag{11-16}$$

Substituting (A + B) for C_0 into equations (11-16) and rearranging the equation gives

$$V_c = \frac{D}{B + A} \tag{11-17}$$

Apparent Volume of Distribution (V_d)

$$V_d = \frac{V_c(K_{12} + K_{21})}{K_{21}} \tag{11-18}$$

Apparent Volume of Tissue Compartment (V_t) Since, $V_d = V_c + V_t$, therefore,

$$V_t = V_d - V_c \tag{11-19}$$

$$V_t = \frac{V_c(K_{12} + K_{21})}{K_{21}} - V_c \tag{11-20}$$

$$V_t = (V_c)\left(\frac{K_{12} + K_{21}}{K_{21}} - 1\right) = \frac{(V_c)(K_{12} + K_{21} - K_{21})}{K_{21}}$$

$$V_t = \frac{(V_c)(K_{12})}{K_{21}} \tag{11-21}$$

Area Under the Curve: Since plasma profile of a two-compartment model is resolved into two linear segments, total area under the curve can be calculated using either of the following equations:

$$AUC_{0\to\infty} = \frac{B}{\beta} + \frac{A}{\alpha} \tag{11-22}$$

$$AUC_{0\to\infty} = \frac{C_0}{K_{10}} \tag{11-23}$$

Example 11-2 Plasma concentration versus time data following administration of a single 250 mg rapid intravenous bolus dose of a drug is shown below. Plot the data and describe the pharmacokinetic model.

Time (h)	Concentration (μg/mL)	Time (h)	Concentration (μg/mL)	Time (h)	Concentration (μg/mL)
0.5	5.571	2.5	2.140	4.5	1.425
1.2	4.258	3.0	1.970	12.0	0.610
1.5	3.356	3.5	1.737	14.0	0.500
2.0	2.729	4.0	1.561	18.0	0.336

Solution

Since, the concentrations range between the values of 0.3 mcg/mL to a high value of 5.6 μg/mL, therefore a 2-cycle semi-logarithmic graph paper should be used to plot the data. A plot of plasma concentration versus time on a semi-logarithmic graph paper is shown in Figure 11-4. This graph shows an initial rapid decline in concentration of drug in plasma, gradually tapering to a relatively slow decline. Since, this graph does not exhibit a linear relationship between concentration and time on the semi-logarithmic graph paper, the data indicate a multi-compartment model. The curve must be stripped (feathered) to determine the number of compartments. The terminal points, which represent elimination as the predominant process are used to obtain the first first-order process. The first-order rate constant of terminal points, β is determined and then equation (11-9) is used to determine y-intercept of this straight line. The y-intercept of this straight line is B.

Rate Constant of Terminal Linear Segment: Depending on the accuracy of data collection, one may either use the last two concentration points to calculate slope (concentration points at 13 and 14 hours in this problem) or determine slope by regression analysis (explained in Chapter 2) using last three concentration points (concentration points at 12, 14 and 18 hours in this problem). Since elimination is predominant only during the terminal phase of bi-exponential curve and distribution is predominant during the earlier segment of plasma profile, including too many data points to determine first-order elimination rate constant would not be desirable. The data collected in this problem appear accurate enough to use the last two points for calculating the first-order rate constant.

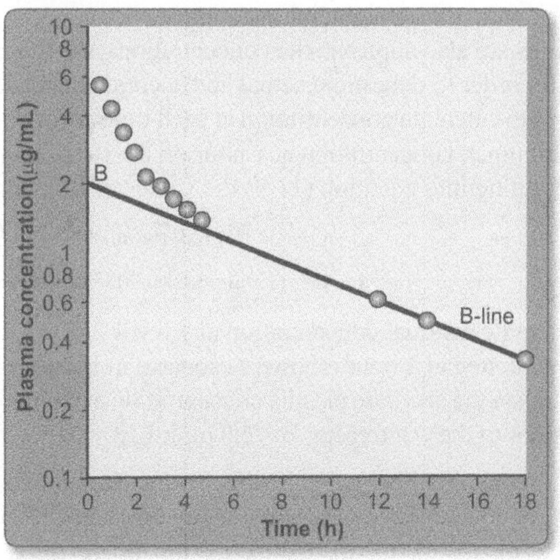

Fig. 11-4 Plot of data in Example 11-2

$$\beta = -\text{slope} = -\frac{\ln 0.500 - \ln 0.336}{(14-18)\text{h}} = -\frac{0.3975}{-4\text{h}} = 0.099/\text{h}$$

Y-Intercept, B: Using equation (11-9), the value of B can be calculated using either one of the terminal data points (concentration point at either 14 hours or at 18 hours in this problem). Using concentration point at 18 hours,

$$C = Be^{-\beta t}$$

$$0.336\ \mu g/mL = Be^{(-0.099/h)(18\ h)}$$

$$= Be^{-1.782} = (B)(0.1683)$$

$$\text{therefore, } B = \frac{0.336\ \mu g/mL}{0.1683} = 2.0\ \mu g/mL$$

Using equation (11-9) for concentration at 14 hour should also yield the same value of B.

$$0.500\ \mu g/mL = Be^{(-0.099/h)(14\ h)}$$

$$= Be^{-1.386} = (B)(0.2500)$$

$$\text{therefore, } B = \frac{0.500\ \mu g/mL}{0.2500} = 2.0\ \mu g/mL$$

A straight line (i.e., B-line) is drawn by joining y-intercept with the terminal concentration point at 14 hour. This straight line represents the first first-order rate process of plasma profile.

To generate the second first-order rate process, the first first-order process is subtracted from the concentration curve. This is accomplished by reading concentration of the first first-order process at each time point and subtracting it from the concentration provided in the data for that time point. The subtracted value at each concentration point represents the residual concentration at that point. The residual concentration is plotted on the graph.

For example, at 0.5 hour, the plasma concentration provided in the data is 5.571 mcg/mL and from the B-line (the straight line having B as the y-intercept), the plasma concentration at 0.5 hour is approximately 1.90 µg/mL. Therefore, the approximate residual plasma concentration at 0.5 hour is:

$$(5.571\ \mu g/mL - 1.90\ \mu g/mL) = 3.671\ \mu g/mL.$$

Reading concentrations on the straight line having y-intercept B poses a serious problem. If all concentrations read from this straight line are approximate concentrations, then the calculated residual concentrations are also approximate concentrations and therefore analysis of the curve is open to question. In order to determine actual and accurate residual concentrations, equation (11-9) should be used to calculate concentration at each time point on the straight line having B as y-intercept. For example, concentration at 1 hour on the straight line having y-intercept B is determined by substituting into equation (11-9) the values of B, β and t (t = 1 hour).

$$C = Be^{-\beta t} = (2.0\ \mu g/mL)(e^{(-0.099/h)(1\ h)})$$

$$C = (2.0\ \mu g/mL)(0.9057) = 1.811\ \mu g/mL$$

Therefore the accurate residual concentration at 1 h = 4.258 – 1.811 = 2.447 µg/mL.

This point is now plotted at 1 hour (shown as squares in Figure 11-5).

Similarly, to calculate the accurate plasma concentration at 2 hour on the straight line having y-intercept B, the values of the y-intercept, B = 2.0 µg/mL, β = 0.099/h and t = 2 h are substituted into equation (11-9).

$$C = Be^{-\beta t} = (2.0\ \mu g/mL)(e^{(-0.099/h)(2\ h)})$$

$$= (2.0\ \mu g/mL)(0.8204) = 1.641\ \mu g/mL$$

Therefore, residual concentration at 2 h = 2.729 μg/mL – 1.641 μg/mL = 1.088 μg/mL

This process of accurately determining concentration at other time points is continued to obtain corresponding accurate residual concentration. The residual concentration values for all data points, which did not fall on the straight line having B as the y-intercept are then plotted on the graph (shown as squares in Figure 11-5).

Table 11-1 shows the data generated by the method of residuals. The residual concentrations in Figure 11-5 exhibit a linear relationship suggesting that the curve consisted of two first-order processes. A straight line is drawn to best represent the residuals either using eye-ball judgment or linear regression analysis (if too much scatter is observed). The straight line representing residual concentrations intersects the y-axis at 5.5 μg/mL and the x-axis at 4.95 hour.

The two y-intercepts are: A = 5.5 μg/mL and B = 2.0 μg/mL.

From the slopes of the two straight lines,

$$\alpha = \frac{\ln 5.5 - \ln 0.1}{(0 - 4.95)\ \text{h}} = -\frac{4.007}{-4.95\ \text{h}} - = 0.81/\text{h}$$

$$\beta = \frac{\ln 2.0 - \ln 0.336}{(0 - 18)\ \text{h}} = -\frac{1.7838}{-18\ \text{h}} - = 0.099/\text{h}$$

Calculation of Parameters

The four values (A, B, α and β) derived from the plot of data shown in Figure 11-5 are used to calculate all parameters in this two-compartment model.

$$C_0 = B + A$$

$$C_0 = 2.0\ \mu\text{g/mL} + 5.5\ \mu\text{g/mL} = 7.5\ \mu\text{g/mL}$$

Biological Half-Life: According to equation (11-11)

$$t_{1/2} = \frac{0.693}{\beta} = \frac{0.693}{0.99/\text{h}} = 0.7\ \text{h}$$

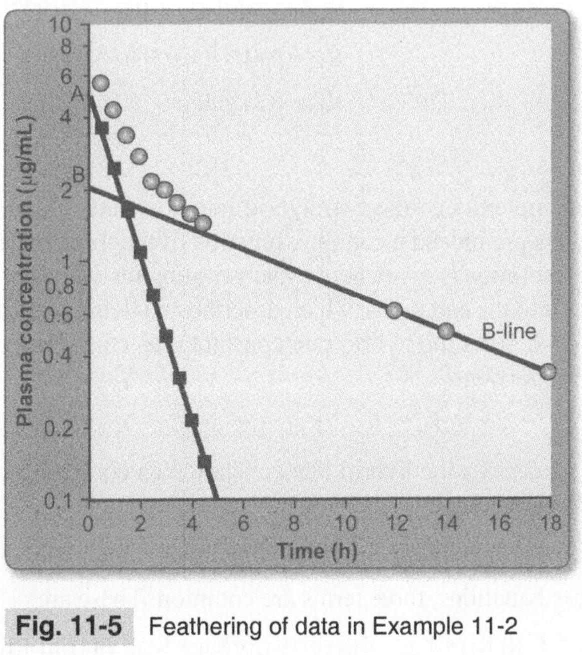

Fig. 11-5 Feathering of data in Example 11-2

Table 11-1 Curve stripping by the method of residuals (for data in Example 11-2)

Time (h)	*Concentration (μg/mL) (data points)** ●	*Data from B-line*	*Residuals (data minus points from B-line)*** ■
0.5	5.571	1.903	5.571 – 1.903 = 3.668
1.0	4.258	1.811	4.258 – 1.811 = 2.447
1.5	3.356	1.724	3.356 – 1.724 = 1.632
2.0	2.729	1.641	2.729 – 1.641 = 1.088
2.5	2.140	1.414	2.140 – 1.414 = 0.726
3.0	1.970	1.486	1.970 – 1.486 = 0.484
3.5	1.737	1.414	1.737 – 1.414 = 0.323
4.0	1.561	1.346	1.561 – 1.346 = 0.215
4.5	1.425	1.281	1.425 – 1.281 = 0.144
12.0	0.610	***	***
14.0	0.500	***	***
18.0	0.336	***	****

*These points are shown as circles in Fig. 11-5

** These points are shown as squares in Fig. 11-5

***These points are not used in determining residuals because these points were already used to draw the B- line.

Rate Constants

$$K_{21} = \frac{A\beta + B\alpha}{B + A} = \frac{0.5445 + 1.62}{2.0 + 5.5}$$

$$K_{21} = \frac{2.1645}{7.5} = 0.2886/\text{h}$$

$$K_{10} = \frac{\alpha\beta}{K_{12}} = \frac{(0.81/\text{h})(0.099/\text{h})}{0.2886/\text{h}}$$

$$K_{10} = \frac{0.0802/\text{h}}{0.2886} = 0.2779/\text{h}$$

$$K_{12} = \alpha + \beta - K_{21} - K_{10}$$

$$K_{12} = 0.81/\text{h} + 0.099/\text{h} - 0.2886/\text{h} - 0.2779/\text{h}$$

$$K_{12} = 0.3425/\text{h}$$

Hybrid Rate Constants α *and* β

To illustrate the complexity of the two hybrid rate constants α and β and to show that these hybrid rate constants are indeed a complex function of the three first-order rate constants (K_{12}, K_{21} and K_{10}), their solution is given here by substituting the values of these three rate constants (K_{10}, K_{12} and K_{21}) into the equations, which describe and define these two hybrid rate constants.

Equation (11-7) defines the hybrid rate constant α as consisting of the three rate constants in the following proportions:

$$\alpha = \tfrac{1}{2}\{K_{12} + K_{21} + K_{10} + [(K_{12} + K_{21} + K_{10})^2 - 4K_{21}K_{10}]^{1/2}\}$$

Equation (11-8) defines the hybrid rate constant β as consisting of the three rate constants in the following proportions:

$$\beta = \tfrac{1}{2}\{K_{12} + K_{21} + K_{10} - [(K_{12} + K_{21} + K_{10})^2 - 4K_{21}K_{10}]^{1/2}\}$$

In both of these equations, three terms are common. These are:

(i) $K_{12} + K_{21} + K_{10}$, (ii) $(K_{12} + K_{21} + K_{10})^2$ and (iii) $4(K_{21})(K_{10})$

Therefore, equations (11-7) and (11-8) may be written in the following forms:

$$\alpha = 1/2\{x + (x^2 - y)^{1/2}\} \quad (11\text{-}7A)$$

$$\beta = 1/2\{x - (x^2 - y)^{1/2}\} \quad (11\text{-}8A)$$

In these equations:

$$x = K_{12} + K_{21} + K_{10}, \text{ and}$$

$$y = 4(K_{21})(K_{10})$$

Substituting the values of the three rate constants (K_{10}, K_{12} and K_{21}) and solving for x and y we get:

$$x = K_{12} + K_{21} + K_{10}, = 0.3425/h + 0.2886/h + 0.2779/h$$

$$x = 0.9090/h$$

$$y = 4(K_{21})(K_{10}) = 4(0.2886/h \times 0.2779/h)$$

$$y = 0.3208/h^2$$

Now substituting these values of x and y into equations 11-7A and 11-7B one can calculate α and β.

$$\alpha = \tfrac{1}{2}[x + (x^2 - y)]^{1/2}$$

$$\alpha = \tfrac{1}{2}\{0.9090/h + [(0.9090/h)^2 - 0.3208/h^2]^{1/2}\}$$

$$\alpha = \tfrac{1}{2}(0.9090/h + [0.8263/h^2 - 0.3208/h^2]^{1/2} = \tfrac{1}{2}[0.9090/h + (0.5055/h^2)^{1/2}]$$

$$\alpha = \tfrac{1}{2}(0.9090/h + 0.711/h) = \tfrac{1}{2} \times 1.62/h$$

$$\alpha = 0.81/h$$

Similarly, $\beta = \tfrac{1}{2}[x - (x^2 - y)]^{1/2}$

$$\beta = \tfrac{1}{2}\{0.9090/h - [(0.9090/h)^2 - 0.3208/h^2]^{1/2}\}$$

$$\beta = \tfrac{1}{2}(0.9090/h - [0.8263/h^2 - 0.3208/h^2]^{1/2} = \tfrac{1}{2}[0.9090/h - (0.5055/h^2)^{1/2}]$$

$$\beta = \tfrac{1}{2}(0.9090/h - 0.711/h) = \tfrac{1}{2} \times 0.198/h$$

$$\beta = 0.099/h$$

Apparent Volume of Distribution

$$V_c = \frac{D}{B + A} = \frac{250 \text{ mg}}{7.5\ \mu\text{g/mL}} = 33.333 \text{ L}$$

$$V_d = \frac{V_c(K_{12} + K_{21})}{K_{21}} = \frac{(33.333 \text{ L})(0.3425/h + 0.2886/h)}{0.2886/h}$$

$$V_d = \frac{21.0365 \text{ L}}{0.2886} = 72.89 \text{ L}$$

$$V_t = V_d - V_c = 72.89 \text{ L} - 33.33 \text{ L} = 39.56 \text{ L}$$

$$\text{or, } V_t = \frac{(V_c)(K_{12})}{K_{21}} = \frac{(33.333\text{L})(0.3425/h)}{0.2886/h} = 39.56 \text{ L}$$

Area Under the Curve

Using equation (11-22):

$$AUC_{total} = \frac{B}{\beta} + \frac{A}{\alpha}$$

$$= \frac{2\ \mu g/mL}{0.099/h} + \frac{5.5\ \mu g/mL}{0.81/h} = 26.99\ \mu g \times h/mL$$

Using equation (11-23):

$$AUC_{total} = \frac{C_0}{K_{10}}$$

$$= \frac{7.5\ \mu g/mL}{0.2779/h}$$

$$= 26.99\ \mu g \times h/mL$$

Description of the Model

Schematic Representation Figure 11-6 is a schematic of the two-compartment model derived from the data in Example 11-2. This schematic shows that a 250 mg bolus dose was given intravenously. The apparent volumes of central and tissue compartments are 33.33 L and 39.56 L, respectively. The first-order rate constant of transfer of drug from central compartment into the tissue compartment is 0.3425/h and the first-order rate constant of transfer of drug from tissue compartment into the central compartment is 0.2886/h. The first-order rate constant of elimination of drug from the central compartment is 0.2779/h.

Description by Equation: From the parameters found in Example 11-2, the plasma profile can be described in the form of equation (11-6) as:

$$C = 5.5(e^{-0.81t}) + 2.0(e^{-0.099t})$$

The two exponents 0.099 and 0.81 represent β and α, respectively. The smaller hybrid rate constant is always β and the hybrid rate constant with the larger value is always α.

Therefore, β = 0.099 and α = 0.81.

Example 11-3 Plasma concentration versus time following administration of a single 250 mg rapid intravenous bolus dose of a drug is represented by the bi-exponential equation:

$$C = 3.5(e^{-0.15t}) + 10.5(e^{-1.2t})$$

Calculate the biological half-life of the drug and total area under the plasma concentration versus time curve, assuming concentrations are in mcg/mL and time is in hours.

Solution

From the bi-exponential equation provided, the following are parameters of the two-compartment model: β = 0.15/h and B = 3.5 μg/mL. Therefore, α must be equal to 1.2/h and A = 10.5 μg/mL.

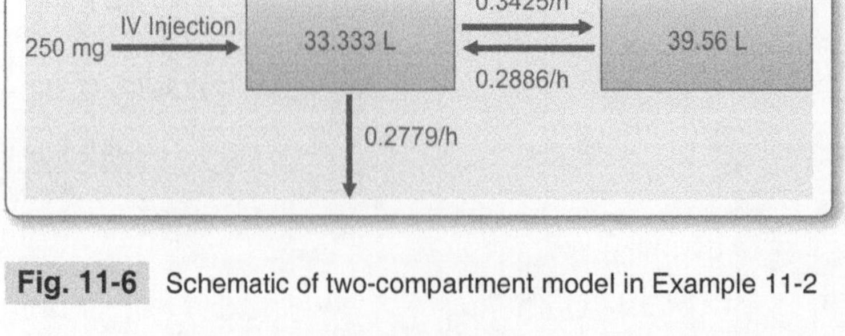

Fig. 11-6 Schematic of two-compartment model in Example 11-2

Biological Half-Life: According to equation (11-11)

$$t_{1/2} = \frac{0.693}{\beta} = \frac{0.693}{0.15/h} = 4.62\ h$$

Area Under the Curve

Using equation (11-22):

$$AUC_{total} = \frac{B}{\beta} + \frac{A}{\alpha}$$

$$= \frac{0.5\ \mu g/mL}{0.15/h} + \frac{10.5\ \mu g/mL}{1.2/h}$$

$$= 23.333\ \mu g \times h/mL + 8.75\ \mu g \times h/mL$$

$$= 32.0833\ \mu g \times h/mL$$

Example 11-4 Plasma concentration versus time following administration of a single 250 mg rapid intravenous bolus dose of a drug is represented by the equation:

$$C = 1.5(e^{-0.13t}) + 12.5(e^{-1.3t})$$

Draw a schematic of the pharmacokinetic model, assuming all concentrations are in μg/mL and time is in hours.

Solution

From the bi-exponential equation, the parameters of the two-compartment model are:

$\beta = 0.13/h$, $B = 1.5\ \mu g/mL$, $\alpha = 1.3/h$ and $A = 12.5\ \mu g/mL$.

To draw a schematic of the pharmacokinetic model, the following parameters are needed: The three rate constants K_{10}, K_{12}, K_{21} and the two apparent volumes of distribution V_c and V_t.

Rate Constants

$$K_{12} = \frac{A\beta + B\alpha}{B + A} = \frac{1.625 + 1.95}{1.5 + 12.5} = \frac{3.575}{14.0} = 0.2554/h$$

$$K_{10} = \frac{\alpha\beta}{K_{21}} = \frac{(1.3/h)(0.13/h)}{0.2554/h} = \frac{0.169/h}{0.2554} = 0.6617/h$$

$$K_{12} = \alpha + \beta - K_{12} - K_{10}$$

$$K_{12} = 1.3/h + 0.13/h - 0.2554/h - 0.6617/h$$

$$K_{12} = 0.5433/h$$

Apparent Volumes of Distribution

$$V_c = \frac{D}{B + A} = \frac{250\ mg}{14\ \mu g/mL} = 17.857\ L$$

$$V_d = \frac{V_c(K_{12} + K_{21})}{K_{21}} = \frac{(17.857\ L)(0.5433/h + 0.2554/h)}{0.2554/h}$$

$$V_d = \frac{14.2624\ L}{0.2554} = 55.843\ L$$

$$V = V - V = 55.843\ L - 17.857\ L = 37.986\ L$$

$$\text{or, } V_t = \frac{(V_c)(K_{12})}{K_{21}} = \frac{(17.857\ L)(0.5433/h)}{0.2554/h} = 37.986\ L$$

Schematic Representation: Schematic representation of the two-compartment model derived from the data given in Example 11-4 is shown in Figure 11-7.

This schematic shows that a 250 mg dose was given intravenously. The apparent volumes of the central and tissue compartments are 17.857 L and 37.986 L, respectively. The first-order rate constant of transfer of drug from central compartment into the tissue compartment is 0.5433/hr and the first-order rate constant of transfer of drug from tissue compartment into the central compartment is 0.2554/h. The first-order rate constant of elimination of drug from the central compartment is 0.6617/h.

THREE-COMPARTMENT MODEL

A three-compartment model is not very common in pharmacokinetic studies. However, the pharmacokinetics of some drugs (e.g., diazepam, digoxin and tubocurarine) is not adequately described by a two-compartment model.

A drug which demonstrates the necessity of a three-compartment model appears to be distributed most rapidly into a highly perfused central compartment, less rapidly into shallow tissue compartment (second compartment) and very slowly into a deep tissue compartment (third compartment).

Plasma Profile

A first-order plot of plasma concentration versus time in a three-compartment model results in a triexponential curve. The initial concentration of drug in the central compartment exhibits a much steeper decline than that seen in a two-compartment model. This is because the loss of drug from the central compartment in three-compartment model is due to more than two first-order processes:

i. Elimination of drug from the central compartment
ii. Transfer of drug between the central compartment and shallow tissue compartment
iii. Transfer of drug between the central compartment and the deep tissue compartment.

In a two-compartment model, the loss of drug from the central compartment is due to elimination and transfer of drug between one tissue compartment. Thus, in three-compartment model, feathering of plasma profile with respect to the back-extrapolated linear terminal portion of plasma profile does not produce linear residuals because these residuals comprise of two first-order processes. The residuals produce a curve which must be feathered again. The feathering of residuals is similar to the feathering of the plasma profile, i.e. residuals obtained after first feathering are feathered with respect to the back-extrapolated terminal linear portion of the residual curve.

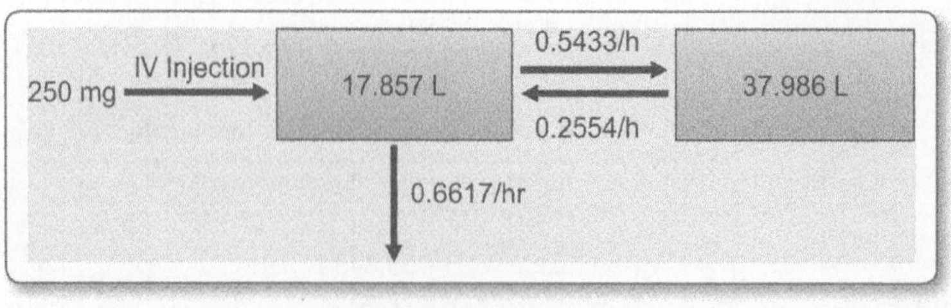

Fig. 11-7 Schematic of two-compartment model in Example 11-4

Tri-exponential Equation

The tri-exponential equation describing the plasma profile of a drug which, when administered as a rapid intravenous dose, confers upon the body the characteristic of a three-compartment model is as follows:

$$C = B(e^{-\beta t}) + A(e^{-\alpha t}) + P(e^{-\pi t}) \tag{11-24}$$

where B, A and P are y-intercepts of back-extrapolated straight lines, and β, α, and π are the respective hybrid rate constants of these straight lines. Hybrid rate constants encompass rate constants of transfer of drug between various compartments and are obtained from slopes of linear segments of the plasma profile. The first hybrid rate constant from the plasma profile is β and it has the smallest value of three hybrid rate constants. Hybrid rate constant obtained from the last linear segment is π and it has the highest value of the three hybrid rate constants.

Equation (11-24) is similar to equation (11-6), except that a third exponential term is added to reflect the third compartment. Since, by definition, $\pi > \alpha > \beta$, it follows that at some time after drug administration, the terms $Ae^{-\alpha t}$ and $Pe^{-\pi t}$ will approach 0 while the term $Be^{-\beta t}$ will still retain some finite value. Equation (11-24) will then reduce to:

$$C = B(e^{-\beta t}) \tag{11-9}$$

Equation (11-9) describes terminal phase of the tri-exponential plasma profile with β as its rate constant, and when back-extrapolated to time 0 it yields the y-intercept = B.

Feathering: A series of residual drug concentration-time values are obtained when one subtracts concentration-time values on back-extrapolated line from the corresponding true plasma concentration-time values (data points). The equation describing time course of these residual concentrations is obtained by subtracting equation (11-9) from equation (11-24). Subtraction gives:

$$C' = A(e^{-\alpha t}) + P(e^{-\pi t}) \tag{11-25}$$

In this equation, C′ is the residual concentration obtained by subtraction. A plot of residual concentrations versus time, described by equation (11-25) yields a bi-exponential curve. Since the value of the hybrid rate constant π is greater than that of the rate constant α, it follows that as t increases, the numerical value of the term $Pe^{-\pi t}$ will approach 0, while the numerical value of the term $Ae^{-\alpha t}$ will still have a finite value. Equation (11-25) will then reduce to:

$$C' = A(e^{-\alpha t}) \tag{11-26}$$

Equation (11-26) describes the terminal linear phase of the residual curve with a rate constant = α and y-intercept = A. The residual concentration curve remaining after terminal linear portion produced this y-intercept can be resolved further. Subtracting residual concentrations, C′, from the corresponding concentration-time values on the back-extrapolated residual straight line having A as the y-intercept yields a second series of residual concentration values. These residuals (C") can be described by an exponential equation obtained by subtracting equation (11-26) from equation (11-25). Subtraction yields:

$$C'' = P(e^{-\pi t}) \tag{11-27}$$

The rate constant of this mono-exponential curve is π and when back-extrapolated to time 0, it will yield a y-intercept = P.

Pharmacokinetic Parameters

The following pharmacokinetic parameters are associated with the drug which, upon administration as a rapid intravenous bolus dose, confers the characteristics of a three-compartment open model on the body:

a. Biological half-life of the drug
b. Rate constant of elimination of drug from the central compartment
c. Rate constants of transfer of drug between the central compartment and the two tissue compartments
d. Apparent volumes of distribution of central and tissue compartments, and therefore, the apparent volume of distribution of the drug
e. Area under the curve. These parameters are determined as follows:

Biological Half-life

The equation describing concentration of drug in the plasma as a function of time is:

$$C = B(e^{-\beta t}) + A(e^{-\alpha t}) + P(e^{-\pi t}) \quad (11\text{-}28)$$

In this equation, it is presumed that $\pi > \alpha > \beta$. Therefore, some time after the distributive phase (i.e. when t becomes large), the last two right-hand side terms, $Ae^{-\alpha t}$ and $Pe^{-\pi t}$, of equation (11-28) will approach a value equal to 0, while the term, $Be^{-\beta t}$, will still have a finite value indicating the end of the distributive phase, but continuation of elimination of drug from the body. At that time, equation (11-28) will be reduced to:

$$C = B(e^{-\beta t}) \quad (11\text{-}9)$$

which, in the logarithmic form is an equation of a straight line. The rate constant of this straight line is β and the biological half-life is given by the following equation:

$$t_{1/2} = \frac{0.693}{\beta} \quad (11\text{-}11)$$

Apparent Volumes of Distribution

The apparent volumes of distribution of the drug in a three-compartment pharmacokinetic model include the following:
a. Apparent volume of the central compartment
b. Apparent volume of the shallow tissue compartment
c. Apparent volume of the deep tissue compartment
d. Apparent total volume of distribution.

The equations used for calculation of apparent volumes of distribution of the two tissue compartments are too complicated and therefore are beyond the scope of this discussion. For this reason, the equation for the apparent total volume of distribution (V_d) is not included here because V_d is the sum of the apparent volumes of distribution of all three compartments.

Volume of Central Compartment

At time t = 0, equation (11-28) becomes

$$C_0 = B + A + P \quad (11\text{-}29)$$

where C_0 is the concentration of drug in plasma immediately after the intravenous administration. Since at this time distribution of drug in tissue compartments has not yet started, C_0, therefore reflects the concentration of the drug dose in the central compartment only.

If D is the dose administered, then

$$C_0 = \frac{D}{V_c} \quad (11\text{-}30)$$

where, V_c is the volume of the central compartment.

Combining equations (11-29) and (11-30),

$$(B + A + P) = \frac{D}{V_c}$$

$$\text{or } V_c = \frac{D}{B + A + P} = \frac{D}{C_0} \quad (11\text{-}31)$$

Rate Constants

There are five first-order rate constants associated with the three-compartment pharmacokinetic model. These are:

a. The first-order rate constant of transfer of drug from central compartment into the shallow tissue compartment (K_{12})
b. The first-order rate constant of transfer of drug from central compartment into the deep tissue compartment (K_{13})
c. The first-order rate constant of transfer of drug from the shallow tissue compartment into the central compartment (K_{21})
d. The first-order rate constant of transfer of drug from the deep tissue compartment into the central compartment (K_{31})
e. The first-order rate constant of elimination of drug from the central compartment (K_{10}).

The equations describing the first-order rate constants of transfer of drug from the deep and the shallow tissue compartments into the central compartment (K_{21} and K_{31}, respectively) are somewhat complex and are best illustrated as follows:

$$K_{21} = 0.5[-x - (x^2 - 4y)^{1/2}] \quad (11\text{-}32)$$

$$K_{31} = 0.5[-x + (x^2 - 4y)^{1/2}] \quad (11\text{-}33)$$

In equations (11-32) and (11-33) the values of x and y are as follows:

$$x = -\frac{\pi B + \pi A + \beta P + \beta A + \alpha P + \alpha B}{B + A + P} \text{ and} \quad (11\text{-}34)$$

$$y = \frac{\alpha\pi B + \pi\beta A + \alpha\beta P}{B + A + P} \quad (11\text{-}35)$$

The equation for the first-order rate constant of elimination of drug from the central compartment (K_{10}) is:

$$K_{10} = \frac{\alpha\beta\pi}{(K_{21})(K_{31})} \quad (11\text{-}36)$$

The equations for the first-order rate constants of transfer of drug from the central compartment to the deep and shallow tissue compartments are:

$$K_{12} = \frac{(\alpha\beta + \alpha\pi + \beta\pi) - (K_{21})(\alpha + \beta + \pi) - (K_{10})(K_{31}) + (K_{21})^2}{(K_{31}) - (K_{21})} \quad (11\text{-}37)$$

$$K_{13} = (\alpha + \beta + \pi) - (K_{10} + K_{21} + K_{31} + K_{12}) \quad (11\text{-}38)$$

Area Under the Curve

The total area under the plasma concentration versus time curve is obtained by using either of the methods described previously. In the three-compartment model, since the plasma profile in effect consists of three linear segments having y-intercepts B, A and P, with respective first-order rate constants equal to β, α and π, the equation for total area under the curve becomes:

$$AUC_{total} = \frac{B}{\beta} + \frac{A}{\alpha} + \frac{P}{\pi} \tag{11-39}$$

The total area under the curve can also be calculated using the following equation:

$$AUC_{total} = \frac{C_0}{K_{10}} \tag{11-40}$$

Example 11-5 Calculate biological half-life, apparent volume of central compartment and total area under the curve from the following plasma concentration versus time data obtained after administration of a single 10 mg intravenous bolus dose of a drug:

Time (h)	*Concentration (µg/L)*	*Time (h)*	*Concentration (µg/L)*	*Time (h)*	*Concentration (µg/L)*
1.5	370.230	7.5	183.265	36.0	95.268
3.0	278.992	9.0	170.444	96.0	43.062
4.5	229.980	10.5	160.643	99.0	41.415
6.0	201.486	30.0	104.291	105.0	38.307

Solution

A plot of data on a three cycle semi-log paper is shown in Figure 11-8 (circles). This plot does not exhibit linearity indicating a multi-compartment model. The plasma profile must be feathered to obtain linear segments. To generate the first linear segment, the terminal two concentration points (at 99 hours and 105 hours) are used to calculate the first-order rate constant and y-intercept of the first linear segment. The rate constant of this straight line is determined from the slope of the two terminal concentration points:

$$\beta = -\text{slope} = -\frac{\ln 41.415 - \ln 38.307}{(99 - 105)\text{ h}} = -\frac{0.7801}{-6\text{ h}} = 0.013/\text{h}$$

The y-intercept, B, of this straight line is calculated by substituting the values of $\beta = 0.013/\text{h}$ and concentration at 105 h = 38.307 µg/L into equation (11-9):

$$38.307\ \mu\text{g/L} = Be^{(-0.013/\text{h})(105\text{ h})} = Be^{-1.365} = (B)(0.2554)$$

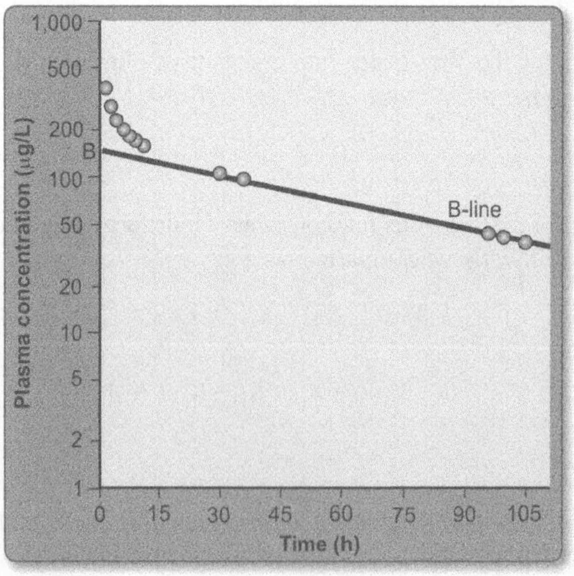

Fig. 11-8 Plot of data in Example 11-5

$$\text{therefore, } B = \frac{38.307 \ \mu g/L}{0.2554} = 150 \ \mu g/L$$

The y-intercept, B, may also be calculated by substituting the values of β (= 0.013/h) and concentration at 99 hour (= 41.415 μg/L) into equation (11-9):

$$41.415 \ \mu g/L = Be^{(-0.013/h)(99\ h)}$$

$$= Be^{-1.365}$$

$$= (B)(0.2761)$$

therefore,

$$B = \frac{41.415 \ \mu g/L}{0.2761}$$

$$B = 150 \ \mu g/L$$

A straight line is drawn by joining 150 μg/L at t = 0 hour and 38.307 μg/L at t = 105 hours. This straight line will be referred to as the B-line.

Feathering of Data

As seen in Figure 11-8, the plasma concentration data points provided in the data from 1.5 hour to 36 hours did not fall on the straight line obtained by joining concentration points 150 μg/L at 0 hour and 38,307 μg/L at 105 hours. (the B-line). These concentration points are now feathered with respect to the straight line B to generate residual concentration points. The feathering technique used for the three-compartment model is similar to the feathering technique used for resolution of data for the two-compartment pharmacokinetic model.

To determine the residual plasma concentration at 1.5 hours, the concentration of drug in plasma at 1.5 hours on the B-line is subtracted from the 1.5 hours concentration of drug in plasma given in the data. The concentration of drug in the plasma on B-Line at 1.5 hour is determined using equation (11-9) as follows:

$$C = Be^{-\beta t}$$

$$= (150 \ \mu g/L)(e^{(-0.013/h)(1.5\ h)})$$

$$= (150 \ \mu g/L)(0.98069)$$

$$= 147.103 \ \mu g/L$$

Therefore, the residual concentration at 1.5 hours is:

$$370.230 \ \mu g/L - 147.103 \ \mu g/L = 223.127 \ \mu g/L.$$

This point is now plotted (as a square) at 1.5 hours on the semi-logarithmic graph paper (Figure 11-9).

Similarly, at 3 hours, data concentration is 278.992 μg/L and concentration on B-line at 3 hours is:

$$C = (150 \ \mu g/L)(e^{(-0.013/h)(3\ h)})$$

$$= (150 \ \mu g/L)(0.9618)$$

$$= 144.263 \ \mu g/L$$

Therefore the residual concentration at 3 hours is:

$$278.992 \ \mu g/L - 144.263 \ \mu g/L = 134.729 \ \mu g/L.$$

This concentration is now plotted at 3 hours in Figure 11-9 (shown as a square).

This process is continued to obtain residual concentrations for data points, which did not fall on the B-line and these concentrations are plotted as squares. The residual concentrations plotted as squares in Figure 11-9 show that residuals do not exhibit linearity, but show a curve. This indicates that, upon administration, the drug does not confer the characteristics of a two-compartment model on the body.

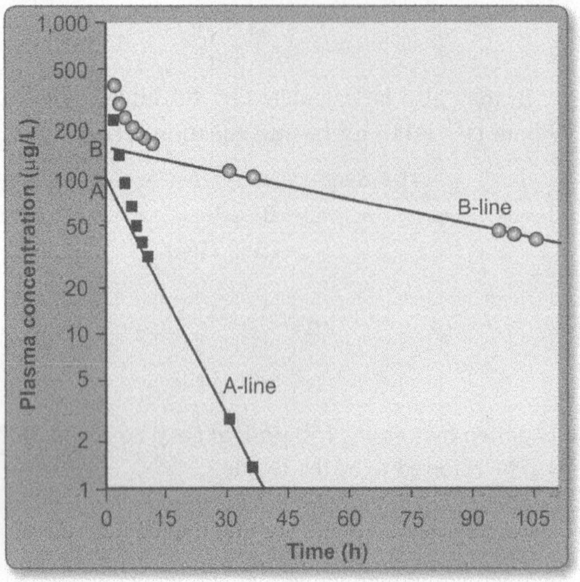

Fig. 11-9 Feathering of data in Example 11-5

Second Feathering

A second feathering is now required to strip the residual concentration curve obtained after the first feathering (squares in Figure 11-9). To obtain the second feathering, the original data points are not used because these points were already used for feathering of the original curve. Similarly, data points on the B-line are not used for the second feathering because these points represent the straight line having the y-intercept B.

The second feathering is similar to the first feathering in the sense that the curve representing the first residual concentrations (shown as squares in Figure 11-9) is feathered with respect to the straight line obtained when the terminal points of this curve are back-extrapolated.

The terminal two points shown as squares in Figure 11-9 are used to determine the first-order rate constant, α and y-intercept, A, of this straight line. This straight line will be referred to as the A-line. The first-order rate constant, α, of this straight line is:

$$\alpha = -\text{slope} = -\frac{\ln 2.732 - \ln 1.330}{(30 - 36)\ \text{h}} = -\frac{0.7199}{-6\ \text{h}} = 0.12/\text{h}$$

The y-intercept, A, of this straight line is determined using equation (11-26). Substituting the concentration at 36 hours into this equation:

$$1.33\ \mu\text{g/L} = \text{A}e^{(-0.12/\text{h})(36\ \text{h})}$$

$$= \text{A}e^{-4.32} = (\text{A})(0.0133)$$

$$\text{therefore, A} = \frac{1.33\ \mu\text{g/L}}{0.0133} = 100\ \mu\text{g/L}$$

The residual concentrations (squares) are now feathered (second feathering) with respect to the straight line having the y-intercept = A and a new set of residuals (second residual concentrations) are obtained. For example, the residual concentration curve (squares in Figure 11-9) shows concentration of drug at 1.5 hours is 223.127 μg/L. The concentration at 1.5 hour on the straight line having y-intercept = A is found using equation (11-26) by substituting the values of the y-intercept (A = 100 mg/L) and the first-order rate constant (α = 0.12/h):

$$C = Ae^{-\alpha t}$$
$$= (100\ \mu g/L)(e^{(-0.12/h)(1.5\ h)})$$
$$= (100\ \mu g/L)(0.83527) = 83.527\ \mu g/L$$

Therefore, the second residual concentration at 1.5 hours is:

$$223.127\ \mu g/L - 83.527\ \mu g/L = 139.600\ \mu g/L.$$

Similarly, concentration at 3 hours on the second curve (squares in Figure 11-9) is 134.729 mcg/L, and at 3 hours, concentration on the straight line having A as the y-intercept is

$$C = (100\ \mu g/L)(e^{(-0.12/h)(3\ h)})$$
$$= (100\ \mu g/L)(0.69768) = 69.768\ \mu g/L$$

Therefore, the second residual concentration at 3 hours is:

$$134.729\ \mu g/L - 69.768\ \mu g/L = 64.961\ \mu g/L.$$

The process of determining the second residual concentrations is continued to obtain second residual concentrations from those first residual concentrations (squares in Figure 11-9), which did not fall on the straight line having the y-intercept = A.

Table 11-2 shows in detail how the concentration points provided in the data were feathered by the method of residuals in order to obtain the first residual concentrations and subsequent feathering of the first residual concentration points to obtain the second residual concentrations. The second set of residual concentrations is plotted as triangles in Figure 11-10.

The residual concentrations generated by the second feathering appear to exhibit a linear relationship. If the second residual concentrations generated by the second feathering process exhibit too much scatter, then one would prefer to use regression analysis to determine if the data can be represented by a linear relationship. If the data indicate a linear relationship, then a straight line can be drawn.

In this Example, the second residual concentrations do not exhibit too much scatter and eyeball judgment may be used. From the graph it is seen that a straight line which best represents the second residual concentration points can be drawn with a y-intercept = P = 300 μg/L.

Table 11-2 Feathering of data in Example 11-5

Time (h)	*Concentration (μg/L)* ●	*1st feathering* ■	*2nd feathering* ▲
1.5	370.230	370.230 – 147.103 = 223.127	223.127 – 83.527 = 139.600
3.0	278.992	278.992 – 144.263 = 134.729	134.729 – 69.768 = 64.961
4.5	229.980	229.980 – 141.477 = 88.503	88.503 – 58.275 = 30.228
6.0	201.486	201.486 – 138.745 = 62.741	62.741 – 48.675 = 14.066
7.5	183.268	183.268 – 136.605 = 47.203	47.203 – 40.657 = 6.546
9.0	170.444	170.444 – 133.438 = 37.006	37.006 – 33.960 = 3.046
10.5	160.643	160.643 – 130.861 = 29.782	39.782 – 28.365 = 1.417
30.0	104.291	104.291 – 101.559 = 2.732	**
36.0	95.268	95.268 – 93.938 = 1.330	**
96.0	43.062	*	**
99.0	41.415	*	**
105.0	38.307	*	**

* Not feathered because these points are found on B-line

** Not feathered because these points are found on A-line

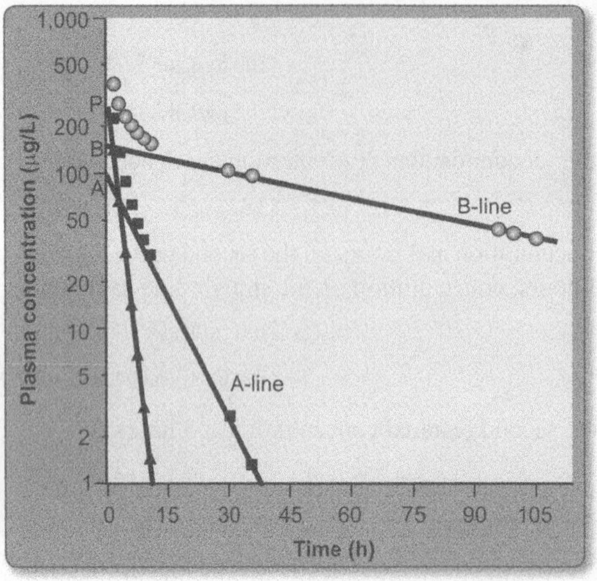

Fig. 11-10 Resolution of plasma profile in Example 11-5.

The first-order rate constant of this straight line, π, can be calculated from the slope by using any two points on this straight line. Sometimes the last terminal point on the final linear segment is rounded off to the nearest approximation because second feathering of the plasma profile results in concentration terms with very low values. Therefore, the last terminal point may not appear to fall on this straight line.

Since the y-intercept of this straight line can be easily read from the graph (300 μg/L) and the second residual concentration at 10.5 hours appears to be on this straight line, therefore, these points are used to calculate the rate constant (π) of this straight line:

$$\pi = -\text{slope} = -\frac{\ln 300 - \ln 1.417}{(0 - 10.5)\ \text{h}} = -\frac{5.35524}{-10.5\ \text{h}} = 0.51/\text{h}$$

The plasma profile of the curve is stripped into three linear segments, yielding the following values. The y-intercepts:

$$B = 150\ \mu g/L,\ A = 100\ \mu g/L \text{ and } P = 300\ \mu g/L$$

and their respective rate constants:

$$\beta = 0.013/\text{h},\ \alpha = 0.12/\text{h} \text{ and } \pi = 0.51/\text{h}$$

These six values are used to calculate various parameters associated with the three-compartment model.

Rate Constants

To determine values of five first-order rate constants (K_{21}, K_{31}, K_{12}, K_{13} and K_{10}), we need to calculate the values of x and y. The value of x is given by equation (11-34) and the value of y is given by equation (11-35). The value of x is obtained by substituting values of the three y-intercepts (B, A, P) and the three hybrid rate constants (β, α and π) into equation (11-34),

$$x = -\frac{\pi B + \pi A + \beta P + \beta A + \alpha P + \alpha B}{B + A + P}$$

$$x = -\frac{(\pi)(B + A) + (\beta)(P + A) + (\alpha)(P + B)}{B + A + P}$$

$$= -\frac{(0.51)(150+100)+(0.013)(300+100)+(0.12)(300+150)}{150+100+300}$$

$$= -\frac{186.7}{550} = -0.3395/\text{h}$$

Similarly, the value of y is obtained by substituting the values of B, A, P, β, α and π into equation (11-35),

$$y = -\frac{a\pi B + \pi\beta A + \alpha\beta P}{B+A+P}$$

$$y = \frac{(0.12)(0.51)(150)+(0.51)(0.013)(100)+(0.12)(0.013)(300)}{150+100+300}$$

$$= \frac{10.311}{550} = 0.01875/\text{h}^2$$

The first-order rate constant of transfer of drug from the first tissue compartment into the central compartment is obtained by substituting the values of x and y into equation (11-32):

$$K_{21} = 0.5[-x - (x^2 - 4y)^{1/2}]$$

$$= 0.5[-(0.3395/\text{h}) - \{(-0.3395/\text{h})^2 - 4(0.01875/\text{h}^2)\}^{1/2}]$$

$$= 0.5[0.3395/\text{h} - (0.11526/\text{h}^2 - 0.075/\text{h}^2)^{1/2}]$$

$$= 0.5(0.3395/\text{h} - 0.2015/\text{h})$$

$$= 0.5(0.138/\text{h}) = 0.069/\text{h}$$

The first-order rate constant of transfer of drug from the second tissue compartment into the central compartment is obtained by substituting the values of x and y into equation (11-33):

$$K_{31} = 0.5[-x + (x^2 - 4y)^{1/2}]$$

$$= 0.5[-(0.3395/\text{h}) + \{(-0.3395/\text{h})^2 - 4(0.01875/\text{h}^2)\}^{1/2}]$$

$$= 0.5[0.3395/\text{h} + (0.11526/\text{h}^2 - 0.075/\text{h}^2)^{1/2}]$$

$$= 0.5(0.3395/\text{h} + 0.2015/\text{h})$$

$$= 0.5(0.541/\text{h}) = 0.2705/\text{h}$$

The first-order rate constant of elimination of drug from the central compartment is calculated using equation (11-36).

Substituting values of α, β, π, K_{21} and K_{31} into the equation:

$$K_{10} = \frac{\alpha\beta\pi}{(K_{21})(K_{31})}$$

$$= \frac{(0.12/\text{h})(0.013/\text{h})(0.51/\text{h})}{(0.069/\text{h})(0.2705/\text{h})}$$

$$= \frac{0.0007956}{0.0186645}$$

$$= 0.042626/\text{h}$$

The rate constant of transfer of drug from the central compartment into the first tissue compartment is determined using equation (11-37):

$$K_{12} = \frac{(\alpha\beta + \alpha\pi + \beta\pi) - (K_{21})(\alpha+\beta+\pi) - (K_{10})(K_{31}) + (K_{21})^2}{(K_{31}) - (K_{21})}$$

The values of terms in the numerator and in the denominator of this equation are calculated to simplify their substitution into equation (11-37):

$$\alpha\beta + \alpha\pi + \beta\pi = (0.12/h)(0.013/h) + (0.12/h)(0.51/h) + (0.013/h)(0.51/h)$$

$$= (0.00156/h^2) + (0.0612/h^2) + (0.00663/h^2)$$

$$= 0.06939/h^2$$

$$(K_{21})(\alpha + \beta + \pi) = (0.069/h)(0.12/h + 0.013/h + 0.51/h)$$

$$= (0.069/h)(0.643/h)$$

$$= 0.04437/h^2$$

$$(K_{10})(K_{31}) + (K_{21})^2 = (0.04263/h)(0.2705/h) + (0.069/h)^2$$

$$= (0.01153/h^2) + (0.004761/h^2)$$

$$= 0.01629/h^2$$

$$(K_{31}) - (K_{21}) = (0.2705/h) - (0.069/h) = 0.2015/h$$

Substituting the appropriate values into equation (11-37):

$$K_{12} = \frac{(0.06939/h^2) - (0.04437/h^2) - (0.01629/h^2)}{0.2015/h}$$

$$= 0.09056/h$$

The first-order rate constant of transfer of drug from the central compartment into second tissue compartment is calculated using equation (11-38). Substituting the values into equation (11-38),

$$K_{13} = (\alpha + \beta + \pi) - (K_{10} + K_{21} + K_{31} + K_{12})$$

$$= (0.12 + 0.013 + 0.51)/h - (0.42626 + 0.069 + 0.2705 + 0.09056)/h$$

$$= 0.643/h - 0.4727/h = 0.17028/h$$

Biological Half-Life: Using equation (11-11)

$$t_{1/2} = \frac{0.693}{\beta}$$

$$= 53.31 \text{ h}$$

Volume of Central Compartment: From equation (11-31),

$$V_C = \frac{D}{B + A + P}$$

$$= \frac{10 \text{ mg}}{150\ \mu g/L + 100\ \mu g/L + 300\ \mu g/L}$$

$$= 18.18 \text{ L}$$

Area Under the Curve: Using equation (11-39)

$$AUC_{total} = \frac{B}{\beta} + \frac{A}{\alpha} + \frac{P}{\pi}$$

$$= \frac{150\ \mu g/L}{0.013/h} + \frac{100\ \mu g/L}{0.12/h} + \frac{300\ \mu g/L}{0.51/h}$$

$$= 12959\ \mu g \times h/L$$

Description of the Model

From the parameters found in Example 11-5, the plasma profile can be described either in the form of equation (11-24) or as a schematic.

Description by Equation: The plasma profile is described in the form of equation (11-24) as:

$$C = 150(e^{-0.013t}) + 100(e^{-0.12t}) + 300(e^{-0.51t}).$$

Schematic Representation: The pharmacokinetic parameters derived from data in Example 11-5 can be represented schematically as shown in Figure 11-11. This schematic shows that a 10 mg dose was administered intravenously. The apparent volume of the central compartment is 18.182 L. The rate constants of transfer of drug from central compartment to the two tissue compartments are 0.09056/h and 0.17028/h, respectively. The respective rate constants of transfer of drug from the two tissue compartments to the central compartment are 0.2705/h and 0.069/h. The rate constant of elimination of drug from the central compartment is 0.042624/h.

Example 11-6 The plasma profile of a drug following administration of a 10 mg rapid intravenous bolus dose is described by the equation:

$$C = 50(e^{-0.13t}) + 35(e^{-0.75t}) + 100(e^{-4.25t}).$$

If concentration is in μg/L and time is in hour, calculate biological half-life, concentration of drug in plasma immediately after administration of the dose, apparent volume of central compartment, rate constant of elimination of drug from the body, and total area under the curve.

Solution

In this three-compartment model, the three y-intercepts and the three rate constants are:

$$B = 50\ \mu g/L,\ A = 35\ \mu g/L \text{ and } P = 100\ \mu g/L$$

$$\beta = 0.13/h,\ \alpha = 0.75/h \text{ and } \pi = 4.25/h$$

Biological Half-Life: Equation (11-11) is used to calculate biological half-life:

$$t_{1/2} = \frac{0.693}{\beta} = \frac{0.693}{0.13/h} = 5.33\ h$$

Concentration at Time Zero: From equation (11-29),

$$C_0 = B + A + P = 50\ \mu g/L + 35\ \mu g/L + 100\ \mu g/L = 185\ \mu g/L$$

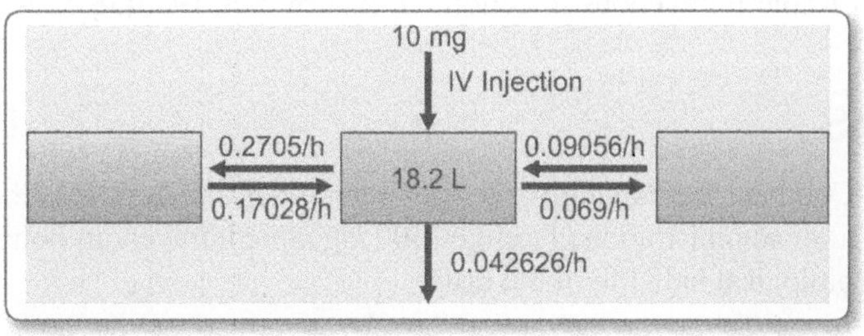

Fig. 11-11 Schematic of the three-compartment model in Example 11-5.

Volume of Central Compartment: From equation (11-31), *D*

$$V_c = \frac{D}{B + A + P}$$

$$= \frac{10 \text{ mg}}{50\ \mu g/L + 35\ \mu g/L + 100\ \mu g/L}$$

$$= \frac{10 \text{ mg}}{185\ \mu g/L}$$

$$= 54.05 \text{ L}$$

Rate Constant of Elimination from the Body

The rate constant of elimination of drug from the body is represented by β, which is 0.13/h.

Total Area Under the Curve

AUC Using equation (11-39)

$$AUC_{total} = \frac{B}{\beta} + \frac{A}{\alpha} + \frac{P}{\pi}$$

$$= \frac{50\ \mu g/L}{0.13/h} + \frac{35\ \mu g/L}{0.75/L} + \frac{100\ \mu g/L}{4.25/h}$$

$$= 384.615\ \mu g \times h/L + 46.667\ \mu g \times h/L + 23.529\ \mu g \times h/L$$

$$= 454.81\ \mu g \times h/L$$

SUGGESTED READING

1. Gibaldi M. Biopharmaceutics and Clinical Pharmacokinetics. Lea and Febiger; 1991.
2. Gibaldi M, Perrier D. Pharmacokinetics, 2nd edition. Marcel Dekker; 1982.
3. Loughman P, Sitar D, Oglivie R and Neims A. The two compartment open system kinetic model: A review of its clinical implications and applications, J. Pediatr., 1976;88:869-73.
4. Madan PL. Bioavailability and Bioequivalence: The Underlying Concepts. US Pharmacist, 1992;17(11):H 10-H 30.
5. Madan PL. Bioavailability and patient variances, US Pharmacist. 1996;21(5):3-14.
6. Madan PL. Introduction to bioavailability and pharmacokinetics. In: Lamba and Walker (eds). Antibiotics and Microbial Transformations. CRC Press, Boca Raton, FL; 1987.
7. Remington: The Science and Practice of Pharmacy, 21st edition. Mack Publishing, 2005.
7. Wagner J. Fundamentals of Clinical Pharmacokinetics, Drug Intell. Publications; 1979.
9. Wagner J, Northam J. Estimation of Volume of Distribution and Half-Life of a Compound After Rapid Intravenous Injection," J. Pharm. Sci. 1975;58:529-31.

PRACTICE PROBLEMS

11-1. Compute the equation and draw the model that describes the plasma profile obtained after administration of a single 300 mg rapid intravenous bolus dose of a drug. Calculate biological half-life of the drug.

Time(h)	1	2	3	4	5	6
Concentration (mg/L)	32.9	18.1	9.9	5.5	3.0	1.6

11-2. The following data were obtained after administration of a single 500 mg intravenous bolus dose of a drug. Calculate biological half-life, concentration of drug in plasma at 15 hours, rate constant of elimination and apparent volume of distribution of the drug.

Time(h)	1	2	3	4	5	6	7
Concentration (μg/mL)	48.5	17.9	17.9	10.8	6.6	4.0	2.4

11-3. The following data were obtained after rapid intravenous bolus administration of a single 30 mg dose of a drug. Calculate biological half-life and apparent volume of central compartment.

Time(h)	1	2	3	4	5	6	7
Concentration (mg/L)	0.58	0.47	0.38	0.31	0.25	0.20	0.17

11-4. Compute the equation and draw a pharmacokinetic model that describes the following plasma concentration data obtained after rapid intravenous administration of a single 100 mg bolus dose of a drug.

Time (h)	*Concentration (μg/L)*	*Time (h)*	*Concentration (μg/L)*	*Time (h)*	*Concentration (μg/L)*
0.25	61.141	3.0	18.133	8.0	5.318
0.50	53.605	4.0	13.172	9.0	4.423
0.75	47.184	5.0	10.058	10.0	3.699
1.0	41.702	6.0	7.962	12.0	2.600
2.0	26.565	7.0	6.457	14.0	1.851

11-5. Draw the pharmacokinetic model and compute the exponential equation, which describes the following data obtained after administration of a single 150 mg rapid intravenous bolus dose of a drug.

Time (h)	*Concentration (μg/L)*	*Time (h)*	*Concentration (μg/L)*	*Time (h)*	*Concentration (μg/L)*
0.25	61.380	1.5	21.624	4.0	7.098
0.50	48.485	2.0	15.937	5.0	5.267
0.75	38.628	2.5	12.396	6.0	3.958
1.0	30.296	3.0	10.041	7.0	3.021

11-6. Compute pharmacokinetic equation and draw pharmacokinetic model that describes the following plasma-drug concentration versus time data obtained after administration of a single 20 mg rapid intravenous bolus dose of an antibiotic. Concentrations are in μg/100 mL and time is in hours.

Time (h)	*Concentration (h)*	*Time (h)*	*Concentration (h)*	*Time (h)*	*Concentration (h)*
0.25	39.222	1.5	15.666	4.0	4.342
0.50	31.087	2.0	10.190	5.0	3.276
0.75	24.924	2.5	7.721	6.0	2.516
1.0	20.236	3.0	6.177	7.0	1.999

11-7. The following data were obtained after a single 250 mg rapid intravenous bolus dose of an antibiotic was administered. Compute the equation, which describes the plasma concentration versus time data and draw the pharmacokinetic model. Concentrations are in μg/100 mL and time is in hours.

Time	Concentration	Time	Concentration	Time	Concentration
0.25	77.086	1.5	43.069	8.0	4.548
0.50	68.398	2.0	34.534	10.0	2.829
0.75	60.781	4.0	15.464	12.0	1.760
1.0	54.097	6.0	7.916	14.0	1.206

11-8. The plasma profile of a drug after administration of a single 100 mg rapid intravenous bolus dose is described by the equation:

$$C = 17(e^{-0.14t}) + 52(e^{-0.39t}).$$

If concentrations are in μg/100 mL and time is in hour, calculate (a) Concentration of drug in plasma at 1.0, 3.5 and 4.5 hours. and (b) Apparent volume of the central compartment.

11-9. A semi-logarithmic plot of concentration versus time after administration of a single 10 mg rapid intravenous bolus dose of a drug produced a bi-exponential curve. Feathering of the plasma profile yielded two straight lines having y-intercepts 10.5 μg/100 mL and 37.5 μg/100 mL. Their respective slopes were –0.03/h and –0.15/h. From the data thus generated, calculate the following parameters: K_{12}, K_{21}, K_{10} and $t_{1/2}$.

11-10. The plasma profile of a drug after administration of a 100 mg intravenous dose can be described by the equation:

$$C = 10(e^{-0.15t}) + 40(e^{-0.49t}).$$

If concentration is in μg/100 mL and time is in hours, calculate the apparent volume of central compartment.

11-11. The plasma profile following intravenous administration of a single 300 mg bolus dose of a drug is described by the mono-exponential equation:

$$C = 92(e^{-0.35t}).$$

If concentration is in mg/L and time is in hours, calculate (a) Biological half-life of the drug, (b) Apparent volume of distribution of the drug, and (c) Concentration of drug in plasma at 6 hr.

11-12. The plasma profile obtained after administration of a 5 mg rapid intravenous. Bolus dose of a drug is described by the following equation:

$$C = 1.2(e^{-0.15t}).$$

If concentration is in mg/L and time is in hours, calculate the following parameters: (a) biological half-life of the drug, (b) apparent volume of distribution, and (c) concentration of drug in plasma at 10 h.

11-13. The plasma profile obtained after administration of a 300 mg rapid intravenous bolus dose of a drug is described by the equation:

$$C = 6(e^{-0.35t}) + 18(e^{-0.87t}).$$

If concentration is in μg/mL and time is in h, calculate (a) Apparent volume of central compartment, (b) Concentration of drug in plasma at 6 hours, and (c) Biological half-life of drug.

11-14. The plasma profile following intravenous administration of 100 mg rapid bolus dose of a drug is described by the equation:

$$C = 1.2(e^{-0.15t}) + 4.8(e^{-0.55t}).$$

If concentration is in mcg/mL and time is in hours, calculate (a) Concentration of drug immediately after administration of the dose, (b) Biological half-life of the drug, (c) Apparent volume of distribution, and (d) Concentration of drug in plasma at 6 hours.

11-15. The following equation describes the plasma profile obtained after rapid intravenous administration of a single 300 mg bolus dose of a drug:

$$C = 10(e^{-0.3t}) + 30(e^{-0.9t}).$$

If concentration of drug in plasma is in μg/mL and time is in hours, calculate the apparent volume of central compartment.

11-16. The plasma profile of a drug following intravenous administration of a single 5 mg bolus dose is given by:

$$C = 165(e^{-0.13t}) + 85(e^{-0.35t}) + 25(e^{-0.85t}).$$

If concentration is in μg/L and t is in hr, calculate: (a) Half-life of the drug, (b) Concentration at time 0, (c) Apparent volume of the central compartment, and (d) Total area under the curve.

11-17. The plasma profile obtained after administration of a single 50 mg intravenous dose is given by the equation:

$$C = 15(e^{-0.15t}) + 55(e^{-0.41t}) + 150(e^{-0.95t}).$$

If concentration is in μg/L and time is in h, calculate:(a) Half-life of the drug, (b) C_0, (c) Apparent volume of the central compartment, and (d) Total area under the curve.

11-18. The following schematic represents the pharmacokinetic model developed from plasma profile of a drug following intravenous administration of a single 50 mg bolus dose. Calculate concentration of drug in plasma immediately following administration of dose.

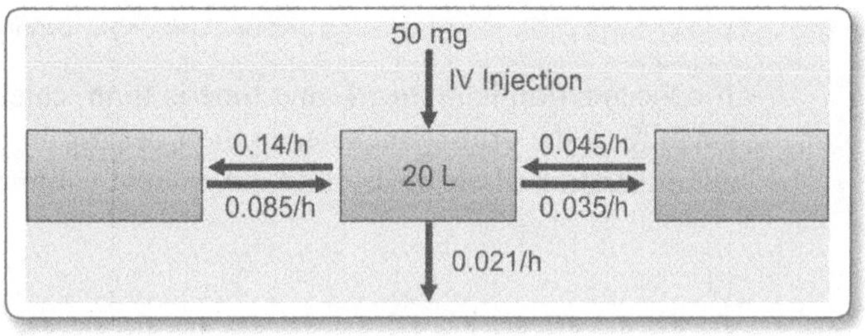

11-19. The plasma profile of a drug following intravenous administration of a single 50 mg bolus dose is given by the equation:

$$C = 10(e^{-0.1t}) + 40(e^{-0.4t}) + 100(e^{-0.9t}).$$

If concentration is in μg/L and time is in h, calculate: (a) Biological half-life, (b) Concentration of drug in plasma immediately after administration of dose, and (c) Volume of central compartment.

11-20. The following schematic represents the pharmacokinetic model developed from plasma profile of a drug following intravenous administration of a single 100 mg bolus dose. Calculate concentration of drug in plasma immediately following administration of dose.

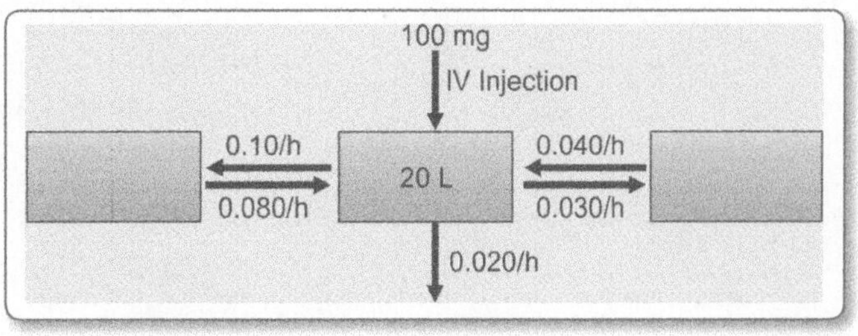

11-21. The plasma profile after intravenous administration of 500 mg rapid bolus dose of a drug is described by the following bi-exponential equation:

$$C = 12(e^{-0.115t}) + 48(e^{-0.755t}).$$

If concentration is in μg/mL and time is in hours, calculate the following: (a) Concentration of drug in plasma immediately after administration, (b) Half-life of the drug, (c) Concentration of drug in plasma 6 hour after administration and (d) Total area under the curve.

11-22. The following schematic represents the pharmacokinetic model developed from plasma profile of a drug following intravenous administration of a single 10 mg bolus dose. Calculate concentration of drug in plasma immediately following administration of the dose.

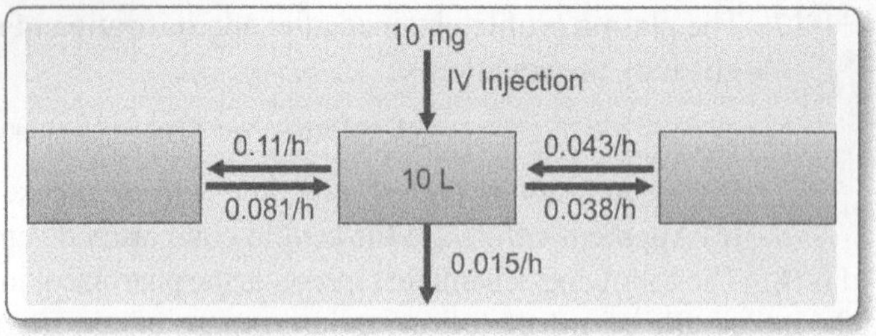

11-23. The plasma profile of a drug following intravenous administration of a single 100 mg bolus dose is given by the equation:

$$C = 10(e^{-0.01t}) + 40(e^{-0.04t}) + 100(e^{-1.09t}).$$

If concentration is in mcg/L and time is in hr, calculate the following; (a) Biological half-life of the drug, (b) Concentration of drug in the plasma immediately following administration of the dose, and (c) Apparent volume of the central compartment.

CHAPTER 12

EXTRAVASCULAR BOLUS DOSE

Administration of a drug by an extravascular route, e.g. oral administration, subcutaneous or intramuscular injection, etc. involves passage of drug by absorption through a biological membrane. Absorption of drugs generally follows first-order drug input. The plasma profile obtained after extravascular administration is different from that obtained after administration of the same dose as a rapid intravenous bolus injection, because the entire administered dose is not absorbed all-at-once. The absorption of drug depends on the rate constant of drug absorption. Thus, the two profiles differ in several respects, but the two more important differences in the plasma profiles from intravenous and extravascular routes of administration are:

Amount of drug in plasma: The amount of drug in plasma immediately after intravenous administration is equal to the amount of dose administered. In extravascular administration, the amount of drug in plasma immediately after administration of the dose is 0, because the drug has to be absorbed before it can appear in plasma. Also, absorption of the entire drug dose is not an instantaneous process.

Concentration of drug in plasma: In rapid intravenous administration, concentration of drug in plasma is at its peak immediately after intravenous injection of the dose. The concentration starts declining (as a function of time) because of elimination of drug (and in multi-compartment model, also due to distribution of drug into the tissues). In extravascular administration, concentration of drug in plasma immediately after administration of the dose is 0, because absorption of drug after administration is not instantaneous. Depending on formulation characteristics of the dosage form and the particular extravascular route of administration, the delay between administration and appearance of drug in plasma may be a few seconds (e.g. buccal administration) or more than an hour (e.g. enteric-coated dosage forms).

PLASMA PROFILE

Most conventional dosage forms are designed to release their active ingredient almost immediately after administration. Therefore, appearance of drug in plasma does not exhibit a significant delay. The plasma drug concentration is a function of rate constants of absorption and elimination in one-compartment model. The time-course of appearance of drug in plasma exhibits the following characteristics:

1. At time 0, the amount of drug in plasma is 0.
2. Soon after administration, the dosage form releases its drug, which dissolves in the biological fluids and the drug is ready for absorption. The exceptions are delayed-release and modified-release dosage forms. The drug from these dosage forms is available for absorption only when the drug starts dissolving in the biological fluids.
3. As soon as the drug becomes available for absorption, the process of absorption begins and the drug starts appearing in plasma. The amount of drug absorbed as a function of time is

directly proportional to the drug's rate constant of absorption (K_a). This is the predominantly absorptive phase.

4. During the predominantly absorptive phase, elimination also begins, but elimination at this stage is less predominant than drug absorption.
5. The absorptive phase continues until most of the drug is absorbed. At the same time elimination, which was very slow at the beginning, now becomes more predominant. When the plasma profile shows peak concentration, the rate of drug absorption is approximately equal to the rate of drug elimination.
6. Soon after peak concentration, absorption starts becoming less predominant, because most of the drug has been absorbed. Elimination now becomes more predominant because a larger amount of drug is now available for elimination. This is the beginning of the post-absorptive phase.
7. The post-absorptive phase is followed by the predominantly elimination phase. Elimination is most predominant during the terminal portion of plasma profile. The last two points on the graph exhibit more predominance in drug elimination than the points previous to the terminal two points. In most conventional dosage forms, the plasma profile during the post-absorptive phase is similar to the plasma profile obtained after intravenous administration of the same drug.

Figure 12-1 is a typical plasma profile of an extravascularly administered drug. In this profile, the segment between time 0 and 2 hours represents predominant absorption, the segment between 2 and 4 hours represents absorption approximately equal to elimination and between the segment between 10 and 13 hour is predominant elimination. Absorption is usually considered to have terminated (for all practical purposes) during the terminal portion of the profile.

ONE-COMPARTMENT MODEL

The plasma profile of many extravascularly administered drugs can be described by one-compartment pharmacokinetic model. Figure 12-2 is a schematic representation of one-compartment model following extravascular administration.

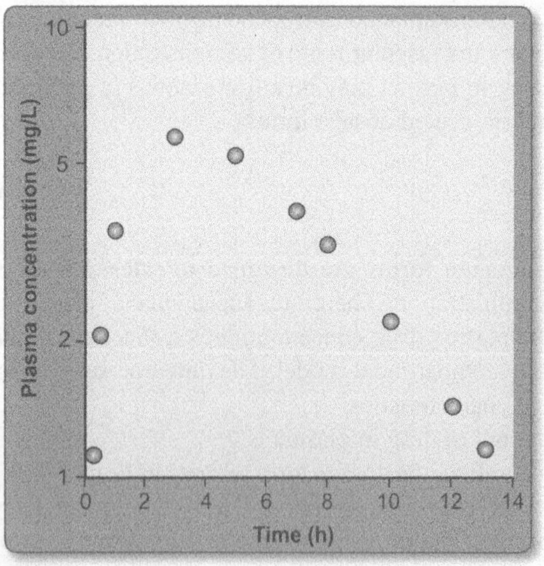

Fig. 12-1 Typical plasma profile of extravascularly administered dose

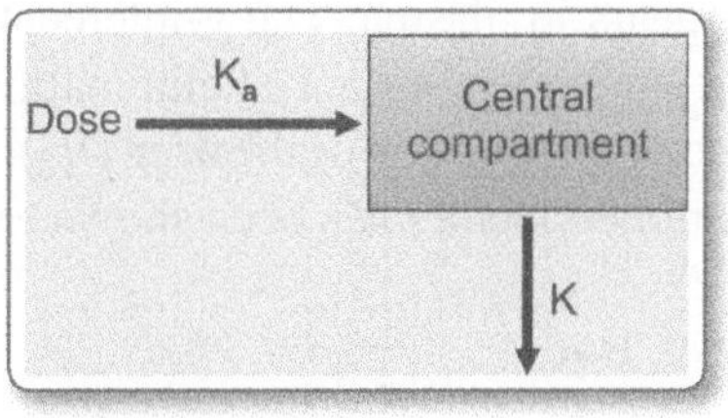

Fig. 12-2 Schematic representation of one-compartment model, extravascular administration

In this model, drug input (absorption) is first-order (K_a = rate constant of absorption), drug output (elimination) is first-order (K = rate constant of elimination) and the drug is distributed in one-compartment, known as the central compartment. The central compartment may be the plasma volume only, or it may include other body fluids and/or tissues. When other body fluids and/or tissues are involved, distribution of drug between plasma and these fluids and/or tissues is considered instantaneous, so that all these components behave as a single unit.

The plasma profile of a drug which, on extravascular administration, confers upon the body the characteristics of one-compartment model, consists of first-order absorption and first-order elimination and is described by the following bi-exponential equation:

$$C = B(e^{-\beta t}) - A(e^{-\alpha t}) \tag{12-1}$$

where,
C = concentration of drug in the plasma,
B = the y-intercept of the back-extrapolated linear segment of the terminal phase,
A = the y-intercept of the mono-exponential absorption phase obtained by the method of residuals,
β = the rate constant of elimination,
$\alpha = K_a$ = rate constant of absorption and
t = time.

In the case of most conventional dosage forms intended to release their contents soon after extravascular administration of the dose, the exponent α is always greater than the exponent β and the two y-intercepts B and A have identical values, i.e. B = A. Under these conditions, equation (12-1) may be written in the following form:

$$C = B(e^{-\beta t}) - B(e^{-\alpha t})$$

$$C = B(e^{-\beta t} - e^{-\alpha t}) \tag{12-2}$$

At time zero (t = 0), the value of the exponential terms is equal to 1 and equation (12-2) becomes

$$C = B(1-1) = 0$$

i.e. no drug appears in plasma at time zero.

Soon after the dose is administered, the concentration of drug in plasma starts increasing according to equation (12-2). Since, by definition, α (the rate constant of absorption) is greater than β (the rate constant of elimination), it follows that as t becomes large, the exponential term $Ae^{-\alpha t}$ will become small. At some time when *t* becomes sufficiently large, the term $Ae^{-\alpha t}$ will approach 0, while the term $Be^{-\beta t}$ will still have a finite value. Equation (12-2) then becomes

$$C = B(e^{-\beta t}) \tag{12-3}$$

This mono-exponential equation describes the elimination phase of the plasma profile, with a rate constant = β and y-intercept = B. During extravascular administration, the y-intercept B obtained by back-extrapolation of the plasma profile does not represent the maximum concentration of drug in plasma because at time zero, absorption of drug has not started and the drug has to be absorbed before it appears in plasma. The y-intercept B is a complex function of the rate constants of absorption (α), the rate constant of elimination (β), the fraction of dose absorbed (F) and the apparent volume of distribution of the drug (V_d). The relationship between the y-intercept B and the above-mentioned factors has been shown to be:

$$B = \frac{(F)(D)(\alpha)}{(V_d)(\alpha - \beta)} \tag{12-4}$$

Therefore, equation (12-2), in its more accurate form is written as follows (*F*)(*D*)(α)

$$C = \frac{(F)(D)(\alpha)}{(V_d)(\alpha - \beta)}\left(e^{-\beta t} - e^{-\alpha t}\right) \tag{12-5}$$

Feathering the Curve

The method of residuals is used to obtain the straight line, which represents the absorption phase. During extravascular drug administration, the concentration of drug in plasma at any time t is given by the bi-exponential equation (12-1):

$$C = B(e^{-\beta t}) - A(e^{-\alpha t})$$

In this equation, the mono-exponential terms $Be^{-\beta t}$ and $Ae^{-\alpha t}$ represent elimination and absorption phases, respectively. To obtain the mono-exponential term $Ae^{-\alpha t}$, equation (12-1) is rearranged to:

$$A(e^{-\alpha t}) = B(e^{-\beta t}) - C \tag{12-6}$$

Therefore, to generate plasma concentration points of the mono-exponential term $Ae^{-\alpha t}$, each plasma concentration point provided in the data must be subtracted from its respective concentration point on the straight line having the y-intercept = B.

Pharmacokinetic Parameters

The pharmacokinetic parameters associated with a drug which, upon extravascular administration, confers the characteristics of one-compartment open model upon the body are: rate constant of elimination (K), rate constant of absorption (K_a), biological half-life ($t_{1/2}$), apparent volume of distribution (V_d) and area under the curve (AUC).

Rate Constant of Elimination: Equation (12-3) represents the terminal phase of concentration of drug in the plasma, which in this case is elimination phase of the plasma profile. The rate constant of this linear portion is the rate constant of elimination, β, which is determined from the slope of the terminal linear portion of the plasma profile.

Rate Constant of Absorption: Application of the method of residuals yields the second linear segment of the biphasic plasma profile. This segment represents the absorption phase and its rate constant ($K_a = \alpha$), is determined either from the slope of the linear segment obtained after feathering of plasma profile, or it may be approximated from the half-life of this linear segment.

Biological Half-Life: The biological half-life ($t_{1/2}$) is determined using the relationship:

$$t_{1/2} = \frac{0.693}{\beta} \tag{12-7}$$

Apparent Volume of Distribution: The apparent volume of distribution (V_d) in one-compartment model following extravascular administration is determined from the y-intercept, B, of the back-extrapolated linear segment of elimination phase. The apparent volume of distribution is calculated by rearranging equation (12-3) as follows:

$$B = \frac{(F)(D)(\alpha)}{(V_d)(\alpha - \beta)}$$

which, upon rearrangement gives:

$$V_d = \frac{(F)(D)(\alpha)}{(B)(\alpha - \beta)} \quad (12\text{-}8)$$

Area Under the Curve: Since the plasma profile of one-compartment model consists of two linear segments having the y-intercepts B and A with rate constants ß and α, respectively, these two linear segments are used to calculate the total area under the curve. Because the concentration of drug in plasma is obtained by subtracting the exponential term representing the absorption phase from the exponential term representing the elimination phase. The equation for calculating the total area under the plasma concentration versus time curve is given by:

$$AUC_{total} = \frac{B}{\beta} - \frac{A}{\alpha} \quad (12\text{-}9)$$

The following Example illustrates plotting the data obtained after extravascular administration of the drug and evaluation of the parameters associated with the one-compartment model after extravascular administration of the drug.

Example 12-1 The following data were obtained when a 500 mg dose of an antibiotic was given orally. Calculate the pharmacokinetic parameters, assuming 100% of the administered dose was absorbed.

Time (h)	Concentration (μg/mL)	Time (h)	Concentration (μg/mL)
1	26.501	6	29.413
2	36.091	8	22.784
3	37.512	16	7.571
4	36.055	18	5.734
5	32.924	20	4.343

Solution

Since the drug is administered by an extravascular route, the plasma profile will have to be feathered to resolve it into linear segments representing the elimination and absorption phases of the drug. To plot the data on a semi-logarithmic graph paper, two cycles will be needed to plot the data and an additional cycle may be needed to plot residual concentrations. Therefore, a three-cycle semi-logarithmic graph paper should be used to plot the data.

A plot of the data on a three-cycle semi-logarithmic graph paper is shown in Figure 12-3. This graph shows initial increase in concentration, followed by a decline, finally tapering to a linear relationship.

Elimination Rate Constant

The rate constant of elimination is calculated from the terminal linear portion of plasma profile. Depending on the accuracy of data collection, one may either use the last two concentration points (concentration points at 18 and 20 hour in this Example), or determine slope by regression analysis using the terminal three concentration points (concentration points at 16, 18 and 20 hours in this Example). Since, the data collected in this Example appear accurate enough to use the last two points, therefore, elimination rate constant is:

$$\beta = -\text{slope} = \frac{\ln 5.734 - \ln 4.343}{(18-20)\text{h}}$$

$$= -\frac{0.2778}{-2\text{h}} = 0.139/\text{h}$$

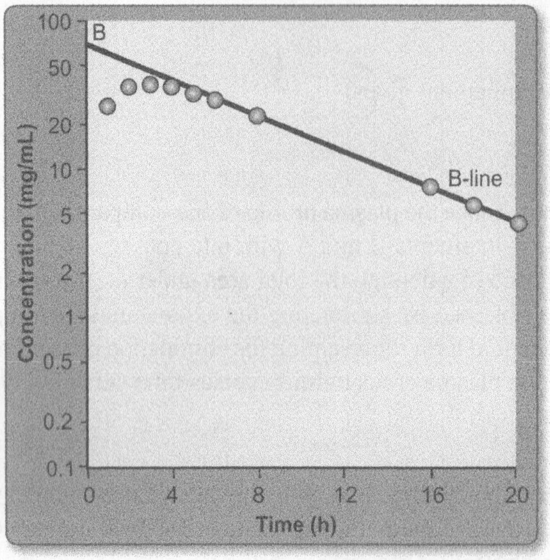

Fig. 12-3 Plot of data in Example 12-1

Biological Half-life

The biological half-life ($t_{1/2}$) is determined using equation (12-7):

$$t_{1/2} = \frac{0.693}{\beta} = \frac{0.693}{0.139/h} = 4.98 \text{ h}$$

Y-intercept, B

The y-intercept of this straight line is B and is determined using equation (12-3):

$$C = B(e^{-\beta t})$$

$$4.343 = B(e^{-(0.139)(20)})$$

$$B = 4.343(e^{(0.139)(20)}) = (4.343)(16.119) = 70 \ \mu g/mL$$

Thus, by joining the y-intercept (70 μg/mL at 0 hour) and the terminal concentration point (4.343 mcg/mL at 20 hr), one obtains the straight line having the y-intercept = B.

Feathering the Curve

To obtain the straight line which represents absorption phase of the drug, the technique of feathering or the method of residuals is used. The feathering technique used for resolution of plasma profile obtained following extravascular administration is similar to the feathering technique used in feathering the plasma profile obtained in a two-compartment model following intravenous administration (see Chapter 10), except that each plasma concentration point provided in the data is subtracted from its respective plasma concentration point on the straight line having the y-intercept = B. The reason for reversing the subtraction procedure is explained to obtain equation (12-1):

$$A(e^{-\alpha t}) = B(e^{-\beta t}) - C$$

Therefore, to generate the plasma concentration points of the mono-exponential term, $Ae^{-\alpha t}$, which describes the absorption phase of the drug, each plasma concentration point provided in the data must be subtracted from its respective plasma concentration point on the straight line having the y-intercept = B.

For example, to feather the first plasma concentration point at 1 hour, the concentration of drug in plasma provided in the data is subtracted from the concentration of drug in plasma at 1 hour on the straight line having the y-intercept = B. The plasma concentration at 1 hour on the straight line having y-intercept = B is determined using the first-order rate equation as follows:

$$\ln C_t = \ln B - \beta t \tag{12-10}$$

Substituting the values of B = 70 μg/mL, β = 0.139/h and t = 1 h, into equation (12-10):

$$\ln C_t = \ln 70 - (0.139)(1) = 4.2485 - 0.139 = 4.1095$$

$$C_t = \text{inverse } \ln 4.1095 = 60.916\ \mu\text{g/mL}$$

The residual concentration at 1 hour is obtained by subtracting from this concentration, the concentration at 1 hour provided in the data. Therefore, residual concentration at 1 hour is:

$$60.916\ \mu\text{g/mL} - 26.501\ \mu\text{g/mL} = 34.415\ \mu\text{g/mL}$$

Similarly, plasma concentration at 2 hour on the straight line having y-intercept = B is determined by substituting the values of B, β and t (= 2 h) into equation (12-10). Substitution yields:

$$\ln C_t = \ln 70 - (0.139)(2) = 4.2485 - 0.278 = 3.9705 = 3.9705$$

$$C_t = \text{inverse } \ln 3.9705 = 53.011$$

Therefore, the residual concentration at 2 hours is:

$$53.011\ \mu\text{g/mL} - 36.091\ \mu\text{g/mL} = 16.920\ \mu\text{g/mL}.$$

The remaining data points that did not fall on the straight line representing the elimination phase are now feathered similarly. The concentration points obtained by the method of residuals (residual concentration points) are plotted as squares in Figure 12-4. If these points indicate a linear relationship then a straight line, which best describes these points is drawn. Depending on the scatter exhibited by the residual concentrations, the straight line may be drawn using eyeball judgment or by using regression analysis. The y-intercept of this straight line is A. If the dosage form released its drug soon after it was administered, the two y-intercepts (B and A) will be identical.

In Example 12-1, both intercepts have the same value (B = A = 70 μg/mL).

Table 12-1 shows the calculations and methodology involved in obtaining residual concentrations using the feathering technique (method of residuals) for the data provided in Example 12-1.

Rate Constant of Absorption

The rate constant of absorption (K_a) is obtained from the slope of straight line, which represents the absorption phase:

$$K_a = \alpha = -\text{ slope}$$

$$= \frac{\ln 70\ \mu\text{g/mL} - \ln 0.1\ \mu\text{g/mL}}{(0 - 9.22)}$$

$$= 0.71/\text{h}$$

Apparent Volume of Distribution

Since 100% of the administered dose was absorbed, therefore F = 1.

Substituting the values of F, B, D, α (= K_a) and β = (K) into equation (12-8), we have

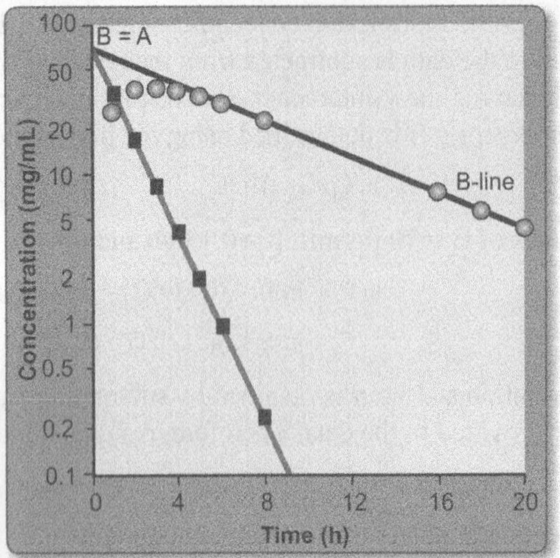

Fig. 12-4 Feathering of data in Example 12-1

Table 12-1 Feathering of data in Example 12-1

Time (h)	*Concentration (data points) (μg/mL)* ●	*(Data from B-line)–(data point) (μg/mL)*	*= New point* (μg/mL)* ■
1	26.501	60.916 – 26.501	= 34.415
2	36.091	53.011 – 36.091	= 16.920
3	37.512	46.131 – 37.512	= 8.319
4	36.055	40.145 – 36.055	= 4.090
5	32.924	34.935 – 32.924	= 2.011
6	29.413	30.402 – 29.413	= 0.989
8	22.784	23.023 – 22.784	= 0.239
16	7.571	**	
18	5.734	**	
20	4.343	**	

* New points are shown as squares in Fig. 12-4

** Not feathered because these points were used to draw the B-line

$$V_d = \frac{(F)(D)(\alpha)}{(B)(\alpha - \beta)}$$

$$= \frac{(1)(500\ \text{mg})(0.71/\text{h})}{(70\ \mu\text{g/mL})(0.71/\text{h} - 0.139/\text{h})}$$

$$= \frac{355{,}000\ \mu\text{g/h}}{39.97\ \mu\text{g/(h} \times \text{mL)}}$$

$$= 8{,}881.66\ \text{mL}$$

Area Under the Curve

According to equation (12-9), total area under the curve is:

$$AUC_{total} = \frac{B}{\beta} - \frac{A}{\alpha}$$

$$= \frac{70\ \mu g/mL}{0.139/h} - \frac{70\ \mu g/mL}{0.71/h}$$
$$= 405.005\ \mu g \times h/mL$$

Description of the Model

This model can be described schematically or by an equation.

Schematic representation: Figure 12-5 shows a schematic of the one-compartment model following extravascular administration of a 500 mg dose. The first-order rate constant of absorption is 0.71/h and the first-order rate constant of elimination is 0.139/h. The apparent volume of the central compartment (which is also the apparent volume of distribution) is 8.88 L.

Description by equation: The plasma profile is described by the equation:

$$C = 70(e^{-0.139t}) - 70(e^{-0.71t})$$

In this equation, B = A = 70, $\beta = 0.139$ and $\alpha = 0.71$

TIME OF MAXIMUM CONCENTRATION (T_{MAX})

The time of maximum concentration of drug in plasma (t_{max}) is that time when the administered drug dose attains its maximum or peak concentration (C_{max}), i.e. T_{max} is the time when C_{max} occurs. In some plasma profiles, a fairly sharp peak is noticed and t_{max} can be estimated easily. Some other plasma profiles may exhibit a plateau rather than a sharp peak, because data points around peak concentration were not obtained in the study. When it is difficult to read t_{max} from the plasma profile, or in the absence of the plasma profile, an equation is used to calculate t_{max}.

Calculation of T_{max}

The equation for calculating the time of maximum concentration of drug in the plasma, t_{max}, can be derived from equation (12-5).

Equation (12-5) may be written as:

$$C = \frac{(F)(D)(\alpha)}{(V_d)(\alpha - \beta)}\left(e^{-\beta t}\right) - \frac{(F)(D)(\alpha)}{(V_d)(\alpha - \beta)}\left(e^{-\beta t}\right) \quad (12\text{-}11)$$

The time at which the concentration of drug in plasma reaches a peak value can be estimated by differentiating equation (12-11) with respect to time. Since the rate constants of absorption (α) and the rate constant of elimination (β) are the only variables in equation (12-11), therefore, differentiation of equation (12-11) yields

$$\frac{dC}{dt} = \frac{(F)(D)(\alpha^2)}{(V_d)(\alpha - \beta)}\left(e^{-\alpha t}\right) - \frac{(F)(D)(\alpha)(\beta)}{(V_d)(\alpha - \beta)}\left(e^{-\beta t}\right) \quad (12\text{-}12)$$

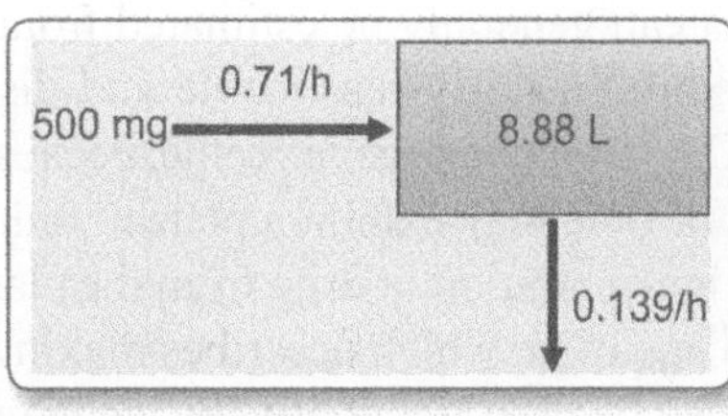

Fig. 12-5 Schematic representation of data in Example 12-1

At t_{max}, the time of maximum concentration, the concentration of drug in the plasma reaches a maximum value. Therefore, at the time of maximum concentration (t_{max}), the value of the function dc/dt is equal to 0.

Setting equation (12-12) equal to 0 and substituting t′ for t_{max} into equation (12-12):

$$0 = \frac{(F)(D)(\alpha^2)}{(V_d)(\alpha - \beta)}(e^{-\alpha t'}) - \frac{(F)(D)(\alpha)(\beta)}{(V_d)(\alpha - \beta)}(e^{-\beta t'})$$

$$\frac{(F)(D)(\alpha^2)}{(V_d)(\alpha - \beta)}(e^{-\alpha t'}) = \frac{(F)(D)(\alpha)(\beta)}{(V_d)(\alpha - \beta)}(e^{-\beta t'}) \tag{12-13}$$

The terms F, D, V_d and $(\alpha - \beta)$ are common to both sides of equation (12-13). Canceling the common terms on both sides, equation (12-13) reduces to

$$(\alpha^2)(e^{-\alpha t'}) = (\alpha)(\beta)(e^{-\beta t'})$$

$$(\alpha)(e^{-\alpha t'}) = (\beta)(e^{-\beta t'})$$

$$\frac{\alpha}{\beta} = \frac{e^{-\beta t'}}{e^{-\alpha t'}} \tag{12-14}$$

Taking natural logarithms on both sides and substituting t_{max} for t′ into equation (12-14),

$$\ln \alpha - \ln \beta = -(\beta)(t_{max}) - (\alpha)(t_{max})$$

$$\ln \alpha - \ln \beta = (t_{max})(\alpha - \beta)$$

$$t_{max} = \frac{\ln \alpha - \ln \beta}{\alpha - \beta} = \frac{\ln K_a - \ln K}{K_a - K} \tag{12-15}$$

Example 12-2 From the data given in Example 12-1, calculate the time when administered drug dose reaches its maximum concentration in plasma.

Solution

From the pharmacokinetic parameters found in Example 12-1, the first-order rate constant of absorption, $\alpha = K_a = 0.71/h$ and the first-order rate constant of elimination, $\beta = K = 0.139/h$.

Substituting these values into equation (12-15), we have

$$t_{max} = \frac{\ln K_a - \ln K}{K_a - K}$$

$$= \frac{\ln 0.71/h - \ln 0.139\ h}{0.71/h - 0.139/h}$$

$$= \frac{(-0.3425) - (-1.9733)}{0.571/h} = \frac{1.6308}{0.571/h} = 2.856\ h$$

MAXIMUM PLASMA CONCENTRATION

The maximum concentration of drug in plasma, C_{max}, is the highest (peak) concentration of drug in the plasma attained by the administered drug dose. In most cases, the highest (peak) concentration of drug in the plasma can generally be estimated from the plasma profile itself, because the plasma profile may exhibit a fairly reasonable and discernible peak. However, sometimes it is difficult to estimate C_{max} from the plasma profile, because the plot of concentration of drug in the plasma as a function of time may exhibit a plateau rather than a sharp peak.

When it is difficult to read peak concentration of drug from the plasma profile, or the plasma profile is not available, one uses an equation, which describes maximum concentration of drug in the plasma. This equation may also be used if a relatively accurate determination of C_{max} is desired. This equation describes C_{max} in terms of plasma concentration at the time of maximum concentration of drug in the plasma (t_{max}).

By definition, t_{max} is the time when drug attains its maximum concentration in plasma. Therefore, concentration of drug in plasma at t_{max} is the maximum concentration of drug in the plasma. Therefore, equation (12-2) can be used to calculate C_{max} as described below.

Calculation of C_{max}

The maximum concentration of drug in plasma, by definition, is the concentration of drug in plasma at t_{max}. Therefore, the maximum concentration of drug in plasma is determined by substituting t_{max} in place of t into equation (12-2). Using t′ to indicate t_{max}, the equation for calculating C_{max} is:

$$C = B(e^{-\beta t'}) - B(e^{-\alpha t'}) = B(e^{-\beta t'} - e^{-\alpha t'}) \tag{12-16}$$

Example 12-3 From the data given in Example 12-1, calculate maximum concentration of drug in plasma attained after administration of the dose.

Solution

The time of maximum concentration, t_{max}, calculated in Example 12-2 was 2.856 hr. Substituting the values of B = 70 μg/mL, α = 0.71/h, β = 0.139/h and t′ = 2,856 h into equation (12-16),

$$\begin{aligned} C &= B(e^{-\beta t'} - e^{-\alpha t'}) \\ &= (70\ \mu g/mL)(e^{-(0.139/h)(2.856\ h)} - e^{-(0.71/h)(2.856\ h)}) = 37.85\ \mu g/mL \end{aligned}$$

LAG-TIME

Lag-time (L) is the time that elapses between administration of the dosage form and the appearance of drug in systemic circulation. Because conventional dosage forms are designed to release the drug soon after administration, the drug starts appearing in plasma exhibiting negligible lag-time. In such cases, the linear segment of absorption phase obtained after resolution of plasma profile is drawn, so as to force the y-intercept of absorption phase to be equal to y-intercept B. A typical plasma profile resolved into elimination and absorption phases exhibiting no lag-time is shown in Example 12-1 (Figure 12-4), as well as in Figure 12-6.

Some dosage forms are designed to release their active ingredient some time after administration of the dosage form (e.g. delayed-release dosage forms). These dosage forms exhibit lag-time. In the case of dosage forms which exhibit lag-time, the linear segment of the absorption phase of the plasma profile obtained after feathering the data produces a y-intercept A, which is greater than the y-intercept of the back-extrapolated elimination phase (y-intercept B). In other words, the two linear segments of the plasma profile obtained after feathering of the plasma profile do not intersect at the y-axis. Instead, the point of intersection lies on the right-hand side of y-axis. The dosage form in such cases is said to exhibit a lag-time.

Figure 12-7 is a typical plasma profile, which exhibits lag-time.

Factors Responsible for Lag-time

By definition, lag-time is the time that elapses between the administration of the drug dose and the appearance of drug in the systemic circulation. Lag-time may be exhibited due to a variety of factors, but most commonly lag-time is exhibited by delayed-release dosage forms. Delayed-release dosage forms are intended to release their contents at a time later than the time

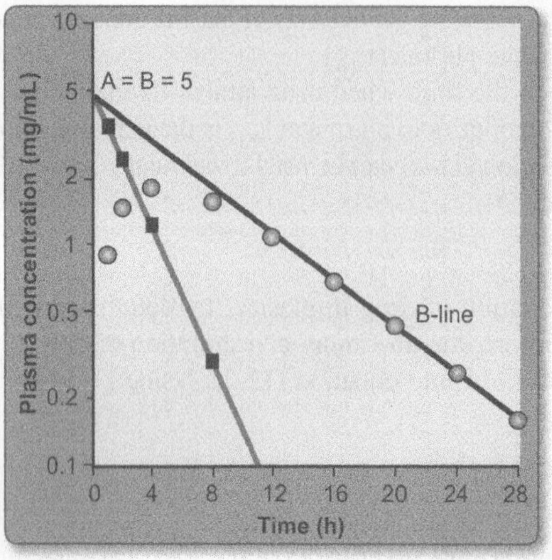

Fig. 12-6 Plasma profile exhibiting no lag-time

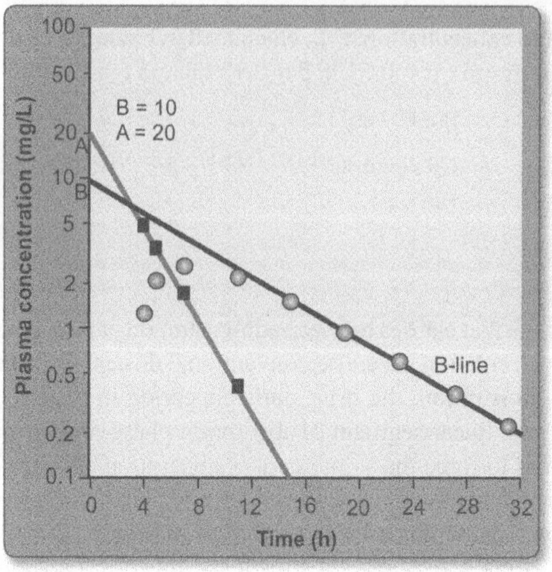

Fig. 12-7 Plasma profile exhibiting lag-time

of administration of the dosage form. However, some conventional dosage forms, although intended to release their drug almost immediately after administration of the drug dose, exhibit delay in the release of drug either in some patients only or in the same patient, but on different occasions. In these situations, the delay in the release of drug from the dosage form delays the appearance of drug in systemic circulation. In some other cases, the dosage form may release the drug soon after administration, but there may be a substantial delay in the appearance of drug in the systemic circulation.

The delayed release of drug from these dosage form and/or delayed appearance of drug in systemic circulation may be due to various reasons, but mainly because of factors, which are related to the dosage form, the patient and/or the drug itself.

Dosage Form-related Factors: Dosage form related factors refer to those factors that are specific to the design of the formulation, which govern the release pattern of the drug from the dosage form. For example, delayed-release dosage forms and enteric-coated dosage forms are designed not to release their drug immediately after administration. The intentional delayed release of drug from these dosage forms is intended to prevent or minimize degradation of drug due to one or more of the following reasons:

i. Prevent drug degradation due to gastric secretions and enzymes
ii. Prevent drug degradation due to the acidic environment of stomach
iii. Prevent release of drug in the stomach when a patient is prone to gastric irritation and/or discomfort by the drug.

Patient-related Factors: Patient-related factors for the delayed release of drug from the dosage form include those instances, where the release of drug from the dosage form is delayed in certain specific situations only. Examples of situations, which may delay the release of drug from the dosage form include the presence of certain disease conditions, or other pathological conditions existing in the patient at the time of drug administration. In these cases, the presence of specific disease condition or a pathological condition may affect release of drug from the dosage form. Once the offending disease or the existing pathological condition becomes non-existent, the drug is then released without exhibiting lag-time.

Drug-related Factors: Some foods and/or other drugs may interact with the administered drug dose or dosage form and consequently delay the release and/or absorption of the administered drug. In these situations, lag-time is exhibited only when the interacting food and/or drug is present at the time when the drug dose is administered and lag-time is not exhibited when the drug is administered in the absence of interacting food and/or drug. Hence, drug absorption in the patient may not be reproducible, because drug absorption becomes dependant on the presence or absence of the interacting foods and/or other drugs.

Calculation of Lag-time

Lag-time (L) may be approximated from the resolved plasma profile by reading the time of intersection of the linear segments of the absorption and elimination phases (the two straight lines having the y-intercept B and y-intercept A). When the plasma profile is not available, but the equation describing the plasma profile is known, lag-time can be calculated as follows:

As mentioned earlier, equation (12-1) describes the plasma profile of an extravascularly administered dose.

$$C = B(e^{-\beta t}) - A(e^{-\alpha t})$$

By definition, lag-time is time that elapses between administration of dosage form and appearance of drug in plasma, i.e. the drug starts appearing in plasma at the end of lag-time. Thus, in the presence of lag-time, time 0 is actually that time when the lag-time ends and not the time of drug administration.

Putting C = 0 and t = L (for lag-time) into equation (12-1), we have

$$0 = B(e^{-\beta L}) - A(e^{-\alpha L})$$

$$B(e^{-\beta L}) = A(e^{-\alpha L}) \quad (12\text{-}17)$$

Taking natural logarithms on both sides of equation (12-17),

$$\ln B - \beta L = \ln A - \alpha L$$

$$\alpha L - \beta L = \ln A - \ln B$$

$$L(\alpha - \beta) = \ln A - \ln B$$

Solving for the lag-time, L, we obtain

$$L = \frac{\ln A - \ln B}{\alpha - \beta} = \frac{\ln A - \ln B}{K_a - K} \quad (12\text{-}18)$$

$$L = \frac{\ln \frac{A}{B}}{\alpha - \beta} = \frac{\ln \frac{A}{B}}{K_a - K} \quad (12\text{-}18)$$

Example 12-4 Calculate lag-time (time between administration of the drug dose and appearance of drug in the systemic circulation) from the plasma profile shown in Figure 12-7.

Solution

From Figure 12-7, B = 10 mg/L and A = 20 mg/L

$$K = \beta = -\frac{\ln 10\text{ mg/L} - \ln 0.2\text{ mg/L}}{(0-32)\text{h}} = \frac{3.9120}{-32\text{h}} = 0.1223/\text{h}$$

$$K_a = \alpha = -\frac{\ln 20\text{ mg/L} - \ln 0.1\text{ mg/L}}{(0-15)\text{h}} = \frac{5.2983}{-15\text{h}} = 0.3532/\text{h}$$

Substituting these values into equation (12-18), lag-time is

$$L = \frac{\ln A - \ln B}{\alpha - \beta} = \frac{\ln 20\text{ mg/L} - \ln 10\text{ mg/L}}{0.3532/\text{h} - 0.1223/\text{h}} = \frac{0.6931}{0.2309/\text{h}} = 3\text{ h}$$

Equation in the Presence of Lag-time

When a dosage form exhibits lag-time, the calculation of plasma drug concentration during lag-time will yield a negative value. Since the drug is not available for absorption during lag-time, the absorption of drug does not begin, until after the lag-time is over and therefore, concentration of drug in the plasma during lag-time is 0. Hence, the true plasma profile of the drug is its plasma profile in the absence of lag-time, i.e. the true plasma profile starts at the end of the lag-time, not at the time of administration of the drug. Therefore, the true plasma profile is obtained if the y-axis is moved to the right-hand side to a point, which represents the start of the absorption of the drug, i.e. if the y-axis starts at the point, of intersection of the two linear segments of the resolved plasma profile. Since lag-time ends at the time indicated by the point of intersection of the two linear segments of the resolved plasma profile, the true plasma profile would start at the end of lag-time rather than at the time of administration of the dosage form (Fig. 12-8).

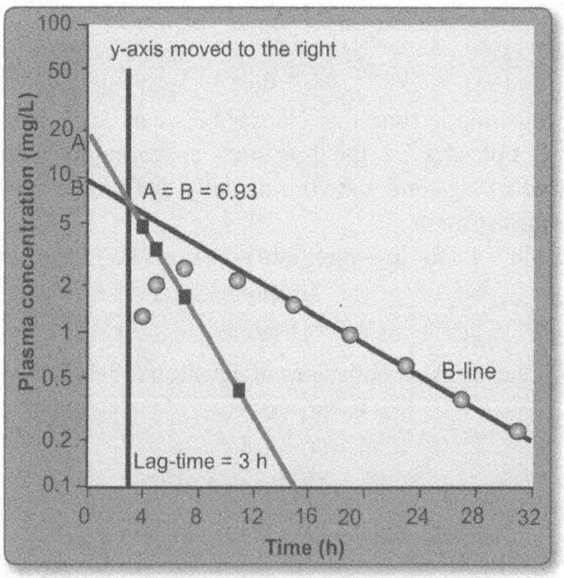

Fig. 12-8 Plasma profile exhibiting lag-time

The y-intercepts A and B obtained after resolution of plasma profile, which exhibits lag-time are not the true y-intercepts, but are apparent y-intercepts of the plasma profile. Since the drug starts appearing in plasma at the end of lag-time, the true (or corrected) y-intercepts A and B are calculated from the apparent y-intercepts A and B using lag-time (L) as the time when the drug starts appearing in the plasma. The corrected y-intercept B, therefore, is equal to the y-intercept at time L and similarly, the corrected y-intercept A is equal to the y-intercept at time L. The corrected y-intercepts B and A can be calculated as follows:

$$\text{Corrected B} = B^* = (\text{apparent B})(e^{-\beta L}) \qquad (12\text{-}19)$$

$$\text{Corrected A} = A^* = (\text{apparent A})(e^{-\alpha L}) \qquad (12\text{-}20)$$

Equations (12-19) and (12-20) can be rearranged as follows:

$$\text{Apparent B} = \frac{B^*}{e^{-\beta L}}, \text{ and Apparent A} = \frac{A^*}{e^{-\alpha L}} \qquad (12\text{-}21)$$

Substituting the values of apparent B and apparent A from equation (12-21) into equation (12-1):

$$C = \frac{(B^*)}{e^{-\beta L}}\left(e^{-\beta t}\right) - \frac{(A^*)}{e^{-\alpha L}}\left(e^{-\alpha t}\right)$$

$$C = B^* e^{-\beta t + \beta L} - A^* e^{-\alpha t + \alpha L} \qquad (12\text{-}22)$$

$$= B^* e^{-\beta(t - L)} - A^* e^{-\alpha(t - L)}$$

Example 12-5 Using the plasma profile shown in Figure 12-7, compute the equation which describes this profile in the presence of lag-time.

Solution

The equation which describes the plasma profile shown in Figure 12-7 is developed from the calculations shown in Example 12-4. According to these calculations

$$C = 10(e^{-0.1223t}) - 20(e^{-0.3532t})$$

Since L = 3 h, the corrected values of B and A are calculated using equations (12-19) and (12-20),

$$\text{Corrected B} = B^* = (\text{apparent B})(e^{-\beta L}) = (10)(e^{-(0.1223/\text{h})(3\text{ h})}) = 6.93\ \mu\text{g/mL, and}$$

$$\text{Corrected A} = A^* = (\text{apparent A})(e^{-\alpha L}) = (20)(e^{-(0.3532/\text{h})(3\text{ h})}) = 6.93\ \mu\text{g/mL}$$

$$\text{Corrected B} = \text{Corrected A} = 6.93\ \mu\text{g/mL}$$

The new equation in the presence of lag-time is

$$C = 6.93(e^{-0.1223(t-3)}) - 6.93(e^{-0.3532(t-3)})$$

Calculation of $T_{max(L)}$

Equation (12-15) cannot be used to calculate the time of maximum concentration of drug in plasma in the presence of lag-time, because this equation calculates the time of maximum concentration when the absorption of drug begins almost immediately after administration. Equation (12-15) drug is based only on the rate constants of absorption and elimination and does not take into account the values of either of the two y-intercepts A and B. Since the actual time of maximum concentration in the presence of lag-time is in effect equal to the time of maximum concentration of drug in plasma in the absence of lag-time (t_{max}) plus the lag-time

(L), the equation for calculating the time of maximum plasma concentration of drug in plasma in the presence of lag-time can be derived as follows:

$$t_{max(L)} = t_{max} + L \tag{12-23}$$

Substituting the value of t_{max} from equation (12-15) and the value of L from equation (12-18) into equation (12-23):

$$t_{max(L)} = \frac{\ln\alpha - \ln\beta}{\alpha - \beta} + \frac{\ln A - \ln B}{\alpha - \beta}$$

$$t_{max(L)} = \frac{\ln\frac{\alpha}{\beta} + \ln\frac{A}{B}}{\alpha - \beta} = \frac{\ln\alpha - \ln\beta + \ln A - \ln B}{\alpha - \beta} \tag{12-24}$$

This equation can also be derived from equation (12-22) using the same rationale, as was used in deriving equation (12-15) for t_{max} from equation (12-5).

Calculation of $C_{max(L)}$

Equation (12-1) can be modified to calculate maximum concentration of drug in the plasma in the presence of lag-time ($C_{max(L)}$) by substituting $t_{max(L)}$ for t. Using t″ to indicate $t_{max(L)}$, equation (12-1) takes the form:

$$C_{max(L)} = B(e^{-\beta t''}) - A(e^{-\alpha t''})$$

Similarly, equation (12-22) can also be modified to calculate $C_{max(L)}$ by substituting $t_{max(L)}$ for t. Using t" to indicate $t_{max(L)}$, equation (12-22) takes the form:

$$C_{max(L)} = (B^*)(e^{-\beta(t''-L)}) - (A^*)(e^{-\alpha(t''-L)}) \tag{12-25}$$

Example 12-6 The following data were obtained when a 500 mg dose of an antibiotic was given orally. Calculate pharmacokinetic parameters, assuming 100% of the administered dose was absorbed.

Time (h)	Concentration (μg/mL)	Time (h)	Concentration (μg/mL)
2	3.915	16	1.814
4	8.005	18	1.344
6	7.321	20	0.996
8	5.803	24	0.546
10	4.403	28	0.300

Solution

The data in this Example range between a low concentration of 0.300 μg/mL at 28 hour and a high concentration of 8.005 mcg/mL at 4 hr. A 2-cycle semi-log paper will be needed to plot the data and an additional cycle may be needed for feathering the data.

The data, plotted on a 3-cycle semi-log paper are shown as circles in Figure 12-9.

The y-intercept, B, of this straight line is determined using the first-order rate equation:

$$B = Ce^{\beta t}$$

$$= (0.3\ \mu g/mL)(e^{(0.15/h)(28\ h)})$$

$$= (0.3\ \mu g/mL)(66.6863) = 20\ \mu g/mL$$

A straight line is drawn by joining the points 20 μg/mL at 0 hour and 0.3 μg/mL at 28 hours. This straight line represents the elimination phase of the plasma profile.

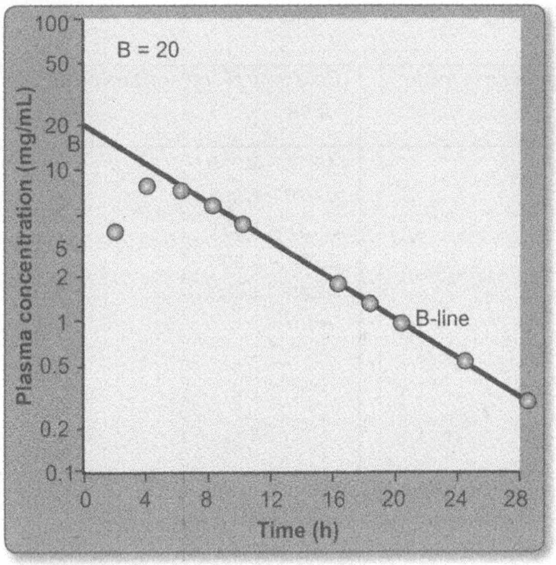

Fig. 12-9 Plot of data in Example 12-6

Feathering the Curve

The plasma profile is feathered with respect to the straight line having the y-intercept = B. To feather the first concentration point, the concentration at 2 hours on the straight line having B as the y-intercept is subtracted from the data concentration at 2 hours. The plasma concentration at 2 hour on the straight line having y-intercept = B is determined using the first-order rate equation:

$$C = Be^{-\beta t} = (20\ \mu g/mL)(e^{-(0.15/h)(2\ h)}) = (20\ \mu g/mL)(0.7408) = 14.816\ \mu g/mL$$

Therefore, residual concentration at 2 hour is the concentration at 2 hour on the straight line having B as the y-intercept minus the 2 hour concentration provided in the data:

$$14.816\ \mu g/mL - 3.915\ \mu g/mL = 10.901\ \mu g/mL$$

Similarly, concentration at 4 hour on the straight line having y-intercept = B is:

$$C = (20\ \mu g/mL)(e^{-(0.15/h)(4\ h)})$$
$$= (20\ \mu g/mL)(0.5488) = 10.976\ \mu g/mL$$

Therefore, residual concentration at 4 hour is the concentration at 4 hours on the straight line having B as the y-intercept minus the 4 hour concentration provided in the data:

$$10.976\ \mu g/mL - 8.005\ \mu g/mL = 2.971\ \mu g/mL$$

The remaining data points that did not fall on the straight line representing the elimination phase are feathered similarly.

The calculations involved in computing the residual concentrations for the data provided in Example 12-6 are shown in Table 12-2. It will be noticed that the concentration terms at 16, 18, 20, 24 and 28 hours were not feathered, because these concentration terms were found on straight line having B as the y-intercept.

The residual concentrations thus obtained represent absorption phase and are plotted as squares in Figure 12-10. The residual concentration points indicate a linear relationship, therefore, a straight line which best describes these points is drawn. This straight line represents absorption.

The y-intercept of this straight line is A (= 40 μg/mL) and rate constant of this straight line is rate constant of absorption, α:

Table 12-2 Feathering of data in Example 12-6

Time (h)	*Concentration (data points) (μg/mL)* ●	*(Data from B-line) – (Data point) (μg/mL)*	*= New point* (μg/mL)* ■
2	3.915	14.816 – 3.915	= 10.901
4	8.005	10.976 – 8.005	= 2.971
6	7.321	8.131 – 7.321	= 0.810
8	5.803	6.024 – 5.803	= 0.221
10	4.403	4.463 – 4.403	= 0.106
16	1.814	**	
18	1.344	**	
20	0.996	**	
24	0.546	**	
28	0.300	**	

* New points are shown as squares in Figure 12-10

** Not feathered because these points were used to draw B-line

$$K_a = \alpha = -\text{ slope}$$

$$= -\frac{\ln 40\ \mu g/mL - \ln 0.221\ \mu g/mL}{(0-8)h} = \frac{5.198}{-8h} - = 0.65/h$$

Pharmacokinetic Parameters

The equation describing the plasma profile in Figure 12-9 is:

$$C = 20(e^{-0.15t}) - 40(e^{-0.65t})$$

The pharmacokinetic parameters associated with this plasma profile are calculated as follows:

Rate Constant of Elimination: The rate constant of elimination is $\beta = 0.15/h$.

Biological Half-life: Biological half-life is calculated using equation (12-7):

$$t_{1/2} = \frac{0.693}{\beta} = \frac{0.693}{0.15/h} = 4.62\ h$$

Rate Constant of Absorption: The rate constant of absorption, α is 0.65/h

Lag-time: The lag-time is calculated using equation (12-18)

$$L = \frac{\ln A - \ln B}{\alpha - \beta} = \frac{\ln 40\ \mu g/mL - \ln 20\ \mu g/mL}{0.65/h - 0.15/h} = \frac{0.693}{0.5/h} = 1.386\ h$$

$t_{max(L)}$: There are two methods that can be used to calculate the time of maximum concentration of drug in plasma in the presence of lag-time.

1. Using equation (12-24): Substituting A = 40 μg/mL, B = 20 μg/mL, $\alpha = 0.65/h$ and $\beta = 0.15/h$ into equation (12-24) gives:

$$t_{max(L)} = \frac{\ln A - \ln B + \ln\alpha - \ln\beta}{\alpha - \beta}$$

$$= \frac{\ln 40\ \mu g/mL - \ln 20\ \mu g/mL + \ln 0.65/h - \ln 0.15/h}{0.65/h - 0.15/h}$$

$$= \frac{2.1595}{0.5/h} = 4.319\ h$$

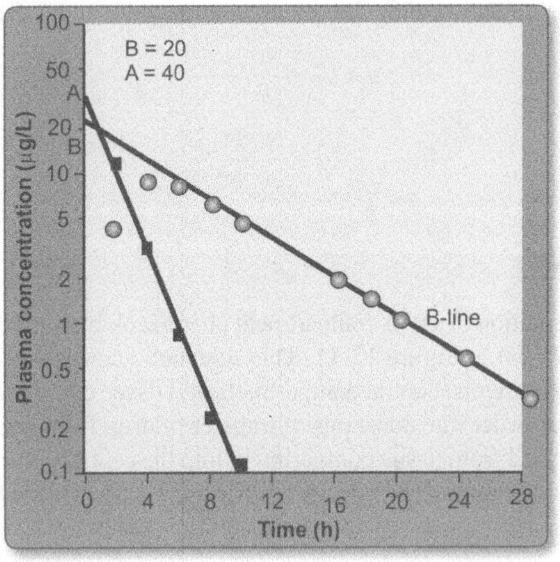

Fig. 12-10 Resolution of data in Example 12-6

2. $t_{max(L)}$ can also be determined by adding lag-time (L) to t_{max}.

$$t_{max(L)} = t_{max} + L = \frac{\ln\alpha - \ln\beta}{\alpha - \beta} + L$$

$$= \frac{\ln 0.65/h - \ln 0.15/h}{0.65 - 0.15/h} + 1.386\ h = 2.933\ h + 1.386\ h = 4.319\ h$$

$C_{max(L)}$: According to equation (12-25), maximum concentration in the presence of lag-time is

$$C_{max(L)} = B(e^{-\beta t''}) - A(e^{-\alpha t''})$$

$$= (20\ \mu g/mL)(e^{-(0.15/h)(4.319\ h)}) - (40\ \mu g/mL)(e^{-(0.65/h)(4.319\ h)})$$

$$= 10.463\ \mu g/mL - 2.415\ \mu g/mL$$

$$= 8.048\ \mu g/mL$$

Apparent Volume of Distribution: To calculate V_d in the presence of lag-time, the corrected values of B and A are determined using equations (12-19) and (12-20) respectively.

$$\text{Corrected B} = B^* = B(e^{-\beta L})$$

$$= (20\ \mu g/mL)(e^{-(0.15/h)}) = 16.25\ \mu g/mL, \text{ and}$$

$$\text{Corrected A} = A^* = B(e^{-\alpha L})$$

$$= (40\ \mu g/mL)(e^{-(0.65/h)(1.386\ h)}) = 16.25\ \mu g/mL$$

$$\text{Corrected B} = \text{Corrected A} = 16.25\ \mu g/mL$$

The apparent volume of distribution can now be determined using equation (12-8):

$$V_d = \frac{(F)(D)(\alpha)}{(B)(\alpha - \beta)}$$

$$= \frac{(1)(500\ mg)(0.65/h)}{(16.25\ \mu g/mL)(0.65 - 0.15)/h} = \frac{325\ mg}{8.125\ mg/L} = 40\ L$$

Area Under the Curve: Substituting the values of corrected B and A, β and α into equation (12-9):

$$AUC_{total} = \frac{B^*}{\beta} - \frac{A}{\alpha}$$

$$= \frac{16.25\ \mu g/mL}{0.15/h} - \frac{16.25\ \mu g/mL}{0.65/h} = 83.33\ \mu g \times h/mL$$

TWO-COMPARTMENT MODEL

A schematic representation of a two-compartment pharmacokinetic model following extravascular administration is shown in Figure 12-11. This schematic consists of two rectangular boxes to represent two-compartments: central compartment and tissue compartment reversibly connected to each other by first-order rate constants of transfer of drug from central compartment into the tissue compartment and from tissue compartment into the central compartment. Drug input takes place in the central compartment and drug elimination also takes place from central compartment.

The Plasma Profile

After first-order absorption, the drug appears in the central compartment, followed by first-order distribution into the tissue compartment and first-order elimination from the central compartment. It is assumed that the rate of absorption of drug is greater than its elimination rate. The plasma profile of the two-compartment pharmacokinetic model following extravascular administration differs from the plasma profile seen in two-compartment model after intravenous administration, in that the extravascular profile shows an absorption phase. Also, the post-absorptive phase is not linear (as was seen in extravascular one-compartment model), but it is biphasic as was seen in two-compartment intravenous model.

Figure 12-12 is a typical plasma profile of a two-compartment model following extravascular administration. This profile consists of the following four segments:

a. The initial portion of the graph reflects absorption, beginning of distribution and elimination. This is followed by distribution of drug between the central and tissue compartments.
b. The peak reflects distribution equilibrium, elimination and beginning of decline of absorption.
c. The middle portion of the biphasic curve represents distribution, predominance of elimination,.and for all practical purposes, termination of absorption.
d. The terminal portion of the plasma profile represents essentially elimination.

This plasma profile therefore, consists of the following first-order processes:

a. First-order absorption of drug.
b. First-order elimination of drug.
c. First-order distribution of drug between the central and the tissue compartment.

The plasma profile of a drug, which confers the characteristics of a two-compartment model upon the body is described by the following tri-exponential equation:

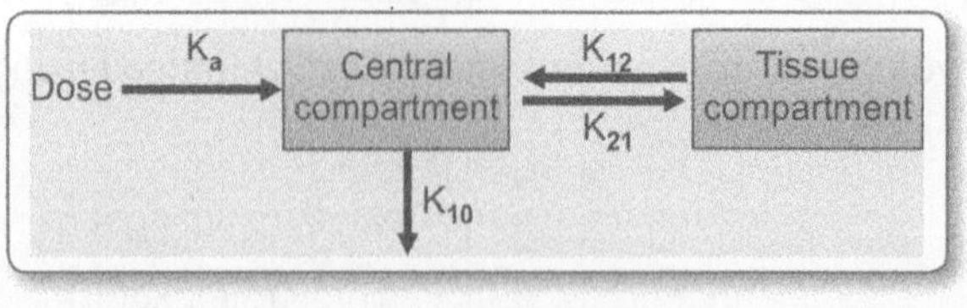

Fig. 12-11 Schematic representation of two-compartment model, extravascular administration

$$C = B(e^{-\beta t}) + P(e^{-\pi t}) - A(e^{-\alpha t}) \quad (12\text{-}26)$$

where,

C = plasma drug concentration

B = the y-intercept of the back-extrapolated terminal phase of plasma concentration data

β = the hybrid micro-constant obtained from the slope of the linear segment having the y-intercept = B

P = the y-intercept of back-extrapolated terminal phase of linear segment obtained after first feathering

π = the hybrid micro-constant obtained from the slope of the linear segment having the y-intercept = P

A = y-intercept of back-extrapolated terminal phase of linear segment obtained after second feathering

α = the hybrid micro-constant obtained from the slope of the linear segment having the y-intercept = A

t = time.

In this equation, $\alpha > \pi > \beta$. The hybrid micro-constant α represents the rate constant of absorption (K_a) and the hybrid micro-constant β represents the rate constants of elimination of drug from the body.

At time 0, the value of each exponential term in equation (12-26) is equal to 1 and equation (12-26) becomes

$$C = B + P - A \quad (12\text{-}27)$$

Also, at time 0, the concentration of drug in plasma is 0 and equation (12-27) becomes

$$0 = B + P - A$$

Therefore,

$$A = B + P \quad (12\text{-}28)$$

For most conventional dosage forms designed to release their active ingredient for immediate and rapid absorption, A is always equal to (B + P). Since, by definition, π and α are greater than β, it follows that some time after drug administration, the two terms, $Pe^{-\pi t}$ and $Ae^{-\alpha t}$, on the right-hand side of equation (12-26) will approach 0, while the first term, $Be^{-\beta t}$, will still retain some finite value. At that time then, equation (12-26) will reduce to equation (12-3) as follows:

$$C = B(e^{-\beta t})$$

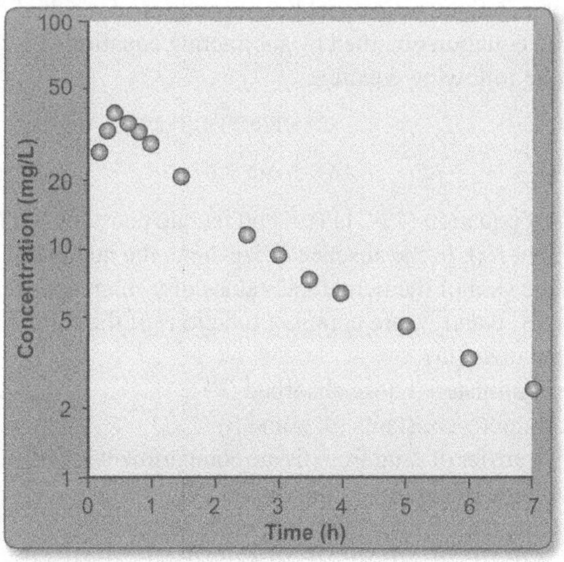

Fig. 12-12 Typical plasma profile of two-compartment model following extravascular administration

Equation (12-3) describes the terminal linear phase of the tri-exponential plasma profile. The rate constant of this linear phase is β and when back-extrapolated to y-axis, it yields a y-intercept = B.

Feathering

A series of residual concentration-time values are obtained when one subtracts concentration-time values on the back-extrapolated line from the corresponding true plasma concentration-time values (data points). Some residual concentration values obtained by subtraction will have a negative value. These are from the data points, which fall below the back-extrapolated straight line. The data points which fall above the back-extrapolated straight line yield positive values.

The equation describing the time course of these residual concentration values (C′) is obtained by subtracting equation (12-3) from equation (12-26):

$$C' = \{B(e^{-\beta t}) + P(e^{-\pi t}) - A(e^{-\alpha t})\} - B(e^{-\beta t})$$

$$C' = P(e^{-\pi t}) - A(e^{-\alpha t}) \quad (12\text{-}29)$$

The subtraction process yields positive residual concentration values when $Pe^{-\pi t}$ values are greater than $Ae^{-\alpha t}$ values and negative values when $Ae^{-\alpha t}$ values are greater than $Pe^{-\pi t}$ values. A plot of the positive residual concentrations (C′) versus time, described by equation (12-29), yields a biexponential curve, because of two monoexponential terms on the right-hand side of equation (12-29). Since the micro-constant α is assumed to be greater than π, it follows that as t increases, the exponential term $Ae^{-\alpha t}$ in equation (12-29) will decrease. When t becomes sufficiently large, $Ae^{-\alpha t}$ will approach 0, while $Pe^{-\pi t}$ will still have a finite value and equation (12-29) will then become

$$C' = P(e^{-\pi t}) \quad (12\text{-}30)$$

Equation (12-30) describes terminal linear phase of the residual curve, with a rate constant = π and when back-extrapolated to time 0, it yields a y-intercept = P. The residual curve remaining after the linear terminal portion produced the y-intercept P can be resolved further. This is accomplished by subtracting residual concentration values C' in equation (12-29) from the corresponding concentration-time values on the straight line, which upon back-extrapolation gave the y-intercept = P. Subtraction yields a second set of residual concentration-time values (C″), described by an equation obtained by subtracting equation (12-29) from equation (12-30). Subtraction yields the following equation:

$$C'' = P(e^{-\pi t}) - \{P(e^{-\pi t}) - A(e^{-\alpha t})\}$$

$$C'' = A(e^{-\alpha t}) \quad (12\text{-}31)$$

The y-intercept of equation (12-31) is A and its rate constant is α (which represents the rate constant of absorption, K_a). In the absence of lag-time, the numerical value of the y-intercept A should be equal to the sum of the numerical values of y-intercepts B and P.

The y-intercepts B, P and A, are complex functions of the following:

a. The administered dose (D)
b. Fraction of the administered dose absorbed (F)
c. The three hybrid micro-constants (α, π and β)
d. Rate constant of transfer of drug from tissue compartment into the central compartment (K_{21})
e. The apparent volume of central compartment (V_c)

The three y-intercepts B, P and A are defined as follows:

$$B = \frac{(F)(D)(\alpha)(K_{21} - \beta)}{(V_c)(\alpha - \beta)(\pi - \beta)} \quad (12\text{-}32)$$

$$B = \frac{(F)(A)(K_{21} - \beta)(\alpha - \pi)}{(A - K_{21})(\beta - \pi)} \quad (12\text{-}33)$$

$$P = \frac{(F)(D)(\alpha)(K_{21} - \pi)}{(V_c)(\alpha - \pi)(\beta - \pi)} \quad (12\text{-}34)$$

$$P = \frac{(F)(A)(K_{21} - \pi)(\alpha - \beta)}{(\beta - \pi)(\alpha - K_{21})} \quad (12\text{-}35)$$

$$A = \frac{(F)(D)(\alpha)(K_{21} - \alpha)}{(V_c)(\alpha - \pi)(\beta - \alpha)} \quad (12\text{-}36)$$

Pharmacokinetic Parameters

Several equations have been proposed to calculate the pharmacokinetic parameters associated with a two-compartment model. Some of these are given here.

Rate Constants

There are four first-order rate constants associated with a two-compartment extravascular pharmacokinetic model. These are:

i. Rate constant of absorption ($K_a = \alpha$)
ii. Rate constant of elimination of drug from the central compartment (K_{10})
iii. Rate constant of transfer of drug from the central compartment into the tissue compartment (K_{12})
iv. Rate constant of transfer of drug from the tissue compartment into the central compartment (K_{21}).

These rate constants are determined using the following equations:

$$K_{21} = \frac{P\beta + \beta\pi}{A} \quad (12\text{-}37)$$

$$K_{10} = \frac{A}{(P/\pi) + (B/B)} = \frac{A\pi\beta}{P\beta + \beta\pi} \quad (12\text{-}38)$$

$$K_{10} = \frac{\pi\beta}{K_{21}} \quad (12\text{-}39)$$

$$K_{12} = \frac{(P\beta)(\beta - \pi)^2}{(A)(P\beta + B\pi)} \quad (12\text{-}40)$$

$$K_{12} = \pi + \beta - K_{21} - K_{10} \quad (12\text{-}41)$$

Biological Half-life

The biological half-life is determined using the hybrid rate constant β and not K_{10}, because the hybrid rate constant β reflects drug elimination from the body, while K_{10} describes elimination of drug from the central compartment:

$$t_{1/2} = \frac{0.693}{\beta} \quad (12\text{-}7)$$

Volumes of Distribution

The apparent volumes of distribution in a two-compartment model are:

i. The apparent volume of central compartment.
ii. The apparent volume of tissue compartment.

The total volume of distribution is the sum total of apparent volumes of distribution of drug in the central and tissue compartments.

$$V_d = V_c + V_t$$

The apparent volume of central compartment and the apparent volume (total) of distribution of the drug are calculated using the following equations and the apparent volume of the tissue compartment is determined by difference:

$$V_d = \frac{(D)(F)(\alpha)(\alpha - K_{21})}{(A)(\alpha - \beta)(\alpha - \pi)} \qquad (12\text{-}42)$$

$$V_d = \frac{(V_c)(K_{12} + K_{21})}{K_{21}} \qquad (12\text{-}43)$$

$$V_d = \frac{(V_c)(\alpha - \beta)}{K_{21} - \beta} \qquad (12\text{-}44)$$

$$V_t = V_d - V_c \qquad (12\text{-}45)$$

Area Under the Curve

The total area under the curve is determined using the equation: *BPA*

$$AUC_{total} = \frac{B}{\beta} + \frac{P}{\pi} - \frac{A}{\alpha} \qquad (12\text{-}46)$$

The following Example illustrates the evaluation of a two-compartment model.

Example 12-7 The following data were obtained after administration of single 500 mg dose of a drug. Plot the data and calculate pharmacokinetic parameters associated with this profile. Describe the pharmacokinetic model that fits these data. Assume F = 1.

Time (h)	*Concentration (mg/L)*	*Time (h)*	*Concentration (mg/L)*	*Time (h)*	*Concentration (mg/L)*
0.2	27.23	0.8	32.24	3.5	7.45
0.3	32.70	1.0	28.70	4.0	6.43
0.4	47.47	1.5	20.86	5.0	4.58
0.5	35.64	2.5	11.94	6.0	3.31
0.6	35.07	3.0	9.5	7.0	2.45

Solution

The concentrations provided in the data range from a low value of 2.45 mg/L at 7 hour to a high value of 47.47 mg/L at 0.4 hour. To plot the data on a semi-logarithmic graph paper, one will need two cycles to plot the concentration terms of the data. The first logarithmic cycle will be used to plot concentrations ranging between 1 mg/L and 10 mg/L. This cycle will accommodate the concentration terms between 2.45 mg/L and 9.5 mg/L. The second logarithmic cycle will be used to plot concentrations ranging between 10 mg/L and 100 mg/L. This cycle will accommodate concentrations between 11.94 mg/L and 47.47 mg/L. An additional logarithmic cycle may be needed to plot residual concentrations generated by the process of feathering. Therefore, a three-cycle semi-logarithmic graph paper should be used to plot the data.

The data would be plotted on the upper two logarithmic cycles (the second and the third logarithmic cycles), leaving the bottom logarithmic cycle (the first logarithmic cycle) to plot the points generated by the process of feathering. This means that the concentration on the bottom cycle (first cycle) of the semi-logarithmic graph paper will begin at 0.1 mg/L. This cycle will end (and the next cycle will begin) at 1 mg/L. The second cycle will end (and the third cycle will begin) at 10 mg/L, and the third cycle will end (top of the semi-logarithmic cycle) at 100 mg/L.

A plot of the data on a three-cycle semi-logarithmic graph paper is shown in Figure 12-13. The plasma profile in Figure 12-13 does not exhibit a smooth curve, indicating that the data do not appear to fit one-compartment model. The plasma profile exhibits a distributive phase. Therefore, this profile may reflect a multi-compartment model and will be feathered according to a multi-compartment model and not according to the method used in one-compartment model.

In order to strip the curve to produce linear segments, the terminal concentration points are used to determine the first-order rate constant and the y-intercept of the first linear segment. The first-order rate constant of this straight line is the hybrid rate constant β and is determined from the slope of the terminal concentration point as follows:

The terminal concentration points are:

$$x_1 = 3.31 \text{ mg/L}, y_1 = 6 \text{ h, and } x_2 = 2.45 \text{ mg/L}, y_2 = 7 \text{ h}$$

A straight line obtained by joining these points will result in a linear segment (i.e. B-line of Figure 12-13) and the rate constant of this linear segment is the hybrid rate constant β.

Using natural logarithms, the hybrid rate constant β is equal to the negative slope of the straight line represented by the terminal concentration points.

$$\beta = -\text{Slope} = -\frac{\ln 3.31 \text{ mg/mL} - \ln 2.45 \text{ mg/mL}}{(6-7)\text{h}}$$

$$\beta = -\text{Slope} = -\frac{1.1969 - 0.8961}{(6-7)\text{h}} = -\frac{0.3}{-1\text{h}} = 0.3/\text{h}$$

The value of the y-intercept of this straight line is determined using the first-order rate constant β and either of the terminal concentration points (concentration 2.45 mg/L at 7 hr, or concentration 3.31 mg/L at 6 hr). The y-intercept of this straight line is B and can be calculated by rearranging equation (12-3) as follows:

$$C = Be^{-\beta t}$$

which upon rearrangement gives

$$B = Ce^{\beta t}$$

Substituting the values of concentration at 7 hours (C = 2.45 mg/L, t = 7 h) into this equation:

$$\text{y-intercept } B = Ce^{\beta t} = (2.45 \text{ mg/L})(e^{(0.3/\text{h})(7 \text{ h})}) = (2.45 \text{ mg/L})(8.1662) = 20 \text{ mg/L}$$

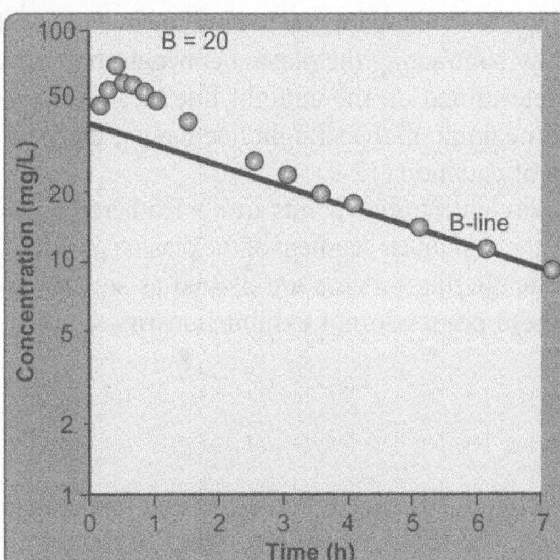

Fig. 12-13 Plot of data in Example 12-7

The y-intercept, B, can also be calculated by substituting C = 3.31 mg/L, the value of concentration at 6 hours.

$$\text{y-intercept, } B = Ce^{\beta t} = (3.31\ \text{mg/L})(e^{(0.3/\text{h})(6\ \text{h})}) = (3.31\ \text{mg/L})(6.0496) = 20\ \text{mg/L}$$

A straight line is now drawn by connecting the two points, 20 mg/L on the y-axis (y-intercept) and 2.45 mg/L at 7 hour (the data point used to determine the first-order rate constant). It is noticed that many concentration points provided in the data did not fall on this straight line. Those concentration points, which did not fall on this straight line are now feathered with respect to this straight line. Feathering of concentration points with respect to this straight line (straight line having y-intercept = B) produces new concentration points (the residual concentration points).

Feathering

It is noticed that many data points did not fall on this straight line. Those concentration points that did not fall on this straight line are now feathered with respect to this straight line (straight line having y-intercept = B, i.e. B-line of Figure 12-13). Feathering produces new concentration points (residual concentrations). The residual concentrations are obtained by subtracting the concentration at each time point on the straight line having the y-intercept = B from the corresponding plasma concentration provided in the data. For example, at 0.2 hr, plasma concentration on the straight line having the y-intercept = B, is calculated using the modified form of equation (12-3):

$$C = Be^{-\beta t} = (20\ \text{mg/L})(e^{-(0.3/\text{h})(0.2\ \text{h})}) = (20\ \text{mg/L})(0.9418) = 18.84\ \text{mg/L}$$

The residual concentration at 0.2 hour is obtained by subtracting concentration at 0.2 hour on the straight line having the y-intercept = B from the 0.2 hour plasma concentration provided in the data:

$$\text{Residual concentration at 0.2 hour} = 27.23\ \text{mg/L} - 18.84\ \text{mg/L} = 8.39\ \text{mg/L}$$

Similarly, concentration at 0.3 hour on the straight line having the y-intercept = B is calculated using the modified form of equation (12-3):

$$C = (2.0\ \text{mg/L})(e^{-(0.3/\text{h})(0.3\ \text{h})}) = (20\ \text{mg/L})(0.9139) = 18.28\ \text{mg/L}$$

And the residual concentration at 0.3 hour is obtained by subtracting the concentration at 0.3 hour on the straight line having the y-intercept = B from the 0.3 hour concentration provided in the data, i.e.

$$\text{Residual concentration at 0.3 hour} = 32.70\ \text{mg/L} - 18.28\ \text{mg/L} = 14.42\ \text{mg/L}$$

The process of determining residual concentrations for the data points, which did not fall on the straight line having the y-intercept = B is continued. The residual concentration at each time point is calculated by subtracting the plasma concentration provided in the data from the plasma concentration determined on the straight line having the y-intercept B. The plasma concentration for each time point on the straight line having the y-intercept B is determined by using the modified form of equation (12-3).

The 6 hours and 7 hours concentration points are not feathered because these two concentration points were used to draw the first linear segment of the plasma profile. The residual concentrations points generated by the feathering process are plotted as squares in Figure 12-14. As can be seen in Figure 12-14, these points do not exhibit linearity, confirming a multi-compartment pharmacokinetic model.

Second Feathering

The feathering process is continued using terminal concentration points of residual concentrations (squares in Figure 12-14). The first-order rate constant of the terminal two points of residual concentrations (shown as squares in Figure 12-14) is π and is determined from the slope of the terminal residual concentration points (squares in Figure 12-14).

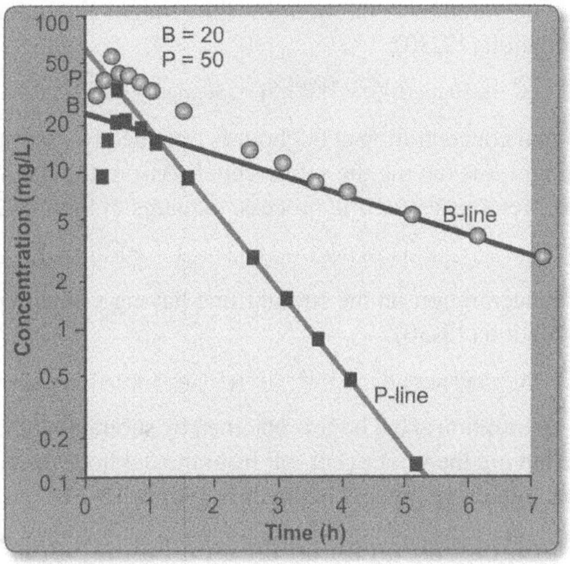

Fig. 12-14 Feathering of data in Example 12-7

The first-order rate constant π is calculated as follows:

$$\pi = -\text{Slope} = -\frac{\ln 0.41\ \text{mg/L} - \ln 0.12\ \text{mg/L}}{(4-5)\text{h}}$$

$$\pi = -\text{Slope} = -\frac{-0.8916-(-2.1203)}{(4-5)\text{h}} = -\frac{1.2}{-1\text{h}} = 1.2/\text{h}$$

The y-intercept, P, of the back-extrapolated straight line, which will be obtained by joining these two residual concentration points is calculated by substituting the values of first-order rate constant, π = 1.2/h and residual concentration = 0.41 mg/L at 4 hours into equation (12-30) as follows:

According to equation (12-30), $C' = P(e^{-\pi t})$, therefore,

$$P = C'(e^{\pi t})$$

Substituting the values of C′ = 0.41 mg/L at t = 4 h and π = 1.2/h, one gets

$$P = C'(e^{\pi t}) = (0.41\ \text{mg/L})(e^{(1.2/\text{h})(4\ \text{h})}) = (0.41\ \text{mg/L})(121.51) = 50\ \text{mg/L}$$

The two points, y-intercept 50 mg/L and concentration 0.41 mg/L at 4 hours are joined to produce a straight line.

The residual concentration points shown as squares are now feathered with respect to the straight line having the y-intercept = P = 50 mg/L (i.e. P-line of Figure 12-14), to obtain a second set of residual concentration points.

The second residual concentration at 0.2 hour is obtained by subtracting concentration at 0.2 hour on the straight line having y-intercept = P from the 0.2 hour plasma concentration obtained during the previous feathering process (squares in Figure 12-14).

At 0.2 hour, the plasma concentration on the straight line having y-intercept = P is calculated using equation (12-30):

$$C = (50\ \text{mg/L})(e^{-(1.2/\text{h})(0.2\ \text{h})}) = (50\ \text{mg/L})(0.7866) = 39.33\ \text{mg/L}$$

Therefore, residual concentration at 0.2 hour is

$$39.33\ \text{mg/L} - 8.39\ \text{mg/L} = 30.94\ \text{mg/L}.$$

Similarly, the concentration at 0.3 hour on the straight line having the y-intercept = P is calculated using equation (12-30):

$$C = (50 \text{ mg/L})(e^{-(1.2/h)(0.3\ h)}) = (50 \text{ mg/L})(0.6977) = 34.88 \text{ mg/L}$$

Therefore, residual concentration at 0.3 hour is obtained by subtracting the concentration at 0.3 hour on the straight line having the y-intercept = P from the 0.3 hour plasma concentration obtained during the previous feathering process, (squares in Figure 12-14):

$$34.88 \text{ mg/L} - 14.42 \text{ mg/L} = 20.46 \text{ mg/L}$$

And at 0.4 hr, concentration on the straight line having y-intercept = P, is calculated using calculated using equation (12-30):

$$C = (50 \text{ mg/L})(e^{-(1.2/h)(0.4\ h)}) = (50 \text{ mg/L})(0.6188) = 30.94 \text{ mg/L}$$

The residual concentration at 0.4 hour is obtained by subtracting the concentration at 0.4 hour on the straight line having the y-intercept = P from the 0.4 hour plasma concentration obtained during the previous feathering process (squares in Figure 12-14):

$$\text{Residual concentration at 0.4 hour} = 43.31 \text{ mg/L} - 29.73 \text{ mg/L} = 13.58 \text{ mg/L}$$

The process of feathering is continued to obtain residual concentrations for all points that did not fall on the straight line having y-intercept = P.

The second set of residual concentrations obtained during the second feathering process is now plotted on the graph paper. These residual concentrations are shown as triangles in Figure 12-15. The residual concentrations plotted as triangles appear to exhibit a fair degree of linearity and a straight line, which best describes these points can be drawn using eyeball judgment.

It should be pointed out that in order to draw the straight line representing the y-intercept = A, more emphasis should be placed on the residual concentrations obtained during the earlier segment of feathering (plasma profile) than those obtained during the terminal segment of feathering. This is because, when the plasma profile is feathered for the first time, some residual concentrations may have been rounded off. If subtraction yielded a large number, rounding it off incorporates a very small error in the residual concentration. But, if subtraction yields a very small number, then rounding it off may incur a significantly large error in the residual concentration generated by the feathering process.

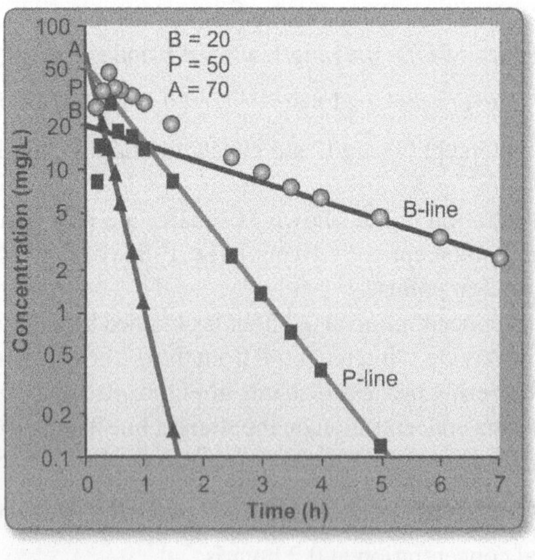

Fig. 12-15 Resolution of data in Example 12-7

For example, if the residual concentration during the first feathering was actually 32 mg/L, but it was rounded off to 30 mg/L (an error of 2 mg/L), the concentration point plotted on the semi-logarithmic graph paper does not pose a significant error, because these two points are so close to each other that either point would not affect the decision of linearity. If all other residual concentration points indicate linearity, then for all practical purposes, either of these two points will be on, or close to, the straight line.

The second feathering process, on the other hand, generates a relatively smaller number of concentration points. For example, some plasma profiles may yield only 3 or 4 concentration points. Also, the residual concentrations are obtained as a result of subtracting a relatively small number from another small number. Therefore, if the residual concentration point during the second feathering was actually 0.1 mg/L, but it got rounded off to 0.3 mg/L (the same error of 2 units), the concentration point plotted on the semi-logarithmic graph paper is more likely to appear non-linear when actually the point may be on the straight line. Therefore, during the second feathering, residual concentrations obtained for the later segment of the plasma profile may not necessarily be accurate, but may exhibit approximate values of the residual concentrations.

The first-order rate constant of the straight line generated during the second feathering is α and the y-intercept of this straight line is A. According to equation (12-28), B + P = A, therefore, y-intercept, A is

$$A = B + P = 20 \text{ mg/L} + 50 \text{ mg/L} = 70 \text{ mg/L}$$

The first-order rate constant, α, of this straight line (having the y-intercept = A) is determined from the slope of this straight line using two points, which fall on this straight line. The y-intercept is chosen as one of these two points.

The first-order rate constant of this linear segment is:

$$\alpha = -\text{slope} = -\frac{\ln 70 \text{ mg/L} - \ln 5.98 \text{ mg/L}}{(0 - 0.6)} = -\frac{2.46}{-0.6\text{h}} = 4.1/\text{h}$$

Table 12-3 details the calculation of residual concentrations for the data.

Table 12-3 Feathering of data in Example 12-7

Time (h)	*C (mg/L) (Data points)* ●	*$Be^{-\beta t}$ (mg/L) (B-line)*	*$C' = C - Be^{-\beta t}$ (mg/L)* ■	*$Pe^{-\pi t}$ (mg/L) (P-line) mg/L*	*$C'' = Pe^{-\pi t} - C' = Ae^{-\alpha t}$ (mg/L)* ▲
0.2	27.23	18.84	8.39	39.33	30.94
0.3	32.70	18.28	14.42	34.88	20.46
0.4	47.47	17.74	29.73	43.31	13.58
0.5	35.64	17.21	18.43	27.44	9.01
0.6	35.07	16.71	18.36	24.34	5.98
0.8	32.24	15.73	16.51	19.14	2.63
1.0	28.70	14.82	13.88	15.06	1.18
1.5	20.86	12.75	8.11	8.26	0.15
2.5	11.94	9.45	2.49	2.49	-
3.0	9.50	8.13	1.37	1.37	-
3.5	7.45	6.70	0.75	0.75	-
4.0	6.43	6.02	0.41	0.41	-
5.0	4.58	4.46	0.12	0.12	-
6.0	3.31	3.31	-	-	-
7.0	2.45	2.45	-	-	-

Resolution of plasma profile in Example 12-7 yields the following y-intercepts and first-order rate constants:

$$B = 20\ mg/L,\ P = 50\ mg/L,\ A = 70\ mg/L,\ \beta = 0.3/h,\ \pi = 1.2/h \text{ and } \alpha = 4.1/h$$

These values are now used to calculate the various pharmacokinetic parameters associated with this model.

Calculation of Parameters

Rate Constants

$$K_a = \alpha = 4.1/h$$

$$K_{21} = \frac{P\beta + B\pi}{A}$$

$$= \frac{(50\ mg/L)(0.3/h) + (20\ mg/L)(1.2/h)}{70\ mg/L}$$

$$= \frac{15/h + 24/h}{70} = \frac{39/h}{70} = 0.5571/h$$

$$K_{21} = \frac{A}{(P/\pi) + (B/\beta)} = 0.6462/h$$

$$K_{10} = \frac{\pi\beta}{K_{21}}$$

$$= \frac{(1.2/h)(0.3/h)}{0.5571/h} = \frac{0.36/h}{0.5571} = 0.6462/h$$

$$K_{12} = \frac{(PB)(\beta - \pi)^2}{A(P\beta + B\pi)}$$

$$= \frac{(50\ mg/L)(20\ mg/L)(0.3/h - 1.2/h)^2}{(70\ mg/L)\{(50\ mg/L)(0.3/h) + (20\ mg/L)(1.2/h)\}}$$

$$= \frac{810/h}{2730} = 0.2967/h$$

$$K_{12} = \pi + \beta - K_{21} - K_{10}$$

$$= 1.2/h + 0.3/h - 0.5571/h - 0.6462/h = 0.2967/h$$

$$t_{1/2} = \frac{0.693}{\beta} = \frac{0.693}{0.3/h} = 2.31\ h$$

$$V_c = \frac{(F)(D)(\alpha)(\alpha - K_{21})}{(A)(\alpha - \pi)(\alpha - \beta)}$$

$$= \frac{(1)(500\ mg)(4.1/h)(4.1/h - 0.5571/h)}{(70\ mg/L)(4.1/h - 1.2/h)(4.1/h - 0.3/h)}$$

$$= \frac{7,262.945\ mg}{771.4\ mg/L} = 9.415\ L$$

$$V_d = \frac{(V_c)(\alpha - \beta)}{K_{21} - \beta} = \frac{(9.415\ L)(4.1/h - 0.3/h)}{0.5571/h - 0.3/h}$$

$$= \frac{35.7770\ L}{0.2571} = 139.156\ L$$

$$V = V_d - V_c$$

$$= 139.156\ L - 9.415\ L = 129.741\ L$$

$$AUC_{total} = \frac{B}{\beta} + \frac{P}{\pi} - \frac{A}{\alpha}$$

$$= \frac{20\ \text{mg/L}}{0.3/\text{h}} + \frac{50\ \text{mg/L}}{1.2/\text{h}} - \frac{70\ \text{mg/L}}{4.1/\text{h}}$$

$$= 66.67\ \text{mg} \times \text{h/L} + 41.67\ \text{mg} \times \text{h/L} - 17.07\ \text{mg} \times \text{h/L} = 91.27\ \text{mg} \times \text{h/L}$$

Description of the Model

The two-compartment model following extravascular administration can be described either schematically or by an equation.

Schematic Representation

A schematic of the data in Example 12-7 is shown in Figure 12-16. This schematic representation shows that a 500 mg dose was administered extravascularly and the drug, upon administration, confers the characteristics of a two-compartment model on the body. From this schematic, the following information is obtained:

a. The rate constant of absorption (K_a) of the drug is 4.1/h.
b. The rate constant of elimination of drug from the central compartment (K_{10}) is 0.6462/h.
c. The rate constant of transfer of drug from central compartment into tissue compartment (K_{12}) is 0.2967/h.
d. The rate constant of transfer of drug from tissue compartment into central compartment (K_{21}) is 0.5571/h.
e. The apparent volume of distribution of the central compartment (V_c) is 9.415 L.
f. The apparent volume of distribution of the tissue compartment (V_t) is 129.741 L.
g. This means that the apparent volume of distribution of the drug (V_d) is 9.415 L + 129.741 L = 139.156 L.

From this schematic, one cannot "read" the biological half-life. It cannot be determined because the rate constant of elimination of drug from the body (K) is not indicated. However, one can compute rate constant of elimination of drug from the body (K) from the parameters derived from this schematic.

Description by Equation

The plasma profile of data in Example 12-7 is described by the equation:

$$C = 20(e^{-0.3t}) + 50(e^{-1.2t}) - 70(e^{-4.1t}).$$

The drug, upon extravascular administration as a bolus dose, confers upon the body the characteristics of a two-compartment pharmacokinetic model. The numerical values of the hybrid rate constants are as follows:

α = exponent with the largest absolute value = 4.1, β = the exponent with the smallest absolute value = 0.3 and π = (by the process of elimination) is the remaining third exponent having a numerical value = 1.2.

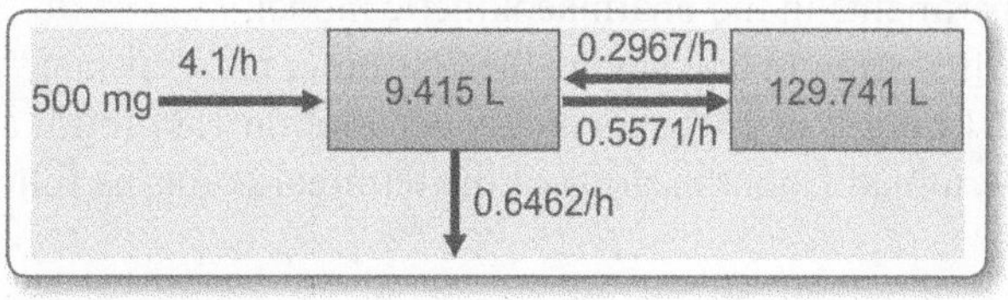

Fig. 12-16 Schematic representation of data in Example 12-7

Similarly, the numerical values of the three y-intercepts are: B, the y-intercept corresponding to the hybrid micro-constant $\beta = 20$, P, the y-intercept corresponding to the hybrid micro-constant $\pi = 50$ and A, the y-intercept corresponding to hybrid micro-constant $\alpha = 70$.

Example 12-7 illustrated the resolution of data of a two-compartment model, where the feathering process yielded positive values for all residual concentration terms. However, in some cases, especially in those cases, where the rate of drug absorption is relatively smaller (although greater than the rate constant of elimination) and the drug distribution into the second compartment is relatively rapid, the feathering process may result in some negative values. In such cases, the negative values are not plotted on the graph paper, but are used in calculations involving feathering.

The following Example illustrates such a case.

Example 12-8 Plasma concentration following administration of a single 500 mg dose of a drug is shown below. Calculate various pharmacokinetic parameters assuming 60% of the administered dose is absorbed.

Time (h)	*Concentration (mg/L)*	*Time (h)*	*Concentration (mg/L)*	*Time (h)*	*Concentration (mg/L)*
0.2	5.31	1.6	17.46	8.0	5.21
0.4	9.25	2.0	16.80	10.0	3.62
0.5	10.80	3.0	14.82	12.0	2.58
12.11	4.0	11.88	13.0	2.14	
15.51	5.0	9.69	14.0	1.84	

Solution

To plot the data provided in this Example on a semi-logarithmic graph paper, a two-cycle semi-logarithmic graph paper will be needed. One logarithmic cycle will run from 1 mg/L to 10 mg/L and the second logarithmic cycle will be from 10 mg/L to 100 mg/L, because:

a. One cycle will be needed to plot concentration points ranging between the values of 17.40 mg/L and 10.80 mg/L. This cycle will have a concentration range from 100 mg/L to 10 mg/L.
b. A second cycle will be needed to plot concentration points ranging between the values of 9.69 mg/L and 1.84 mg/L. This cycle will have a concentration range from 10 mg/L to 1 mg/L.

However, a three-cycle semi-logarithmic graph paper is used here, because a third cycle may be needed to plot those residual concentrations, which may have values less than 1 mg/L. Since the highest concentration is 17.40 mg/L, one does not expect that any of the y-intercepts will have values greater than 100 mg/L. If it was expected that one of the y-intercept may have a value greater than 100 mg/L, then a four-cycle semi-logarithmic graph paper would be used in order to "read" the y-intercept on the fourth cycle (the cycle at the top of the paper). The data would be plotted on the second and third cycle, leaving the first cycle (on the bottom of the paper) to plot residual concentrations.

A plot of data on a three-cycle semi-logarithmic graph paper is shown in Figure 12-17. This plasma profile shows extravascular administration and since the plasma profile did not result in a smooth curve, it appears that this profile may not reflect a simple one-compartment model, but a multi-compartment pharmacokinetic model. It should be realized that the nature of the plot (smooth curve or not-so-smooth curve) does not necessarily provide an indication as to the number of compartments in the pharmacokinetic model.

To obtain the first straight line having the first-order rate constant = β, the terminal two points (concentration 2.14 mg/L at 13 hours and concentration 1.84 mg/L at 14 hours) are used. The value of β is determined from the slope of the terminal points as follows:

$$\beta = -\text{slope} = -\frac{\ln 2.14\ \text{mg/L} - \ln 1.84\ \text{mg/L}}{(13-14)\text{h}} = \beta = -\frac{0.151}{-1\ \text{h}} - = 0.151/\text{h}$$

The y-intercept of this straight line, B, is determined using the first-order rate equation (12-3) in its modified form.

$$B = C(e^{\beta t}) = (1.84\ \text{mg/L})(e^{(0.151/\text{h})(14\ \text{h})}) = (1.84\ \text{mg/L})(8.28) = 15\ \text{mg/L}$$

A straight line is drawn by joining the two points: y-intercept (15 mg/L at time 0) and concentration at 14 hours (1.84 mg/L at 14 hours).

Feathering

Curve stripping by feathering the data with respect to the straight line having y-intercept = B gives new points. As can be seen from Figure 12-17, some data points (concentration points from time 0 to 0.6 hour in this Example) are found below the back-extrapolated straight line (straight line having the y-intercept = B, i.e. B-line of Figure 12-17).

Subtraction of data points, which are found below the straight line (having B as the y-intercept), from the calculated concentration points, on the straight line having y-intercept = B will result in negative residual concentration points.

For example, the residual concentration at 0.2 hour is determined by subtracting the concentration at 0.2 hour on the straight line having B as the y-intercept (B-line) from the concentration provided in the data at 0.2 hour (5.31 mg/L):

$$\text{Residual concentration at 0.2 hour} = (5.31\ \text{mg/L}) - (15\ \text{mg/L})(e^{-(0.151/\text{h})(0.2\ \text{h})})$$

$$\text{Residual concentration at 0.2 hour} = (5.31\ \text{mg/L}) - (14.55\ \text{mg/L}) = -9.24\ \text{mg/L}$$

Similarly, residual concentration at 0.4 hour is:

$$\text{Residual concentration at 0.4 hour} = (9.25\ \text{mg/L}) - (15\ \text{mg/L})(e^{-(0.151/\text{h})(0.4\ \text{h})})$$

$$\text{Residual concentration at 0.4 hour} = (9.25\ \text{mg/L}) - (14.12\ \text{mg/L}) = -4.87\ \text{mg/L}$$

And, residual concentration at 0.5 hour is

$$\text{Residual concentration at 0.5 hour} = (10.08\ \text{mg/L}) - (15\ \text{mg/L})(e^{-(0.151/\text{h})(0.5\ \text{h})})$$

$$\text{Residual concentration at 0.5 hour} = (10.08\ \text{mg/L}) - (13.91\ \text{mg/L}) = -3.83\ \text{mg/L}$$

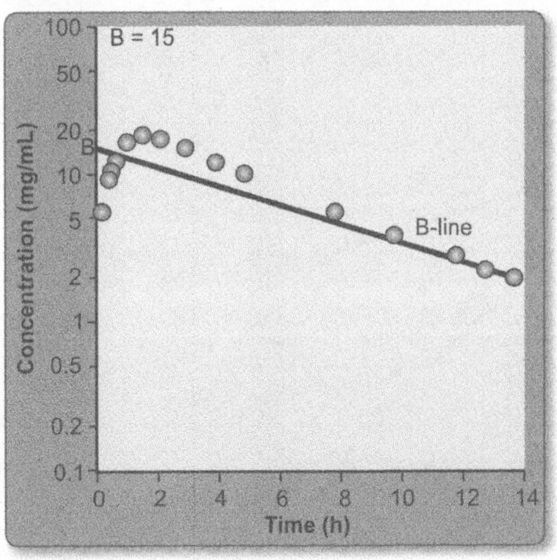

Fig. 12-17 Plot of data in Example 12-8

Since negative values cannot be plotted on a semi-logarithmic graph paper, therefore, residual concentration points having negative values will not be plotted, but will be used for determining second residual concentration points in the next feathering process. Hence, only those points, which have positive values (after the 0.6 hour concentration point) will be plotted.

The residual concentrations from 1 hour through 12 hours are calculated as follows:

$$\text{Residual concentration at 1.0 hour} = (15.51 \text{ mg/L}) - (15 \text{ mg/L})(e^{-(0.151/\text{h})(1.0 \text{ h})})$$

$$\text{Residual concentration at 1.0 hour} = (15.51 \text{ mg/L}) - (12.90 \text{ mg/L}) = 2.61 \text{ mg/L}$$

The residual concentrations yielding positive values are plotted as squares in Figure 12-18. As can be seen, the residual concentration points obtained by the feathering process did not result in a linear relationship. Therefore, the residual concentration points obtained during this feathering must be feathered again in order to develop the multi-compartment pharmacokinetic model.

The terminal points of the newly generated residual concentrations (second set of residual concentrations plotted as squares in Figure 12-18) are now used to draw the straight line with a first-order rate constant = π. The value of the first-order rate constant, π, is determined from the slope of the terminal two points obtained after the first feathering process as follows:

$$\pi = -\text{ slope} = -\frac{\ln 0.31 \text{ mg/L} - \ln 0.13 \text{ mg/L}}{(10-12)\text{h}} = -\frac{0.869}{-2\text{ h}} \quad -\pi = 0.435/\text{h}$$

The y-intercept of this straight line, P, is calculated by substituting concentration at either 12 hours or at 10 hours into the modified form of equation (12-30) as follows: substituting the relevant values for concentration at 12 hours (concentration = 0.13 mg/L and time = 12 hours):

$$P = C'(e^{\pi t}) = (0.13 \text{ mg/L})(e^{(0.435/\text{h})(2 \text{ h})}) = (0.13 \text{ mg/L})(184.93) = 24 \text{ mg/L}$$

Similarly, substituting the relevant values for concentration at 10 hours:

$$P = (0.31 \text{ mg/L})(e^{(0.435/\text{h})(10 \text{ h})}) = (0.31 \text{ mg/L})(77.478) = 24 \text{ mg/L}$$

Second Feathering

A second feathering process is needed to generate a new set of concentration points, which will be second residual concentration points. Residual concentrations having negative values obtained

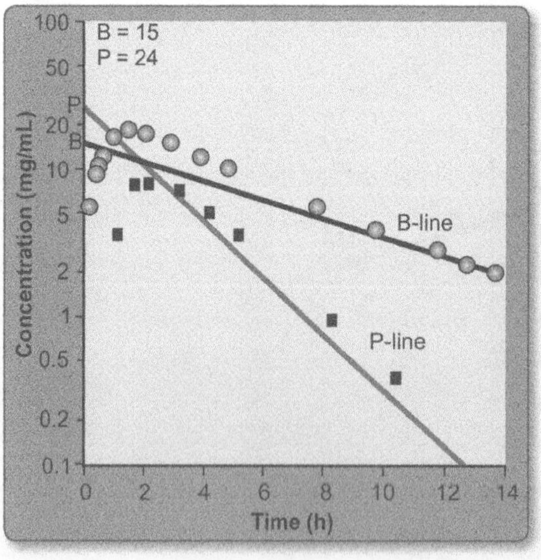

Fig. 12-18 Feathering of data in Example 12-8

during the first feathering process (not plotted on the graph, because negative concentration points cannot be plotted on a semi-logarithmic paper) are now used to calculate the new residual concentration points. For example, at 0.2 hour, the concentration on the straight line having the y-intercept = P, is calculated using equation (12-30):

$$C = P(e^{-\pi t}) = (24 \text{ mg/L})(e^{-(0.435/\text{hr})(0.2 \text{ hr})}) = 21.10 \text{ mg/L}$$

The second residual concentration at 0.2 hour is obtained by subtracting first residual concentration from the concentration at 0.2 hour on the straight line having y-intercept = P.

The second residual concentration at 0.2 hour = 21.10 mg/L – (– 9.24 mg/L) = 30.34 mg/L. This concentration point has a positive value and therefore, this point can now be plotted on the graph. Similarly, concentration at 0.4 hour on the straight line having y-intercept = P, is:

$$C = (24 \text{ mg/L})(e^{-(0.435/\text{h})(0.4 \text{ h})}) = 19.36 \text{ mg/L}$$

Therefore, the second residual concentration at 0.4 hour is obtained by subtracting first residual concentration from the concentration at 0.4 hour on the straight line having the y-intercept = P, i.e., second residual concentration at 0.4 hour = 19.36 mg/L – (– 4.87 mg/L) = 24.23 mg/L. This concentration point also has a positive value; therefore, this concentration point can also be plotted on the graph.

As shown above, subtraction of negative residual concentration points (obtained during the first feathering process of the plasma profile) from the concentration points on the straight line having P as the y-intercept, now become positive residual concentration points during the second feathering process. These residual concentration points having positive values can be plotted on the graph paper.

The process of second feathering is continued to generate a second set of residual concentration and the residual concentrations thus generated are plotted on the graph paper. The second set of residual concentration points are shown as triangles in Figure 12-19.

These residual concentration points (triangles) appear to exhibit linearity and therefore, no further feathering process is involved in resolution of the data. Thus, the plasma profile of the data given in this Example is completely resolved into three linear segments.

Since this is the final linear segment of the plasma profile, the rate constant of this straight line, by tradition, is α. This is the rate constant of absorption (K_a). The y-intercept of the straight line, which best describes the second set of residual concentration points (triangles) is A. The value of this intercept, according to equation (12-28) is:

$$A = B + P = 15 \text{ mg/L} + 24 \text{ mg/L} = 39 \text{ mg/L}$$

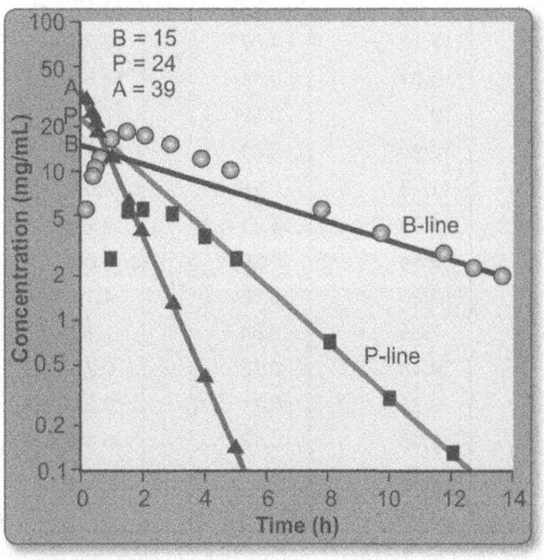

Fig. 12-19 Resolution of data in Example 12-8

In this Example, the second set of residuals does not exhibit too much scatter and therefore, eyeball judgment can be used to draw the best straight line that represents these points. The y-intercept of this straight line must have a value = A = 39 mg/L.

The first-order rate constant of this straight line, α, can be calculated using any two points, which fall on this straight line. Since the y-intercept of this straight line is known (39 mg/L) and residual concentration at 4 hour appears to be on this straight line, therefore, these two points (39 mg/L at time 0 and 0.42 mg/mL at 4 hr) are used to calculate the rate constant α of this straight line:

$$\alpha = -\text{slope} = -\frac{\ln 39\ \text{mg/L} - \ln 0.42\ \text{mg/L}}{(0-4)\,\text{hr}} = -\frac{4.53}{-4\ \text{h}} = 1.133/\text{h}$$

Feathering of the plasma profile yield the following information:

B = 15 mg/L, P = 24 mg/L, A = 39 mg/L; and

β = 0.151/h, π = 0.431/h, α = 1.133/h

These six values are used to calculate the various pharmacokinetic parameters associated with this model. The calculations involved in the process of obtaining first residual concentrations (squares) and second residual concentrations (triangles) are shown in Table 12-4.

Calculation of Pharmacokinetic Parameters

Rate Constants

$$K_a = \alpha = 1.133/\text{h}$$

$$K_{21} = \frac{P\beta + B\pi}{A}$$

$$= \frac{(24\ \text{mg/L})(0.151/\text{h}) + (15\ \text{mg/L})(0.431/\text{h})}{39\ \text{mg/L}}$$

Table 12-4 Feathering of data in Example 12-8

Time (h)	*C (mg/L) (Data Points)* ●	*$Be^{-\beta t}$ (mg/L) (B-line)*	*$C' = C - Be^{-\beta t}$ (mg/L)* ■	*$Pe^{-\pi t}$ (mg/L) (P-line) mg/L*	*$C'' = Pe^{-\pi t} - C' = Ae^{-\alpha t}$ (mg/L)* ▲
0.2	5.31	14.55	– 9.24*	21.10	30.34
0.4	9.25	14.12	– 4.87*	19.36	24.23
0.5	10.80	13.91	– 3.11*	18.54	21.65
0.6	12.11	13.70	– 0.59*	17.76	18.35
1.0	15.51	12.90	2.61	14.95	12.34
1.6	17.46	11.78	5.68	12.04	6.36
2.0	16.80	11.09	5.71	9.71	4.00
3.0	14.82	9.54	5.28	6.59	1.31
4.0	11.88	8.20	3.68	4.10	0.42
5.0	9.69	7.05	2.64	2.78	0.14
8.0	5.21	4.48	0.73	0.73	-
10.0	3.62	3.31	0.31	0.31	-
12.0	2.58	2.45	0.13	0.13	-
13.0	2.14	2.14	-	-	-
14.0	1.84	1.84	-	-	-

* Negative residuals are not plotted on the graph, but are used to calculate C″.

$$K_{21} = \frac{10.149/h}{39} = 0.2602/h$$

$$K_{10} = \frac{A}{(P/\pi) + (B/\beta)}$$

$$= \frac{39\ mg/L}{(24\ mg/L)/(0.435/h) + (15\ mg/L)/(0.151/h)}$$

$$= \frac{39\ mg/L}{154.510\ mg \times h/L} = 0.2524/h$$

$$K_{10} = \frac{\pi\beta}{K_{21}}$$

$$= \frac{(0.435/h)(0.151/h)}{0.2602/h} = \frac{0.06568/h}{0.2602} = 0.2524/h$$

$$K_{12} = \frac{(PB)(\beta - \pi)^2}{A(P\beta + B\pi)}$$

$$= \frac{(24\ mg/L)(15\ mg/L)(0.151/h - 0.435/h)^2}{(39\ mg/L)\{(24\ mg/L)(0.151/h) + (15\ mg/L)(0.435/h)\}} = 0.0734/h$$

$$t_{1/2} = \frac{0.693}{\beta} = \frac{0.693}{0.151/h} = = 4.59\ h$$

$$V_c = \frac{(F)(D)(\alpha)(\alpha - K_{21})}{(A)(\alpha - \pi)(\alpha - \beta)}$$

$$= \frac{(0.6)(500\ mg)(1.133/h)(1.133/h - 0.2602/h)}{(39\ mg/L)(1.133/h - 0.435/h)(1.133/h - 0.151/h)}$$

$$= \frac{296.222\ mg}{26.732\ mg/L} = 11.081\ L$$

$$V_d = \frac{(V_c)(\alpha - \beta)}{K_{21} - \beta}$$

$$= \frac{(11.081\ L)(1.133/h - 0.151/h)}{0.2602/h - 0.151/h} = \frac{10.881\ L}{0.1092} = 99.642\ L$$

$$V_t = V_d - V_c$$

$$= 99.642\ L - 11.081\ L = 88.561\ L$$

$$AUC_{total} = \frac{B}{\beta} + \frac{P}{\pi} - \frac{A}{\alpha}$$

$$= \frac{15\ mg/L}{0.151/h} + \frac{24\ mg/L}{0.435/h} - \frac{39\ mg/L}{1.133/h}$$

$$= 99.338\ mg \times h/L + 55.172\ mg \times h/L - 34.422\ mg \times h/L$$

$$= 120.088\ mg \times h/L$$

Description of the Model

The two-compartment model can be described either schematically or by an equation.

Schematic representation

The resolution of the data in Example 12-8 can be represented schematically as shown in Figure 12-20. The description of this schematic is similar to the description of the schematic given in Example 12-7, except for the values of the rate constants and the apparent volumes of distribution.

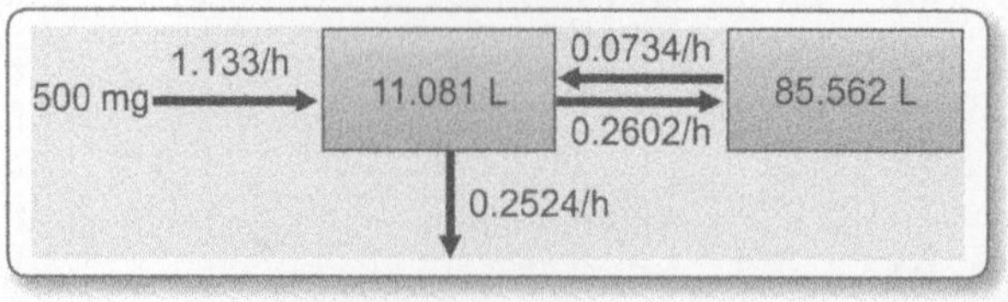

Fig. 12-20 Schematic representation of data in Example 12-8

Description by equation

The equation describing the plasma profile in Example 12-8 is:

$$C = 15(e^{-0.151t}) + 24(e^{-0.435t}) - 70(e^{-1.133t})$$

The explanation of the various values is similar to the explanation given for the equation that describes the plasma profile of data in Example 12-7.

The numerical values of the hybrid rate constants are:

α = the rate constant with the highest value = 1.133

β = the rate constant with the smallest value = 0.15, and

π = determined by the process of elimination. It is the remaining third rate constant having a numerical value = 0.435.

The numerical values of the three y-intercepts are:

B = y-intercept corresponding to hybrid micro-constant β = 15

P = y-intercept corresponding to hybrid micro-constant π = 24, and

A = y-intercept corresponding to hybrid micro-constant α = 39.

SUGGESTED READING

1. Benet L. Pharmacokinetics: A Modern View. Plenum Press; 1984.
2. Gibaldi M. Biopharmaceutics and Clinical Pharmacokinetics. 4th edition. Lea and Febiger; 1991.
3. Gibaldi M, Perrier D. Pharmacokinetics. 2nd edition. Marcel Dekker; 1982.
4. Madan PL. Bioavailability and Bioequivalence: The Underlying Concepts. US Pharmacist. 1992;**17**(11):H 10-H 30.
5. Madan PL. Introduction to bioavailability and pharmacokinetics. In: SS Lamba, CA walker (eds). Antibiotics and Microbial Transformations. Boca Raton, Florida: CRC Press; (1987).
6. Prescott P, W.S. Nimmo. Drug Absorption: Proceedings of the Edinburgh International Conference. ADIS Press; 1981.
7. Remington: The Science and Practice of Pharmacy. 21st edition. Mack Publishing; 2005.
8. Rowland and Tozer. Clinical Pharmacokinetics: Concepts and Applications. 3rd edition. Williams and Wilkins; 1995.
9. Wagner. Biopharmaceutics and Relevant Pharmacokinetics. Drug Intelligence Publications; 1971.
10. Wagner J. Fundamentals of Clinical Pharmacokinetics. Drug Intelligence Publications; 1979.

PRACTICE PROBLEMS

12-1. The following data were obtained following the administration of a single 100 mg dose of an experimental drug. Plot the data on a graph paper and compute the equation, which describes the plasma profile of this drug. Calculate the apparent volume of distribution, if the fraction of dose absorbed is 0.7.

Time (h)	Concentration (μg/L)	Time (h)	Concentration (μg/L)	Time (h)	Concentration (μg/L)
0.5	5.310	2.5	11.034	9.0	3.029
1.0	8.490	3.0	10.705	10.0	2.336
1.5	10.212	4.0	9.405	12.0	1.393
2.0	10.948	6.0	6.313	14.0	0.810

12-2. The following data were obtained following the administration of a 500 mg dose of an antibiotic. Compute the equation, which describes the plasma profile.

Time (h)	Concentration (μg/mL)	Time (h)	Concentration (μg/mL)	Time (h)	Concentration (μg/mL)
0.5	11.042	4.0	22.524	10.0	9.097
1.0	17.845	5.0	20.005	12.0	6.501
1.5	21.766	6.0	17.365	14.0	4.628
2.0	23.743	7.0	14.887		
3.0	24.259	8.0	12.675		

12-3. The following data were obtained following the administration of a single 1 g dose of a drug. If the extent of absorption of the drug is 60%, calculate all pharmacokinetic parameters associated with this plasma profile.

Time (h)	Concentration (mg/L)	Time (h)	Concentration (mg/L)	Time (h)	Concentration (mg/L)
1	11.075	5	14.654	12	5.581
2	15.503	6	13.091	14	4.110
3	16.553	8	10.032		
4	15.965	10	7.503		

12-4. The following data showing plasma concentration as a function of time were obtained following the administration of a single 500 mg dose of an antibiotic. Calculate all pharmacokinetic parameters associated with this pharmacokinetic compartment model. Assume that the fraction of administered dose absorbed is 0.8.

Time (h)	Concentration (mg/L)	Time (h)	Concentration (mg/L)	Time (h)	Concentration (mg/L)
2	1.905	6	6.462	10	3.654
3	5.887	7	5.712	11	3.060
4	7.091	8	4.948	12	2.601
5	7.038	9	4.239	13	2.188

12-5. The plasma profile obtained after administration of a single 500 mg oral dose of a drug is described by the following equation:

$$C = 30(e^{-0.02t}) - 30(e^{-0.15t}).$$

Calculate the concentration of drug in the plasma at $t = 5$.

12-6. The following data were obtained following the administration of a single 1,000 mg dose of a drug. Plot the data on a graph paper and determine the equation, which describes the plasma profile of the drug.

Time (h)	Concentration (mg/L)	Time (h)	Concentration (mg/L)	Time (h)	Concentration (mg/L)
1	26.44	4	36.02	10	17.38
2	36.02	6	29.40	12	13.20
3	37.76	8	22.78	14	10.00

12-7. The following data were obtained after the administration of a single 1,000 mg dose of an antibiotic. Determine the equation, which describes the concentration of drug in plasma as a function of time and calculate the following pharmacokinetic parameters: rate constant of absorption (K_a), rate constant of elimination (K), biological half-life of the drug ($t_{1/2}$) and apparent volume of distribution (V_d) of the drug. Assume that the fraction of administered drug dose absorbed into the systemic circulation is 0.81.

Time (h)	Concentration (mg/L)	Time (h)	Concentration (mg/L)	Time (h)	Concentration (mg/L)
2	9.63	10	11.97	20	7.51
4	12.83	14	10.02	24	6.17
6	12.56	18	8.27	28	5.07

12-8. A single 500 mg oral dose of a drug provided the following data. Compute the equation that describes the plasma profile.

Time (h)	Concentration (mg/L)	Time (h)	Concentration (mg/L)	Time (h)	Concentration (mg/L)
0.2	7.69	2.0	23.67	7.0	8.81
0.4	13.34	3.0	20.38	8.0	7.24
0.5	15.54	4.0	16.61	10.0	5.01
0.75	16.61	5.0	13.38	12.0	3.31
1.0	22.11	6.0	10.81	14.0	2.45

12-9. Compute the equation that describes the following plasma profile obtained after administration of a single 1,000 mg dose of an antibiotic.

Time (h)	Concentration (mg/L)	Time (h)	Concentration (mg/L)	Time (h)	Concentration (mg/L)
0.5	19.50	2.25	32.25	12.0	7.28
0.75	25.30	3.0	29.57	15.0	5.01
1.5	32.38	6.0	17.73	18.0	3.45
2.0	31.94	9.0	11.00	21.0	2.48

12-10. The plasma profile of a single 500 mg oral dose of a drug is described by the following equation:

$$C = 60(e^{-0.02t}) - 60(e^{-0.12t})$$

Calculate the concentration of drug in plasma at t = 3.

12-11. The plasma profile of a single 300 mg oral dose of a drug is described by the following equation:

$$C = 42.7(e^{-0.03t}) - 42.7(e^{-0.15t})$$

Calculate t_{max}, C_{max} and concentration of drug in plasma at t = 2, t = 4, t = 8 and t = 10.

12-12. The following model has been proposed for a drug:

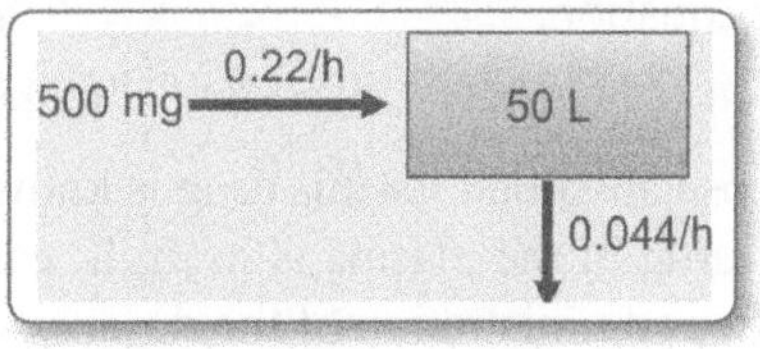

Assuming no lag-time and F = 1, calculate: (a) the time of maximum concentration, (b) the maximum concentration of drug in the plasma and (c) the concentration of drug in plasma at 5 hr.

12-13. The plasma profile of a drug is given by the equation (t is in hour):

$$C = 25(e^{-0.102t} - e^{-0.402t})$$

Calculate the concentration of drug in the plasma at 1, 4, 10 and 14 hours.

12-14. The plasma profile of a drug following the administration of a 2,000 mg dose is given by the following equation:

$$22(e^{-0.131t} - e^{-0.433t})$$

If concentration is in μg/mL and time is in hours, calculate the plasma concentration of drug at 1, 2, 8 and 12 hours, assuming F = 0.47.

12-15. The plasma profile of a drug following administration of a 300 mg dose is given by the following equation:

$$C = 15(e^{-0.33t}) - 35(e^{-1.03t})$$

If time is in hours and concentration is in mg/100 mL, calculate the lag-time, the apparent volume of distribution and concentration of drug in the plasma at 2 hours, assuming the fraction of dose absorbed is 0.75.

12-16. The plasma profile of a drug following administration of a 250 mg dose is given by the following equation:

$$C = 35(e^{-0.33t}) - 35(e^{-1.03t})$$

If time is in hours and concentration is in mg/100 mL, calculate the concentration of drug in plasma at 2 hr, assuming the fraction of dose absorbed is 0.75.

12-17. The plasma profile of a drug following administration of a 500 mg dose is given by the following equation:

$$C = 15(e^{-0.151t}) + 24(e^{-0.435t}) - 39(e^{-1.133t}).$$

The fraction of dose absorbed after oral administration for this drug is known to be 0.75. If time is in hours and concentration is in mg/100 mL, calculate the rate constant of absorption and biological half-life of the drug.

12-18. The plasma profile of a drug following administration of a 1,000 mg dose is given by the following equation:

$$C = 25(e^{-0.015t}) + 40(e^{-0.043t}) - 65(e^{-0.335t}).$$

The fraction of dose absorbed for this drug is known to be 0.85. If time is in hours and concentration of drug in plasma is in mg/L, calculate the rate constant of absorption and biological half-life of the drug.

12-19. The plasma profile of a drug following administration of a 100 mg dose is given by the following equation:

$$C = 15(e^{-0.02t}) + 30(e^{-0.05t}) - 45(e^{-0.15t}).$$

The fraction of dose absorbed for this drug is known to be 0.80. If time is in hours and concentration of drug in plasma is in mg/L, calculate the rate constant of absorption and biological half-life of the drug.

12-20. The plasma profile of a drug following administration of a single 100 mg dose is given by the following equation.

$$C = 15(e^{-0.02t}) + 30(e^{-0.05t}) - 45(e^{-0.15t}).$$

The fraction of dose absorbed for this drug is known to be 0.80. If time is in hours and concentration of drug in the plasma is in μg/L, calculate concentration of drug in the plasma 4 hour after administration of the dose.

12-21. The following data were obtained when a 500 mg dose of an antibiotic was administered orally. Compute the equation that describes this plasma profile, assuming 100% of the administered dose was absorbed.

Time (h)	Concentration (μg/mL)	Time (h)	Concentration (μg/mL)
1	3.915	8	1.814
2	8.005	9	1.344
3	7.321	10	0.996
4	5.803	12	0.546
5	4.403	14	0.300

12-22. The following data were obtained when a single 500 mg dose of an antibiotic was administered orally. Calculate the pharmacokinetic parameters, assuming 100% of the administered dose was absorbed.

Time (h)	Concentration (μg/mL)	Time (h)	Concentration (μg/mL)
2	9.7875	16	2.9600
4	20.0125	18	3.3600
6	18.3025	20	2.4900
8	14.5075	24	1.3650
10	11.0075	28	0.7500

12-23. The plasma profile of a drug following administration of a 1,000 mg dose is given by the following equation:

$$C = 25(e^{-0.02t}) + 40(e^{-0.043t}) - 65(e^{-0.35t}).$$

The fraction of dose absorbed for this drug is known to be 0.77. If time is in hours and concentration of drug in plasma is in mg/L, calculate the rate constant of absorption and biological half-life of the drug.

12-24. The following data were obtained when a 750 mg dose of an antibiotic was administered orally. Compute the equation that describes this plasma profile, assuming 100% of the administered dose was absorbed.

Time (h)	Concentration (μg/mL)	Time (h)	Concentration (μg/mL)
2	5.873	16	2.721
4	12.001	18	2.016
6	10.982	20	1.494
8	8.705	24	0.819
10	6.605	28	0.450

12-25. The following data were obtained following the administration of a single 750 mg dose of an antibiotic. Calculate the pharmacokinetic parameters, assuming 100% of the administered dose was absorbed.

Time (h)	Concentration (μg/mL)	Time (h)	Concentration (μg/mL)
1	39.7515	6	44.1195
2	54.1365	8	34.1760
3	56.2680	16	11.6265
4	54.0825	18	8.6010
5	49.3860	20	6.5145

12-26. The following data were obtained following the oral administration of a single 500 mg dose of an antibiotic. Calculate the pharmacokinetic parameters, assuming 50% of the administered dose was absorbed.

Time (h)	*Concentration (μg/mL)*	*Time (h)*	*Concentration (μg/mL)*
0.5	26.501	3.0	29.413
1.0	36.091	4.0	22.784
1.5	37.512	8.0	7.571
2.0	36.055	9.0	5.734
2.5	32.924	10.0	4.343

12-27. The plasma profile of a drug following administration of a 100 mg dose is given by the following equation:

$$C = 15(e^{-0.02t}) + 40(e^{-0.05t}) - 75(e^{-0.15t}).$$

The fraction of dose absorbed for this drug is known to be 0.80. If time is in hours and concentration of drug in plasma is in mg/L, calculate the total area under the curve.

12-28. The plasma profile of a drug following administration of a 100 mg dose is given by the equation:

$$C = 25(e^{-0.02t}) + 50(e^{-0.05t}) - 85(e^{-0.15t}).$$

The fraction of dose absorbed for this drug is known to be 0.95. If time is in hours and concentration is in μg/L, calculate biological half-life of the drug.

12-29. The plasma profile of a drug following administration of a 250 mg dose is given by the following equation:

$$C = 75(e^{-0.15t}) - 75(e^{-1.33t})$$

If time is in hours and concentration is in mg/100 mL, calculate biological half-life of the drug, assuming the fraction of dose absorbed is 0.75.

CHAPTER 13

MULTIPLE DOSING

A single dose of a drug is usually administered in order to attain therapeutic concentration of drug in the plasma for a very brief period of time. For instance, a single dose of an analgesic (e.g. aspirin, ibuprofen or acetaminophen) is usually sufficient to treat an acute condition such as an occasional headache. It is also not uncommon for a therapeutic agent to be administered in more than just one dose, but for a relatively short period of time, e.g. if the condition being treated persists for 2 or 3 days. However, in most clinical situations it is necessary that the drug be administered for relatively longer periods of time (i.e. on a chronic basis) in order to maintain therapeutic plasma concentrations for prolonged periods. Examples of these situations include treatments that last a few weeks (e.g. antibiotics and sulfonamides) or a few months, (e.g. hormones) or for periods extending into years (e.g. anti-diabetics and anticoagulants). While in most cases the therapeutic concentration of the medicinal agent in the plasma must be maintained, in the case of some drugs, however, fluctuations between high and low levels of drug concentration with respect to minimum effective concentration may in fact be preferred, e.g. in the case of treatment with penicillins.

During multiple dosing, when therapeutic levels of the drug must be maintained above a certain concentration, the recommended dose of the drug is generally administered at the drug's biological half-life intervals. For example, if the biological half-life of a drug is about 6 hours, then each dose of the drug is administered every 6 hours. Since each succeeding dose is administered, when about one-half of the preceding dose is still in the body, the amount of drug remaining in the body from each successive dose accumulates. Assuming that the dosing interval is kept constant and the size of dose is not changed during the course of therapy, the extent of accumulation of drug in the body then depends on the dosing interval. (It is also assumed that the drug follows linear pharmacokinetics and other pharmacokinetic parameters, such as the volume of distribution, rate constant of elimination and therefore, the clearance of drug does not change during the course of therapy). Obviously, a larger amount of drug will accumulate with each administered dose if the dosing interval is less than the biological half-life of the drug, than when the dosing interval is greater than the biological half-life of the drug. The following discussion examines the effect of dosing interval on the accumulation and subsequent plasma concentration of drug in the body during multiple dosing.

INTRAVENOUS ADMINISTRATION

The simplest case is a drug, which when administered intravenously as a single bolus dose, follows linear pharmacokinetic and confers upon the body the characteristics of one-compartment open model. As mentioned earlier, it is assumed that during multiple dosing, administration of earlier doses of the drug do not affect the pharmacokinetics of subsequent doses, i.e. elimination, metabolism, clearance, etc. of the drug remain unchanged. When administered intravenously, the entire drug dose appears in plasma immediately after the dose is administered and drug elimination begins according to first-order kinetics. If the dosing interval between each dose is such that the previous dose is virtually eliminated before the next dose is administered (e.g. if the biological half-life of the drug, $t_{1/2}$, is 3 hours and the drug is administered every 24 hours), then the concentration of drug in plasma just before the administration of the next dose will be virtually zero. That means, there will be no accumulation of drug from each dose administered. In such cases, administration of the second dose will yield a plasma profile virtually identical to the plasma profile obtained after the administration of the first dose, because, during multiple dosing the amount of drug remaining in the body from the first dose is virtually zero. Therefore, the concentration of drug in plasma versus time plot will exhibit a series of single-dose profiles as shown in Figure 13-1.

If the dosing interval is relatively shorter than the time for virtual elimination of each dose (e.g. if the biological half-life of the drug is 3 hours and the drug is administered every 9 hours), then the fraction of dose not eliminated from each previous dose accumulates as subsequent doses are administered. Thus, if a second bolus dose is administered before the first dose is virtually eliminated, then the concentration of drug in plasma immediately after administration of the second dose is equal to the plasma concentration of drug due to second dose plus the plasma concentration of drug due to the drug still remaining to be eliminated from the first dose. Obviously, this plasma concentration will be greater than that obtained immediately after the first dose.

Similarly, when the third bolus dose is administered, the fraction of dose still remaining to be eliminated from the first two doses adds to the plasma concentration of drug due to administration of the third dose. Consequently, the concentration of drug in plasma immediately after administration of the third dose will be greater than the plasma drug concentration achieved immediately after administration of the second dose (which, it will be recalled, was greater than the plasma concentration immediately after the first dose was administered). Thus, a fraction of each administered dose accumulates in the body as subsequent doses are administered

Since most drugs are usually administered at dosing intervals, which are approximately equal to their biological half-life, it follows that during a given dosing interval, approximately one-half of the administered dose is eliminated and approximately one-half of the administered drug dose persists in the body before the next dose is administered. Thus, when the second dose is administered, the amount of drug in the body is increased due to the presence of approximately one-half of the first dose persisting in the body. Similarly, just before administration of the third dose, approximately 25% of the drug is still remaining to be eliminated from the first dose and about 50% of the drug is still remaining to be eliminated from the second dose. Thus, with the administration of subsequent doses, the fraction of each drug dose that persists in the body from

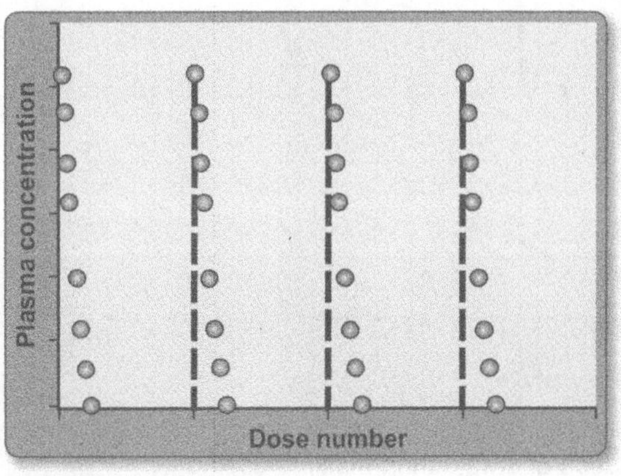

Fig. 13-1 Plasma profile when dosing interval is too large

the administration of previous doses accumulates. If the dosing interval between each dose is less than the biological half-life of the drug, a substantial accumulation of each drug dose occurs at the time of administration of the next dose.

Figure 13-2 shows the accumulation of drug in plasma, when dosing interval is equal to the biological half-life of the drug.

Drug Accumulation

To appreciate the extent of drug accumulation in the body following each dose, consider the case of a drug, which is administered as a 400 mg dose (D = 400 mg) at its biological half-life intervals (Dosing Interval is equal to biological half-life of the drug, i.e. $\tau = t_{1/2}$). If the biological half-life of this drug is 6 hours, then the dosing interval τ is also 6 hours. Since, $t_{1/2}$ = 6 hours, therefore the rate constant of elimination, K is:

$$K = \frac{0.693}{t_{1/2}}$$

$$= \frac{0.693}{6\text{ h}} = 0.1155\text{ h}$$

The mathematics of drug accumulation as each constant dose (400 mg) is administered at the fixed dosing interval of 6 hours is as follows: When the first dose is administered, the amount of drug in the body is equal to the dose, i.e. 400 mg. After 6 hours, just before the second dose is given, 50% of the first dose is eliminated and the amount of drug in the body is reduced to (0.5)(400 mg) = 200 mg, i.e. amount of drug in the body ranged between 400 mg (maximum amount) and 200 mg (minimum amount) during the first dose period. When the second dose is administered, the amount of drug in the body is increased to 200 mg + 400 mg = 600 mg and 6 hour after the administration of the second dose, 50% of the amount of drug in the body is eliminated, i.e. the amount of drug in the body is reduced to (0.5)(600) mg = 300 mg. That is, the amount of drug in the body ranges between 600 mg (maximum amount during the second dose period) and 300 mg (minimum amount during the second dose period). For the first three doses the following happens:

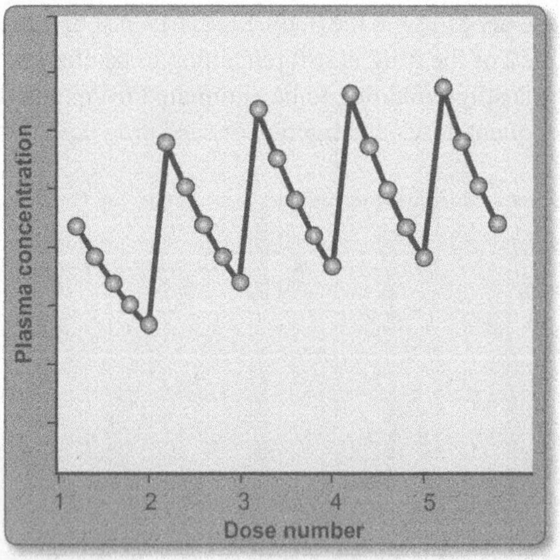

Fig. 13-2 Accumulation of drug during multiple dosing

During the first dose,

Amount administered = 400 mg

Amount eliminated = 200 mg

Amount persisting in the body = 400 mg – 200 mg = 200 mg

During the second dose,

Amount from the first dose = 200 mg

Amount administered = 400 mg

Amount in the body = 600 mg

(200 mg from the first dose and 400 mg from second dose)

Amount eliminated = 300 mg

(100 mg from first the dose and 200 mg from second dose)

Amount now persisting in the body = 600 mg – 300 mg = 300 mg

(100 mg from the first dose and 200 mg from the second dose)

During the third dose,

Amount from the first two doses = 300 mg

(100 mg from the first dose and 200 mg from the second dose) amount administered = 400 mg amount in the body = 700 mg (100 mg from first dose, 200 mg from second dose, 400 mg from third dose) amount eliminated = 350 mg (50 mg from first dose, 100 mg from second dose, 200 mg from third dose) amount now persisting in the body = 700 mg – 350 mg = 350 mg (50 mg from first dose, 100 mg from second dose, 200 mg from third dose)

Thus, during the first dose, the amount of drug in the body ranged between a maximum of 400 mg to a minimum of 200 mg and during the second dose, the range was between a maximum of 600 mg to a minimum of 300 mg and the maximum and minimum amounts of drug in the body during the third dose ranged between a high of 700 mg to a low of 350 mg. Comparing the maximum and minimum amounts of drug in the body during the first three doses, one finds that the maximum amounts were 400 mg, 600 mg and 700 mg for the first, second and third dose, respectively, i.e. showing an increase of 200 mg between the first and second dose, but an increase of only 100 mg between the second and third dose. Similarly, the minimum amounts of drug in the body during the first three doses were 200 mg, 300 mg and 350 mg, respectively, indicating an increase of 100 mg between the first two doses, but an increase of only 50 mg between the second and third dose. The increase in the amount of drug in the body becomes successively smaller with each dose administered. This pattern indicates that with each successive dose, the maximum amount of drug in the body increased 50% of the previous increase. For a comprehensive look at the amount of drug in the body during multiple dosing of similar doses administered at fixed dosing intervals, let us consider the elimination and persistence of the drug in terms of the percentage of each administered dose. Table 13-1 lists the percentage of drug in the body following the administration of each dose.

In Table 13-1 the first column is dose number, i.e. the first dose, the second dose, the third dose, etc. The second column shows the breakdown of the amount of drug persisting in the body for each dose. Column 3 indicates the cumulative total amount of drug in the body. The first line for each dose is amount of drug in the body immediately after the dose is administered and this represents the maximum amount of drug at the time of administration of that dose. The second line for each dose is the amount of drug in the body just before administration of the next dose and therefore this line represents the minimum amount of drug up to the time of administration of the next dose. The last column (column 4) is the range of amount of drug in the body (maximum and minimum amount of drug in the body) for each dose.

For the sake of simplicity, the decimal fractions are avoided in this tabulation. The fractional percentages in Table 13-1 have been rounded to the nearest whole numbers. For example, the percentage of first dose remaining in the body just before the administration of the fourth dose is actually 12.5, but this number is rounded off to 13. Similarly, the percentage of the first dose remaining in the body just before the the administration of the fifth dose is rounded off to 6 (instead of the actual number, which is calculated to be 6.125). For each of the doses listed in Table 13-1, the actual numbers representing the percentage of first dose remaining in the body just before the next dose is administered should be: 50, 25, 12.5, 6.25, 3.125, 1.562, 0.781, 0.391, 0.195, etc., but these are rounded off to: 50, 25, 13, 6, 3, 2, 1, 0, 0 and 0, respectively.

It should be remembered; however, that the percentage of first dose remaining in the body never attains a value of zero, i.e. the drug, theoretically, is never completely eliminated from the body. This is because elimination is a first order process, meaning that the amount of drug eliminated is always a fraction of the amount of drug remaining to be eliminated from the body. However, when the amount of drug remaining in the body becomes very small, so small that it may be difficult to detect the presence of drug in the body or in the plasma, then, for all practically purposes, the drug is considered to have been completely eliminated.

Table 13-1 shows that approximately 95% of the first dose is eliminated after about 4 or 5 doses and the first dose is virtually eliminated after about 8 doses. After 8 doses, the amount of drug appears to reach a plateau, the maximum and minimum amounts (or concentrations) ranging between 200% and 100% of the dose. Comparing the breakdown for the 9th dose with the breakdown for the 8th dose, one finds that the numbers in both rows of the second column are identical except that a zero is added for the first dose in each row. Similarly, comparing the breakdown for the 10th dose with that of the 9th dose, the numbers are again the same except that another zero is added (for the second dose).

If one continued to compare the breakdown for the 11th, 12th 13th and the *n*th dose, one will finds that the numbers in both rows of the second column will be identical except that a zero will be added for the first dose in each row. Thus, the breakdown for each successive dose will be identical to that of the preceding dose except that the numbers in the rows representing the succeeding dose will be shifted one step to the right, i.e. the maximum and minimum amounts

Table 13-1 Percent drug in the body following each dose

Dose #	*Percent drug in the body** *Percent drug persisting for each dose*	*Total*	*Range*
I	100 50	100 50	max min
II	50 + 100 25 + 50	150 75	max min
III	25 + 50 + 100 13 + 25 + 50	175 88	max min
IV	13 + 25 + 50 + 100 6 + 13 + 25 + 50	188 94	max min
V	6 + 13 + 25 + 50 + 100 3 + 6 + 13 + 25 + 50	194 97	max min
VI	3 + 2 + 6 + 13 + 25 + 50 + 100 3 + 6 + 13 + 25 + 50	199 97	max min
VII	2 + 1 + 3 + 2 + 6 + 13 + 25 + 50 + 100 3 + 6 + 13 + 25 + 50	202 100	max min
VIII	1 + 0 + 2 + 1 + 3 + 2 + 6 + 13 + 25 + 50 + 100 3 + 6 + 13 + 25 + 50	200 100	max min
IX	0 + 0 + 1 + 0 + 2 + 1 + 3 + 2 + 6 + 13 + 25 + 50 + 100 3 + 6 + 13 + 25 + 50	200 100	max min
X	0 + 0 + 0 + 0 + 1 + 0 + 2 + 1 + 3 + 2 + 6 + 13 + 25 + 50 + 100 3 + 6 + 13 + 25 + 50	200 100	max min

* See text for explanation

(column 4) for all successive doses would remain the same, as long as the drug is administered at the same dose level and at the same dosing interval.

From the data shown in Table 13-1, the following observations can be made:

a. When the drug is administered at its biological half-life intervals ($\tau = t_{1/2}$), one-half of each administered dose is eliminated (lost) between the administration of each dose and one-half of the administered dose persists in the body.
b. When subsequent doses are administered, the fraction of each dose remaining in the body from the previous doses undergoes persistence and elimination in the same manner as did the previous doses, when these doses were administered (Fig. 13-2), i.e. one-half of the dose remaining in the body from each dose is eliminated and one-half persists in the body.
c. Thus, a portion of each administered dose is lost (elimination) from the body and a portion of each administered dose persists in the body. During administration of subsequent doses, the portion of each dose not eliminated (i.e. persisting in the body) accumulates.

Therefore, during multiple dosing, concentration of drug in the body depends on the following three factors:

1. The fraction of each dose persisting in the body, known as the Persistence Factor,
2. The fraction of each dose eliminated (lost) from the body, known as the Loss Factor
3. The fraction of each dose accumulating in the body, known as the Accumulation Factor.

Persistence Factor

As defined above, persistence factor represents the fraction of each dose that persists in the body during multiple dosing. This is the fraction that was not eliminated. Therefore, the fraction of dose persisting in the body can be determined from the equation describing the first-order rate process because elimination is a first-order process. The first-order equation describing concentration of drug in the body after administration of a dose is:

$$C = C_0(e^{-Kt}) \qquad (13\text{-}1)$$

In equation (13-1), C is the concentration of drug at time t,, C_0 is the concentration of drug at time 0, K is the first-order rate constant of elimination and t is the time.

During multiple dosing, the first-order rate constant K is first-order rate constant of elimination and time t is dosing interval (τ). Substituting τ for t into equation (13-1), we have:

$$C = C_0(e^{-K\tau}) \qquad (13\text{-}2)$$

Since, concentration = $\dfrac{\text{amount of drug}}{\text{volume of distribution}}$, equation (13-2) may be written as

$$\frac{D}{V_d} = \frac{D_0}{V_d}\left(e^{-K\tau}\right) \qquad (13\text{-}3)$$

where,
D is the amount of drug in the body,
D_0 is the amount of drug in the body at time 0 = Dose and
V_d is the apparent volume of distribution.

Dividing both sides of equation (13-3) by D_0 yields the following equation.

$$\frac{D}{V_0} = e^{-K\tau} \qquad (13\text{-}4)$$

In equation (13-4), the ratio $\dfrac{D}{V_0}$ represents the fraction of dose in the body at the end of the dosing interval, i.e. this ratio is the fraction of dose persisting in the body during the dosing interval, τ. Equation (13-4) is therefore equivalent to:

$$\text{Persistence Factor} = P = e^{-K\tau} \qquad (13\text{-}5)$$

According to equation (13-5), persistence factor depends only on two factors:

i. K, the rate constant of elimination
ii. τ, the dosing interval.

Example 13-1 The half-life of a drug is 6 h. Calculate persistence factor if the dose is administered:

a. Every 6 hours, and
b. Every 12 hours.

Solution

Since $t_{1/2} = 6$ h, therefore $K = 0.693/t_{1/2} = 0.693/6\text{ h} = 0.1155/\text{h}$

a. When $\tau = 6$ h, $P = e^{-K\tau}$

$$P = e^{-(0.1155/\text{hr})(6\text{ hr})} = e^{-0.693} = 0.5$$

That is 50% of each dose will persist in the body before the next dose is administered at 6 hours intervals.

b. When $\tau = 12$ hours, $P = e^{-K\tau}$

$$P = e^{-(0.1155/\text{h})(12\text{ h})} = e^{-1.386} = 0.25$$

This means that when the dosing interval is 12 hours, 25% of each dose will persist in the body before the next dose is administered.

Loss Factor

Loss of drug from the body refers to drug elimination. The fraction of each dose not persisting in the body represents the fraction of each dose that is lost, i.e. eliminated from the body. Since the amount of drug lost from the body (eliminated) plus the amount of drug still in the body (persistence) is equal to the amount of dose administered, it follows that the fraction of dose lost plus the fraction of dose persisting should be equal to one. In other words,

$$\text{Loss Factor} = E = 1 - \text{Persistence Factor}$$

$$\text{Loss Factor} = E = 1 - P = 1 - e^{-K\tau} \qquad (13\text{-}6)$$

Example 13-2 If the biological half-life of a drug is 6 h, calculate the Loss Factor if identical doses are administered

a. Every 6 hours.
b. Every 12 hour.

Solution

$$\text{Since } t_{1/2} = 6\text{ h, therefore, } K = 0.693/t_{1/2} = 0.693/6\text{ h} = 0.1155/\text{h}$$

a. When $\tau = 6$ h, the Loss Factor, according to equation (13-6) is: $E = 1 - e^{-K\tau} = 1 - e^{-(0.1155)(6)} = 0.5$ Thus, 50% of each dose will be eliminated before the next dose is administered.
b. Similarly, in Example 13-1 it was found that when the drug is administered every 12 hours, Persistence Factor = 0.25. Using equation (13-6) to calculate the Loss Factor,

$$E = 1 - P = 1 - 0.25 = 0.75$$

Thus, 75% of each dose will be eliminated before the next dose is administered.

Accumulation Factor

Accumulation of drug during multiple dosing is due to accumulation of each successive dose of drug that persists in the body. The Accumulation Factor, S, after administration of n doses is determined using the following ratio:

$$\text{Accumulation Factor} = S = \frac{1 - e^{-nK\tau}}{1 - e^{-K\tau}} \qquad (13\text{-}7)$$

After a large number of doses are administered, i.e. when n becomes sufficiently large and the value of the exponential term $nK\tau$ increases, the term $e^{-nK\tau}$ approaches 0. The Accumulation Factor, S, then becomes

$$S = \frac{1}{1 - e^{-K\tau}} = \frac{1}{\text{Loss Factor}} \tag{13-8}$$

Example 13-3 If the biological half-life of a drug is 6 h and identical doses are administered every 6 hours, calculate the Accumulation Factor after (a) 3 doses and (b) after 20 doses.

Solution

Since $t_{1/2} = 6$ h, therefore K = 0.693/6 h = 0.1155/h,

(a) Accumulation Factor after 3 doses:

From equation (13-7)

$$S = \frac{1 - e^{-nK\tau}}{1 - e^{-K\tau}}$$

$$= \frac{1 - e^{-(3)(0.1155/hr)(6\,hr)}}{1 - e^{-(0.1155/hr)(6\,hr)}} = \frac{1 - 0.125}{1 - 0.5} = \frac{1}{0.5} = 1.75$$

The accumulation of drug after 3 doses is (1.75)(Dose) or 175% of the dose.

(b) Accumulation Factor after 20 doses:

Equation (13-8) may be used to calculate Accumulation Factor after 20 doses,

$$S = \frac{1 - e^{-nK\tau}}{1 - e^{-K\tau}}$$

$$= \frac{1 - e^{-(20)(0.1155/h)(6\,h)}}{1 - e^{-(0.1155/h)(6\,h)}} = \frac{1 - 0}{1 - 0.5} = \frac{1}{0.5} = 2$$

After administration of 20 doses, each dose administered at 6 hours intervals, the accumulation of the drug will be (2)(Dose) or 200% of the dose.

Mathematical Treatment

If the drug follows first-order elimination, then the concentration of drug in plasma during multiple dosing can be predicted from the concentration of drug in plasma after the first dose, as long as the size of each subsequent dose and the dosing intervals are held constant. Figure 13-3 shows a typical plasma profile after administration of the first dose. In this profile, the y-intercept is C_0 and the first-order rate constant of elimination (K) is obtained from the slope of the straight line.

The first-order equation for concentration of drug in plasma at any time t is equation (13-1)

$$C = C_0(e^{-Kt})$$

In this equation the exponential term represents fraction of dose persisting in the body, i.e. $e^{-K\tau}$ and C_0 is concentration just after administration of the dose. Equation (13-1) may be written as equation (13-2)

$$C = C_0(e^{-K\tau})$$

First Dose

Since, plasma concentration immediately after administration of the first dose (C_0) is the maximum plasma drug concentration for the first dose,

$$C_{max1} = C_0 \tag{13-9}$$

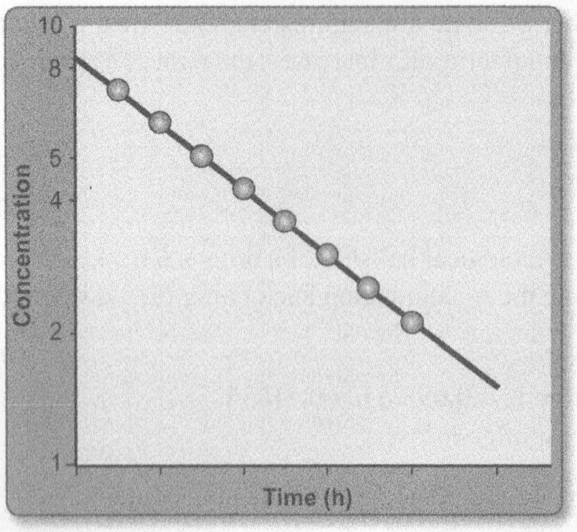

Fig. 13-3 Typical plasma profile after administration of first dose

Just before the second dose is administrated (at time = τ), the plasma drug concentration is the minimum concentration of drug in plasma for the first dose. Since, equation (13-1) predicts drug concentration at any time t after the first dose, it follows that at time t = τ,

$$C_{min\ 1} = C_0(e^{-K\tau}) \quad (13\text{-}10)$$

Second Dose

When the second dose is administered, the maximum concentration of drug in plasma, $C_{max\ 2}$, is the sum of minimum plasma drug concentration after the first dose, $C_{min\ 1}$ and concentration of drug provided by the second dose. Since the same dose is given again, the second dose provides the same concentration of drug as was obtained, when the first dose was administered, i.e. C_0. Therefore,

$$C_{max\ 2} = C_0 + C_{min\ 1} \quad (13\text{-}11)$$

Substituting the value of $C_{min\ 1}$ from equation (13-10) into equation (13-11), we have:

$$C_{max\ 2} = C_0 + C_0(e^{-K\tau}) \quad (13\text{-}12)$$

$$C_{max\ 2} = C_0(1 + e^{-K\tau})$$

Just before administration of the third dose, concentration of drug in plasma is the minimum plasma concentration after the second dose, i.e. $C_{min\ 2}$. This concentration can be determined using the same rationale that was used for obtaining minimum concentration of drug in plasma after the first dose. The minimum concentration after the second dose is obtained by multiplying plasma drug concentration at the time of administration of the second dose ($C_{max\ 2}$) with the Persistence Factor ($e^{-K\tau}$), i.e.

$$C_{min\ 2} = (C_{max\ 2})(e^{-K\tau}) \quad (13\text{-}13)$$

Substituting the value of $C_{max\ 2}$ from equation (13-12) into equation (13-13),

$$C_{min\ 2} = C_0(1 + e^{-K\tau})(e^{-K\tau}) \quad (13\text{-}14)$$

Third Dose

When the third dose is given, the maximum concentration in plasma is minimum concentration after the second dose ($C_{min\ 2}$) plus the concentration provided by the third dose. Since the same dose is administered, the third dose provides the same concentration that was obtained when the first dose was administered, i.e. C_0. Therefore maximum concentration of drug after the third dose is

$$C_{max\,3} = C_0 + C_{min\,2} \quad (13\text{-}15)$$

Substituting the value of $C_{min\,2}$ from equation (13-14) into equation (13-15), one gets:

$$C_{max\,3} = C_0 + C_0(1+e^{-K\tau})(e^{-K\tau}) \quad (13\text{-}16)$$

$$C_{max\,3} = C_0(1+e^{-K\tau}+e^{-2K\tau})$$

The minimum concentration of drug in plasma after the third dose is obtained in a manner similar to the one used for determining the minimum plasma drug concentration after the second dose, i.e.

$$C_{min\,3} = (C_{max\,3})(e^{-K\tau}) \quad (13\text{-}17)$$

Substituting the value of $C_{max\,3}$ from equation (13-16) into equation (13-17),

$$C_{min\,3} = C_0(1+e^{-K\tau}+e^{-2K\tau})(e^{-K\tau}) \quad (13\text{-}18)$$

Fourth Dose

Similarly, the maximum concentration of drug in plasma after the fourth dose should be

$$C_{max\,4} = C_0(1+e^{-K\tau}+e^{-2K\tau}+e^{-3K\tau}) \quad (13\text{-}19)$$

and the minimum concentration after administration of the fourth dose of the drug should be

$$C = C_0(1+e^{-K\tau}+e^{-2K\tau}+e^{-3K\tau})(e^{-K\tau}) \quad (13\text{-}20)$$

General Equations

A close examination of equations describing maximum and minimum concentrations of drug in plasma after the administration of each of first four doses reveals that these equations follow a specific pattern. To illustrate this pattern, equations (13-9), (13-12), (13-16) and (13-19), which describe the maximum concentration after each of the first four doses are shown in a simplified form in Table 13-2.

These equations exhibit a geometric progression. According to geometric progression, each term, after the first term, is a obtained by multiplying the preceding term with a constant, called common ratio. The first term in this series is C_0 and the common ratio is $e^{-K\tau}$. Therefore, the second term in this series is C_0 multiplied by $e^{-K\tau} = C0\, e^{-K\tau}$. Similarly, the third term is obtained by multiplying the second term, $C_0\, e^{-K\tau}$, with the common ratio, $e^{-K\tau}$ and the third term is $(C_0\, e^{-K\tau})(e^{-K\tau}) = C_0\, e^{-2K\tau}$.

Similarly, equations (13-10), (13-14), (13-18) and (13-20) which describe minimum concentration of drug in plasma after each of the first four doses are shown in the simplified form in Table 13-3.

Comparing this series (Table 13-3) with the series describing the maximum the concentrations of drug in plasma after each of the first four doses (Table 13-2), one finds a similarity and a difference. The similarity is that the common ratio, $e^{-K\tau}$ is the same in both cases. The difference is that the first term is different in the two series. The first term in the series in Table 13-3 is not C_0 as seen in Table 13-2, but it is $C_0\, e^{-K\tau}$. Thus, the second term in this series is $(C_0\, e^{-K\tau})(e^{-K\tau})$, which is equal to $C_0\, e^{-2K\tau}$. The third term, by definition, is the second term (which is $C_0\, e^{-2K\tau}$) multiplied by the constant (which is $e^{-K\tau}$), i.e. the third term is $(C_0\, e^{-2K\tau})(e^{-K\tau}) = (C_0)(e^{-3K\tau})$.

Maximum Plasma Concentration, C_{max}

The maximum concentration of drug in plasma, after the first, second, third and the fourth dose is described by Equations (13-9), (13-12), (13-16) and (13-19), respectively. These equations are

Table 13-2 Simplified form of equations describing C_{max}

Dose #	Equation	Simplified form of equation
1	(13-9)	C_0
2	(13-12)	$C_0 + C_0\, e^{-K\tau}$
3	(13-16)	$C_0 + C_0\, e^{-K\tau} + C_0\, e^{-2K\tau}$
4	(13-19)	$C_0 + C_0\, e^{-K\tau} + C_0\, e^{-2K\tau} + C_0\, e^{-3K\tau}$

Table 13-3 Simplified form of equations describing C_{min}

Dose #	Equation	Simplified form of equation
1	(13-10)	$C_0\, e^{-K\tau}$
2	(13-14)	$C_0\, e^{-K\tau} + C_0\, e^{-2K\tau}$
3	(13-18)	$C_0\, e^{-K\tau} + C_0\, e^{-2K\tau} + C_0\, e^{-3K\tau}$
4	(13-20)	$C_0\, e^{-K\tau} + C_0\, e^{-2K\tau} + C_0\, e^{-3K\tau} + C_0\, e^{-4K\tau}$

shown in a simplified form in Table 13-2. As can be seen, these equations exhibit the development of a generalized form. According to the development of this generalized form (Table 13-2), the maximum concentration of drug in plasma after the administration of n doses can be expressed by the equation:

$$C_{max\,n} = C_0 + C_0e^{-K\tau} + C_0e^{-2K\tau} + C_0e^{-3K\tau} + C_0e^{-4K\tau} + \ldots\ldots\ldots + C_0e^{-(n-1)K\tau} \quad (13\text{-}21)$$

In this equation, $C_{max\,n}$ is maximum concentration of drug in plasma after administration of the nth dose. Equation (13-21) is a general expression equation that can be simplified by mathematical procedures to express maximum concentration of drug in the plasma after n number of doses as follows:

First, multiply both sides of equation (13-21) with ($e^{-K\tau}$) to obtain equation (13-22). One writes these two equations as follows:

$$C_{max\,n} = C_0 + C_0e^{-K\tau} + C_0e^{-2K\tau} + C_0e^{-3K\tau} + C_0e^{-4K\tau} + \ldots\ldots + C_0e^{-(n-1)K\tau} \quad (13\text{-}21)$$

$$(e^{-K\tau})C_{max\,n} = C_0e^{-K\tau} + C_0e^{-2K\tau} + C_0e^{-3K\tau} + C_0e^{-4K\tau} + \ldots\ldots + C_0e^{-(n-1)K\tau} + Ce^{-(n)K\tau} \quad (13\text{-}22)$$

Equation (13-22) is obtained from equation (13-21) by multiplying each member of the equation (13-21) by $e^{-K\tau}$. Writing like terms of the right hand side members of both equations one under the other and subtracting equation (13-22) from equation (13-21) one obtains

$$C_{max\,n} - (e^{-K\tau})C_{max\,n} = C_0\,(1 - e^{-nK\tau})$$

or,

$$C_{max\,n}\,(1 - e^{-K\tau}) = C_0\,(1 - e^{-nK\tau})$$

$$C = \frac{C_0\left(1 - e^{-nK\tau}\right)}{1 - e^{-K\tau}} \quad (13\text{-}23)$$

Equation (13-23) describes maximum concentration of drug in plasma after the administration of *n* doses.

Minimum Plasma Concentration, C_{min}

As was seen earlier in the case of equations describing the maximum concentration of drug in the plasma after the first four doses, one also sees the development of a similar pattern when one examines equations (13-10), (13-14), (13-18) and (13-20), each of which describes the minimum concentration of drug in plasma after the first, second, third and the fourth dose, respectively.

These equations, shown in a simplified form in Table 13-3, also exhibit the development of a similar generalized pattern. According to the development of this generalized form (Table 13-3), the minimum concentration of drug after administration of *n* doses can be expressed by the equation:

$$C_{min\ n} = C_0e^{-K\tau} + C_0e^{-2K\tau} + C_0e^{-3K\tau} + C_0e^{-4K\tau} + ... + C_0e^{-(n)K\tau} \quad (13\text{-}24)$$

where,
$C_{min\ n}$ is concentration of drug in plasma at the end of dosing interval of the nth dose, and $C_{min\ n-1}$ is the concentration of drug in plasma just before the beginning of dosing interval of the nth dose.

Equation (13-24) can also be simplified by mathematical procedures similar to those used to simplify equation (13-21).

The simplified equation that expresses the minimum concentration of drug in plasma after n number of doses is derived by writing the two equations as follows:

$$C_{min\ n} = C_0e^{-K\tau} + C_0e^{-2K\tau} + C_0e^{-3K\tau} + C_0e^{-4K\tau} + ... + C_0e^{-(n)K\tau} \quad (13\text{-}24)$$

$$(e^{-K\tau})C_{min\ n} = C_0e^{-2K\tau} + C_0e^{-3K\tau} + C_0e^{-4K\tau} + ... + C_0e^{-(n)K\tau} + C_0e^{-(n+1)K\tau} \quad (13\text{-}25)$$

Equation (13-25) is obtained from equation (13-24) by multiplying each member of the equation (13-24) by $e^{-K\tau}$ and writing the like terms of the right hand side members of the equations one under the other. Subtraction of equation (13-25) from equation (13-24) gives

$$C_{min\ n} - (e^{-K\tau})C_{min\ n} = C_0e^{-K\tau} - C_0e^{-(n+1)K\tau} \quad (13\text{-}26)$$

Equation (13-26) can be simplified to

$$C_{min\ n}(1 - e^{-K\tau}) = C_0(e^{-K\tau} - e^{-(n+1)K\tau})$$

or

$$C_{min\ n}(1 - e^{-K\tau}) = C_0e^{-K\tau}(1 - e^{-nK\tau})$$

and

$$C_{min\ n} = \frac{C_0e^{-K\tau}(1 - e^{-nK\tau})}{1 - e^{-K\tau}}$$

This equation can be written as follows.

$$C_{min\ n} = \frac{C_0(1 - e^{-nK\tau})}{1 - e^{-K\tau}}(e^{-K\tau}) \quad (13\text{-}27)$$

Substituting $C_{max\ n}$ for its value from equation (13-23) into equation (13-27), one gets

$$C_{max\ n} = C_{max\ n}(e^{-K\tau}) \quad (13\text{-}28)$$

The relationship shown in equation (13-28) can also be established when equations shown in Table 13-2 are compared with those shown in Table 13-3. The equations shown in Table 13-3 are identical to those shown in Table 13-2, except that each member of right-hand side of equation in Table 13-3 is multiplied by the term $e^{-K\tau}$, i.e. minimum concentration of drug in plasma after each dose is equal to the product of maximum concentration of drug in plasma after that dose and $e^{-K\tau}$, as shown in Table 13-4.

According to this pattern, the minimum concentration of drug in plasma after n doses will be equation (13-28):

$$C_{max\ n} = C_{max\ n}(e^{-K\tau})$$

From equations (13-23) and (13-27) it is seen that one can calculate maximum and minimum drug plasma concentrations after administration of any number of equal doses given at fixed time intervals, provided the following parameters are known: C_0 (initial concentration), K (rate constant of elimination), τ (dosing interval) and n (number of doses administered).

Table 13-4 Minimum concentration after each IV dose

Dose	*Minimum plasma drug concentration*
First	$(C_{max\,1})(e^{-K\tau})$
Second	$(C_{max\,2})(e^{-K\tau})$
Third	$(C_{max\,3})(e^{-K\tau})$
Fourth	$(C_{max\,4})(e^{-K\tau})$
Fifth	$(C_{max\,5})(e^{-K\tau})$

Example 13-4 Calculate maximum plasma drug concentration after the administration of fourth dose, if 50 mg bolus doses are given intravenously every 4 hour. Given: C_0 = 3 mg/L and K = 0.2/h.

Solution

Using equation (13-23), the maximum plasma drug concentration after the fourth dose is

$$C_{max\,4} = \frac{C_0\left(1-e^{-nK\tau}\right)}{1-e^{-K\tau}} = \frac{(3\ \text{mg/L})\left(1-e^{-(4)(0.2/\text{h})(4\text{h})}\right)}{1-e^{-(0.2/\text{h})(4\,\text{h})}}$$

$$= \frac{(3\ \text{mg/L})(1-0.04076)}{1-0.4493} = \frac{3\ \text{mg}\times 0.95924}{0.55067} = 5.226\ \text{mg/L}$$

Example 13-5 Calculate the maximum and minimum plasma concentrations of a drug after administration of the fourth dose, if 50 mg bolus dose is given intravenously every 4 hours. The volume of distribution of the drug is 40 L and the rate constant of elimination is 0.07/h.

Solution

Since, dose = 50 mg and apparent volume of distribution = 40 L, therefore

$$C_0 = \frac{\text{Dose}}{\text{Volume of distribution}} = \frac{50\ \text{mg/L}}{40\ \text{L}} = 1.25\ \text{mg/L}$$

a. Using equation (13-23), the maximum concentration of drug after the fourth dose is

$$C_{max\,4} = \frac{C_0\left(1-e^{-nK\tau}\right)}{1-e^{-K\tau}} = \frac{(1.25\ \text{mg/L})\left(1-e^{-(4)(0.07/\text{h})(4\,\text{h})}\right)}{1-e^{-(0.07/\text{h})(4\,\text{h})}}$$

$$= \frac{(1.25\ \text{mg/L})(0.6737)}{0.2442} = 3.45\ \text{mg/L}$$

b. Using equation (13-28), the minimum concentration of drug after the fourth dose is:

$$C_{max\,4} = (C_{max\,4})(e^{-K\tau}) = (3.45\ \text{mg/L})(e^{-(0.07/\text{h})(4\,\text{h})}) = (3.45\ \text{mg/L})(0.7558) = 2.61\ \text{mg/L}$$

STEADY-STATE CONCENTRATIONS

The steady-state concentration of drug in plasma (or the plateau level) is reached, when the values of the maximum concentration of drug in plasma (C_{max}) and the minimum concentration of drug in plasma (C_{min}) become constant for each successive dose. This can happen only, when the equations describing the maximum concentration of drug in plasma (C_{max}) and the minimum concentration of drug in plasma are not affected by n (the number of dose). In other words, the equations describing the maximum and minimum concentrations of drug in the plasma at steady-state do not include a term containing n. This would be case, when the value of the exponential term $e^{-nK\tau}$ in these equations approaches a value of zero. At that time the equations describing the maximum and minimum plasma concentrations will exhibit a plateau. In order for the value of $e^{-nK\tau}$ to approach a value of 0, n must have a sufficiently large value. When this happens, the amount of drug eliminated from the body becomes equal to the amount of drug administered into the body and equilibrium is reached between drug input and drug output.

Maximum Concentration, $C_{max\ ss}$

According to equation (13-23), the maximum concentration of drug in the plasma at steady-state is the maximum concentration drug plasma concentration after the administration of a large number of doses, i.e. $C_{max\ ss}$ is $C_{max\ n}$ when n (number of doses administered) becomes very large. At very large values of n, the exponential term ($e^{-nK\tau}$) in the numerator of equation (13-23) approaches a value of zero and the numerator now becomes equal to $C_0\ (1 - 0) = C_0$. Therefore, equation (13-23) is reduced to

$$C_{max\ ss} = \frac{C_0}{1 - e^{-K\tau}} \qquad (13\text{-}29)$$

Minimum Concentration, $C_{min\ ss}$

The minimum concentration of drug in the plasma at steady-state ($C_{min\ ss}$) can be derived from equations (13-27) and (13-28). When n becomes very large (after administration of a large number of doses), the exponential term ($e^{-nK\tau}$) in the numerator of equation (13-27) approaches a value of 0. Therefore, at large values of n, the numerator in equation (13-7) is equal to $C_0\ (1 - 0) = C_0\ e^{-K\tau}$. Therefore, equation (13-27) becomes

$$C_{min\ ss} = \frac{C_0}{1 - e^{-K\tau}}(e^{-K\tau}) = C_{max\ ss}\ (e^{-K\tau}) \qquad (13\text{-}30)$$

Example 13-6

From the data provided in Example 13-5, calculate $C_{max\ ss}$ and $C_{min\ ss}$.

Solution

From the data provided in Example 13-5:

$$C_0 = 1.25 \text{ mg/L},\ K\tau = 0.28 \text{ and } e^{-K\tau} = 0.756$$

a. Using equation (13-29), the maximum concentration of drug in plasma at steady-state is

$$C_0\ C_{max\ ss} = \frac{C_0}{1 - e^{-K\tau}}$$

$$= \frac{(1.25 \text{ mg/L})}{1 - e^{-(0.07/\text{h})(4\text{h})}} = \frac{(1.25 \text{ mg/L})(0.6737)}{0.244} = 5.12 \text{ mg/L}$$

b. Using equation (13-30), the minimum concentration of drug in plasma at steady-state is

$$C_{min\ ss} = (C_{max\ ss})(e^{-K\tau})$$

$$= (5.12 \text{ mg/L})(e^{-(0.07/\text{h})(4\text{ h})})$$

$$= (5.12 \text{ mg/L})(0.756) = 3.87 \text{ mg/L}$$

Example 13-7 The following data were obtained after administration of a 300 mg intravenous bolus dose of an antibiotic. Calculate $C_{max\ ss}$ and $C_{min\ ss}$ if a 300 mg dose is given every 6 hourly.

Time(h):	1	2	3	4	6	8	10	12
Concentration (μg/mL):	36	33	29	26	20	16	13	10

Solution

A plot of the data is shown in Figure 13-4.

This graph shows that upon administration, the drug confers upon the body the characteristics of one-compartment pharmacokinetic model.

From Figure 13-4, $C_0 = 41$ μg/mL and $t_{1/2} = 6$ h.

Therefore, $K = \dfrac{0.693}{6\text{ h}} = 0.1155/\text{h}$ and $e^{-K\tau} = e^{-0.693} = 0.5$

Substituting these values into equation (13-29):

$$C_{max\ ss} = \frac{C_0}{1 - e^{-K\tau}}$$

$$= \frac{41\ \mu g/mL}{1 - e^{-(0.1155/h)(6h)}} \frac{41\ mg/L}{1 - 0.5} = 82\ \mu g/mL$$

Similarly, substituting the values of $C_{max\ 11}$, K and τ into equation (13-30):

$$C_{min\ ss} = (C_{max\ ss})(e^{-K\tau})$$

$$= (82\ mg/L)(e^{-(0.1155/h)(6\ h)}) = (82\ mg/L)(0.5) = 41\ mg/L$$

Example 13-8 A 300 mg bolus dose of an antibiotic administered intravenously gave the following data. Calculate the maximum and minimum concentration of drug in the plasma at steady-state if a 300 mg dose is given intravenously every 6 hours.

Time (h):	2	4	6	8	10	12
Concentration (μg/mL)	25.2	19.9	17.8	15.8	12.5	11.2

Solution

A plot of the data is shown in Figure 13-5

This plot shows that upon administration the drug confers the characteristics of one-compartment pharmacokinetic model on the body.

From this graph, $C_0 = 30$ μg/mL and $t_{1/2} = 8$ h.

$$K = \frac{0.693}{t_{1/2}} = \frac{0.693}{8\text{ h}} = 0.0866\text{ h}$$

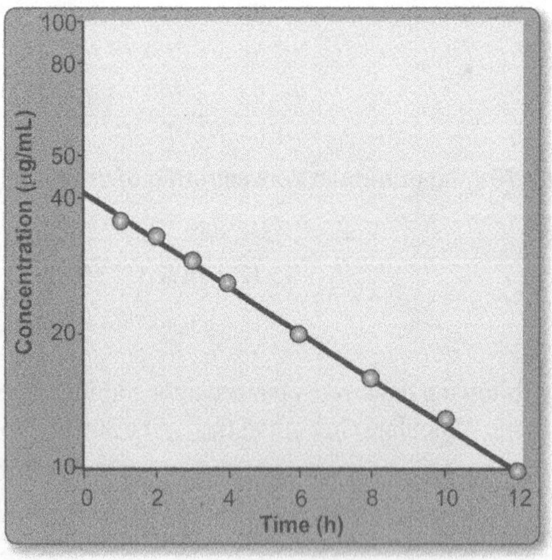

Fig. 13-4 Plot of data in Example 13-7

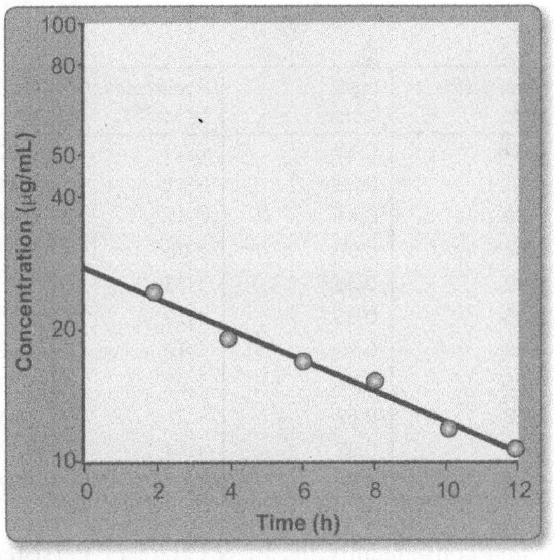

Fig. 13-5 Plot of data in Example 13-8.

$$K\tau = (0.0866/h)(6\ h) = 0.5196,$$

$$\text{therefore } e^{-K\tau} = e^{-0.5196} = 0.595.$$

Substituting these values into equation (13-29):

$$C_{min\ ss} = \frac{C_0}{1-e^{-K\tau}} = \frac{30\ \mu g/mL}{1-e^{-(0.0866/h)(8h)}} = \frac{30\ \mu g/mL}{1-0.595} = 74.1\ \mu g/mL$$

Similarly, substituting the values into equation (13-30):

$$C_{min\ ss} = (C_{max\ ss})e^{-K\tau} = (74.1\ \mu g/mL)e^{-(0.0866/h)(8\ h)} = (74.1\ \mu g/mL)(0.595) = 44.1\ \mu g/mL$$

Effect of Dosing Interval

Comparing the values of the maximum and minimum concentrations of drug in the plasma at steady-state found in Examples 13-7 and 13-8, one finds that the value of $C_{min\ ss}$ was equal to the value of C_0 in Example 13-7, but the value of $C_{min\ ss}$ was greater than the value of C_0 in Example 13-8. Also, it is seen that in Example 13-7, $C_{max\ ss}$ was equal to twice the value of C_0, but $C_{max\ ss}$ was greater than two-times the value of C_0 in Example 13-8. This is because in Example 13-7, the dosing interval was equal to the biological half-life of the drug and in Example 13-8 the dosing interval was less than the biological half-life of the drug, which was responsible for the difference in the accumulation of the drug in the body. Table 13-5 shows the effect of dosing interval on drug accumulation.

The following explanation clarifies the difference in the values of maximum and minimum steady-state concentrations of drug in plasma found in Examples 13-7 and 13-8:

a. Dosing interval = biological half-life
When dosing interval is equal to biological half-life of the drug, i.e. when $\tau = t_{1/2}$,
Persistence Factor = $P = e^{-K\tau} = e^{-0.695} = 0.5$,
Loss Factor = 1 − Persistence Factor = 1 − 0.5 = 0.5 and

$$\text{Accumulation factor} = \frac{1}{1-\text{Persistance factor}} = \frac{1}{1-0.5} = \frac{1}{0.5} = 2$$

b. Dosing interval less than biological half-life
But when dosing interval is less than biological half-life of the drug, the term $K\tau$ becomes small and the exponential term $e^{-K\tau}$ will have a larger value. Therefore, Persistence Factor

Table 13-5 Effect of dosing interval on $C_{max\ ss}$ and $C_{min\ ss}$

Dosing interval	*Persistence factor*	*Loss factor*	*Accumulation factor*	$C_{max\ ss}$	$C_{min\ ss}$
$\tau = 0.25t_{1/2}$	0.84	0.16	6.29	$6.29C_0$	$5.29C_0$
$\tau = 0.50t_{1/2}$	0.71	0.29	3.41	$3.41C_0$	$2.41C_0$
$\tau = 0.75t_{1/2}$	0.59	0.41	2.47	$2.47C_0$	$1.47C_0$
$\tau = 1.00t_{1/2}$	0.50	0.50	2.00	$2.00C_0$	$1.00C_0$
$\tau = 1.25t_{1/2}$	0.42	0.58	1.73	$1.73C_0$	$0.73C_0$
$\tau = 1.50t_{1/2}$	0.35	0.65	1.55	$1.55C_0$	$0.55C_0$
$\tau = 1.75t_{1/2}$	0.30	0.70	1.42	$1.42C_0$	$0.42C_0$
$\tau = 2.00t_{1/2}$	0.25	0.75	1.33	$1.33C_0$	$0.33C_0$
$\tau = 2.50t_{1/2}$	0.18	0.82	1.21	$1.21C_0$	$0.21C_0$
$\tau = 3.00t_{1/2}$	0.13	0.87	1.14	$1.14C_0$	$0.14C_0$
$\tau = 4.00t_{1/2}$	0.06	0.94	1.07	$1.07C_0$	$0.07C_0$

$(e^{-K\tau})$ is increased and consequently the Loss Factor (1-Persistence Factor) is decreased. Decrease in Loss Factor will increase Accumulation Factor, which indicates increased accumulation of drug in the body and accounts for larger values of $C_{max\ ss}$ and $C_{min\ ss}$.

c. Dosing interval greater than biological half-life

If, on the other hand, the dosing interval is greater than biological half-life of the drug, then the term $K\tau$ will become large and hence $e^{-K\tau}$ will have a smaller value. Therefore, Persistence Factor will decrease, the Loss factor will increase and consequently the Accumulation Factor will decrease, indicating less accumulation of drug in the body and the $C_{min\ ss}$ and $C_{max\ ss}$ values will also decrease.

Example 13-9 From the data given in Example 13-8, calculate the maximum and minimum concentrations at steady-state ($C_{max\ ss}$ and $C_{min\ ss}$) if τ was made 12 hours.

Solution

When $\tau = 12$ h, $K\tau = (0.0866)(12) = 1.0392$ and $e^{-K\tau} = e^{-1.0392} = 0.3537$.
Therefore,

$$C_{max\ ss} = \frac{C_0}{1-e^{-K\tau}}$$

$$= \frac{30\ \mu g/mL}{1-e^{-(0.0866/h)(12h)}} = \frac{30\ \mu g/mL}{1-0.354} = \frac{30\ \mu g/mL}{0.646} = 46.44\ \mu g/mL$$

$$C_{min\ ss} = C_{max\ ss}\,(e^{-K\tau})$$

$$= (46.44\ \mu g/mL)(e^{-(0.0866/h)(12\ h)})$$

$$= (46.44\ \mu g/mL)(0.354) = 16.44\ \mu g/mL$$

Relationship Between $C_{max\ ss}$ and $C_{min\ ss}$

During multiple dosing, when equal doses are given at fixed dosing intervals, the difference between maximum and minimum concentrations of drug at steady-state ($C_{max\ ss} - C_{min\ ss}$) is always equal to C_0. This can be seen if we subtract equation (13-30), equation for the minimum concentration of drug at steady-state from equation (13-29), equation for maximum steady-state concentration of drug. Subtraction yields:

$$C_{max\ ss} - C_{min\ ss} = \frac{C_0}{1-e^{K\tau}} - \frac{C_0}{1-e^{-K\tau}} - \frac{C_0}{1-e^{-K\tau}}\left(e^{-K\tau}\right) = \frac{C_0\left(1-e^{-K\tau}\right)}{1-\left(e^{-K\tau}\right)} = C_0 \qquad (13\text{-}31)$$

In linear pharmacokinetics, since C_0 is a function of dose and apparent volume of distribution, the only factors that will influence C_0 are the dose and the apparent volume of distribution. Thus, if the dose and apparent volume of distribution do not change during multiple dosing, the difference between maximum and minimum concentrations of drug in plasma at steady-state will be always equal to C_0.

Factors Influencing Steady-State Concentration

Equations (13-29) and (13-30) describe steady-state concentrations of drug. These equations show that $C_{max\ ss}$ and $C_{min\ ss}$ depend on C_0, K and τ. In linear pharmacokinetics C_0 is proportional to D (because C_0 = Dose/V_d) and if the volume of distribution (V_d) and rate constant of elimination (K) do not change during the course of therapy, then the maximum and minimum concentrations at steady-state will depend only on dose (D) and dosing interval (τ).

Effect of Dose

According to equation (13-29),

$$C_{max\ ss} = \frac{C_0}{1-e^{-K\tau}}, \text{ and since, } C_0 = \frac{D}{V_d}, \text{ therefore,}$$

$$C_{max\ ss} = \frac{D}{V_d\left(1-e^{-K\tau}\right)} \tag{13-32}$$

If a dose D" (instead of the dose D) is administered and assuming no change in dosing interval, apparent volume of distribution and rate constant of elimination of the drug, then the maximum concentration at steady-state ($C_{max\ ss''}$) is given by

$$C_{max\ ss''} = \frac{D''}{V_d\left(1-e^{-K\tau}\right)} \tag{13-33}$$

Dividing equation (13-32) by equation (13-33),

$$\frac{C_{max\ ss}}{C_{max\ ss''}} = \frac{\dfrac{D}{V_d\left(1-e^{-K\tau}\right)}}{\dfrac{D''}{V_d\left(1-e^{-K\tau}\right)}}$$

$$\frac{C_{max\ ss}}{C_{max\ ss''}} = \frac{D}{D''} \tag{13-34}$$

Using the same rationale for minimum concentrations at steady-state, it can be shown that

$$\frac{C_{max\ ss}}{C_{max\ ss''}} = \frac{D}{D''} \tag{13-35}$$

Thus, changes in the size of the drug dose administered will correspondingly increase or decrease the steady-state maximum and minimum concentration of drug in the plasma. The following Example illustrates the effect of dose on steady-state concentrations.

Example 13-10 Administration of a single 50 mg intravenous bolus dose of a drug gave the following data: one-compartment model with C_0 = 2 mcg/mL and K = 0.1125/hr. Calculate steady-state concentrations in two patients:

a. One patient is administered a 50 mg dose every 8 hours and
b. The second patient receives a 35 mg dose (instead of 50 mg dose) every 8 hours from the start of the treatment.

Solution

a. $K\tau = (0.1125/h)(8\ h) = 0.9,\ e^{-K\tau} = e^{-0.9} = 0.4066\ C_0$

$$C_{min\ ss} = \frac{C_0}{1-e^{-K\tau}}\left(e^{-K\tau}\right)$$

$$= \frac{2\ \mu g/mL}{1-e^{-(0.1125/h)(8\ h)}}(0.4066)\ (1-e^{-(0.1125/h)(8\ h)})$$

$$= \frac{2\ \mu g/mL}{1-0.4066}(0.4066) = 1.37\ \mu g/mL$$

$$C_{max\ ss} = \frac{C_0}{1-e^{-K\tau}} = \frac{2\ \mu g/mL}{1-e^{-(0.1125/h)(8\ h)}} = \frac{2\ \mu g/mL}{1-0.4066} = 3.37\ \mu g/mL$$

b. Since only the dose is changed, K and τ are unchanged. Therefore the values of $e^{-K\tau}$ and $(1-e^{-K\tau})$ remain unchanged. The value of C_0, however, will change because dose is changed. Assuming linear pharmacokinetics, since $C_0 = D/Vd$, therefore

$$\text{new } C_0 = \frac{(\text{old } C_0)(\text{new dose})}{\text{old dose}} = \frac{(2\ \mu g/mL)(35\ mg)}{50\ mg} = 1.4\ \mu g/mL$$

$$\text{new } C_{min\ ss} = \frac{C_0}{1-e^{-K\tau}}\left(e^{-K\tau}\right)$$

$$= \frac{1.4\ \mu g/mL}{1-e^{-(0.1125/h)(8\ h)}}(1-e^{-(0.1125/h)(8\ h)})$$

$$= \frac{1.4\ \mu g/mL}{1-0.4066}(0.4066) = 0.96\ \mu g/mL$$

$$\text{new } C_{max\ ss} = \frac{C_0}{1-e^{-K\tau}}$$

$$= \frac{1.4\ \mu g/mL}{1-e^{-(0.1125/h)(8h)}} = \frac{1.4\ \mu g/mL}{1-0.4066} = 2.36\ \mu g/mL$$

From Example 13-10, comparing the maximum and minimum concentrations of drug in plasma at steady-state, it is seen that

$$\frac{\text{old } C_{min\ ss}}{\text{new } C_{min\ ss}} = \frac{1.37\ \mu g/mL}{0.96\ \mu g/mL} = 1.43$$

$$\frac{\text{old } C_{max\ ss}}{\text{new } C_{max\ ss}} = \frac{3.37\ \mu g/mL}{2.36\ \mu g/mL} = 1.43$$

$$\text{and } \frac{\text{old dose}}{\text{new dose}} = \frac{50\ mg}{35\ mg} = 1.43$$

which is in agreement with equations (13-34) and (13-35).

Effect of Dosing Interval

The effect of dosing interval on the steady-state minimum and maximum concentrations of drug in the plasma is not as simple and straight-forward as the effect of dose. This is because in linear pharmacokinetics, the size of dose is directly proportional to the value of C_0 and any change in the size of dose has a linear effect on the concentration of drug in the plasma at steady-state. Dosing interval is not related in a similar linear manner to the terms used to calculate minimum and maximum concentrations of drug in plasma at steady-state. In equations used for calculating steady-state concentrations of drug, dosing interval appears in the exponential terms.

Therefore, the relationship between dosing interval and steady-state concentrations becomes more complicated and it is not possible to relate the effect of dosing interval on steady-state concentrations with a simple relationship.

EXTRAVASCULAR ADMINISTRATION

Extravascular administration, particularly administration by the oral route is the more popular route used during multiple dosing. Although, accumulation of drug during extravascular administration is very similar to that found during intravenous administration, the magnitude of accumulation of drug is not similar in both cases. In extravascular administration, immediately after the administration of the drug dose, the concentration of drug in plasma first increases (due to absorption), reaches its peak and then decreases (due to very little absorption). In intravenous administration, the concentration of drug in plasma is at its peak at the time of administration, but peak concentration in extravascular administration is usually less than that seen in intravenous administration, because the entire drug-dose is not placed in the blood stream all at once. The drug appears in plasma because of absorption and the magnitude of increase in concentration of drug in plasma depends upon the rates of absorption, distribution and elimination of the drug. Thus, the steady-state concentrations of drug during multiple dosing following extravascular administration depend on the rates of absorption, distribution and elimination of the drug.

The simplest case is a drug which, when administered extravascularly as a single bolus dose, confers upon the body the characteristics of one-compartment model. It is assumed that during multiple dosing, earlier doses of the drug do not affect pharmacokinetics of subsequent doses, that is, the processes of absorption, elimination, metabolism and clearance, etc. of the drug remain unchanged and the apparent volume of distribution of the drug also remains unchanged. It is also assumed that the entire administered drug dose is completely absorbed ($F = 1$) and following absorption, elimination begins according to first-order kinetics. If the dosing interval between doses is such that the previous dose is virtually eliminated before the next dose is administered (e.g. if biological half-life of the drug is 3 hours and the drug is administered once a day), then the plasma concentration versus time plot will exhibit a series of single-dose profiles. But, if the dosing interval is approximately equal to half-life of the drug, the drug accumulates in the body as each successive dose is administered.

Accumulation of the drug during multiple dosing in extravascular administration is similar to accumulation of drug during intravenous administration. The main difference between the two is absorption of the drug. If the drug is absorbed rapidly and completely, then the plasma profiles are very similar except that the graph depicting extravascular administration exhibits the absorption phase. For most conventional formulations, except those intended to provide delayed or modified release of the active ingredient (sustained or prolonged release and enteric-coated dosage forms), the extravascular dosage form is formulated to provide rapid absorption. Therefore, the terminal portion of plasma profile (which exhibits predominantly elimination) following extravascular administration is very similar to the terminal portion of the graph obtained following intravenous administration of the drug.

Thus, determination of plateau levels during multiple dosing of extravascularly administrated dosage forms is similar to the determination of plateau levels attained during multiple dosing by intravenous administration, except that during extravascular administration, K_a, the rate constant of absorption must be taken into consideration. During extravascular administration, the y-intercept B (obtained by back-extrapolating the terminal linear portion of elimination phase) is used in place of C_0 (the y-intercept used during intravenous administration). It should be mentioned, however, that the numerical value of the y-intercept B obtained during extravascular administration is usually less than the numerical value of the y-intercept C_0 obtained following intravenous administration.

Steady-State Concentrations

Since the minimum concentration of drug in plasma during a dosing period is the concentration just prior to the administration of the next dose and if dosing interval is such that the next dose is administered in the postabsorptive phase of the previous dose, then one can assume that most of the drug from each dose was absorbed before the next dose was administered. Therefore the rate of drug absorption would not affect the minimum concentration attained during each dose, as well as at the steady-state ($C_{min\ ss}$). However, since the maximum concentration attained after each dose occurs at the time of maximum concentration (t_{max}) and tmax is a complex function of absorption and elimination rate constants, the utilization of maximum concentration values after each dose to determine the maximum plasma concentration at steady-state ($C_{max\ ss}$) becomes relatively complicated. A simpler relationship is given here.

Maximum Concentration, $C_{max\ ss}$

The maximum drug plasma concentration at steady-state is calculated using the equation:

$$C_{max\ ss} = \frac{(B)}{1 - e^{-K\tau}}(e^{-R}) \tag{13-36}$$

In this equation B is the y-intercept obtained by back-extrapolating the terminal linear portion of plasma profile to time zero following the administration of the first dose, K and τ have been defined previously and R is a factor, which accounts for the absorption and elimination rate constants of the drug. The factor R is calculated using the relationship:

$$R = K(t_{max}) \tag{13-37}$$

In equation (13-37), t_{max} is the time of peak concentration after the first dose. For all practical purposes, if K_a >>> K, i.e. K_a is at least five-times greater than K, the plasma profile shows a distinct and sharp peak enabling one to read t_{max} from the graph as a good approximation. However, if the plasma profile does not exhibit a sharp peak and/or if it is difficult to read t_{max} from the graph, it can be calculated using the equation:

$$t_{max} = \frac{\ln K_a - \ln K}{K_a - K} \tag{13-38}$$

$$t = \frac{\ln \alpha_a - \ln \beta}{\alpha_a - \beta} \tag{13-38}$$

Minimum Concentration, $C_{min\ ss}$

The minimum concentration of drug in plasma following extravascular administration of n doses is described by the equation

$$C_{min\ n} = (B)\frac{(1 - e^{-nK\tau})(e^{-K\tau})}{1 - e^{-K\tau}} - \frac{(1 - e^{-nG})(e^{-G})}{1 - e^{-G}} \tag{13-39}$$

where,

$C_{min\ n}$ = minimum concentration of drug in plasma during the nth dose,
B = back-extrapolated y-intercept of the terminal linear phase after the first dose,
K = elimination rate constant, τ = dosing interval,
$G = K_a\tau$ and
K_a = absorption rate constant.

By setting n = 1 in equation (13-39) an expression for the minimum plasma concentration of drug following the first dose ($C_{min\ 1}$) can be obtained. When n = 1, equation (13-39) becomes:

$$C = (B)\frac{\left(1-e^{-K\tau}\right)\left(e^{-K\tau}\right)}{1-e^{-K\tau}} - \frac{\left(1-e^{-G}\right)\left(e^{-G}\right)}{1-e^{-G}}$$

$$C_{min\,1} = (B)(e^{-K\tau} - e^{-G}) \qquad (13\text{-}40)$$

When n becomes large, i.e. when steady-state is attained, an expression for minimum plasma concentration of drug at steady-state is obtained from equation (13-39). When n becomes large, the exponential terms $e^{-nK\tau}$ and e^{-nG} approach 0 and equation (13-39) becomes

$$C = (B)\left(\frac{e^{-K\tau}}{1-e^{-K\tau}} - \frac{e^{-G}}{1-e^{-G}}\right) \qquad (13\text{-}41)$$

In the postabsorptive phase, G (the product of K_a and τ) becomes large and therefore, the exponential term e^{-G} approaches 0. Equation (13-41) is then reduced to

$$C_{min\,ss} = \frac{(B)\left(e^{-K\tau}\right)}{1-e^{-K\tau}} \qquad (13\text{-}42)$$

Example 13-11 From the following data obtained after oral administration of a single 500 mg dose of an antibiotic, calculate maximum and minimum steady-state concentrations of the drug if a 500 mg oral dose is administered every 4 hourrly.

Time (h)	*Concentration (μg/mL)*	*Time (h)*	*Concentration (μg/mL)*	*Time (h)*	*Concentration (μg/mL)*
0.5	19.8	2.0	28.0	5.0	16.7
1.0	27.0	3.0	23.7	6.0	14.0
1.5	28.3	4.0	20.0	7.0	12.0

Solution

A plot of concentration of drug in plasma as a function of time is shown in Figure 13-6.

Back-extrapolation of the terminal linear portion gives B = 40 μg/mL. The initial data points representing the predominantly absorption phase are feathered to yield the absorption phase. The graph shows that the drug confers the characteristics of one-compartment model on the body. From the graph,

$$K = \frac{\ln 40 - \ln 20}{(0-4)h} = -\frac{0.6931}{-4\ h} = 0.1733/h$$

$$K\tau = (0.1733/h)(4\ h) = 0.6932,\ \text{therefore, } e^{-K\tau} = e^{-0.693} = 0.5$$

$$K_a = -\frac{\ln 40 - \ln 1}{(0-2.1)h} = -\frac{3.6889}{-2.1\ h} = 1.7567/h$$

$$G = (Ka)(\tau) = (1.757/h)(4\ h) = 7.028,\ \text{therefore, } e^{-G} = e^{-7.028}$$

From the graph it appears that the time of maximum concentration of drug in the plasma, tmax, is about 1.5 hour. According to equation (13-38), tmax is: $\ln K_a - \ln K$

$$t_{max} = \frac{\ln K_a - \ln K}{K_a - K}$$

$$= \frac{\ln 1.7567 - \ln 0.1733}{1.7567/h - 0.1733/h} = \frac{2.3162}{1.5834/h} = 1.463\ h$$

$$R = (K)(t_{max}) = (0.1733/h)(1.463h) = 0.2535,$$

Therefore, $e^{-R} = e^{-0.2535} = 0.776$.

Substituting the values of B, e^{-R}, e^{-G} and $e^{-K\tau}$ into equations (13-36) and (13-41),

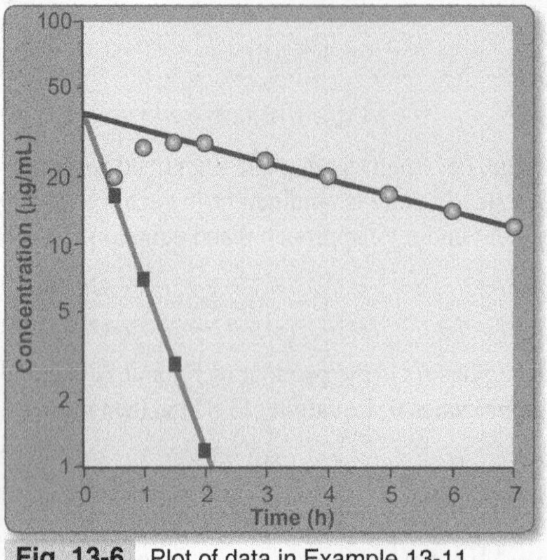

Fig. 13-6 Plot of data in Example 13-11

$$C_{max\ ss} = \frac{B}{1-e^{-K\tau}}\left(e^{-R}\right)$$

$$= \frac{40\ \mu g/mL}{1-0.5}(0.776) = \frac{31.04\ \mu g/mL}{0.5} = 62.08\ \mu g/mL \text{ and}$$

$$C_{min\ ss} = (B)\left(\frac{e^{-K\tau}}{1-e^{-K\tau}} - \frac{e^{-G}}{1-e^{-G}}\right)$$

$$= (40\ \mu g/mL)\left(\frac{0.5}{1-0.5} - \frac{0}{1-0}\right) = (40\ \mu g/mL)(1-0) = 40\ \mu g/mL$$

If the approximate values of K_a and t_{max} were used in calculating Cmax ss and $C_{min\ ss}$, the answers obtained are not likely to be significantly different from the answers obtained using the more accurate values, because, the approximate values of the rate constant of absorption and the time of maximum concentration are not significantly different from their accurate values.

For example, using Ka = 1.7325/h and t_{max} = 1.5 h,

$$R = (K_e)(t_{max}) = (0.1733/h)(1.5\ h) = 0.25995, \text{ therefore,}$$

$$e^{-R} = e^{-0.2599} = 0.771$$

$$G = (K_a)(\tau) = (1.7325/h)(4\ h) = 6.93, \text{ therefore,}$$

$$e^{-G} = e^{-6.93} = 0.001$$

Substituting the values into equations (13-36) and (13-41),

$$C_{max\ ss} = \frac{B}{1-e^{-K\tau}}\left(e^{-R}\right)$$

$$= \frac{40\ \mu g/mL}{1-0.5}(0.771) = \frac{3084\ \mu g/mL}{0.5} = 61.68\ \mu g/mL \text{ and}$$

$$C_{min\ ss} = (B)\left(\frac{e^{-K\tau}}{1-e^{-K\tau}} - \frac{e^{-G}}{1-e^{-G}}\right)$$

$$= (40\ \mu g/mL)\left(\frac{0.5}{1-0.5} - \frac{0.001}{1-0.001}\right) = (40\ \mu g/mL)(1-0.001) = 39.96\ \mu g/mL$$

It will be noticed that in this Example, the dosing interval (τ) was equal to the biological half-life ($t_{1/2}$) of the drug; therefore the minimum plasma concentration of drug at steady-state

($C_{min\ ss}$) was approximately equal to the y-intercept B (Fig. 13-6). However, the maximum concentration of drug at steady-state ($C_{max\ ss}$) was not equal to twice the value of B, because administration of drug via extravascular route requires time for absorption.

Relationship Between $C_{max\ ss}$ and $C_{min\ ss}$: It was shown in equation (13-34) that during intravenous multiple dosing the difference between the maximum and minimum concentrations of drug in plasma at steady-state was always equal to C_0 (as long as there is no change in the dose, volume of distribution and dosing interval). In extravascular administration the difference between maximum and minimum concentrations of drug in plasma at steady-state, obtained by subtracting equation (13-41) from equation (13-36) is not, as simple as was seen during intravenous administration, but is a complex function of the factors that determine these concentrations.

Factors Influencing Steady-State Concentration

From equations (13-36) and (13-41) it is seen that during extravascular administration, the minimum concentration of drug in the plasma at steady-state depends on three factors: the y-intercept B, the rate constant of elimination K and the dosing interval τ. On the other hand, maximum concentration of drug in the plasma at steady-state depends on four factors: the y-intercept B, the rate constant of elimination K, the dosing interval τ and the rate constant of absorption K_a. The factors influencing $C_{min\ ss}$ are similar to those seen during intravenous administration, because the parameter B in the extravascular administration (the y-intercept of the resolved plasma profile after administration of the first dose) is similar to the parameter C_0 in the intravenous administration (the y-intercept of the plasma profile after administration of the first dose). However, the factors affecting the maximum concentration at steady-state differ in the two cases, because, during extravascular administration, there is an added factor, K_a. In linear pharmacokinetics, B is directly proportional to Dose (D), because equation (12-5) of Chapter 12:

$$B = \frac{(F)(D)(K_a)}{(V_d)(K_a - K)} \tag{12-5}$$

and it is assumed that the values of F, V_d, K_a and K do not change during the course of therapy. The steady-state maximum and minimum concentrations of drug in the plasma therefore depend only on Dose (D) and Dosing Interval (τ).

Effect of Dose: According to equation (13-41),

$$C_{min\ ss} = (B)\left(\frac{e^{-K\tau}}{1-e^{-K\tau}} - \frac{e^{-G}}{1-e^{-G}}\right)$$

$$\text{Since, } B = \frac{(F)(D)(K_a)}{(V_d)(K_a - K)}\text{, therefore,}$$

$$C_{min\ ss} = \frac{(F)(D)(K_a)}{(V_d)(K_a - K)}\left(\frac{e^{-K\tau}}{1-e^{-K\tau}} - \frac{e^{-G}}{1-e^{-G}}\right) \tag{13-43}$$

The minimum concentration of drug in plasma at steady-state ($C_{min\ ss''}$) following the administration of a Dose D″ (assuming no change in dosing interval, volume of distribution, rate constant of absorption, elimination rate constant and the fraction of dose absorbed) is given by

$$C_{min\ ss''} = \frac{(F)(D'')(K_a)}{(V_d)(K_a - K)}\left(\frac{e^{-K\tau}}{1-e^{-K\tau}} - \frac{e^{-G}}{1-e^{-G}}\right) \tag{13-44}$$

Dividing equation (13-43) by equation (13-44),

$$\frac{C_{min\ ss}}{C_{min\ ss''}} = \frac{D}{D''} \tag{13-45}$$

Similarly, using the same rationale, it can be shown that

$$\frac{C_{max\ ss}}{C_{max\ ss''}} = \frac{D}{D''} \tag{13-46}$$

Thus, an increase or decrease in the dose will correspondingly increase or decrease the steady-state concentrations. The following Example illustrates the effect of dose on steady-state maximum and minimum concentrations of drug in the plasma.

Example 13-12 Administration of 500 mg oral dose of an antibiotic gave the following data: B = 70 μg/mL, K_a = 0.71/h and K = 0.139/h. Calculate steady-state maximum and minimum plasma concentration of drug if:

a. 500 mg dose is administered every 6 hourly
b. 400 mg dose is administered every 6 hour.

Solution

a. From the data provided:

$$t_{max} = \frac{\ln K_a - \ln K}{K_a - K}$$

$$= \frac{\ln 0.71 - \ln 0.139}{0.71/h - 0.139/h} = \frac{1.6308}{0.571/h} = 2.856\ h$$

$$R = (K)(t_{max}) = (0.139/h)(2.856\ h) = 0.397, \text{ therefore,}$$

$$e^{-R} = e^{-0.397} = 0.6723$$

$$K\tau = (0.139/h)(6\ h) = 0.834, \text{ therefore,}$$

$$e^{-K\tau} = e^{-0.834} = 0.4343$$

$$(1 - e^{-K\tau}) = (1 - 0.4343) = 0.5657$$

$$G = (0.71/h)(6\ h) = 4.26, \text{ therefore,}$$

$$e^{-G} = e^{-4.26} = 0.0141$$

Substituting these values into equation (13-36):

$$C_{max\ ss} = \frac{B}{1 - e^{-K\tau}}\left(e^{-R}\right)$$

$$= \frac{70\ \mu g/mL}{1 - 0.4343}(0.6723) = \frac{47.061\ \mu g/mL}{0.5657} = 83.19\ \mu g/mL$$

Similarly, substituting these values into equation (13-41),

$$C_{min\ ss} = (B)\left(\frac{e^{-K\tau}}{1 - e^{-K\tau}} - \frac{e^{-G}}{1 - e^{-G}}\right)$$

$$= (70\ \mu g/mL)\left(\frac{0.4343}{1 - 0.4343} - \frac{0.0141}{1 - 0.0141}\right) = (70\ \mu g/mL)\left(\frac{0.4343}{0.5657} - \frac{0.0141}{0.9859}\right)$$

$$= (70\ \mu g/mL)(0.7677 - 0.01430) = 52.73\ \mu g/mL$$

Using equation (13-43), the minimum concentration at steady-state is

$$C_{min\ ss} = \frac{B}{1 - e^{-K\tau}}\left(e^{-K\tau}\right)$$

$$= \frac{70\ \mu g/mL}{1 - 0.4343} \times 0.4343 = \frac{30.401\ \mu g/mL}{0.5657} = 53.74\ \mu g/mL$$

It is seen that the minimum concentration of drug in plasma at steady-state obtained using equation (13-41) is slightly larger than that obtained using equation (13-43). This is because the factor e^{-G} did not approach 0. Therefore the second exponential term on the right-hand side of equation (13-41) still had a finite value. The value of minimum concentration of drug in the plasma at steady-state obtained using equation (13-41) is more accurate than the value obtained using equation (13-43).

b. When the dose is changed from 500 mg to 400 mg, the values of P(?) and R are not changed, because the factors affecting P and R (D, K and K_a) are not affected. Therefore, $e^{-K\tau}$ and e^{-R} are also unchanged. The value of y-intercept, B will change because of change in dose. Assuming linear pharmacokinetics,

$$\text{new B} = \frac{(\text{old B})(\text{new dose})}{\text{old dose}} = \frac{(70\ \mu g/mL)(400\ mg)}{500\ mg} = 56\ \mu g/mL$$

$$C_{max\ ss} = \frac{B}{1-e^{-K\tau}}\left(e^{-R}\right) = \frac{56\ \mu g/mL}{1-0.4343}(0.4343) = \frac{37.65\ \mu g/mL}{0.5657} = 66.55\ \mu g/mL$$

$$C_{max\ ss} = \frac{B}{1-e^{-K\tau}}\left(e^{-K\tau}\right) = \frac{56\ \mu g/mL}{1-0.4343}(0.4343) = \frac{24.32\ \mu g/mL}{0.5657} = 42.99\ \mu g/mL$$

From Example 13-12 it is seen that

$$\frac{\text{old } C_{min\ ss}}{\text{new } C_{min\ ss}} = \frac{53.74\ \mu g/mL}{66.55\ \mu g/mL} = 1.25$$

$$\frac{\text{old } C_{max\ ss}}{\text{new } C_{max\ ss}} = \frac{83.19\ \mu g/mL}{66.55\ \mu g/mL} = 1.25$$

$$\text{and} \quad \frac{\text{old dose}}{\text{new dose}} = \frac{500\ mg}{400\ mg} = 1.25$$

which is in agreement with equations (13-45) and (13-46).

Effect of Dosing Interval: It was mentioned earlier (in the section dealing with intravenous administration of bolus doses), that the effect of dosing interval on the plasma minimum and maximum concentrations of drug at steady-state ($C_{min\ ss}$ and $C_{max\ ss}$) is not simple and straight-forward. During extravascular administration, the same reasoning holds true. In linear pharmacokinetics, the size of dose is directly proportional to the value of B-intercept of the plasma concentration vs time plot and any change in the size of dose has a linear effect on the concentration of drug in the plasma at steady-state. Dosing interval is not related in a similar linear manner to the terms used in calculating the minimum and maximum concentrations of drug in plasma at steady-state. In equations used for calculating steady-state concentrations of drug, dosing interval appears in the exponential terms. Therefore, the relationship between dosing interval and steady-state concentrations becomes more complicated and it is not possible to relate the effect of dosing interval on steady-state concentrations with a simple relationship.

SUGGESTED READING

1. Evans WE, Schentag JJ and Jusko WJ (eds). Applied Pharmacokinetics: Principles of Therapeutic Drug Monitoring, 3rd edition, Applied Therapeutics; 1995.
2. Benet L. Pharmacokinetics: A Modern View. Plenum Press; 1984.
3. Gibaldi M, Perrier D. Pharmacokinetics, 2nd edition. Marcel Dekker; 1982.
4. Mungall D (ed). Applied Clinical Pharmacokinetics. Raven Press; 1983.
5. Remington: The Science and Practice of Pharmacy, 20th edition. Mack Publishing; 2000.
6. Ritschel WA. Handbook of Basic Pharmacokinetics, 3rd edition. Drug Intelligence Publications; 1986.

PRACTICE PROBLEMS

13-1. The biological half-life of a drug is 5 h. Calculate the persistence factor if identical doses are administered: (a) Every 6 hours or (b) Every 12 hours.

13-2. The biological half-life of a drug is 4 h. Calculate the loss factor if identical doses are administered: (a) Every 6 hours, or (b) Every 12 hours.

13-3. The biological half-life of a drug is 4 h and identical doses are administered every 6 hours. Calculate the accumulation factor after the administration of: (a) Two doses, (b) Three doses, (c) Four doses, (d) Five doses, and (e) Twenty doses.

13-4. Calculate the maximum and minimum plasma concentrations of a drug after the administration of the fourth dose. The drug, upon administration, confers the characteristics of one-compartment pharmacokinetic model on the body. Each dose is 80 mg administered intravenously as a bolus injection every 4 hours, the apparent volume of distribution of the drug is 40 L and the rate constant of elimination is 0.07/h.

13-5. Calculate the maximum and minimum plasma concentrations of a drug after the administration of the third dose. The drug confers the characteristics of one-compartment pharmacokinetic model on the body. Each dose is 50 mg administered intravenously as a bolus injection every 4 hours, the apparent volume of distribution of the drug is 40 L and the rate constant of elimination is 0.07/h.

13-6. Calculate the maximum and minimum plasma concentrations of a drug after administration of the thirty-sixth dose of the drug. The drug confers the characteristics of one-compartment model on the body. Each dose is 50 mg administered intravenously as a bolus injection every 4 hours, the apparent volume of distribution of the drug is 40 L and the rate constant of elimination is 0.07/h.

13-7. The following table details the concentration of drug in the plasma, as a function of time after the administration of a single 300 mg intravenous bolus dose of an antibiotic. Calculate the minimum and maximum steady-state concentrations of drug in the plasma if a 300 mg rapid intravenous bolus dose is given: (a) Every 12 hours, (b) Every 8 hours, or (c) Every 4 hours

Time (h)	*Concentration (mg/L)*	*Time (h)*	*Concentration (mg/L)*
0.5	0.925	4.0	0.500
1.0	0.845	5.0	0.420
2.0	0.710	6.0	0.352
3.0	0.595	8.0	0.250

13-8. The following table details the concentration of drug in the plasma, as a function of time after the administration of a single intravenous bolus dose of an antibiotic. Calculate the minimum and maximum concentrations of drug in the plasma at the plateau level if the same dose is administered: (a) Once a day, (b) Every 10 hours, or (c) Every 3 hours.

Time (h)	*Concentration (μg/mL)*	*Time (h)*	*Concentration (μg/mL)*
2.0	455	8.0	195
4.0	345	10.0	150
6.0	260	12.0	115

13-9. The following table details the concentration of drug in the plasma as a function of time after the administration of a single 500 mg oral dose of an antibiotic. Calculate the maximum and minimum concentrations of the drug at steady-state if a 500 mg dose of the antibiotic is administered: (a) Every 8 hours, (b) Every 16 hours, or (c) Every 24 hours.

Time (h)	Concentration (mg/L)	Time (h)	Concentration (mg/L)	Time (h)	Concentration (mg/L)
1	2.88	8	2.00	20	0.73
2	3.25	12	1.45	24	0.53
4	2.85	16	1.02	28	0.38

13-10. Blood level data following a single 300 mg oral dose of a drug are shown below. Calculate the maximum and minimum concentrations at steady-state if the patient is given a 300 mg bolus dose every 6 hours.

Time (h)	Concentration (μg/L)	Time (h)	Concentration (μg/L)
0.5	650	6.0	585
1.0	900	8.0	425
2.0	1100	10.0	310
4.0	800	12.0	255

13-11. Blood level data following a single intravenous dose of an antibiotic are shown below. Calculate the minimum and maximum concentrations of drug in plasma at plateau level if the same dose is administered: (a) Once a day, (b) Every 10 hours, or (c) Every 3 hours.

Time (h)	Concentration (μg/L)	Time (h)	Concentration (μg/L)
2.0	546	8.0	234
4.0	414	10.0	180
6.0	312	12.0	138

13-12. Blood level data following intravenous administration of a 500 mg bolus dose of an antibiotic are shown below. Calculate the minimum and maximum steady-state concentrations of the drug in the plasma if a 300 mg intravenous bolus dose is given (a) Every 12 hours, (b) Every 8 hours, or (c) Every 4 hours.

Time (h)	Concentration (mg/L)	Time (h)	Concentration (mg/L)
0.5	1.4800	4.0	0.8000
1.0	1.3520	5.0	0.6720
2.0	1.1360	6.0	0.5632
3.0	0.9520	8.0	0.4000

13-13. Blood level data following intravenous administration of a single 450 mg dose of an antibiotic are shown below. Calculate the minimum and maximum steady-state concentrations of drug in plasma if a 300 mg rapid intravenous bolus dose is given: (a) Every 12 hours, (b) Every 8 hours, or (c) Every 4 hours.

Time (h)	Concentration (mg/L)	Time (h)	Concentration (mg/L)
0.5	1.295	4.0	0.700
1.0	1.183	5.0	0.588
2.0	0.994	6.0	0.493
3.0	0.833	8.0	0.350

13-14. Blood level data following intravenous administration of a single 550 mg bolus dose of an antibiotic are shown below. Calculate the minimum and maximum steady-state concentrations of drug in plasma if a 300 mg rapid intravenous bolus dose is given: (a) Every 12 hours, (b) Every 8 hours, or (c) Every 4 hours.

Time (h)	*Concentration (mg/L)*	*Time (h)*	*Concentration (mg/L)*
0.5	1.6650	4.0	0.9000
1.0	1.5210	5.0	0.7560
2.0	1.2780	6.0	0.6336
3.0	1.0710	8.0	0.4500

CHAPTER 14

LOADING DOSE

Most drugs for chronic conditions are prescribed in a dosage regimen, which is based on the administration of a fixed constant dose of drug administered at fixed regular dosing intervals (τ) for relatively long periods of time. The size of the dose and dosing interval recommended by the manufacturer is based on effective therapeutic concentration of drug in the plasma needed to treat the chronic condition. The dosing interval suggested by the manufacturer is based on the rate constant of elimination of the drug. In the majority of situations, the dosing interval is approximately equal to the biological half-life ($t_{1/2}$) of the drug, i.e. $\tau = t_{1/2}$.

As pointed out earlier in the discussion dealing with multiple dosing of intravenously administered drugs (Chapter 13), which, upon administration, confer upon the body the characteristics of one-compartment model, the steady-state concentration of drug in plasma during multiple dosing is given by the equations (13-29) and (13-30):

$$C_{max\ ss} = \frac{C_0}{1 - e^{-K\tau}}$$

$$C_{min\ ss} = \frac{C_0}{1 - e^{-K\tau}}(e^{-K\tau}) = C_{max\ ss}(e^{-K\tau})$$

It will be recalled that in these two equations, C_0 is the back extrapolated y-intercept after administration of a single dose (the size of this dose is equal to the size of maintenance dose) and $e^{-K\tau}$ is persistence factor.

It is clear from equations (13-29) and (13-30) that the concentration of drug in plasma at steady-state depends on the following three factors:

a. C_0, concentration of drug in plasma immediately after administration of maintenance dose
b. K, rate constant of elimination of drug (therefore, biological half-life of the drug)
c. τ, the dosing interval.

In linear pharmacokinetics, C_0 obtained after the administration of a single dose is directly proportional to the size of the dose, i.e. if the dose was reduced 25%, then C_0 will also reduce 25% and if the dose was doubled, then C_0 will also be doubled. If we assume that the rate constant of elimination of drug does not change during the course of therapy and a fixed, constant maintenance dose of the drug, D, is administered at fixed dosing intervals, τ, then the time required for the drug to accumulate to a steady-state concentration in plasma will depend only on the rate constant of elimination (therefore, the biological half-life of the drug). If the dosing interval is equal to the biological half-life of drug, then the time to reach steady-state concentration of drug in the plasma will be approximately 7 or 8 half-lives of the drug. In other words, for a drug with a half-life of 6 hours, it would take approximately 2 days before the concentration of drug in the plasma attains a steady-state level. Similarly, for a drug with a half-life of 24 hours, it would take approximately 1 week before concentration of drug in the plasma reaches steady-state levels.

If the time to reach steady-state concentration of drug in the plasma represents an unacceptable delay (e.g. in the case of serious illness and/or with drugs having a long biological half-life), then a loading dose is usually recommended. This dose has also been known as the priming dose or initial dose. The concept of loading dose is especially useful in those cases, where therapeutic plasma concentration range of the drug has been identified and established.

The primary purpose of using loading dose in therapeutic treatment is to attain steady-state concentration of drug as quickly as possible, usually right from the start of treatment. This approach has the added advantage that it may also reduce the time of onset of drug action, i.e. the time it takes to achieve the minimum effective concentration. Since the purpose of administering loading dose is to reduce the time needed for drug to accumulate to steady-state levels in the plasma, i.e. accelerate accumulation of drug in plasma, the size of loading dose is therefore always larger than the size of maintenance dose. Obviously, the size of loading dose will depend upon the dosing interval of the maintenance dose.

INTRAVENOUS ADMINISTRATION

The simplest case is a drug which, when administered intravenously as a single rapid bolus dose, confers the characteristics of one-compartment model on the body. As mentioned above, the main purpose of administering loading dose is to provide a concentration of drug in the plasma (as soon as therapy is initiated), which is equal to steady-state concentration of drug in plasma during multiple dosing, i.e. attain steady-state plasma concentration with the administration of the very first dose (loading dose). The size of loading dose needed to achieve steady-state plasma levels of the drug can be calculated based upon either the maximum concentration at steady-state or the minimum concentration at steady-state.

Loading Dose Based on $C_{max\ ss}$

As mentioned above, the maximum concentration of drug in the plasma at steady-state, $C_{max\ ss}$, is given by equation (13-29)

$$C_{max\ ss} = \frac{C_0}{1 - e^{-K\tau}}$$

In this equation, C_0 is the concentration of drug in plasma immediately after administration of a single dose (the size of this dose is equal to the size of maintenance dose) and $e^{-K\tau}$ is the persistence factor. If the drug follows linear pharmacokinetics then C_0 obtained after administration of a rapid intravenous bolus dose is directly proportional to the size of dose, D. Equation (13-29) is therefore analogous to

$$C_{max\ ss} \propto \frac{D}{1 - e^{-K\tau}} \qquad (14\text{-}1)$$

where D = dose (maintenance dose)

Since the purpose of loading dose is to attain maximum concentration of drug in the plasma at steady-state ($C_{max\ ss}$) as soon as treatment is initiated, the size of the loading dose should be such that administration of its 1-time single dose will provide an initial concentration, C_0, which is equal to the value of $C_{max\ ss}$. In other words, $C_{max\ 1}$ after the administration of loading dose (D*) should be equal to $C_{max\ ss}$ attained at steady-state with the dose (D) administered at a regular dosing interval = τ.

From equation (13-29), the maximum concentration at steady-state is

$$C_{max\ ss} = \frac{C_0}{1 - e^{-K\tau}}$$

Since, in single dose intravenous bolus administration of drugs which confer upon the body the characteristics of one-compartment model, concentration of drug in the plasma immediately after administration of the first dose is given by the relationship:

$$C_0 = \frac{D}{V_d}$$

where, D = dose (maintenance dose) and V_d = apparent volume of distribution.

Therefore, equation (13-29) may be written as:

$$C = \frac{D}{V_d\left(1 - e^{-K\tau}\right)} \qquad (14\text{-}1)$$

The maximum concentration after the first dose is

$$C_{max\,1} = C_0 = \frac{D}{V_d}$$

Since the loading dose, D*, should provide $C_{max\,1} = C_{max\,ss}$, the concentration of drug in plasma immediately after the administration of the loading dose, $^*C_0$, is given by

$$^*C_0 = \frac{D^*}{V_d} \qquad (14\text{-}2)$$

By definition, the purpose of administering the loading dose is that $^*C_0$ obtained with the administration of the loading dose must be equal to $C_{max\,ss}$ obtained during multiple dosing. This means that $C_{max\,ss}$ in equation (13-29) should be equal to $^*C_0$ in equation (14-2), i.e.,

$$^*C = C_{max\,ss} \qquad (14\text{-}3)$$

Substituting the value of $^*C_0$ from equation (14-2) and the value of $C_{max\,ss}$ from equation (14-1) into equation (14-3) gives

$$\frac{D^*}{V_d} = \frac{D}{V_d\left(1 - e^{-K\tau}\right)}$$

Canceling the common term V_d from the denominator on both sides of the equation yields

$$D^* = \frac{D}{1 - e^{-K\tau}} \qquad (14\text{-}4)$$

Thus, the size of loading dose is a function of maintenance dose, D and persistence factor, $e^{-K\tau}$.

Since persistence factor is a function of rate constant of elimination and dosing interval, it follows that the size of loading dose depends on the following three factors:

a. Maintenance dose, D
b. Elimination rate constant, K (therefore biological half-life of drug)
c. Dosing interval, τ.

Example 14-1 Calculate the size of loading dose to attain steady-state maximum concentration of drug in plasma at the start of therapy for an antibiotic having a maintenance dose of 300 mg. The dose is administered intravenously every 9 hours and the biological half-life of the antibiotic is 9 hours.

Solution

Since $t_{1/2}$ = 9 hours, therefore K = 0.693/9 h = 0.077/h.

Substituting the values of maintenance dose = 300 mg, elimination rate constant = 0.077/h and dosing interval = 9 h into equation (14-4), one gets,

$$D^* = \frac{D}{1 - e^{-K\tau}} = \frac{300\text{ mg}}{1 - e^{-(0.077/\text{h})(9\text{ h})}} = \frac{300\text{ mg}}{1 - e^{-(0.693)}} = \frac{300\text{ mg}}{1 - 0.5} = 600\text{ mg}$$

In this example, the dosing interval was equal to biological half-life of the drug and the size of loading dose is found to be twice the size of maintenance dose. If dosing interval is not equal to biological half-life of the drug, then the size of loading dose is also not equal to twice the size of the maintenance dose. The following two examples illustrate the effect of dosing interval on the size of loading dose.

Example 14-2 Calculate the size of loading dose to attain the steady-state maximum concentration of drug in plasma at the start of therapy for an antibiotic having a maintenance dose of 300 mg. The dose is administered intravenously every 8 hours and the biological half-life of the antibiotic is 9 hours.

Solution

Substituting the values of maintenance dose = 300 mg, elimination rate constant = 0.077/h and dosing interval = 8 h into equation (14-4):

$$D^* = \frac{D}{1-e^{-K\tau}} = \frac{300\text{ mg}}{1-e^{-(0.077/\text{h})(8\text{ h})}} = \frac{300\text{ mg}}{1-e^{-(0.616)}} = \frac{300\text{ mg}}{1-0.54} = \frac{300\text{ mg}}{0.46} = 652\text{ mg}$$

Example 14-3 Calculate the size of loading dose to attain steady-state maximum concentration of drug in plasma at the start of therapy for an antibiotic having a maintenance dose of 300 mg administered intravenously every 10 hr. The biological half-life of the antibiotic is 9 hours.

Solution

Substituting the values of maintenance dose = 300 mg, elimination rate constant = 0.077/h and dosing interval = 10 h into equation (14-4): *D* 300 mg 300 mg

$$D^* = \frac{D}{1-e^{-K\tau}} = \frac{300\text{ mg}}{1-e^{-(0.077/\text{h})(10\text{ h})}} = \frac{300\text{ mg}}{1-e^{-(0.77)}}$$

$$= = \frac{300\text{ mg}}{1-0.463} = \frac{300\text{ mg}}{0.537} = 559\text{ mg}$$

From these three examples, it is seen that the size of the loading dose is different in each case. In Example 14-1 the size of the loading dose is 600 mg, which is twice the size of the 300 mg maintenance dose; but the size of loading dose needed for data given in Example 14-2 is 652 mg (which is more than twice the size of the 300 mg maintenance dose) and the size of loading dose is 559 mg in Example 14-3 (which is less than twice the size of the 300 mg maintenance dose). Since the only variable in these three examples is the dosing interval, the difference in the size of loading dose in each of these three instances is therefore only due to the different dosing intervals in each of these three examples.

Loading Dose Based on $C_{min\ ss}$

It was shown in Chapter 13 and earlier in this Chapter that during multiple dosing, the minimum concentration of drug in plasma at steady-state, $C_{min\ ss}$, is given by the equation (13-30):

$$C_{min\ ss} = \frac{C_0}{1-e^{-K\tau}}(e^{-K\tau}) = C_{min\ ss}(e^{-K\tau})$$

If the drug follows linear pharmacokinetics then C_0 obtained after administration of a single dose (maintenance dose, D) is directly proportional to the size of maintenance dose. Equation (13-30) is therefore analogous to

$$C_{min\ ss} \propto \frac{D}{1-e^{-K\tau}}(e^{-K\tau})$$

The purpose of loading dose is to attain the steady-state minimum concentration of drug in plasma ($C_{min\ ss}$) right from the start of treatment, i.e. the minimum concentration of drug in plasma just before administration of second dose should be equal to minimum concentration of drug in plasma attained at the steady-state. That is, the size of loading dose should be such that administration of loading dose will provide $C_{min\ 1}$, which is equal to $C_{min\ ss}$, i.e. $C_{min\ 1}$ after administration of loading dose (D*) should be equal to $C_{min\ ss}$ at steady-state with maintenance dose (D) administered at a fixed dosing interval = τ.

From equation (13-30):

$$C_{min\ ss} = \frac{C_0}{1-e^{-K\tau}}(e^{-K\tau})$$

In linear pharmacokinetics, when a single bolus dose of the drug is administered intravenously,

$$C_0 = \frac{D}{V_d}$$

Therefore, equation (13-30) may be written as

$$C_{min\ ss} = \frac{D}{V_d\left(1-e^{-K\tau}\right)}(e^{-K\tau}) \qquad (14\text{-}5)$$

The minimum concentration of drug in the plasma after administration of the first dose (maintenance dose) is given by the following equation:

$$C = (C_0)(e^{-K\tau}) = \frac{D}{V_d}(e^{-K\tau})$$

For the loading dose (D*), we need $C_{min\ 1} = ({}^*C_0)(e^{-K\tau})$, which should be equal to $C_{min\ ss}$, i.e.

$$({}^*C_0)(e^{-K\tau}) = \frac{D^*}{V_d}(e^{-K\tau}) \qquad (14\text{-}6)$$

where, the terms C_0, D* and V_d have previously been defined in equation (14-2).

Since the product $({}^*C_0)(e^{-K\tau})$ must be equal to $C_{min\ ss}$, equations (14-6) and (13-30) are combined to yield the following relationship:

$$({}^*C_0)(e^{-K\tau}) = C_{min\ ss}$$

$$\text{i.e., } (e^{-K\tau}) = \frac{D}{V_d\left(1-e^{-K\tau}\right)}(e^{-K\tau}) \qquad (14\text{-}7)$$

The two common terms ($e^{-K\tau}$ in the numerator and V_d in the denominator) on both sides of equation (14-7) can be canceled and equation (14-7) is therefore simplified to yield:

$$D^* = \frac{D}{1-e^{-K\tau}}$$

It will be noticed that this equation is identical to the equation (14-4) used for calculating loading dose based on the maximum concentration of drug in the plasma at steady-state.

Factors Affecting Size of Loading Dose

Equation (14-4) relates the size of loading dose with the following factors:

a. Size of the maintenance dose
b. Dosing interval
c. Rate constant of elimination of the drug.

It is assumed in this equation that all doses and all dosing intervals are kept constant during multiple dosing. As can be seen from this equation, if all doses and all dosing intervals are kept constant, then the size of loading dose depends on the size of maintenance dose, dosing interval and elimination rate constant of the drug. Since the rate constant of elimination of a drug in a given individual is assumed to be constant and assuming that it does not change during the course of therapy, the size of loading dose is therefore dependant only on dosing interval and maintenance dose.

Effect of Dosing Interval

Everything else being equal, i.e. if the size of maintenance dose is kept constant and biological half-life of the drug (rate constant of elimination of the drug) does not change during the course of therapy, then the size of the loading dose for a given treatment (assuming one-compartment model) depends entirely on the dosing interval of the given drug. If the dosing interval is much greater than the biological half-life of the drug ($\tau > t_{1/2}$), i.e. the drug is administered at relatively longer intervals, then a large fraction of the administered dose is lost from the body due to elimination before the next dose is administered. Since a large fraction of each administered dose is eliminated before the administration of the next dose, accumulation of drug in the body is slow, i.e. $C_{max\ ss}$ does not attain a relatively high value. Therefore, the size of loading dose needed to achieve $C_{max\ ss}$ is small. If, on the other hand, the dosing interval is less than the biological half-life of the drug ($\tau < t_{1/2}$), i.e. the drug is administered more frequently, then the accumulation of drug due to more frequent administration of the dose maintains high plasma levels of drug and therefore the size of loading dose required to achieve the high levels of $C_{max\ ss}$ is also large.

Table 14-1 summarizes the effect of dosing interval on the size of loading dose needed to achieve steady-state concentrations of drug in the plasma from the time the treatment is initiated.

The fact that the size of loading dose (D*) is equal to twice the size of the maintenance dose, when dosing interval $\tau = t_{1/2}$, can be easily shown if one uses the same rationale that was used to calculate the persistence of each dose during multiple dosing (see Table 13-1).

Table 14-2 shows the breakdown of the percentage of each administered dose persisting in body, when therapy is initiated with a loading dose the size of which is equal to two-times the size of the maintenance dose, i.e. D* = (2)(D). The loading dose, D* is followed by each maintenance dose (D) given at a dosing interval (τ) which is equal to biological half-life ($t_{1/2}$) of the drug ($\tau = t_{1/2}$). In this Table, the first line for each dose represents percentage of dose in the body immediately after administration of the dose and the second line for each dose represents percentage of dose in the body just before the administration of next dose.

From the data shown in Table 14-2, it is seen that the maximum and minimum amounts of drug persisting in the body after the administration of each dose attain a steady-state (plateau level) immediately after administration of the initial dose (loading dose). Since, in linear pharmacokinetics, the amount of drug in the body is proportional to the concentration of drug in the plasma, one can say that the maximum concentration of drug in the plasma (C_{max}) and the

Table 14-1 Effect of dosing interval on the size of loading dose

Dosing interval	*Persistence factor*	*Loss factor*	*Accumulation factor*	*Loading dose*
$\tau = 0.25t_{1/2}$	0.84	0.16	6.29	6.29D
$\tau = 0.50t_{1/2}$	0.71	0.29	3.41	3.41D
$\tau = 0.75t_{1/2}$	0.59	0.41	2.47	2.47D
$\tau = 1.00t_{1/2}$	0.50	0.50	2.00	2.00D
$\tau = 1.25t_{1/2}$	0.42	0.58	1.73	1.73D
$\tau = 1.50t_{1/2}$	0.35	0.65	1.55	1.55D
$\tau = 1.75t_{1/2}$	0.30	0.70	1.42	1.42D
$\tau = 2.00t_{1/2}$	0.25	0.75	1.33	1.33D
$\tau = 2.50t_{1/2}$	0.18	0.82	1.21	1.21D
$\tau = 3.00t_{1/2}$	0.13	0.87	1.14	1.14D
$\tau = 4.00t_{1/2}$	0.06	0.94	1.07	1.07D

Table 14-2 Percent drug in the body following each dose

Dose	Percent drug persisting for each dose	Total	Range
D*	200 100	200 100	max min
D-1	100 + 100 50 + 50	200 100	max min
D-2	50 + 50 + 100 25 + 25 + 50	200 100	max min
D-3	25 + 25 + 50 + 100 12.5 + 12.5 + 25 + 50	200 100	max min
D-4	12.5 + 12.5 + 25 + 50 + 100 6.25 + 6.25 + 12.5 + 25 + 50	200 100	max min

Explanation of Symbols
D* = Loading dose (equal to twice the maintenance dose. The loading dose is given as the initial priming dose)
D-1 = First maintenance dose (actually the second dose during treatment)
D-2 = Second maintenance dose (actually the third dose during treatment)
D-3 = Third maintenance dose (actually the fourth dose during treatment)
D-4 = Fourth maintenance dose (actually the fifth dose during treatment)

minimum concentration of drug in the plasma (C_{min}) attain a steady-state level from the time the therapy is initiated, i.e. C_{max} and C_{min} values from the start of the treatment are equal to the $C_{max\ ss}$ and $C_{min\ ss}$ values found in Table 13-1 after approximately 8 doses of the drug are administered.

The data presented in Table 14-2 are generated using calculations based on a dosing interval equal to the elimination half-life of the drug. When the dosing interval is not equal to the biological half-life of the drug, the maximum and minimum amounts of drug in the body after each dose will be different from the data shown in Table 14-2.

In order to calculate the maximum and minimum amounts of drug in the body after the administration of each dose, when the dosing interval is not equal to the biological half-life of the drug, one can use the rationale similar to the one used for calculating the amount of drug in the body when dosing interval was equal to the biological half-life of drug. Thus, one can calculate the size of the loading dose needed to attain steady-state concentration of drug in the plasma when dosing interval is less than the biological half-life of the drug or when the interval between doses is greater than the biological half-life of the drug.

From these calculations it can be shown that following the administration of the loading dose (which will be the first drug dose administered at the initiation of the treatment), the values of the maximum and minimum concentrations of drug in the plasma after the first dose ($C_{max\ 1}$ and $C_{min\ 1}$, respectively) are similar to the maximum and minimum concentrations of drug in the plasma attained at the steady state ($C_{max\ ss}$ and $C_{min\ ss}$, respectively) during multiple dosing when no loading dose was used, i.e. when the size of all doses (maintenance doses as well as the initial dose) were identical.

Example 14-4

The concentration of drug in plasma as a function of time following intravenous administration of a single 300 mg rapid bolus dose of an antibiotic is shown below. Calculate the size of loading dose that should be administered so as to attain $C_{max\ ss}$ and $C_{min\ ss}$ from the start of therapy, if 300 mg doses of the drug will be administered intravenously: (a) Every 12 hours, (b) Every 8 hours or (c) Every 4 hours.

Time (h):	0.5	1.0	2.0	3.0	4.0	5.0	6.0
Concentration (mg/L):	0.925	0.845	0.710	0.595	0.500	0.420	0.354

Solution

A plot of concentration versus time on a semi-logarithmic graph paper is shown in Figure 14-1. The data points exhibit linearity indicating that upon administration, the drug confers upon the body the characteristics of one-compartment pharmacokinetic model.

Since the data do not exhibit too much scatter, a straight line can be drawn using eye-ball judgment. The y-intercept of this straight line is C_0 and the elimination rate constant of the drug can be determined from the slope of this straight line.

From Figure 14-1, C0 = 1.0 mg/L, and

$$K = -\text{slope} = -\ -\frac{\ln 1.0 - \ln 0.42}{(0-5)\text{h}} = -\ -\frac{0.8675}{-5} = 0.1735/\text{h}$$

Therefore, biological half-life of the drug is:

$$t_{1/2} = \frac{0693}{K} = \frac{0.693}{0.1735/\text{h}} = 4\ \text{h}$$

Alternatively, the rate constant of elimination can be determined by reading biological half-life of the drug from the graph, i.e. one reads the time, when C_0 becomes one-half of C_0.

Since $C_0 = 1.0$ mg/L, the time when C_0 becomes one-half of 1.0 mg/L = 0.5 mg/L is read from Figure14-1. From Figure 14-1, $t_{1/2} = 4$ h, therefore,

$$K = \frac{0.693}{t_{1/2}} = \frac{0.693}{4\text{h}} = K = 0.1735/\text{h}$$

(a) To calculate loading dose when the drug is administered every 12 hours, substituting the values of maintenance dose (= 300 mg), elimination rate constant (= 0.1735/h) and dosing interval (= 12 h) into equation (14-4),

$$D^* = \frac{D}{1-e^{-K\tau}}$$

$$= \frac{300\ \text{mg}}{1-e^{-(0.1735/\text{h})(12\text{h})}} = \frac{300\ \text{mg}}{1-e^{-(2.082)}} = \frac{300\ \text{mg}}{1-0.125} = \frac{300\ \text{mg}}{0.875} = 342.86\ \text{mg}$$

The value of loading dose obtained is similar to the approximate value of the loading dose shown in Table 14-1:

$$\text{when } \tau = 3t_{1/2},\ D^* = 1.14D = (1.14)(300) = 342\ \text{mg}$$

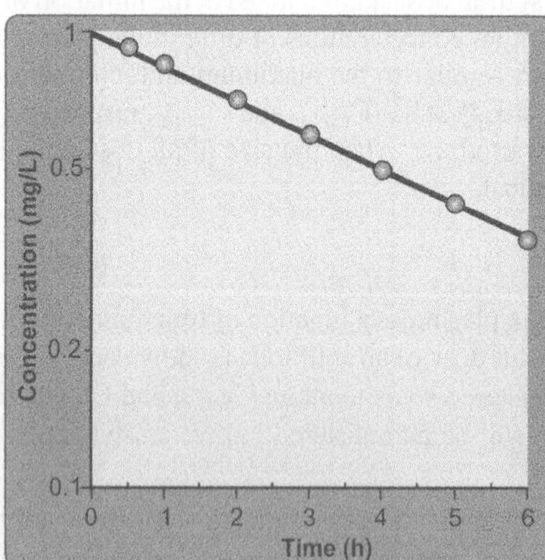

Fig. 14-1 Plot of data in Example 14-4

(b) If the dose is given every 8 hours, because of change in τ, substituting the values of maintenance dose (= 300 mg), elimination rate constant (= 0.1735/h) and dosing interval (= 8 h) into equation (14-4),

$$D^* = \frac{D}{1-e^{-K\tau}}$$

$$= \frac{300\text{ mg}}{1-e^{-(0.1735/h)(8h)}} = \frac{300\text{ mg}}{1-e^{-(1.388)}} = \frac{300\text{ mg}}{1-0.25} = \frac{300\text{ mg}}{0.75} = 400\text{ mg}$$

The value obtained is similar to the approximate value of the loading dose shown in Table 14-1:

$$\text{when } \tau = 2t_{1/2},\ D^* = 1.33D = (1.33)(300) = 399\text{ mg}$$

(c) If the dose is given every 4 hr, because of change in τ, substituting the values of maintenance dose (= 300 mg), elimination rate constant (= 0.1735/h) and dosing interval (= 4 h) into equation (14-4),

$$D^* = \frac{D}{1-e^{-K\tau}}$$

$$= \frac{300\text{ mg}}{1-e^{-(0.1735/h)(4h)}} = \frac{300\text{ mg}}{1-e^{-(0.694)}}$$

$$D^* = \frac{300\text{ mg}}{1-0.5} = \frac{300\text{ mg}}{0.5} = 600\text{ mg}$$

The value obtained here is similar to the value of loading dose shown in Table 14-1:

$$\text{when } \tau = t_{1/2},\ D^* = 2D = (2)(300) = 600\text{ mg}$$

EXTRAVASCULAR ADMINISTRATION

For the determination of loading dose during extravascular administration, the simplest case is a drug which, when administered extravascularly, confers upon the body characteristics of one-compartment open model and does not exhibit lag-time.

Similar to the discussion dealing with intravenous administration, the size of loading dose needed to attain steady-state concentration of drug in plasma (after extravascular administration) from the time the therapy is initiated, can be considered based upon: maximum concentration of drug in plasma at steady-state, $C_{max\ ss}$ or minimum concentration of drug in plasma at steady-state $C_{min\ ss}$.

Loading Dose Based on $C_{max\ ss}$

It was shown in Chapter 13 that during multiple dosing via extravascular administration, the maximum concentration of drug in plasma at steady-state ($C_{max\ ss}$) is given by the equation (13-36):

$$C_{max\ ss} = \frac{(B)}{1-e^{-K\tau}}\left(e^{-R}\right)$$

In this equation, B = the back extrapolated y-intercept of the linear terminal portion of the elimination phase after administration of a single dose (the size of this dose is equal to the size of maintenance dose, D), K = the rate constant of elimination of the drug, τ = the dosing interval and R = (K)(t_{max}), where t_{max} = time of maximum concentration.

Thus, the maximum concentration of drug in the plasma at steady-state is a function of B (which is a function of dose, fraction of dose absorbed, apparent volume of distribution, and the rate constants of absorption and elimination as described in equation (12-4) of Chapter 12), dosing interval, rate constant of elimination, and time of maximum concentration of drug in the plasma.

The time of maximum concentration following single dose extravascular administration of drug is a simple function of the rate constants of absorption and elimination, and can be determined rather easily and relatively accurately using equation (12-15). However, the determination of time of maximum concentration during multiple dosing becomes more complex, because during multiple dosing, the time of maximum concentration becomes a complex function of the rate constants of absorption and elimination. Hence, utilization of steady-state maximum concentration of drug in plasma to estimate loading dose also becomes complicated. Therefore, for the sake of convenience and understanding, the derivation of equation used for calculating loading dose based upon maximum concentration of drug in plasma at steady-state is not presented here.

It was shown in the derivation of equations dealing with loading dose following intravenous administration of the drug that the equation derived for calculating loading dose based on the maximum plasma drug concentration at steady-state is identical to that derived on the basis of the minimum concentration of drug in the plasma at steady-state. Therefore, derivation of the equation for calculating the loading dose presented here is based on the minimum concentration of drug in the plasma at steady-state.

Loading Dose Based on $C_{min\ ss}$

The minimum concentration of drug following extravascular administration of n doses ($C_{min\ n}$) is described by the equation (13-39) in Chapter 13:

$$C_{min\ n} = (B)\frac{\left(1-e^{-nK\tau}\right)\left(e^{-K\tau}\right)}{1-e^{-K\tau}} - \frac{\left(1-e^{-nG}\right)\left(e^{-G}\right)}{1-e^{-G}}$$

In this equation, B = back-extrapolated y-intercept of the terminal linear phase, K = rate constant of elimination, τ = dosing interval and G = $(K_a)(\tau)$, where K_a is absorption rate constant.

The factor G takes into account the delay in accumulation due to the absorptive phase and this factor depends only on rate constant of absorption, Ka and dosing interval, τ.

If the drug follows linear pharmacokinetics then B obtained after the administration of a single dose (maintenance dose, D) is directly proportional to the size of the dose, because, by definition (12-4),

$$B = \frac{(F)(D)(K_a)}{(V_d)(K_a - K)}$$

It is assumed that the fraction of dose absorbed, F, apparent volume of distribution, V_d and the rate constants of absorption and elimination, K_a and K, respectively, remain unchanged during the course of therapy. Thus, if the maintenance dose, D was doubled, then the value of the y-intercept B will also double. Similarly, if the maintenance dose, D, was made 50%, then the value of B will also become 50%.

By setting n equal to 1 in equation (13-39), an expression for $C_{min\ 1}$, minimum concentration of drug in the plasma following the first dose (maintenance dose, D) can be obtained. This expression is

$$C_{min1} = (B)\frac{\left(1-e^{-K\tau}\right)\left(e^{-K\tau}\right)}{1-e^{-K\tau}} - \frac{\left(1-e^{-G}\right)\left(e^{-G}\right)}{1-e^{-G}}$$

Canceling common terms in the numerator and denominator of the right-hand side of above equation yields the simplified relationship:

$$C_{min1} = (B)(e^{-K\tau} - e^{-G}) \qquad (14\text{-}8)$$

Similarly, when n becomes sufficiently large, i.e., when steady-state is attained after the administration of a large number of doses, an expression for the minimum concentration of drug in the plasma at steady-state can be obtained from equation (13-39). When n becomes large, the two exponential terms, $e^{-nK\tau}$ and e^{-nG}, in equation (13-39) approach zero, and equation (13-39) becomes

$$C_{\text{min ss}} = (B)\left(\frac{e^{-K\tau}}{1-e^{-K\tau}} - \frac{e^{-G}}{1-e^{-G}}\right) \tag{14-9}$$

Since the y-intercept, B, obtained after the administration of the first dose is directly proportional to the dose, D, equations (14-8) and (14-9) may be written as

$$C_{\text{min1}} \propto (D)(e^{-K\tau} - e^{-G}) \tag{14-10}$$

$$\text{and, } C_{\text{min ss}} \propto (D)\left(\frac{e^{-K\tau}}{1-e^{-K\tau}} - \frac{e^{-G}}{1-e^{-G}}\right) \tag{14-11}$$

If a loading dose (D*) is administered as the first dose, then equation (14-10) becomes

$$C_{\text{min1}} \propto (D^*)(e^{-K\tau} - e^{-G}) \tag{14-12}$$

The loading dose required to achieve steady-state plasma concentration levels of drug upon administration of the first dose may be determined by letting equation (14-12) for $C_{\text{min 1}}$ equal to equation (14-11) for $C_{\text{min ss}}$, i.e.,

$$(D^*)(e^{-K\tau} - e^{-G}) = (D)\left(\frac{e^{-K\tau}}{1-e^{-K\tau}} - \frac{e^{-G}}{1-e^{-G}}\right) \tag{14-13}$$

Bringing the right-hand side of equation (14-13) to a common denominator, we have

$$(D^*)(e^{-K\tau} - e^{-G}) = (D)\left(\frac{\left(e^{-K\tau}\right)\left(1-e^{-G}\right) - \left(e^{-G}\right)\left(1-e^{-K\tau}\right)}{\left(1-e^{-K\tau}\right)\left(1-e^{-G}\right)}\right)$$

$$(D^*)(e^{-K\tau} - e^{-G}) = (D)\left(\frac{e^{-K\tau} - e^{-K\tau}e^{-G} - e^{-G} + e^{-K\tau}e^{-G}}{\left(1-e^{-K\tau}\right)\left(1-e^{-G}\right)}\right)$$

which upon simplification gives

$$(D^*)(e^{-K\tau} - e^{-G}) = (D)\left(\frac{e^{-K\tau} - e^{-G}}{\left(1-e^{-K\tau}\right)\left(1-e^{-G}\right)}\right) \tag{14-14}$$

By canceling the common term $(e^{-K\tau} - e^{-G})$ from the numerator on both sides of equation (14-14), one obtains:

$$D^* = \frac{D}{\left(1-e^{-K\tau}\right)\left(1-e^{-G}\right)} \tag{14-15}$$

Thus, the equation used for calculating loading dose during extravascular administration (assuming maintenance doses, D, and dosing intervals, τ, are not changed during the course of treatment) for drugs which are absorbed rapidly (i.e., where rate constant of absorption, K_a is much greater than the rate constant of elimination, K) is similar to the equation used for intravenous administration, except that a factor, G, is incorporated into the equation. This factor G takes into account the delay in accumulation of drug due to the absorptive phase of the drug. It will be recalled that this factor is a function of dosing interval, τ, and rate constant of absorption, Ka, of the drug. In the case of drugs which are absorbed extremely rapidly and are administered at sufficiently large dosing intervals, i.e., those drugs whose rate constant of absorption and dosing interval are very large, the product of rate constant of absorption and dosing interval ($K_a \times \tau$, which is equal to the factor G) becomes very large, and, the value of the exponential term (e^{-G}) approaches a value of 0. The value of the exponential term e^{-G} also approaches zero if the maintenance doses are administered in the post-absorptive phase of the preceding dose. In either case, when the value of the exponential term e^{-G} approaches zero, equation (14-15) becomes equation (14-4):

$$D^* = \frac{D}{1 - e^{-K\tau}}$$

The following Examples illustrate the use of equation (14-15) in the determination of loading dose of a drug during extravascular administration.

Example 14-5 From the blood level data obtained after extravascular administration of a single 250 mg dose of an antibiotic, the following information was obtained: B = 6 mg/L, $t_{1/2}$ = 5 h, and K_a = 0.3 h^{-1}.

Calculate the size of loading dose needed to provide steady-state plasma concentration if 250 mg maintenance dose is given every 6 hours.

Solution

Since $t_{1/2}$ = 5 h, therefore

$$K = \frac{0.693}{t_{1/2}} = \frac{0.693}{5\,h} = 0.1386/h$$

$$G = (K_a)(\tau) = (0.3/h)(6\,h) = 1.8$$

Substituting the values of maintenance dose, D (= 250 mg), elimination rate constant (= 0.1386/h), dosing interval (= 6 h), and G (= 1.8) into equation (14-15):

$$D^* = \frac{D}{\left(1 - e^{-K\tau}\right)\left(1 - e^{-G}\right)} = \frac{250\text{ mg}}{1 - e^{-(0.1386/h)(6h)}\left(1 - e^{-(1.8)}\right)}$$

$$= \frac{250\text{ mg}}{\left(1 - e^{-(0.8316)}\right)(1 - 0.165)} = \frac{250\text{ mg}}{(1 - 0.435)(1 - 0.165)}$$

$$= \frac{250\text{ mg}}{(0.565)(0.825)}\ 530\text{ mg}$$

Example 14-6 Blood level data following administration of a single 300 mg dose of a drug are shown below. Calculate the loading dose if maintenance dose is 300 mg and the dose is administered every 6 hours.

Time (h)	*Concentration (μg/mL)*	*Time (h)*	*Concentration (μg/mL)*
0.5	0.63	4.0	0.74
1.0	0.89	6.0	0.53
1.5	0.97	8.0	0.38
2.0	0.97	10.0	0.27
3.0	0.87	12.0	0.19

Solution

A plot of plasma concentration as a function of time is shown in Figure 14-2. This profile indicates that upon administration, the drug confers the characteristics of one-compartment pharmacokinetic model on the body.

Since the terminal portion of the profile does not exhibit too much scatter, a straight line is drawn using eye-ball judgment. This straight line best represents the elimination phase of the plasma profile.

It is seen that the plasma concentration points at 6 hours, 8 hours, 10 hours, and 12 hours fall on this straight line. No attempt is made to accommodate the plasma concentration points at 4 hours, 3 hours, or 2 hours to fall on this straight line. From this straight line, one reads that the y-intercept, B is 1.5 μg/mL. The first-order rate constant of elimination, K, is determined from the slope this straight line as follows:

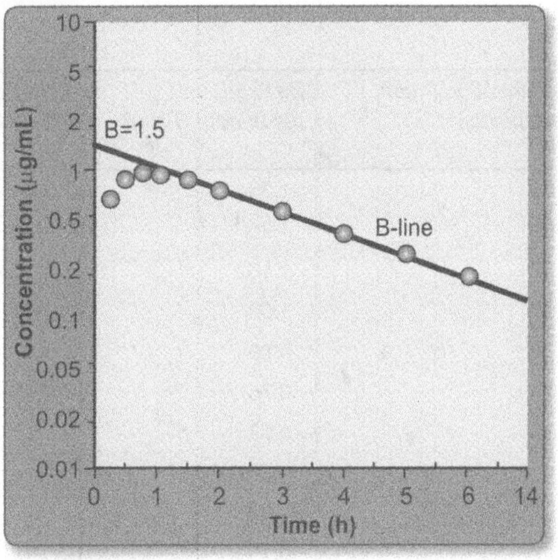

Fig. 14-2 First-order plot of data in Example 14-6 on a semi-logarithmic graph paper

To calculate the slope, one chooses two points, as far apart as possible. Suppose we choose the following two points:

$$x_1 = 0 \text{ h}, y_1 = 1.5 \ \mu\text{g/mL}; \text{ and } x_2 = 12 \text{ h}, y_2 = 0.19 \ \mu\text{g/mL}$$

The rate constant of elimination, K, of the straight line is:

$$K = -\text{slope} = -\frac{\ln 1.5 - \ln 0.19}{(0-12)\text{h}} \; K = -\frac{2.066}{-12\text{h}} = 0.172/\text{h}$$

The plasma profile is feathered to obtain the absorption phase and the rate constant of absorption.

Feathering

Those concentration points, which did not fall on the straight line having y-intercept = B (concentration points at 0.5, 1.0, 1.5, 2.0, 3.0 and 4.0 hours) are now feathered.

For example, the residual concentration at 0.5 hour is calculated as follows:

Concentration at 0.5 hr on the straight line having y-intercept = B is calculated using the first-order equation:

$$C = B(e^{-Kt})$$

$$= (1.5 \ \mu\text{g/mL})(e^{-(0.172/\text{h})(0.5 \text{ h})}) = (1.5 \ \mu\text{g/mL})(0.9176) = 1.38 \ \mu\text{g/mL}$$

Therefore, the residual concentration at 0.5 hour is:

$$C' = 1.38 \ \mu\text{g/mL} - 0.63 \ \mu\text{g/mL} = 0.75 \ \mu\text{g/mL}$$

Table 14-3 shows the calculations involved in the determination of residual concentration values for the absorption phase obtained by the feathering process.

The residual concentration points are plotted as triangles in Figure 14-3. The residual concentration points appear linear and do not exhibit too much scatter. Therefore, a straight line which best represents these points can be drawn using eyeball judgment. This straight line represents the absorption phase.

Rate Constant of Absorption

Since the linear phase of the absorption phase does not appear to exhibit a lag-time, therefore, the straight line representing the absorption phase is drawn so as to have the value of its y-intercept

Table 14-3 Feathering of data in Example 14-6

Time (hour)	*Concentration (μg/mL) (Data points)** ●	$Be^{-\beta t}$ *(μg/mL) (Data from B-line)*	*C′ =* $Be^{-\beta t}$ *– C (μg/mL) (Points from B-line minus data)*** ▲
0.5	0.63	1.38	1.38 – 0.63 = 0.75
1.0	0.89	1.26	1.26 – 0.89 = 0.37
1.5	0.97	1.16	1.16 – 0.97 = 0.19
2.0	0.97	1.06	1.07 – 0.97 = 0.10
3.0	0.87	0.89	0.89 – 0.87 = 0.02
4.0	0.74	0.75	0.75 – 0.74 = 0.01
6.0	0.53	0.53	–
8.0	0.38	0.38	–
10.0	0.27	0.27	–
12.0	0.19	0.19	–

* These points are shown as circles in Figure 14-3 ** These points are shown as triangle in Figure 14-3

equal to the value of the y-intercept of the straight line representing the elimination phase. The value of the y-intercept of both linear segments = 1.5 μg/mL.

The rate constant of absorption is determined by using the slope of the straight line representing the absorption phase.

$$K_a = -\text{slope} = -\frac{\ln 1.5 - \ln 0.1}{(0-2)\,h} = -\frac{2.708}{-2\,h} = 1.354/h$$

Calculation of Loading Dose

To calculate the loading dose, one needs to know the value of the factor G. The value of the factor G is calculated as follows:

$$G = (K_a)(\tau) = (1.354/hr)(6\ hr) = 8.124$$

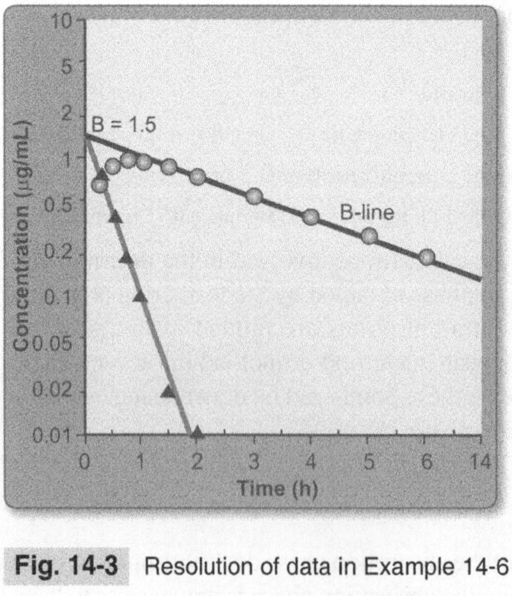

Fig. 14-3 Resolution of data in Example 14-6

The size of the loading dose (D*) is calculated by substituting the following values into equation (14-15): maintenance dose D = 300 mg, elimination rate constant K = 0.172/h, dosing interval τ = 6 h and G = 8.124.

$$D^* = \frac{D}{\left(1-e^{-K\tau}\right)\left(1-e^{-G}\right)}$$

$$= \frac{300\text{ mg}}{\left(1-e^{-(0.172/h)(6\,h)}\right)\left(1-e^{-(8.124)}\right)}$$

$$= \frac{300\text{ mg}}{\left(1-e^{-(1.032)}\right)(1-0.0003)} = \frac{300\text{ mg}}{(1-0.3563)(1-0)} = \frac{300\text{ mg}}{0.6437} = 466\text{ mg}$$

SUGGESTED READING

1. Benet L, Massoud N and Gambertoglio J (eds). Pharmacokinetic Basis for Drug Treatment. Raven Press; 1984.
2. Evans WE, Schentag JJ and Jusko WJ (eds). Applied Pharmacokinetics: Principles of Therapeutic Drug Monitoring, 3rd edition. Applied Therapeutics; 1995.
3. Gibaldi M and D. Perrier. Pharmacokinetics, 2nd edition. Marcel Dekker; 1982.
4. P. Welling, "Pharmacokinetics: Process and Mathematics," American Chemical Society, 1986.
5. Rowland and Tozer. Clinical Pharmacokinetics: Concepts and Applications, 3rd edition. Williams and Wilkins; 1995.
6. Sadee W. Pharmacokinetics: Drug Level Monitoring. John Wiley & Son; 1980.
7. Wagner J. Fundamentals of Clinical Pharmacokinetics. Drug Intelligence Publications; 1979.

PRACTICE PROBLEMS

14-1. The plasma drug concentration versus time following administration of a single 10 mg intravenous bolus dose is shown below. Calculate the loading dose needed to attain plateau levels from the start of therapy if a 10 mg dose is administered: (a) Every 6 hours, and (b) Every 4 hours.

Time (h)	*Concentration (μg/L)*	*Time (h)*	*Concentration (μg/L)*
0.5	925	4.0	500
1.0	845	5.0	420
2.0	710	6.0	352
3.0	595	8.0	250

14-2. The plasma data following oral administration of a single 30 mg dose of a drug are shown below. Assuming the fraction of dose absorbed = 1.0, calculate the priming dose needed to attain plateau levels if the patient receives a 30 mg dose:
(a) Every 4 hours, or (b) Every 8 hours.

Time (h)	*Concentration (mg/L)*	*Time (h)*	*Concentration (mg/L)*
0.5	7.0	6.0	6.6
1.0	10.5	8.0	4.5
2.0	12.0	10.0	3.0
4.0	9.4	12.0	2.0

14-3. The plasma data following a 300 mg intravenous bolus dose of an antibiotic is shown below. Calculate the size of initial dose that must be administered to attain plateau levels if a 300 mg dose will be administered:
(a) Every hour, or (b) Every 3 hours.

Time (h)	Concentration (mg/L)	Time (h)	Concentration (mg/L)	Time (h)	Concentration (mg/L)
0.5	42.0	2.0	18.0	5.0	4.1
1.0	31.0	3.0	11.0	6.0	2.2
1.5	24.0	4.0	6.4	7.0	1.35

14-4. The following information was gathered from the blood level data obtained after extravascular administration of a single 500 mg dose of an antibiotic:

$$B = 8 \text{ mg/L}, t1/2 = 6 \text{ h, and } K_a = 0.3 \text{ h}^{-1}$$

Calculate the size of loading dose needed to provide steady-state plasma concentration, if a 500 mg maintenance dose is given every 6 hours.

14-5. From the blood level data after extravascular administration of a single 500 mg dose of an antibiotic, the following information was obtained:

$$B = 8 \text{ mg/L}, t_{1/2} = 6 \text{ h, and Ka} = 0.35 \text{ h}^{-1}$$

Calculate the size of loading dose needed to provide steady-state plasma concentration of drug if a 500 mg maintenance dose is administered every 8 hours.

14-6. The plasma profile following administration of a 500 mg dose is described by the equation:

$$C = 10(e^{-0.1t}) - 10(e^{-0.9t}).$$

If concentration is in mg/L, time is in hr and $\tau = 6$ hr, calculate the size of loading dose needed to achieve steady-state levels soon after initiation of the treatment.

14-7. The plasma profile following administration of a 250 mg dose is described by the equation:

$$C = 20(e^{-0.03t}) - 10(e^{-0.25t}).$$

If concentration is in mg/L, time is in hr and $\tau = 24$ h, calculate loading dose needed to achieve steady-state plasma levels soon after initiation of the treatment.

14-8. The plasma profile following administration of a 300 mg dose is described by the equation:

$$C = 20(e^{-0.04t}) - 20(e^{-0.35t}).$$

If concentration is in mg/L, time is in hr and $\tau = 24$ h, calculate the size of loading dose needed to achieve steady-state plasma levels very soon after initiation of the treatment.

14-9. The plasma drug concentration versus time following administration of a single 15 mg intravenous bolus dose is shown below. Calculate the loading dose needed to attain plateau levels from the start of therapy if a 10 mg dose is administered:
(a) Every 6 hours, and (b) Every 4 hours.

Time (h)	Concentration (μg/L)	Time (h)	Concentration (μg/L)
0.5	740.0	4.0	400.0
1.0	676.0	5.0	336.0
2.0	568.0	6.0	281.6
3.0	476.0	8.0	200.0

14-10. The following information was gathered from the blood level data obtained after extravascular administration of a single 450 mg dose of a drug:

$$G = 8.124, K = 0.172/\text{h, and } K_a = 1.354 \text{ h}^{-1}$$

Calculate the size of loading dose needed to provide steady-state plasma concentration, if a 450 mg maintenance dose is given every 6 hours.

14-11. The plasma concentration vs time after administration of a 12 mg IV dose is shown below. Calculate loading dose if a 10 mg dose is administered:
(a) Every 6 hours, and (b) Every 4 hours.

Time (h)	*Concentration (μg/L)*	*Time (h)*	*Concentration (μg/L)*
0.5	555.0	4.0	300.0
1.0	507.0	5.0	252.0
2.0	426.0	6.0	211.2
3.0	357.0	8.0	150.0

CHAPTER 15

CONTINUOUS INTRAVENOUS INFUSION

Continuous intravenous infusion of drugs is an important method of drug administration. For obvious reasons, this method of drug administration has traditionally been restricted within the hospital setting, where the drug may generally be infused for as little as 15 to 30 minutes, to as long as 24 hours or longer. The continuous intravenous infusion was recently gaining popularity in the home health care industry, where the patient was taught self-administration of drug by intravenous route as a continuous intravenous infusion. In this setting, the drug was infused for a short period of time, usually 30 minutes to about 1 hour. In particular, this method of self-administration was limited to the treatment of the lyme disease.

In the hospitals and nursing homes, continuous intravenous infusion has been used for administration of fluids (for fluid replacement), nutrients (to provide nourishment in emergency situations or in situations involving patients who cannot be fed by normal routes) and/or in the treatment with drugs during the critical stages of illness. For example, glucose and saline solutions are routinely infused in large amounts (usually in liter-doses) over 24 hours periods. These solutions are also used as vehicles to administer such drugs as theophylline, aminophylline and lidocaine to provide consistent plasma concentration of drug for maximum benefit to the patient. Table 15-1 lists examples of solutions used for fluid replacement and electrolyte management.

Some of these solutions are also used as vehicles for continuous intravenous infusion, e.g. 5% dextrose in water (5%D/W) and 0.9% sodium chloride. For example, in the treatment of an acute asthmatic condition, aminophylline is infused in 100 or 200 mL of either 5% dextrose solution for injection or 0.9% sodium chloride solution for injection at a rate not exceeding 25 mg/min. Thereafter, maintenance therapy is administered by a large volume infusion to deliver the desired amount of drug each hour. Similarly, for the treatment of cardiac arrhythmias in patients in whom arrhythmia tends to recur and who are incapable of receiving oral antiarrhythmic therapy, intravenous infusion of lidocaine is administered usually in 5% dextrose solution at the rate of about 1 to 4 mg/min (the usual dose is 20 to 50 μg per kilogram body weight per min). The solution

Table 15-1 Solutions used as vehicles for intravenous infusion

Solution	*Osmolarity (mOsm/kg)*	*Glucose (g/liter)*	*Na (mEq/liter)*	*Cl*
5% D/W	252	50	-	-
10% D/W	505	100	-	-
50% D/W	2525	500	-	-
0.45% NaCl	154	-	77	77
0.45% NaCl with 5% dextrose	408	50	77	77
0.9% NaCl	308	-	154	154
0.9% NaCl with 5% dextrose	560	50	154	154
3% NaCl	1026	-	513	513
Ringer lactate	272	-	130	109
Ringer lactate with 5% dextrose	524	50	130	109

for infusion is prepared by the addition of infusion dosage form available as lidocaine solution without sodium chloride or preservative to 1 liter of 5% dextrose in water using aseptic technique. The infusion dosage form is available in a variety of dosage forms and dosage strengths, such as:

a. A 25 mL single use vial
b. A 5 mL additive syringe containing 1 gram of lidocaine hydrochloride
c. A 50 mL single use vial
d. A 10 mL additive syringe containing 2 gram of lidocaine hydrochloride.

It should be mentioned here that in emergency situations, continuous intravenous infusion of lidocaine is preceded by a bolus dose of lidocaine to rapidly achieve an effective concentration of the drug. Although the infusion achieves the objective of maintaining the plasma concentration of lidocaine, it is unable to match the decline in plasma concentration of lidocaine due to distribution of the drug into the tissues. This has a potential of ineffective lidocaine plasma concentration for a period of time. Although a larger bolus dose may overcome this problem, it has the potential of toxicity due to higher initial concentration of the drug. In practice, the problem is solved either by administering supplementary bolus doses or an initially higher infusion rate.

Table 15-2 lists some examples of drugs that are frequently used for continuous intravenous infusion.

Table 15-2 Drugs commonly used in continuous intravenous infusion

Drug	*Diluent**	*Concentration*
Aminocaproic acid	D5W	5 g/250 mL = 20 mg/mL
Amrinone	NS only	200 mg/200 mL = 1 mg/mL
		500 mg/200 mL = 2.5 mg/mL
Bretylium	NS, D5W	2 g/500 mL = 4 mg/mL
Dilitiazem	NS, D5W	125 mg/125 mL = 1 mg/mL
Dobutamine	NS, D5W	250 mg/500 mL = 0.5 mg/mL
		500 mg/500 mL = 1 mg/mL
Dopamine	NS, D5W	400 mg/500 mL = 0.8 mg/mL
		800 mg/500 mL = 1.6 mg/mL
Epinephrine	NS, D5W	8 mg/500 mL = 16 μg/mL
Esmolol	NS, D5W	5 g/500 mL = 10 mg/mL
Famotidine	NS, D5W	40 mg/250 mL = 0.16 mg/mL
Heparin	NS, D5W	12,500 units/250 mL = 50 units/mL
Insulin, Regular	NS	50 units/250 mL = 0.2 units/mL
Isoproterenol	NS, D5W	2 mg/500 mL = 4 μg/mL
Labetalol	NS, D5W	200 mg/200 mL = 1 mg/mL
Lidocaine	NS, D5W	2 g/500 mL = 4 mg/mL
Magnesium sulfate	NS, D5W	50 g/500 mL = 100 mg/mL (OB/GYN)
		16 g/250 mL = 64 mg/mL (cardiac)
Milrinone	NS, D5W	50 mg/250 mL = 0.2 mg/mL
Morphine sulfate	D5W	62.5 mg/250 mL = 0.25 mg/mL
		125 mg/250 mL = 0.5 mg/mL
Nitroglycerine**	NS, D5W	50 mg/250 mL = 200 μg/mL
Nitroprusside	D5W only	50 mg/250 mL = 200 μg/mL
Norepinephrine	D5W only	8 mg/500 mL = 16 μg/mL
Phenylephrine	NS, D5W	10 mg/250 mL = 40 μg/mL
Procainamide	NS, D5W	2 g/500 mL = 4 mg/mL
Theophylline	NS, D5W	1 g/500 mL = 2 mg/mL
Vasopressin	NS, D5W	200 units/250 mL = 0.8 units/mL
Vecuronium	NS' D5W	100 mg/500 mL = 0.2 mg/mL

*NS = normal saline; D5W = 5% dextrose in water

**only glass bottles and special nitroglycerin tubing should be used

PLASMA PROFILE

The plasma profile resulting from continuous intravenous infusion of a drug differs from the plasma profile obtained following a rapid intravenous bolus dose of the same drug in various respects. The major difference is that when the drug is administered as a rapid bolus dose, the entire drug dose is placed in plasma all at once. Therefore, the concentration of drug in the plasma is at its peak level immediately after administration of the entire drug dose (Chapter 11). The concentration of drug in plasma then begins to decline due to elimination of the drug. During continuous intravenous infusion, on the other hand, the concentration of drug in plasma is not at its peak when infusion is started because the entire drug dose is not administered all at once. The concentration of drug in plasma starts to build up and continues to increase (instead of showing a decline) because the drug is being administered continuously as a function of time (assuming that infusion rate is greater than elimination rate of the drug). If the drug is infused for a relatively long period of time, the build up in concentration continues until the plasma concentration reaches a steady-state (Fig. 15-1).

Upon termination of infusion, the concentration of drug in the plasma starts to decline (according to first-order elimination of the drug) because now there is no further input of the drug, but elimination continues to remove the drug from the plasma.

The concentration of drug in plasma at any time after termination of the infusion can be calculated using the basic first-order equation described in equation (3-27):

$$C = C_0(e^{-Kt})$$

where, C is concentration of drug in plasma at any time after termination of infusion, C_0 is concentration of drug in plasma at steady-state, K is first-order rate constant of elimination of the drug and t is time elapsed since the termination of infusion. If the infusion is terminated before reaching the steady-state concentration of drug in plasma (intermittent infusion or short infusion), then the concentration of drug in plasma begins to decline according to first-order elimination of drug at the time of termination of infusion, because now there is no further input of the drug, but drug elimination continues to remove the drug from plasma. Figure 15-2 shows the plasma profile of a short infusion and subsequent decline in plasma concentration following the termination of the infusion.

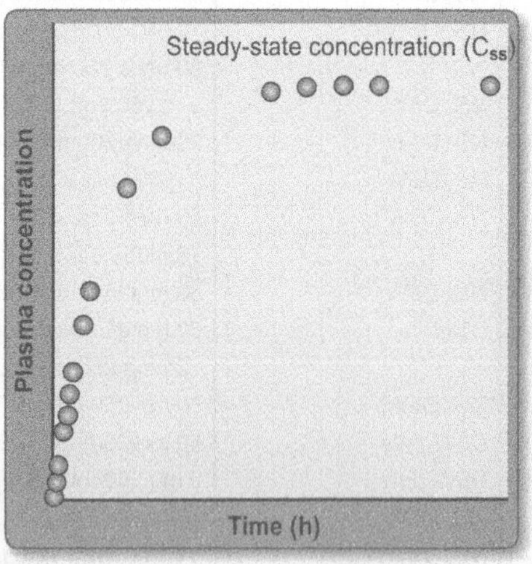

Fig. 15-1 Plasma drug concentration as a function of time during continuous intravenous infusion

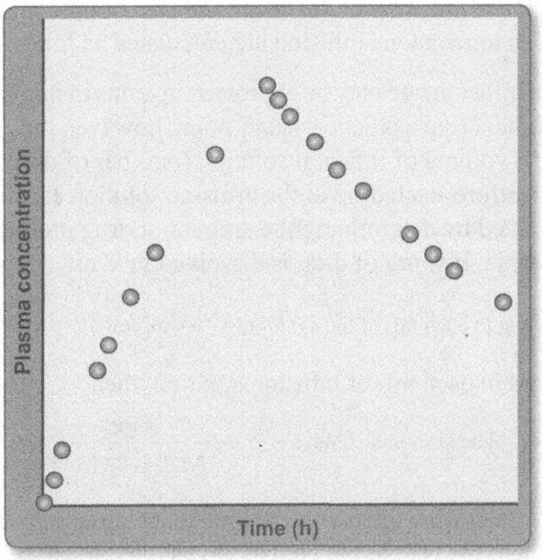

Fig. 15-2 Plasma drug concentration as a function of time during short intravenous infusion

Extent of Drug Accumulation

The extent of accumulation of drug in plasma during continuous intravenous infusion may be considered as a result of administration of a very large number of small intravenous bolus doses of the drug at very short dosing intervals. Providing the rate of drug output (elimination) is less than the rate of drug input, the build-up of concentration of drug in plasma during continuous intravenous infusion will depend on the rate at which the drug is infused (infusion rate of drug). Therefore, the equations used for calculating the maximum and minimum concentrations of drug in plasma after administration of n doses during multiple dosing ($C_{max\ n}$ and $C_{min\ n}$), discussed in Chapter 13, can be used to determine concentration of drug in plasma at any given time during the period of continuous intravenous infusion.

Determination of Plasma Concentration

For the sake of convenience, it is assumed that the apparent volume of distribution and overall rate constant of elimination of drug do not change during the course of therapy. As shown in Chapter 13, accumulation of drug during multiple dosing by intravenous bolus administration depends on three factors: concentration of drug in plasma immediately after the administration of the first dose (C_0), the overall rate constant of elimination (K) and the dosing interval (τ).

In linear pharmacokinetics, since C_0 is a function of dose and apparent volume of distribution, the following four factors therefore determine the extent of drug accumulation during multiple dosing:

a. The size of dose
b. The apparent volume of distribution
c. The overall rate constant of elimination (or biological half-life)
d. The dosing interval.

The apparent volume of distribution and overall rate constant of elimination of the drug are considered constant in a given patient. If it is assumed that these two factors remain unchanged during the course of therapy, then of the four factors mentioned above, the size of dose and the dosing interval (infusion rate or drip rate) are the only two parameters that are responsible for accumulation of drug in the body. Therefore, only these two parameters are used to determine the rate and duration of infusion of the drug. The size of dose and the dosing interval (infusion rate) for continuous intravenous infusion are calculated as follows:

Size of Dose: The infusion rate may be expressed in terms of amount of drug to be infused over a certain length of time. From a practical stand-point, however, the practitioner calculates infusion rate in terms of the volume of infusion solution (number of drops) to be administered per unit time (minute). Therefore, each drop of the infusion solution constitutes a dose. The size of each dose is thus calculated by determining the amount of drug present in each drop of the infusion solution. For example, if w mg of drug is dissolved in V mL of the infusion solution, then

$$\text{The amount of drug in each mL of the solution} = \frac{w}{V}\ (\text{mg/mL}) \tag{15-1}$$

If there are m drops in each mL of infusion solution, then

$$\text{The size of each dose is} = \frac{\text{w mg}}{(\text{V mL})(\text{m drops/mL})} \tag{15-2}$$

Dosing Interval: The dosing interval is the time that elapses between the administration of each drop of the infusate. This is determined as follows:

If the infusion rate is x drops per minute, then one can set-up the following proportionality for the dosing interval, τ:

$$\frac{\text{x drops}}{\text{1 min}} = \frac{\text{1 drop}}{\tau\ \text{min}} \tag{15-3}$$

$$\text{Therefore, } \tau = \frac{1}{x}\ (\text{min}) \tag{15-4}$$

The following Example illustrates application of this concept in determination of size of dose and dosing interval from the infusion rate.

Example 15-1 A 72 kg adult patient is administered aminophylline by continuous intravenous infusion at the rate of 0.5 mg aminophylline/kg/h for 4 hours. If the drug is dissolved in 1 liter of normal saline solution and each mL of infusate measures 30 drops, calculate:

i. The size of each dose, and

ii. The dosing interval during infusion period.

Solution

i. *Size of Each Dose*

$$\text{The amount of drug administered per hour} = \left(\frac{0.5\ \text{mg}}{\text{kg}}\right)(72\ \text{kg}) = 36\ \text{mg}$$

$$\text{Amount of drug administered in 4 hours} = \left(\frac{36\ \text{mg}}{1\ \text{h}}\right)(4\ \text{h}) = 145\ \text{mg}$$

The volume of infusate administered in 4 hours = 1,000 mL

Since there are 30 drops in each mL of the infusate, the size of each dose may be determined using equation (15-2):

$$\text{The size of each dose} = \frac{145\ \text{mg}}{(1{,}000\ \text{mL})(30\ \text{drops/mL})} = 0.0048\ \text{mg / drop}$$

ii. *Dosing Interval During Infusion Period*

Since there are 30 drops/mL of the infusion solution, therefore, 1,000 mL of the infusate contains

$$(1{,}000)(30) = 30{,}000\ \text{drops.}$$

Since the 30,000 drops of the infusate are administered in 4 hours, therefore,

$$\text{Infusion rate} = \frac{30{,}000 \text{ drops}}{4 \text{ h}} = \frac{7{,}500 \text{ drops}}{\text{h}}$$

$$\text{Infusion rate} = \frac{7{,}500 \text{ drops}}{60 \text{ min}} = 125 \text{ drops/min}$$

The dosing interval is determined using equation (15-4)

$$\text{The dosing interval} = \tau = \frac{1 \text{ drop}}{125 \text{ drops/min}} = 0.008 \text{ min}$$

Once the size of dose and dosing interval are known, one then uses the concepts of multiple dosing (explained in Chapter 13) to determine concentration of drug in plasma during the infusion period. The following Example illustrates the methodology involved in these calculations.

Example 15-2 A 72 kg adult male patient is administered aminophylline by continuous intravenous infusion at the rate of 0.5 mg/kg/h for 8 hours. Calculate the concentration of aminophylline in plasma during infusion period if the drug is dissolved in 960 mL of infusate and each mL of infusion solution measures 20 drops. Assume that the apparent volume of distribution of aminophylline in this patient is 30 liters and the biological half-life of aminophylline in this patient is 8 hours.

Solution

Aminophylline is the soluble form of theophylline. It is prepared by combining 80 parts by metric weight of theophylline with 20 parts by metric weight of ethylenediaminetetraacetic acid (EDTA). The EDTA-complex of theophylline has better water-solubility than theophylline itself. Therefore, plasma concentration of aminophylline is equivalent to 80% concentration of theophylline.

To determine the concentration of aminophylline in plasma during the 8-hour infusion period, first we need to determine the following three quantities:

i. The amount of drug needed to be dissolved in 960 mL of the infusion solution.
ii. The size of each dose (amount of drug in each drop), and finally
iii. The dosing interval (rate of infusion). These are calculated as follows:

i. *Amount of Drug Needed*

In the adult male patient weighing 72 kg, the amount of aminophylline that should be administered is:

$$(0.5 \text{ mg/kg/h})(72 \text{ kg}) = 36 \text{ mg/h}.$$

Since the solution will be infused over an 8-hr period, the amount of drug to be infused is:

$$(38 \text{ mg/h})(8 \text{ h}) = 288 \text{ mg}$$

Thus, 288 mg of aminophylline is dissolved in the infusion solution to prepare 960 mL of the infusate and the patient receives the infusion over an 8-hour period.

ii. *Size of Dose*

Since 960 mL of solution is infused over 8 hours, the rate of infusion in terms of mL per min is calculated as follows:

$$\frac{960 \text{ mL}}{8 \text{ h}} = \frac{120 \text{ mL}}{\text{h}} = \frac{120 \text{ mL}}{60 \text{ min}} = 2 \text{ mL/min}$$

If 1 mL of the infusate measures 20 drops, then the 2 mL/min rate of infusion in terms of drops per minute is calculated using the following proportionality:

$$\left(\frac{2 \text{ mL}}{\text{min}}\right)\left(\frac{20 \text{ drops}}{\text{mL}}\right) = \frac{40 \text{ drop}}{\text{min}}$$

Since 288 mg of aminophylline was dissolved in 960 mL of the infusate, the quantity of drug in each drop of the infusion solution is:

$$\frac{288\text{ mg}}{960\text{ mL}} = \frac{0.3\text{ mg}}{1\text{ mL}} = \frac{0.3\text{ mg}}{20\text{ drops}} = 0.015\text{ mg/drops}$$

iii. *Dosing Interval*

Since the patient receives 40 drops/min, the patient receives 40 doses per min. Therefore, dosing interval is calculated by setting up the proportionality:

$$\frac{40\text{ doses}}{1\text{ min}} = \frac{1\text{ dose}}{x}\text{, therefore, } x = \frac{1}{40} = 0.025\text{ min}$$

Thus, continuous intravenous infusion of 288 mg/L of aminophylline over an 8-hour period is in effect administration of multiple dosing of 0.015 mg of bolus doses of aminophylline administered every 0.025 min, i.e. D = 0.015 mg and τ = 0.025 min. The total number of doses received in 8 hours is, therefore:

$$\left(\frac{40\text{ doses}}{\text{min}}\right)\left(\frac{60\text{ min}}{\text{h}}\right)(8\text{ h}) = \left(\frac{2,400\text{ doses}}{\text{h}}\right)(8\text{ h}) = 19,200\text{ doses}$$

Since elimination half-life of aminophylline in this patient is 8 h, the rate constant of elimination is:

$$K = \frac{0.693}{t_{1/2}} = \frac{0.693}{8\text{ h}} = \frac{0.086625}{\text{h}} = \frac{0.086625}{60\text{ min}} = 0.00144375/\text{min}$$

iv. *Aminophylline Concentration During Infusion*

Now that we know D, τ and K, we can use equations (13-23) and (13-28) to determine maximum and minimum concentrations of aminophylline at any time during infusion period. For example, C_0 after administration of the first dose is:

$$C_0 = \frac{D}{V_d} = \frac{0.015\text{ mg}}{30\text{ L}} = 0.0005\text{ mg/L}$$

Since, K = 0.00144375/min and τ = 0.025 min,

therefore $(K)(\tau) = (0.00144375/\text{min})(0.025\text{ min}) = 0.0000361$

Thus, knowing C_0 = 0.0005 mg/L and $(K)(\tau)$ = 0.0000361, the maximum and minimum concentrations after the first dose are:

$$C_{max\,1} = C_0 = 0.0005\text{ mg/L},$$

$$\text{and } C_{min\,1} = (C_0)(e^{-K\tau}) = (0.0005\text{ mg/L})(e^{-0.0000361}) = 0.0005\text{ mg/L}$$

Similarly, after 100 doses (i.e. after 0.025 min × 100 = 2.5 min), the maximum concentration of drug in the plasma can be calculated using equation (13-23):

$$C_{max\,n} = \frac{C_0\left(1 - e^{-nK\tau}\right)}{1 - e^{-K\tau}}$$

$$C_{max\,100} = \frac{(0.0005\text{ mg/L})\left(1 - e^{-(100)(0.0000361)}\right)}{1 - e^{-(0.0000361)}} = 0.0499\text{ mg/L}$$

and the minimum concentration can be calculated using equation (13-28):

$$C_{min\,100} = (C_{max\,100})(e^{-K\tau}) = (0.0499\text{ mg/L})(e^{-(0.0000361)}) = 0.0499\text{ mg/L}$$

After 1,000 doses (i.e. after 0.025 min × 1,000 = 25 min), the maximum and minimum concentrations are:

$$C_{max\ 1,000} = \frac{(0.0005\ mg/L)\left(1 - e^{-(1,000)(0.0000361)}\right)}{1 - e^{-(0.0000361)}} = 0.491\ mg/L$$

$$C_{min\ 1,000} = (C_{max\ 1,000})(e^{-K\tau})$$

$$= (0.491\ mg/L)(e^{-(0.0000361)}) = 0.491\ mg/L$$

Similarly, after 6,000 doses (i.e. after 0.025 min × 6,000 = 2.5 h),

$$C_{max\ 6,000} = \frac{(0.0005\ mg/L)\left(1 - e^{-(6,000)(0.0000361)}\right)}{1 - e^{-(0.0000361)}} = 2.697\ mg/L$$

$$C_{min\ 6,000} = (C_{max\ 6,000})(e^{-K\tau}) = (2.697\ mg/L)(e^{-(0.0000361)}) = 2.697\ mg/L$$

And, after 10,000 doses (i.e. after 0.025 min × 10,000 = 4.17 h),

$$C_{max\ 10,000} = \frac{(0.0005\ mg/L)\left(1 - e^{-(10,000)(0.0000361)}\right)}{1 - e^{-(0.0000361)}} = 4.197\ mg/L$$

$$C_{min\ 10,000} = (C_{max\ 10,000})(e^{-K\tau}) = (4.197\ mg/L)(e^{-(0.0000361)})$$

$$C_{min\ 10,000} = 2.697\ mg/L$$

Since the patient receives a total of 19,200 doses in 8 hr, the maximum and minimum concentrations of aminophylline at the end of 19,200 doses (at the termination of infusion) are:

$$C_{max\ 19,200} = \frac{(0.0005\ mg/L)\left(1 - e^{-(19,200)(0.0000361)}\right)}{1 - e^{-(0.0000361)}} = 6.926\ mg/L$$

$$C_{min\ 19,200} = (C_{max\ 19,200})(e^{-K\tau}) = (6.926\ mg/L)(e^{-(0.0000361)}) = 6.926\ mg/L$$

Using the calculations shown above, one can determine the concentration of drug in plasma at any given time during continuous intravenous infusion. Also, one can calculate the amount of drug administered and the amount of drug in the body at any time during the infusion period, as shown in Table 15-3.

It is seen from the calculations shown above (and summarized in Table 15-3) that the calculated values of maximum and minimum concentrations of drug in plasma at various times during the infusion period are identical in each case. This is because the value of Persistence Factor, $e^{-K\tau}$, is approximately equal to 1 and since $C_{min\ n} = (C_{max\ n})(e^{-K\tau})$, therefore multiplication of C_{max} with the Persistence Factor is essentially equal to $C_{max\ n}$. Also, of the total amount of drug

Table 15-3 Plasma concentration of drug (data in Example 15-2) during continuous intravenous infusion

Dose #	*Time (min)*	*Amount of drug administered (mg)*	*C_{max} (mg/L)*	*C_{min} (mg/L)*	*Amount in Body (mg) (C_{min} × Vd)*
1	0.025	0.015	0.00055	0.00055	0.015
100	2.5	1.5	0.0499	0.0499	1.497
1,000	25	15.0	0.491	0.491	14.73
2,000	50	30.0	0.965	0.965	28.97
5,000	125	75.0	2.287	2.287	68.62
6,000	150	90.0	2.697	2.697	80.92
8,000	200	120.0	3.474	3.474	104.23
10,000	250	150.0	4.197	4.197	125.91
15,000	378	225.0	5.792	5.792	173.74
19,200	480	288.0	6.926	6.926	207.76

infused over an 8-hour period (288 mg), the amount of drug in the body at the end of infusion period is 208 mg, (which is about 72% of the administered dose). If this patient was given 288 mg of aminophylline as a single bolus dose instead of the continuous intravenous infusion, the concentration of drug in the body after 8 hr can be calculated using equation (3-27):

$$C_t = C_0(e^{-Kt})$$

$$= \frac{288\text{ mg}}{30\text{ L}}\left(e^{-(0.086625/\text{hr})(8\text{ hr})}\right)$$

$$= \left(\frac{288\text{ mg}}{30\text{ L}}\right)\left(e^{-0.693}\right) = (9.6\text{ mg/L})(0.5) = 4.8\text{ mg/L}$$

and amount of drug in the body would be:

$$(4.8\text{ mg/L})(30\text{ L}) = 145\text{ mg}$$

This is 50% of the administered dose.

Example 15-3 The half-life of aminophylline in a patient is 6 hr and the apparent volume of distribution of the drug is 30 L. If this patient is administered 360 mg of aminophylline by continuous intravenous infusion in 2,000 mL of normal saline over an 8 hours period at a rate of 125 drops/min (assume 1 mL of the infusate = 30 drops), calculate the concentration of aminophylline in the plasma in this patient at (a) 1 hour after the infusion is started, (b) 3 hours after the infusion is started, (c) 6 hours after the infusion is started, and (d) 8 hours after the infusion is started.

Solution

$$\text{Infusion rate} = \frac{2{,}000\text{ mL}}{8\text{ h}} = \frac{250\text{ mL}}{\text{h}} = \left(\frac{150\text{ mL}}{60\text{ min}}\right)\left(\frac{30\text{ drops}}{1\text{ mL}}\right) = 125\text{ drops/min}$$

$$\text{Amount of drug per drop} = \frac{360\text{ mg}}{2{,}000\text{ mL}} = \frac{0.18\text{ mg}}{\text{mL}} = \frac{0.18\text{ mg}}{30\text{ drops}} = 0.006\text{ mg/drop}$$

$$\text{Dose} = 0.006\text{ mg},\ C_0 = \frac{0.006\text{ mg}}{30\text{ L}} = 0.002\text{ mg/L and } \tau = \frac{1\text{ min}}{125} = 0.008\text{ min}$$

Since $t_{1/2} = 6$ h, therefore

$$K = 0.693/6\text{ h} = 0.1155/\text{h} = 0.001925/\text{min}$$

$$(K)(\tau) = (0.001925/\text{min})(0.008\text{ min}) = 0.0000154,\text{ therefore,}$$

$$e^{-K\tau} = 0.9999846$$

a. *Concentration at 1 hour:*

$$n = \text{infusion rate} \times \text{time} = \left(\frac{125\text{ drops}}{\text{min}}\right)(60\text{ min}) = 7{,}500\text{ drops} = 7{,}500\text{ doses}$$

From equation (13-23)

$$C_{\max n} = \frac{C_0\left(1 - e^{-nK\tau}\right)}{1 - e^{-K\tau}}$$

$$C_{\max 7{,}500} = \frac{(0.0002\text{ mg/L})\left(1 - e^{-(7{,}500)(0.0000154)}\right)}{1 - e^{-(0.0000154)}} = 1.4166\text{ mg/L}$$

b. *Concentration at 3 hours:*

$$n = \text{infusion rate} \times \text{time} = \left(\frac{125\text{ drops}}{\text{min}}\right)(180\text{ min}) = 22{,}500\text{ drops} = 22{,}500\text{ doses}$$

$$C_{max\ 22,500} = \frac{(0.0002\ \text{mg/L})\left(1 - e^{-(22,500)(0.0000154)}\right)}{1 - e^{-(0.0000154)}} = 3.803\ \text{mg/L}$$

c. *Concentration at 6 hours*

$$n = \text{infusion rate} \times \text{time} = \left(\frac{125\ \text{drops}}{\text{min}}\right)(360\ \text{min}) = 45,000\ \text{drops} = 45,000\ \text{doses}$$

$$C_{max\ 45,000} = \frac{(0.0002\ \text{mg/L})\left(1 - e^{-(45,000)(0.0000154)}\right)}{1 - e^{-(0.0000154)}} = 6.49\ \text{mg/L}$$

d. *Concentration at 8 hours*

$$n = \text{infusion rate} \times \text{time} = \left(\frac{125\ \text{drops}}{\text{min}}\right)(480\ \text{min}) = 60,000\ \text{drops} = 60,000\ \text{doses}$$

$$C_{max\ 60,000} = \frac{(0.0002\ \text{mg/L})\left(1 - e^{-(60,000)(0.0000154)}\right)}{1 - e^{-(0.0000154)}} = 7.832\ \text{mg/L}$$

Concentration after Termination of Infusion

When continuous intravenous infusion is terminated, the concentration of drug in the plasma declines according to first-order kinetics, because from this point onward there is no drug input, but the elimination of drug continues. To determine concentration of drug in plasma at any time after termination of infusion, one can modify the first-order rate equation discussed in Chapter 3. The first-order rate equation describing concentration of drug in plasma after a rapid intravenous bolus dose is given by equation (3-22):

$$C_t = C_0(e^{-Kt})$$

where, C_t is concentration of drug in plasma at time t, C_0 is concentration of drug in plasma immediately after administration of the intravenous bolus dose, t is the time after administration of the intravenous bolus dose and K is elimination rate constant of the drug.

When continuous intravenous infusion is terminated, the concentration of drug in plasma at the time of termination (C_t) may be considered to be equal to the concentration C_0 in equation (3-22). Thus, equation (3-22) may be written as

$$C = C_t(e^{-Kt}) \qquad (15\text{-}5)$$

In equation (15-5),
C = concentration of drug in plasma at any time t after the infusion is terminated,
C_t = concentration of drug in the plasma immediately after termination of infusion,
K = the elimination rate constant of the drug and
t = time after infusion.

Example 15-4 From the data given in Example 15-3, calculate concentration of aminophylline in plasma 3 hr after the termination of the infusion.

Solution

The concentration of aminophylline in plasma 3 hr after termination of continuous intravenous infusion of the drug is obtained by substituting the values of C_t = 7.832 mg/L, K = 0.1155/h and t = 3 h into equation (15-5). Substitution yields:

$$C = (7.832\ \text{mg/L})(e^{-(0.1155/\text{h})(3\ \text{h})}) = (7.832\ \text{mg/L})(0.707) = 5.537\ \text{mg/L}$$

STEADY-STATE CONCENTRATION

The steady-state concentration of a drug in the plasma is achieved when:

a. The drug is infused for a sufficient length of time, so that eventually the rate of infusion (rate of drug input) becomes equal to the rate of drug output (i.e. the rate of infusion becomes equal to the rate of elimination of the drug).
b. A loading dose is administered by a rapid intravenous bolus dose of the drug so as to bring the concentration of drug in plasma at the desired level of steady-state concentration and at the same time continuous intravenous infusion is started simultaneously. In this case, the rate at which continuous intravenous infusion is infused should be such that the rate of infusion is equal to rate of elimination of the drug.

Prolonged Intravenous Infusion

The term prolonged intravenous infusion as used here refers to the administration of continuous intravenous infusion to start the treatment, i.e. the patient does not receive a loading dose (either intravenously or extravascularly), but the steady-state concentration of drug in plasma is achieved by continuous intravenous infusion of the drug for a prolonged period of time.

Concentration of Drug in Plasma

As shown earlier, the concentration of drug in the plasma during prolonged continuous intravenous infusion may be calculated using equations (13-23) and (13-28). For instance, using the data given in Example 15-2, one can determine the concentration of drug in plasma using equations (13-23) and (13-28), if the patient continued to receive intravenous infusion for a very long period of time. The concentration of drug in the plasma increases somewhat rapidly soon after the infusion is started and then the increase in plasma concentration of the drug slows down as infusion of the drug progresses. After some time, the concentration of drug in plasma starts approaching steady-state and at this stage the increase in the concentration of drug in the plasma is extremely slow. As shown in Table 15-4, it would take a long time to reach steady-state concentration.

It should be realized that, theoretically, the steady-state may never be reached, because the value of the term $e^{-nK\tau}$ in equation (13-23) does not equal zero even after a very long time. However, as the exponent $nK\tau$ in equation (13-23) becomes very large, the value of the term $e^{-nK\tau}$ approaches zero and for all practical purposes, steady-state is considered to have been reached. In this particular instance, approximately 99.5% of the steady-state concentration is reached after about 8 or 9 half-lives. If the drug was administered as an intravenous bolus dose (288 mg every 8 hours) rather than continuous intravenous infusion, one would expect to attain similar steady-state concentration in approximately the same length of time (8 hours × 9 half-lives = 72 hours), i.e. 3 days after initiation of drug therapy. This is because, as shown in Chapter 13, the dosing interval in this case is equal to the biological half-life of the drug (i.e. $\tau = t_{1/2}$).

It should be remembered that if a higher infusion rate had been used, for example, 0.8 mg/kg/h instead of 0.5 mg/kg/h, the time to reach steady-state concentration would not change. It would still take the same time (in minutes and hours) to reach steady-state concentration of drug in the plasma, but the magnitude of the steady-state concentration attained (concentration of drug in the plasma) would be increased proportionately.

Effect of Infusion Rate and Elimination Rate Constant

The steady-state concentration and time of attainment of steady-state concentration of drug in plasma depends on many factors. If the drug follows linear pharmacokinetics, the two most important factors that determine the steady-state concentration and time when steady-state concentration of drug in plasma will be achieved are:

(a) rate of infusion, and (b) rate constant of elimination of drug (i.e. biological half-life of the drug). The effect of infusion rate on attainment of steady-state concentration of drug in plasma is shown in Figure 15-3.

As can be seen from Figure 15-3, the effect of infusion rate on attainment of steady-state concentration of drug in the plasma is similar to the effect of maintenance dose on attaining steady-state concentration of drug in plasma during multiple dosing by rapid intravenous bolus injection (Chapter 13). In continuous intravenous infusion also, the concentration of drug in

Table 15-4 Plasma concentration of drug (data in Example 15-2) during prolonged intravenous infusion

Dose #	*Time (h)*	*# Of $t_{1/2}$*	*Amount of drug administered (mg)*	*C_{max} (mg/L)*	*C_{min} (mg/L)*	*Amount in body (mg) ($C_{min} \times V_d$)*
100	2.5 min	0.005	1.5	0.0499	0.0499	1.5
1,000	25 min	0.05	15	0.491	0.491	14.73
6,000	2.5	0.31	90	2.697	2.697	81
10,000	4.3	0.54	150	4.197	4.197	126
19,200	8.0	1.0	288	6.926	6.926	208
38,400	16.0	2.0	576	10.389	10.389	312
57,600	24.0	3.0	864	12.121	12.121	364
115,200	48.0	6.0	1,728	13.634	13.634	409
134,400	56.0	7.0	2,016	13.745	13.745	412
153,600	64.0	8.0	2,304	13.799	13.799	414
172,800	72.0	9.0	2,592	13.826	13.826	415
230,400	96.0	12.0	3,456	13.850	13.850	415
259,200	108.0	13.5	3,888	13.852	13.852	415
288,000	120.0	15.0	4,320	13.852	13.852	415

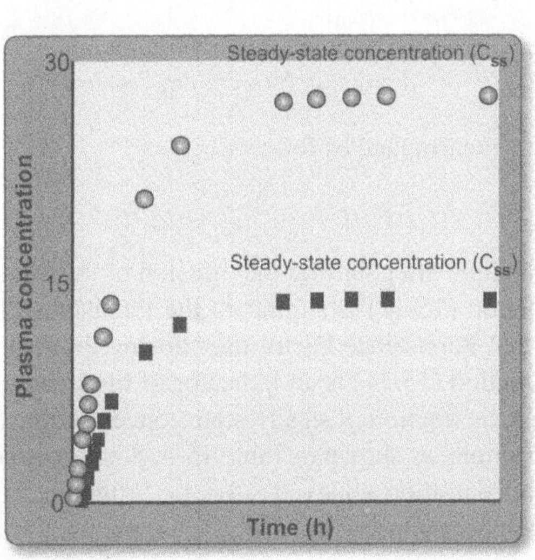

Fig. 15-3 Effect of infusion rate on steady-state concentration

(symbols ● represent an infusion rate that is twice the infusion rate represented by the symbols ■)

plasma attains more than 90% of steady-state concentration after a period of time equal to about four times the biological half-life of the drug and more than 99% of plateau levels are reached after about 7 biological half-lives of the drug. It takes approximately 8 or 9 biological half-lives for the drug to approximate its steady-state concentration in plasma. In other words, drugs having long half-lives take longer to attain steady-state concentration and drugs having short half-lives reach plateau levels relatively rapidly.

The plasma concentration resulting from continuous infusion of a drug depends on:

a. Rate of infusion, i.e. rate of zero-order drug input
b. Apparent volume of distribution of the drug
c. Rate constant of drug elimination
d. Time of drug infusion.

A simpler equation describing the relationship among these parameters for drug infusion may be derived as follows.

Constant intravenous infusion of a drug is a zero-order rate process in which the drug is infused into systemic circulation at a constant rate. Since elimination of most drugs follows first-order process, therefore, constant intravenous infusion is described as a zero-order input and a first-order output model. Thus, change in the amount of drug in the body at any time t during infusion period is given by the rate of input minus the rate of output.

$$\text{Rate of drug input} = \text{infusion rate} = K_0 \quad (15\text{-}6)$$

$$\text{Rate of drug output} = (A_t)(K) \quad (15\text{-}7)$$

In equation (15-7), A_t is amount of drug in the body and K is first-order rate constant of elimination of the the drug.

Therefore, the change in the amount of drug in the body at any time t during the infusion period is given by the following relationship:

$$\frac{dA_t}{dt} = K_0 - (K)(A_t) \quad (15\text{-}8)$$

Equation (15-8) upon integration yields the following equation.

$$A_t = \frac{K_0}{K}(1 - e^{-Kt}) \quad (15\text{-}9)$$

Since the amount of drug in the body at any time t is equal to concentration of drug in the body at time t multiplied by the apparent volume of distribution of the drug, equation (15-9) becomes K

$$(C)(V_d) = \frac{K_0}{K}(1 - e^{-Kt}) \quad (15\text{-}10)$$

Equation (15-10) can be rearranged as follows:

$$C = \frac{K_0}{(V_d)(K)}(1 - e^{-Kt}) \quad (15\text{-}11)$$

In equation (15-11) t is time after starting the infusion of the drug.

The term e^{-Kt} in equation (15-11) is similar to the Persistence Factor ($e^{-K\tau}$) used during multiple dosing, except that Persistence Factor uses dosing interval (τ) instead of the time, t. The term $(1 - e^{-Kt})$ in equation (15-11) is an indicator of the steady-state concentration in the sense that this factor gives the fraction of steady-state concentration achieved at time t after the infusion is started. For example, as shown in Table 15-4, 8 hours after starting the infusion, the fraction of steady-state concentration achieved is 0.5, i.e., after 8 hr of infusion, one has reached 50% of the steady-state concentration of drug in the plasma. The value of the factor $(1 - e^{-K\tau})$ after 8 hr of infusion is:

$$(1 - e^{-Kt}) = (1 - e^{-(0.086625)(8)}) = (1 - e^{-(0.693)}) = 0.5$$

This indicates that after 8 hr of infusion, one has reached 50% of the steady-state concentration of drug in the plasma. The value of this factor, if infusion was continued beyond 8 hr, will also increase and consequently the concentration of drug in plasma will increase (Table 15-4). One may consider this factor as an indicator of relative distance to attaining the steady-state concentration. When t is a very low number, e.g. soon after infusion is begun, the value of the factor $(1 - e^{-Kt})$ is very small and it approaches a value near to a value of zero. When t is very large, the value of the factor $(1 - e^{-Kt})$ approaches a value equal to one and there is no further increase in the concentration of drug in plasma, i.e. steady-state concentration is attained. At that time, equation (15-11) becomes:

$$C_{ss} = \frac{K_0}{(V_d)(K)} \tag{15-12}$$

Equation (15-12) can also be derived if one considers that, by definition, steady-state is attained when the rate of infusion equals rate of elimination of the drug, i.e. at steady-state, the rate of drug input is equal to the rate of drug output. Since the rate of drug input is the amount of drug administered per unit time, the rate of drug input is the infusion rate, i.e.

$$\text{Rate of drug input} = K_0 \tag{15-6}$$

$$\text{Rate of drug output} = \text{amount of drug eliminated per unit time} \tag{15-13}$$

$$\text{Since, amount} = (\text{concentration})(\text{volume})$$

therefore,

$$\text{Amount eliminated} = (\text{plasma concentration})(\text{volume of distribution}) \tag{15-14}$$

$$\text{Amount eliminated} = (C_{ss})(V_d) \tag{15-15}$$

$$\text{Amount eliminated/unit time} = (C_{ss})(V_d)(\text{elimination rate constant})$$

therefore,

$$\text{Rate of drug output} = (C_{ss})(V_d)(K) \tag{15-16}$$

When the rate of drug input equals the rate of drug output, the right-hand side of equation (15-6) equals the right-hand side of equation (15-16), i.e.

$$K_0 = (C_{ss})(V_d)(K) \tag{15-17}$$

which upon rearrangement yields equation (15-12).

From equation (15-12), it is seen that steady-state concentration of drug in plasma is directly proportional to the rate of infusion of the drug (K_0) and inversely proportional to apparent volume of distribution (V_d) and elimination rate constant (K) of the drug. This equation assumes that volume of distribution and rate constant of elimination of the drug do not change during the infusion period.

Since the denominator in equation (15-12) is clearance of the drug, equation (15-12) may be written as follows:

$$C_{ss} = \frac{K_0}{Cl} \tag{15-18}$$

where Cl is the clearance of the drug.

Example 15-5

The half-life of aminophylline in an adult patient is 6 h and apparent volume of distribution is 30 L. If this patient is administered aminophylline by continuous intravenous infusion at a rate of 45 mg/h, calculate the concentration of aminophylline in plasma at the following time periods;

(a) 1 hour after the infusion is started, (b) 3 hours after the infusion is started, (c) 6 hours after the infusion is started, (d) 8 hours after the infusion is started.

Solution

Since $t_{1/2}$ = 6 h, therefore K = 0.693/6 h = 0.1155/h

a. *Concentration at 1 hour*

From equation (15-11)

$$C = \frac{K_0}{(V_d)(K)}(1 - e^{-Kt})$$

$$= \frac{45 \text{ mg/h}}{(30 \text{ L})(0.1155/\text{h})}(1 - e^{-(0.1155/\text{h})(1 \text{ h})})$$

$$C = 1.4166 \text{ mg/L}$$

b. *Concentration at 3 hours*

$$C = \frac{45 \text{ mg/h}}{(30 \text{ L})(0.1155/\text{h})}(1 - e^{-(0.1155/\text{h})(3 \text{ h})})$$

$$C = 3.803 \text{ mg/L}$$

c. *Concentration at 6 hours*

$$C = \frac{45 \text{ mg/h}}{(30 \text{ L})(0.1155/\text{h})}(1 - e^{-(0.1155/\text{h})(6 \text{ h})})$$

$$C = 6.49 \text{ mg/L}$$

d. *Concentration at 8 hours*

$$C = \frac{45 \text{ mg/h}}{(30 \text{ L})(0.1155/\text{h})}(1 - e^{-(0.1155/\text{h})(8 \text{ h})})$$

$$C = 7.832 \text{ mg/L}$$

Example 15-6 A patient was administered 200 mg of aminophylline in 1 liter of 5% glucose solution by continuous intravenous infusion over an 8 hours period. If the apparent volume of distribution of aminophylline in this patient is 30 L and the biological half-life of aminophylline in this patient is 6 h, calculate the concentration of aminophylline in the plasma at following time periods after initiation of the infusion: (a) 1 hour, (b) 4 hours, (c) 6 hours and (d) 8 hours.

Solution

Since $t_{1/2}$ = 6 h, therefore

$$K = \frac{0.693}{6 \text{ h}} = 0.1155/\text{h and infusion rate} = \frac{20 \text{ mg}}{8 \text{ h}} = 25 \text{ mg/h}$$

a. *Concentration at 1 hour*

From equation (15-11)

$$C = \frac{K_0}{(V_d)(K)}(1 - e^{-Kt})$$

$$= \frac{25 \text{ mg/h}}{(30 \text{ L})(0.1155/\text{h})}(1 - e^{-(0.1155/\text{h})(1 \text{ h})})$$

$$C = 0.7865 \text{ mg/L}$$

b. *Concentration at 4 hours*

$$C = \frac{25 \text{ mg/h}}{(30 \text{ L})(0.1155/\text{h})}(1 - e^{-(0.1155/\text{h})(4 \text{ h})})$$

$$C = 2.669 \text{ mg/L}$$

c. *Concentration at 6 hours*

$$C = \frac{25\ \text{mg/h}}{(30\ \text{L})(0.1155/\text{h})}(1 - e^{-(0.1155/\text{h})(6\ \text{h})})$$

$$C = 3.608\ \text{mg/L}$$

d. *Concentration at 8 hours*

$$C = \frac{25\ \text{mg/h}}{(30\ \text{L})(0.1155/\text{h})}(1 - e^{-(0.1155/\text{h})(8\ \text{h})})$$

$$C = 4.351\ \text{mg/L}$$

Example 15-7 The half-life of aminophylline in a patient receiving continuous intravenous infusion of aminophylline is 6 h. If the apparent volume of distribution of aminophylline is 30 L, calculate the steady-state plasma concentration of aminophylline for a continuous intravenous aminophylline infusion of 40 mg/h.

Solution

The steady-state plasma concentration of aminophylline is calculated by substituting the following values into equation (15-12):

$$K_0 = 40\ \text{mg/h},\ V_d = 30\ \text{L and } K = 0.63/6\ \text{h} = 0.1155/\text{h}$$

$$C_{ss} = \frac{K_0}{(V_d)(K)} = \frac{40\ \text{mg/h}}{(30\ \text{L})(0.1155/\text{h})} = \frac{40\ \text{mg/h}}{3.465\ \text{L/h}} = 11.54\ \text{mg/L}$$

Infusion Rate to Reach Steady-State

Equation (15-12) shows that steady-state concentration is directly proportional to infusion rate. Assuming no change in the elimination rate constant (biological half-life) of aminophylline and apparent volume of distribution of the drug during therapy, equation (15-12) may be rearranged as follows:

$$C_{ss} = \frac{K_0}{(V_d)(K)}$$

$$K_0 = (C_{ss})(V_d)(K) \tag{15-19}$$

Equation (15-19) describes the infusion rate (as the amount of drug to be administered per unit time) needed to attain steady-state concentration.

Example 15-8 A patient is to be administered aminophylline by continuous intravenous infusion. The half-life of aminophylline in this patient is 8 hr and the apparent volume of distribution is 30 L. Calculate the infusion rate that should be used to attain the desired steady-state plasma level of aminophylline at 20 μg/mL.

Solution

$$\text{Since } t_{1/2} = 8\ \text{h, therefore, } K = 0.693/8\ \text{h} = 0.086625/\text{h}$$

The infusion rate to attain the desired steady-state plasma level is calculated using equation (15-19):

$$K_0 = (C_{ss})(V_d)(K) = (20\ \mu\text{g/mL})(30\ \text{L})(0.086625/\text{h}) = 51.975\ \text{mg/h}$$

Example 15-9 A physician orders continuous aminophylline infusion for a patient. The half-life of aminophylline in this patient is 6 h and volume of distribution is 30 L. Calculate the amount of aminophylline that must be dissolved in a liter of 5% glucose solution for continuous infusion over a 6 hours period to attain steady-state plasma concentration of 20 μg/mL of aminophylline.

Solution

$$\text{Since } t_{1/2} = 6\text{ h, therefore } K = 0.693/6\text{ h} = 0.1155/\text{h}$$

Substituting values of C_{ss} = 20 µg/mL, V_d = 30 L and K = 0.1155/h into equation (15-19):

$$K_0 = (C_{ss})(V_d)(K) = (20\ \mu g/mL)(30\ L)(0.1155/h) = 69.3\ mg/h$$

Since infusion is for 6 hr, the amount of drug needed to provide an infusion rate of 69.3 mg/h is:

$$\text{Amount needed} = (\text{infusion rate})(\text{time})$$

$$\text{Amount needed} = (69.3\ mg/h)(6\ h) = 415.8\ mg$$

Example 15-10 The half-life of aminophylline in a patient is 6 h and the volume of distribution is 30 L. Calculate concentration of aminophylline in plasma after 6 hours if this patient is administered

a. A single 300 mg intravenous bolus dose, or
b. A 300 mg dose by continuous intravenous infusion over a 6-hour period.

Solution

$$\text{Since } t_{1/2} = 6\text{ h, therefore}$$

$$K = 0.693/t_{1/2} = 0.693/6\ h$$

$$K = 0.1155/h$$

a. *Intravenous Bolus Dose*

The equation (3-27) describing concentration of drug in plasma after an intravenous bolus dose is

$$C_t = C_0(e^{-Kt})$$

$$\text{where } C_0 = \frac{\text{Dose}}{\text{Volume of distribution}} = \frac{300\ mg}{30\ L} = 10\ mg/L$$

$$C_t = C_0(e^{-Kt})$$

$$= (10\ mg/L)(e^{-(0.1155/h)(6\ h)})$$

$$= (10\ mg/L)(0.5) = 5\ mg/L$$

b. *Continuous Intravenous Infusion*

Equation (15-11) is used to determine concentration of aminophylline in plasma after 6 hours infusion period.

Here K_0 = 300 mg/6 h = 50 mg/h

$$C_t = \frac{K_0}{(V_d)(K)}\left(1-e^{-Kt}\right)$$

$$= \frac{50\ mg/h}{(30\ L)(0.1155/h)}\ 1-(e^{-(0.1155/h)(6\ h)}) = \frac{50\ mg/L}{3.465\ L/h}(0.5) = 7.215\ mg/L$$

It is seen from Example 15-10 that although the same dose is administered in both cases (bolus as well as infusion), the concentration of drug in plasma at 6 hr is higher during continuous intravenous infusion than when the drug is administered as a single bolus dose. The reason for this is that when the drug is administered as a bolus dose, a large amount of drug is available for elimination immediately after drug administration and, according to first-order kinetics; a large amount of the administered dose undergoes elimination when a large amount of the drug is available for elimination. This continues during the 6-hour period. However, when the drug is administered as an infusion, the amount of drug available for elimination is very small immediately after the infusion is begun, therefore only a small amount of the drug is eliminated after infusion is started. The amount of drug in plasma increases as a function of time, but since the drug is administered continuously; the loss of drug due to elimination is relatively small.

Time to Reach a Certain Level of Steady-State

The steady-state plasma drug concentration during continuous intravenous infusion is given by equation (15-12):

$$C_{ss} = \frac{K_0}{(V_d)(K)}$$

This equation is derived from the following equation (15-11), which is used to calculate concentration of drug in plasma at any time t during the infusion period:

$$C = \frac{K_0}{(V_d)(K)}\left(1 - e^{-Kt}\right)$$

As mentioned earlier, the derivation of equation (15-12) from equation (15-11) is based upon the fact that when t becomes very large, the value of the exponential term, e^{-Kt}, in equation (15-11) becomes very small. With the increasing value of t, the value of the exponential term becomes so small that it approaches a value of 0 and equation (15-11) is then reduced to equation (15-12). It should be remembered that even after an infinitely long period of time, i.e. when t becomes extremely large, the value of exponential term e^{-Kt} does not actually become zero (because the exponential term represents first-order kinetics), but the value of the exponential term becomes so small that for all practical purposes it may be considered to be equal to zero. Since, theoretically, the value of the exponential term can never attain a value of zero, it is quite acceptable in actual practice to reach near 100% of steady-state concentration and consider it as having reached the steady-state concentration.

The equation to calculate the time needed to achieve a certain level of the steady-state concentration (e.g. 95%, 99% or 99.9%) can be derived as follows:

To determine the time to reach plasma concentration equal to x% of the steady-state concentration, one substitutes x% C_{ss} as the concentration term into equation (15-11): xK

$$\left(\frac{x}{100\%}\right)(C_{ss}) = \frac{K_0}{(V_d)(K)}\left(1 - e^{-Kt}\right) \quad (15\text{-}20)$$

Dividing equation (15-20) by equation (15-12),

$$\frac{\left(\frac{x}{100\%}\right)(C_{ss})}{Css} = \frac{\left(\frac{K_0}{(V_d)(K)}\right)\left(1 - e^{-Kt}\right)}{\frac{K_0}{(V_d)(K)}} \quad (15\text{-}21)$$

which, upon simplification yields the following equation:

$$\frac{x}{100\%} = 1 - e^{-Kt} \quad (15\text{-}22)$$

$$e^{-Kt} = 1 - \frac{x}{100\%} \quad (15\text{-}23)$$

Taking natural logarithms on both sides of equation (15-23),

$$-Kt = \ln\left(1 - \frac{x}{100\%}\right)$$

$$Kt = -\ln\left(1 - \frac{x}{100\%}\right)$$

$$t = -\frac{1}{K}\ln\left(1-\frac{x}{100\%}\right) \quad (15\text{-}24)$$

For example, to calculate the time required to attain 99.9% of the steady-state concentration during prolonged intravenous infusion, equation (15-24) becomes

$$t = -\frac{1}{K}\ln\left(1-\frac{99.9\%}{100\%}\right)$$

$$= -\frac{1}{K}\ln(0.001)$$

$$= -\frac{1}{K}(-6.9078) = \frac{6.9087}{K}$$

Equation (15-24) may also be written in terms of biological half-life of the drug as follows:

$$t = -\frac{t_{1/2}}{0.693}\ln\left(1-\frac{x}{100\%}\right)$$

$$t = -(1.443)(t_{1/2})\ln\left(1-\frac{x}{100\%}\right)$$

Using the concepts and equations given above, one can calculate time needed to attain a given level of steady-state concentration during continuous intravenous infusion. Table 15-5 shows the calculated values of time (both, in terms of biological half-life of the drug, as well as in terms of the overall rate constant of elimination) needed to attain a given level of steady-state concentration of drug in the plasma.

As can be seen from the data presented in Table 15-5, it takes only one biological half-life for the drug to attain 50% of steady-state concentration in plasma. In less than four half-lives, the drug reaches 95% of steady-state concentration in plasma. More than six half-lives are required to approach (not even reach) 99% of the steady-state concentration. The number of half-lives required to attain the last 1 percent of steady-state concentration increases dramatically.

Table 15-5 Time to attain a given level of steady-state concentration

x or $\%C_{ss}$	$1-\frac{x}{100\%}$ *or* $1-\frac{\%C_{ss}}{100\%}$	$\ln\left(1-\frac{x}{100\%}\right)$ *or* $\ln\left(1-\frac{\%C_{ss}}{100\%}\right)$	*Time to attain steady-state concentration* (C_{ss})	
			In Terms of K	*In Terms of* $t_{1/2}$
50	0.5	–0.6931	0.6931/K	1.0002
75	0.25	–1.3863	1.3863/K	2.0004
80	0.20	–1.6094	1.6094/K	2.3224
90	0.1	–2.3026	2.3026/K	3.3226
95	0.05	–2.9957	2.9957/K	4.3228
96	0.04	–3.2189	3.2189/K	4.6458
97	0.03	–3.5066	3.5066/K	5.0599
98	0.02	–3.9120	3.9120/K	5.6450
99	0.01	–4.6052	4.6052/K	6.6453
99.50	0.005	–5.2983	5.2983/K	7.6455
99.90	0.001	–6.9078	6.9078/K	9.9679
99.950	0.0005	–7.6009	7.6009/K	10.9681
99.9950	0.00005	–9.9035	9.9035/K	14.2907
99.9990	0.00001	–11.5129	11.5129/K	16.6132
99.99990	0.000001	–13.8155	13.8155/K	19.9358
99.999990	0.0000001	–16.1181	16.1181/K	23.2584
99.9999990	0.00000001	–18.4207	18.4207/K	26.5810

Example 15-11 The desired steady-state plasma concentration of aminophylline in a patient is 10 mg/L. Calculate the time needed to achieve 99% of this steady-state plasma concentration if the drug is administered at a rate of 35 mg/h. The rate constant of elimination of aminophylline in this patient is 0.1155/h and the apparent volume of distribution is 30 L.

Solution

From equation (15-24), time to achieve x% of steady-state concentration is

$$t = \frac{1}{K} \ln\left(1 - \frac{X}{100\%}\right)$$

Substituting x = 99% into equation (15-24),

$$t = -\frac{1}{0.1155/h} \ln\left(1 - \frac{99\%}{100\%}\right)$$

$$= - -\frac{1}{0.1155/h} \ln(0.01) = -\frac{1}{0.1155/h} (-4.6052) = 39.87 \text{ h}$$

Almost 40 hours or 7 half-lives will be needed to reach 99% of steady-state plasma concentration.

Example 15-12 Calculate the time needed to achieve plasma concentration within 2% of the steady-state concentration of 15 mg/L of aminophylline, if the drug is administered at a rate of 30 mg/h to an adult patient having K = 0.099/h and V_d = 28 L.

Solution

To achieve within 2% of steady-state concentration means to attain 98% of steady-state concentration. That is, here, x = 100% – 2% = 98%. Substituting x = 98% into equation (15-24),

$$t = -\frac{1}{0.099/h} \ln\left(1 - \frac{98\%}{100\%}\right)$$

$$= -\frac{1}{0.099/h} \ln(0.02) = -\frac{1}{0.099/h} (-3.912) = 39.52 \text{ h}$$

Infusion Rate for Concentration in Specified Time

In some cases it may be desired to attain a specified concentration of drug in plasma (which in most cases is the desired steady-state concentration) within a specific period of time. In such cases, infusion of the drug is started at a higher rate for a specific period of time so as to attain desired concentration quickly. It should be pointed out that if the specified time to attain a certain concentration of drug in plasma is less than the time necessary to attain steady-state concentration, then continuation of infusion beyond the specified time will result in further increase in concentration of drug in plasma. It may therefore be judicious to modify infusion rate (in order to sustain the concentration of drug in plasma at the attained level) once the desired concentration of drug in the plasma has been achieved.

Once the desired level of drug concentration in plasma is reached, the infusion is then continued at a relatively slower rate so that the rate of drug input (infusion rate) is equal to the rate of drug output (elimination rate of the drug). This maintains the concentration of drug at the desired level during the remainder of infusion period. Hence, one needs to determine initial infusion rate in order to achieve the desired concentration of drug in plasma within the specified time period and then again a second infusion rate to maintain the desired concentration during the remainder of infusion period.

Initial Infusion Rate: The initial infusion rate needed to achieve the desired concentration of drug in plasma within a short period of time is determined by rearranging equation (15-11) and solving for K_0 as follows:

According to equation (15-11)

$$C = \frac{K_0}{(V_d)(K)}(1 - e^{-Kt})$$

which, upon rearrangement gives

$$K_0 = \frac{(C)(V_d)(K)}{(1 - e^{-Kt})} \tag{15-25}$$

Equation (15-25) is used to calculate initial infusion rate needed to achieve the desired concentration of drug in plasma within a short period of time.

Maintenance Infusion Rate: The infusion rate necessary to maintain and sustain the concentration of drug during remainder of infusion period is determined using equation (15-17).

$$K_0 = (C_{ss})(V_d)(K)$$

Example 15-13 It is desired to reach 10 mg/L steady-state concentration of aminophylline in a patient. The half-life of aminophylline in this patient is 8 h and the volume of distribution is 30 L. Calculate: (a) Infusion rate that must be used to achieve the desired concentration in 30 minutes, and (b) Infusion rate to sustain this concentration during the remainder of infusion period.

Solution

$$\text{Since } t_{1/2} = 8 \text{ h, therefore } K = 0.693/8 \text{ h} = 0.086625/\text{h}$$

a. *Infusion rate to achieve a concentration of 10 mg/L*

Substituting the values of K, C, V_d and t = 0.5 hr into equation (15-25),

$$K_0 = \frac{(C)(V_d)(K)}{(1 - e^{-Kt})}$$

$$= \frac{(10 \text{ mg/L})(30 \text{ L})(0.086625/\text{h})}{\left(1 - e^{-(0.086625/\text{h})(0.5\text{h})}\right)} = \frac{25.9875 \text{ mg/h}}{0.04239} = 613 \text{ mg/h}$$

Thus, the patient receives 613 mg/h of drug during the initial 30 minutes of continuous intravenous infusion, i.e. 306.5 mg in the first 30 minutes.

b. *Infusion rate to sustain a concentration of 10 mg/L*

Infusion rate after 30 minutes should be reduced in order to sustain the attained 10 mg/L concentration of drug in the plasma. The infusion rate for the remainder of infusion period is determined using equation (15-17).

Substituting the values of C_{ss}, K and V_d into equation (15-17), one obtains

$$K_0 = (10 \text{ mg/L})(30 \text{ L})(0.086625/\text{h})$$

$$K_0 = 25.9875 \text{ mg/h}$$

LOADING DOSE FOLLOWED BY CONTINUOUS INFUSION

During continuous intravenous infusion, a period of time elapses before steady-state concentration of drug is attained in the plasma (Fig. 15-1). Also, as indicated earlier and shown in Table 15-4, it would take a relatively long time to reach steady-state concentration, because the value of the term $e^{-nK\tau}$ in equation (13-23) does not equal zero even after a very long time. However, as the exponent nKτ becomes very large, the value of $e^{-nK\tau}$ approaches zero and for all practical purposes, steady-state is considered to have been reached.

If the time required for reaching steady-state concentration is quite long, especially for drugs which have a long half-life, it is often convenient to administer an intravenous bolus dose as the loading dose. The intent of administering a loading in the form of a simultaneous bolus injection is to bring the plasma concentration of drug to the desired level as soon as continuous intravenous infusion is started and therefore sustain the steady-state level during the infusion period.

Plasma Profile

The plasma profile exhibiting simultaneous injection of an intravenous bolus dose (given as the loading dose) and initiation of constant intravenous infusion of drug can be obtained from the equations describing these two processes. The equation that describes the time course of amount (or concentration) of drug in the body (or plasma) after simultaneous administration of a single bolus dose and initiation of constant intravenous infusion is the sum of the two equations describing these two processes individually.

Rapid Bolus Injection

The amount of drug in the body as a function of time following a rapid bolus injection of the drug is given by the first-order rate equation. The first-order rate equation describing the concentration of drug in the plasma as a function of time using equation (3-27) is:

$$C_t = C_0(e^{-Kt})$$

By definition, concentration = amount/volume and the volume here is apparent volume of distribution of drug.

Multiplying both sides of equation (3-27) with the apparent volume of distribution gives

$$(C_t)(V_d) = (C_0)(V_d)(e^{-Kt}) \tag{15-26}$$

$$A_t = (A_0)(e^{-Kt}) \tag{15-27}$$

where A_t is amount of drug in the body at time t, A_0 is amount of drug in the body at time 0, K is first-order rate constant of elimination of the drug and t is time.

Since A_0 is the amount of drug in the body at time zero, therefore, A_0 represents the intravenous bolus dose, D*. Hence, equation (15-27) may be written as

$$A_t = (D^*)(e^{-Kt}) \tag{15-28}$$

Continuous Infusion

The amount of drug in the body as a function of time following continuous intravenous infusion is given by equation (15-9), i.e.

$$A_t = \frac{K_0}{K}(1 - e^{-Kt})$$

Bolus Injection and Continuous Infusion

The equation describing time course of amount of drug in the body after simultaneous administration of a bolus dose and constant intravenous infusion is the sum of the two equations describing these two processes individually. Combining equations (15-28) and (15-9), we have,

$$A_t = (D^*)(e^{-Kt}) + \frac{K_0}{K}(1 - e^{-Kt})$$

$$A_t = (D^*)(e^{-Kt}) + \frac{K_0}{K} - \frac{K_0}{K}(e^{-Kt})$$

and upon rearrangement yields

$$A_t = \frac{K_0}{K} + (D^*)(e^{-Kt}) - \frac{K_0}{K}(e^{-Kt})$$

$$A_t = \frac{K_0}{K} + \left(D^* - \frac{K_0}{K}\right)\left(e^{-Kt}\right) \quad (15\text{-}29)$$

If the patient is administered a loading dose sufficient to provide C_{ss} at the time of bolus injection, then

$$D^* = (C_{ss})(V_d)$$

Substituting D* for $(C_{ss})(V_d)$ into equation (15-12) gives

$$D^* = \frac{K_0}{K} \quad (15\text{-}30)$$

Substituting equation (15-30) into equation (15-29) we get

$$A_t = \frac{K_0}{K} + \left(\frac{K_0}{K} - \frac{K_0}{K}\right)\left(e^{-Kt}\right)$$

$$A_t = \frac{K_0}{K} + (0)\left(e^{-Kt}\right)$$

$$A_t = \frac{K_0}{K} \quad (15\text{-}31)$$

Since, the amount of *drug = (concentration of drug)(volume of distribution)*, equation (15-31) may be written as:

$$(C_t)(V_d) = \frac{K_0}{K}$$

which upon rearrangement gives

$$C_t = \frac{K_0}{(V_d)(K)} \quad (15\text{-}32)$$

Since the right-hand side of equation (15-32) is identical to right-hand side of equation (15-12), it follows that the term C_t in equation (15-32) is identical to the term C_{ss} in equation (15-12), i.e. following an intravenous loading dose and simultaneous constant intravenous infusion, the concentration of drug in plasma remains constant from time zero until infusion is terminated. Figure 15-4 compares plasma drug concentration in the presence and in the absence of the administration of the loading dose.

If the size of the loading dose is chosen so as to provide plasma drug concentration equal to the desired steady-state concentration of drug in the plasma, one attains steady-state concentration (plateau levels) right from the start of the continuous infusion. This is because administration of the bolus dose at the initiation of the continuous infusion brings the plasma concentration of drug at the desired level and simultaneous administration of continuous infusion provides drug input equal to drug output (elimination). This approach is useful not only in maintaining plasma concentration at steady-state level, but also assures continuous therapy without having to wait for the attainment of steady-state concentration of drug in the plasma.

Size of Loading Dose

The size of loading dose needed to attain initial concentration of drug equal to the steady-state concentration may be determined as follows:

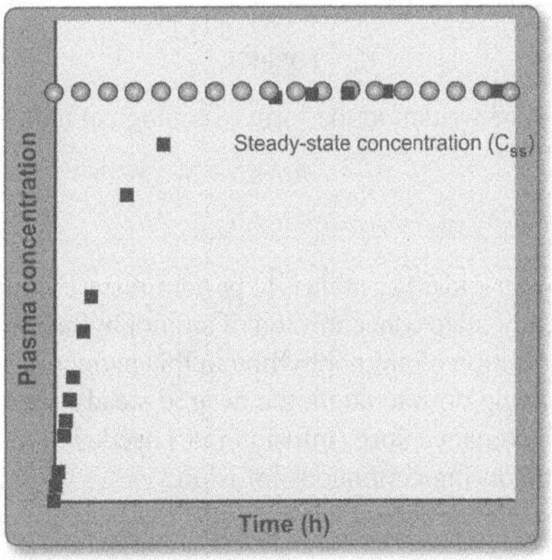

Fig. 15-4 Effect of loading dose on plasma concentration during continuous intravenous infusion

■ Continuous infusion in the absence of loading dose
● Simultaneous administration of loading dose and continuous infusion)

Since loading dose of the drug is administered as a intravenous bolus dose, its concentration in plasma at the time of injection is given by:

$$\text{Concentration} = \frac{\text{Dose}}{\text{Apparent volume of distribution}}$$

$$\text{Dose} = (\text{Concentration})(\text{Apparent volume of distribution}) \quad (15\text{-}33)$$

The concentration in equation (15-33) should be equal to steady-state concentration of drug in plasma during continuous intravenous infusion. Thus, equation (15-33) becomes

$$\text{Loading dose} = D^* = (C_{ss})(V_d) \quad (15\text{-}34)$$

Example 15-14 A patient is ordered aminophylline by intravenous infusion. If the desired steady-state concentration of aminophylline is 15 mg/L and the apparent volume of distribution of aminophylline is 35 L, calculate the size of loading dose needed to attain the desired concentration at the time of initiating the infusion.

Solution

According to equation (15-34),

$$\text{Loading dose} = D^* = (C_{ss})(V_d) = (15\text{ mg/L})(35\text{ L}) = 525\text{ mg}$$

Maintenance Dose (Infusion Rate)

Maintenance dose or infusion rate of this dose depends on the desired steady-state concentration of drug in plasma. Since the size of loading dose was based on steady-state concentration, therefore, rate of administration of maintenance dose depends on the size of the loading dose. Once the size of loading dose is determined, the size of maintenance dose is approximated using equation (15-17):

$$K_0 = (C_{ss})(V_d)(K)$$

Since $(C_{ss})(V_d) = D^*$, equation (15-17) becomes

$$K_0 = (D^*)(K) \tag{15-35}$$

Equation (15-35) may also be written in the form of biological half-life of the drug as follows:

$$K_0 = \frac{(D^*)(0.693)}{t_{1/2}} = \frac{(C_{ss})(V_d)(0.693)}{t_{1/2}} \tag{15-36}$$

Example 15-15 A 72-year-old 60 kg male is to be administered aminophylline by continuous infusion. The desired steady-state concentration of aminophylline in this patient is 16 mg/L. If apparent volume of distribution of aminophylline in this patient is 35 L and K = 0.1155/h and the patient receives a loading dose to attain the desired steady-state concentration at the start of infusion, calculate maintenance dose (infusion rate) needed to maintain the desired plasma steady-state concentration during continuous infusion.

Solution

According to equation (15-34) the size of loading dose is:

$$\text{Loading dose} = (C_{ss})(V_d) = (16\text{ mg/L})(35\text{ L}) = 560\text{ mg}$$

Therefore, the size of maintenance dose needed is given by equation (15-35):

$$K_0 = (D^*)(K) = (560\text{ mg})(0.1155/\text{h}) = 64.88\text{ mg/h}$$

Example 15-16 A 70-year-old 65 kg female is to be administered an antibiotic by continuous infusion. The desired steady-state concentration of the antibiotic in this patient is 20 mg/L. The apparent volume of distribution of the antibiotic in this patient is 1.6 L/kg body weight and the rate constant of elimination of the antibiotic is 0.1155/h. The patient received a loading dose to attain the desired steady-state concentration at the start of infusion. Calculate the maintenance dose (infusion rate) needed to maintain the desired plasma steady-state concentration during continuous infusion.

Solution

According to equation (15-34) the size of loading dose is:

$$\text{Loading dose} = (C_{ss})(V_d) = (20\text{ mg/L})(1.6\text{ L} \times 65) = 2080\text{ mg}$$

Therefore, the size of maintenance dose needed is given by equation (15-35):

$$K_0 = (D^*)(K) = (2080\text{ mg})(0.1155/\text{h}) = 240.24\text{ mg/h}$$

SUGGESTED READING

1. Mitenko P and Ogilvie R. Rapidly achieved plasma concentration plateaus with observations on the theophylline kinetics. Clin Pharmacol Ther. 1972;13(3):325-29.
2. Schumacher, (ed). Therapeutic Drug Monitoring. Appleton and Lange; 1995.
3. Wagner J. A safe method for rapidly achieving plasma concentration plateaus. Clin Pharmacol. Ther. 1974;16:691–700.

PRACTICE PROBLEMS

15-1. A 75 kg adult male patient receives aminophylline by continuous intravenous infusion at the rate of 0.8 mg aminophylline/kg/h for 6 hours. The drug is dissolved in 1 liter of normal saline solution and each mL of the infusate measures 30 drops. Calculate: (a) The size of each dose, and (b) The dosing interval during infusion period.

15-2. A 45-year-old adult male weighing 70 kg is administered aminophylline at the rate of 0.6 mg/Kg/h for 8 hours. Calculate the concentration of aminophylline in plasma at 2.5 hours during the infusion period if the drug is dissolved in 960 mL of the infusate and each mL of the infusion solution measures 20 drops. Assume the biological half-life of aminophylline in this patient is 8 hr and the volume of distribution is 30 L.

15-3. The biological half-life of aminophylline in a patient is 6 h and the volume of distribution of aminophylline in this patient is known to be 30 L. If this patient is administered 300 mg of aminophylline by continuous infusion in 2,000 mL of normal saline over an 8-hr period at a rate of 125 drops/min, calculate the concentration of aminophylline in the plasma at the following time periods after the start of the infusion: (a) 1 hour, (b) 3 hours, (c) 6 hours, and (d) 8 hours. Assume that each mL of the infusion solution delivers 30 drops.

15-4. A 45-year-old adult female weighing 60 kg is administered aminophylline at the rate of 0.7 mg/kg/h for 6 hours. Calculate the concentration of aminophylline in the plasma 2 hours after the termination of infusion. Aminophylline is dissolved in 1000 mL of the infusion solution and each mL of the solution measures 20 drops. Assume that the biological half-life of aminophylline in this patient is 6 h and the volume of distribution of aminophylline in this patient is 0.5 L/kg of body weight.

15-5. The half-life of aminophylline in a patient is 6 h and the apparent volume of distribution is 30 L. If this patient is administered aminophylline by continuous infusion at the rate of 45 mg/hours, calculate the concentration of aminophylline at (a) 2 hours, (b) 4 hours and (c) 5 hours after the infusion is started.

15-6. A patient was administered 300 mg of aminophylline (dissolved in 900 mL of 5% glucose solution) by continuous intravenous infusion over an 8 hours period. If the volume of distribution of aminophylline in this patient is 35 L, the half-life is 6 h and the infusate measures 30 drops/mL, calculate the concentration of aminophylline in the plasma at (a) 1 hour, (b) 4 hours, (c) 6 hours, and (d) 8 hours.

15-7. The biological half-life of aminophylline in a patient receiving continuous intravenous infusion of aminophylline is 8 h. If the apparent volume of distribution of aminophylline in this patient is 30 L, calculate steady-state plasma concentration for a continuous aminophylline infusion of 35 mg/h.

15-8. A patient is to be given aminophylline by continuous intravenous infusion. If the half-life of aminophylline is 8 h and the volume of distribution of aminophylline is 30 L, what infusion rate would you recommend if the desired steady-state plasma level of aminophylline 15 μg/mL?

15-9. A physician orders continuous aminophylline infusion for a 70-year-old male weighing 75 kg. The half-life of aminophylline in this patient is 6 h and the volume of distribution is 0.4 L/kg of body weight. Calculate the amount of aminophylline that must be dissolved in a liter of 5% glucose solution for continuous infusion over a 6 hours period to attain steady-state aminophylline plasma concentration of 18 μg/mL.

15-10. The biological half-life of a new antibiotic in adult patients is 8 h and the apparent volume of distribution of the antibiotic is reported to be 30 L. Calculate the concentration of this antibiotic in plasma after 6 hours if an adult patient is administered: (a) A 300 mg single intravenous bolus dose, or (b) 300 mg by continuous intravenous infusion over a 6 hours period.

15-11. A 72-year-old, 70 kg female is to be administered aminophylline by continuous intravenous infusion. If the desired steady-state concentration of aminophylline in this patient is 12 mg/L and the apparent volume of distribution of aminophylline is 0.5 L/kg of body weight, calculate the size of the loading dose needed to attain the desired concentration at the time of initiating infusion.

15-12. A 42-year-old female weighing 60 kg is to be administered aminophylline by continuous intravenous infusion. The desired steady-state plasma concentration of aminophylline is 16 mg/L. The apparent volume of distribution of the drug is 0.5 L/kg of body weight and the rate constant of elimination of aminophylline is 0.086625/h. This patient received a loading dose to attain the desired steady-state plasma concentration of aminophylline at the start of infusion. Calculate the rate of infusion needed to maintain the steady-state plasma concentration during continuous infusion.

15-13. Calculate the time needed to achieve 99.5% of steady-state plasma concentration of an investigational new drug if the drug is administered at a rate of 35 mg per hour to an adult patient. The rate constant of elimination rate of the drug is 0.1155/h and the apparent volume of distribution of the drug in this patient is 30 L.

15-14. It is desired to maintain a 12 mg/L plasma concentration of aminophylline in a patient. If the half-life of aminophylline in this patient is 8 h and the apparent volume of distribution was determined to be 30 L, calculate the following: (a) Infusion rate that must be used to achieve the desired concentration of aminophylline in the plasma in 30 minutes, and (b) the rate at which aminophylline should be infusion to sustain this concentration during the remainder of infusion period.

15-15. A 58-year-old female patient weighing 64 kg is to receive aminophylline by continuous intravenous infusion for 24 hours. The desired steady-state plasma concentration of aminophylline in this patient is 125 μg/kg of body weight per liter. If the half-life of aminophylline in this patient is 6 h and the volume of distribution is 25 L, calculate: (a) Infusion rate that must be used to achieve the plasma steady-state concentration of aminophylline in 20 minutes, and (b) Infusion rate for the remainder of the infusion period to maintain the steady-state aminophylline concentration in the plasma.

15-16. It is desired to reach 10 mg/L steady-state plasma concentration of aminophylline in a 48-year-old female patient weighing 70 kg. The half-life of aminophylline is 6 h and the apparent volume of distribution is 0.4 L/kg of body weight. Calculate (a) the aminophylline infusion rate that must be used to achieve the desired aminophylline concentration in the plasma in 30 minutes, and (b) aminophylline infusion rate to sustain this concentration during the remainder of infusion period.

15-17. It is desired to reach 15 mg/L steady-state plasma concentration of aminophylline in a 50-year-old male patient weighing 70 kg. The half-life of aminophylline is 6 hr and the volume of distribution is 30 L. Calculate: (a) infusion rate that must be used to achieve the desired concentration in 30 minutes, and (b) infusion rate to sustain this concentration during the remainder of infusion period.

15-18. It is desired to reach 15 mg/L steady-state concentration of aminophylline in a old female patient weighing 60 kg. The half-life of aminophylline in this patient is 6 hr and the volume of distribution is 37 L. Calculate: (a) infusion rate that must be used to achieve the desired concentration in 45 minutes, and (b) infusion rate to sustain this concentration during the remainder of infusion period.

15-19. It is desired to reach 12 mg/L steady-state plasma concentration of aminophylline in a patient. The half-life of aminophylline in this patient is 6 hr and the apparent volume of distribution of aminophylline is 37 L. Calculate: (a) the rate of infusion of aminophylline that must be used to achieve the desired plasma aminophylline concentration in 40 minutes, and (b) the rate of infusion that will sustain this concentration during the remainder of the infusion period.

15-20 A 60-year-old weighing 92.5 kg male is to be administered aminophylline by continuous infusion. The desired steady-state plasma concentration of aminophylline in this patient is 15 mg/L. The apparent volume of distribution of aminophylline in this patient is 0.4 L per kg of body weight and the rate constant of elimination of aminophylline is 0.1155/h.

If the patient received a loading dose to attain the desired steady-state concentration at the start of infusion, calculate the aminophylline maintenance dose (infusion rate) needed to maintain the desired plasma steady-state concentration during continuous infusion.

15-21. A 60-year-old weighing100 kg male is to be administered aminophylline by continuous infusion. The desired steady-state concentration of aminophylline in the plasma in this patient is 15 mg/L. The apparent volume of distribution of aminophylline in this patient is 0.3 L per kg of body weight and the rate constant of elimination is 0.099/h. If this patient received a loading dose to attain the desired steady-state concentration of aminophylline in the plasma at the start of infusion, calculate the maintenance dose (infusion rate) needed to maintain desired plasma steady-state concentration during continuous infusion.

15-22. A patient is ordered aminophylline by intravenous infusion. If the desired steady-state concentration of aminophylline is 12 mg/L and the apparent volume of distribution of aminophylline is 30 L, calculate the size of loading dose needed to attain the desired concentration at the time of initiating the infusion.

15-23. A patient is ordered aminophylline by intravenous infusion. If the desired steady-state concentration of aminophylline is 10 mg/L and the apparent volume of distribution of aminophylline is 37 L, calculate the size of loading dose needed to attain the desired concentration at the time of initiating the infusion.

15-24. A patient is to be administered aminophylline by continuous intravenous infusion. The half-life of aminophylline in this patient is 8 hr, the apparent volume of distribution is 37 L and the desired steady-state concentration of aminophylline is 15 μg/mL. Calculate the infusion rate that should be used to attain the desired steady-state plasma level of aminophylline.

15-25. Calculate the time needed to achieve plasma concentration within 5% of the plasma steady-state concentration of 10.8 mg/L of aminophylline, if the drug is administered at a rate of 30 mg/h to an adult patient having $K = 0.099/h$ and $V_d = 28$ L.

15-26. It is desired to reach 8 mg/L steady-state concentration of aminophylline in a patient. The half-life of aminophylline in this patient is 8 h and the apparent volume of distribution is 30 L. Calculate:

(a) Aminophylline infusion rate that must be used to achieve the desired concentration in 30 minutes, and (b) Infusion rate to sustain this concentration during the remainder of infusion period.

CHAPTER 16

RENAL IMPAIRMENT

Renal impairment signifies reduction in kidney function. Patients with renal impairment pose a special problem in the evaluation of their pharmacokinetic data because kidneys play a major role in a variety of functions associated with the amount and concentration of drug in the body. These functions include drug elimination, metabolite removal, regulation of body fluids and electrolyte balance. Thus, administration of a drug to patients with impaired renal function becomes complicated. Some of the factors, which cause complication in drug therapy include the following:

1. Presence of other medical and/or physiological problems associated with the patient.
2. The type and number (quantity) of drugs received by the patient.
3. Possible alteration in disposition and elimination of the drug due to disease state or other drugs ingested by the patient.
4. Protein binding of drugs in the plasma.

Various conditions may cause acute and/or chronic renal impairment. These include disease state (e.g. pyelonephritis, hypertension, diabetes, etc.), presence of nephrotoxic agents (e.g. nephrotoxic drugs or metals) and traumatic injury. In hypertension, for example, the body has a tendency to retain fluids and electrolytes and leads to chronic overloading of the kidney with the electrolytes and fluid, which may lead to kidney insufficiency. Similarly, in the case of diabetes mellitus, the disturbance of sugar metabolism and acid-base balance is very common. This may predispose or lead a patient to degenerative renal disease. Irreversible kidney damage may also be caused by certain drugs taken chronically (e.g. aminoglycosides and phenacetin). Chronic consumption of small doses of heavy metals (e.g. mercury and lead), may also cause irreversible kidney damage. Under normal conditions, kidneys are highly perfused and receive a large blood supply via the renal artery. The blood supply received by normal kidneys (in the absence of renal impairment) is approximately 20 to 25% of the cardiac output, which represents the rate of blood flow through the kidney at approximately 850 L to 1000 L per day. Any condition causing reduction in renal blood flow will eventually lead to renal ischemia and damage. Also, certain compounds may produce an immune type of sensitivity reaction with nephritic syndrome thus causing kidney failure. Renal impairment alters kidney function and generally reduces glomerular filtration rate. Therefore, during renal impairment there always exists a possibility of decreased ability of the kidneys to remove waste, such as unchanged drugs, metabolites of drugs and urea.

Another consequence of renal impairment, important from the standpoint of pharmacokinetics, is the possible decrease in plasma protein binding of drugs and therefore the apparent volume of distribution of the drug. However, it should be remembered that, in renal disease, alteration in protein binding is seen only in the case of acidic or neutral drugs in plasma. Basic drugs are either not affected at all or are affected only slightly. Some of the reasons that explain changes in protein binding of drugs during renal impairment include the following:

1. Changes in conformation of albumin that result in decreased affinity for binding sites.
2. Competition for protein binding sites by the accumulating metabolite waste (e.g. urea, the drug and its biotransformation products) that may have ability to displace the parent drug from proteins.
3. Competition for protein binding sites with small acidic molecules that accumulate in uremia
4. Hypoalbuminemia that occurs as a result of protein loss in the urine.

Regardless, of what causes changes in protein binding, there is a potential for changes in plasma protein binding. For some drugs these changes may be somewhat small and not very critical, but for other drugs these changes may be potentially significant. Therefore, care must be exercised in interpreting concentration of drug in plasma whenever changes in protein binding are suspected.

Renal impairment does not affect elimination of all drugs. For drugs, which do not depend heavily on renal elimination, even complete anuria may not have a significant effect on their elimination from the body. Yet, there are a number of drugs, which depend primarily on renal elimination and therefore, even mild renal impairment may necessitate adjustment in the dosage regimen. Table 16-1 is a partial listing of values of normal and anephric elimination rate constants of some drugs.

DOSAGE ADJUSTMENT IN RENAL IMPAIRMENT

Dosage adjustment in patients with renal impairment, discussed in this Chapter, is based on certain assumptions, which may or may not be valid for each and every patient under treatment. Therefore, caution must be exercised in using the concepts presented here for determining dosage regimen in patients with impaired renal function, i.e. the concepts presented here can only be used if the following assumptions are valid for the particular patient.

1. The desired concentration of drug in plasma at steady-state in the renally impaired patient should be the same as that for a non-renally impaired patient.
2. Drugs which are primarily eliminated by renal excretion (e.g. gentamicin) are affected more in renal impairment than drugs, which are eliminated primarily by a nonrenal mechanism such as elimination by biotransformation (e.g. theophylline).
3. It is presumed that the presence of renal impairment does not affect majority of pharmacokinetic parameters. These include binding of drug to plasma proteins, the apparent volume of distribution and non-renal elimination or biotransformation of the drug.
4. It is also assumed that unless glomerular filtration rate falls significantly below normal, the dosage may not need adjustment for a patient with minor renal impairment.

The methodology used for dosage adjustment for renally impaired patients is based on the extent of kidney damage involved in the process of renal elimination of the drug, i.e. on the estimation of fraction of total body clearance remaining available for elimination of the drug. From the knowledge of clearance described in Chapter 7, total body clearance (Cl) is the sum total of renal and nonrenal clearance, i.e.

$$Cl = Cl_r + Cl_{nr}$$

where, Cl_r is renal clearance and Cl_{nr} is nonrenal clearance of drug from the body.

Since clearance values are obtained by multiplying the overall rate constant of elimination, K and apparent volume of distribution, V_d, of the drug, i.e.

$$Cl = (K)(V_d)$$

Therefore,

$$(K)(V_d) = (K_r)(V_d) + (K_{nr})(V_d) \quad (16\text{-}1)$$

where, K is the apparent first-order rate constant for the overall removal of drug from the body in the absence of renal impairment, K_r is the apparent first-order rate constant for renal excretion of unmetabolized drug in the absence of renal impairment and K_{nr} is the sum of all first-order rate constants for the nonrenal elimination of drug (e.g. metabolism, biliary excretion, hepatic excretion, salivary excretion, biotransformation, etc.) in the absence of renal impairment.

If the apparent volume of distribution of drug during renal impairment is assumed to be identical to apparent volume of distribution of drug in the absence of renal impairment, equation (16-1) becomes

$$K = K_r + K_{nr} \tag{16-2}$$

Table 16-1 Elimination rate constants in normal and anephric patients

Drug	*Normal K_{el} (h^{-1})*	*Anephric K_{el} (h^{-1})*
Alpha-methyldopa	0.17	0.03
Amikacin	0.40	0.04
Amoxicillin	0.70	0.10
Amphotericin B	0.04	0.02
Ampicillin	0.70	0.10
Carbenicillin	0.60	0.05
Cefazolin	0.40	0.04
Cephacetrile	0.70	0.03
Cephalexin	1.00	0.03
Cephalothin	1.40	0.04
Cephaloridine	0.50	0.03
Chloramphenicol	0.30	0.20
Chlorpropamide	0.02	0.008
Chlortetracycline	0.10	0.10
Clindamycin	0.47	0.10
Cloxacillin	1.40	0.35
Colistimethate	0.20	0.04
Digitoxin	0.004	0.003
Digoxin	0.017	0.006
Erythromycin	0.50	0.14
Ethambutol	0.58	0.09
Fluorocytosine	0.24	0.01
Gentamicin	0.30	0.01
Isoniazid (fast acetylators)	0.60	0.20
(slow acetylators)	0.20	0.08
Kanamycin	0.40	0.01
Lidocaine	0.40	0.36
Lincomycin	0.15	0.06
Methicillin	1.40	0.17
Minocycline	0.05	0.03
Nafcillin	1.20	0.48
Oxacillin	1.40	0.35
Oxytetracycline	0.08	0.02
Penicillin G	1.40	0.05
Polymyxin B	0.16	0.02

Contd...

Contd...

Drug	Normal K_{el} (h^{-1})	Anephric K_{el} (h^{-1})
Procainamide	0.22	0.01
Propranolol	0.20	0.16
Quinidine	0.07	0.06
Rifampin	0.25	0.25
Streptomycin	0.27	0.01
Sulfadiazine	0.08	0.03
Sulfamethoxazole	0.70	0.70
Tetracycline	0.08	0.01
Ticarcillin	0.60	0.06
Tobramycin	0.36	0.01
Trimethoprim	0.60	0.02
Vancomycin	0.12	0.003

Thus, for patients exhibiting renal impairment, the overall rate constant of elimination of drug, K, may change if a significant fraction of the drug undergoes either renal elimination in the unchanged form or the drug undergoes tubular reabsorption to a significant extent. The overall elimination rate constant K in the renally-impaired patient is usually termed K_{ri} (overall rate constant of elimination of drug in renally-impaired patient). For the renally impaired patient, equation (16-2) may be written as

$$K_{ri} = K_r + K_{nr} \tag{16-3}$$

DETERMINATION OF K_{ri}

The method for determination of rate constant of elimination of drug in the renally-impaired patient, K_{ri}, is based on body creatinine clearance, which is an easily measured clinical laboratory parameter. Since the rate constant for excretion of the unchanged drug, K_r, is directly proportional to creatinine clearance, Cl_{cr}, i.e.

$$K_r \propto Cl_{cr} \tag{16-4}$$

therefore,

$$K_r = (m)(Cl_{cr}) \tag{16-5}$$

where m is a proportionality constant and represents the degree of renal elimination of drug.

For example, if the rate constant of renal elimination of a drug, K_r, is 50% of the overall rate constant of elimination, K, of the drug, i.e. if

$$\frac{K_r}{K} = 0.5$$

then m = 0.5, i.e. elimination of 50% of the unchanged drug depends upon the kidneys for its removal from the body. Similarly, if K_r is one-fourth that of K, then m = 0.25 and if the drug is eliminated unchanged entirely via renal elimination, i.e. if

$$\frac{K_r}{K} = 1.0$$

then m = 1.0, meaning that elimination of 100% of the unchanged drug depends upon the kidneys for its removal from the body.

Hence, the proportionality constant m may be defined as:

$$m = \frac{K_r}{K} \tag{16-6}$$

Substituting equation (16-5) into equation (16-3), gives

$$K_{ri} = (m)(Cl_{cr}) + K_{nr} \quad (16\text{-}7)$$

where K_{ri} is overall first-order rate constant of elimination of drug in the presence of renal impairment.

If, both K_{ri} and K_{nr}, are expressed as a fraction of the overall rate constant of elimination of the drug, K, the equation (16-7) then becomes:

$$\frac{K_{ri}}{K} = (m)(Cl_{cr}) + \frac{K_{nr}}{K} \quad (16\text{-}8)$$

Substituting the value of m from equation (16-6) into equation (16-8), we obtain the expression:

$$\frac{K_{ri}}{K} = \frac{K_r}{K}(Cl_{cr}) + \frac{K_{nr}}{K} \quad (16\text{-}9)$$

Equation (16-9) may be written as:

$$\%K_{ri} = (\%K_r)(Cl_{cr}) + \%K_{nr} \quad (16\text{-}10)$$

In equation (16-10) the symbol % before each term indicates the percentage of K, i.e. percentage of the overall rate constant of elimination of drug in normal patients. Thus, $\%K_{ri}$ is the rate constant of overall elimination of drug in the presence of renal impairment, expressed as a percentage of the overall rate constant of elimination of drug in the normal patients; $\%K_r$ is percentage of renal elimination of drug in normal patients, expressed as a percentage of overall rate constant of elimination of drug in normal patients and $\%K_{nr}$ is percentage of non-renal elimination of drug in normal patients, expressed as percentage of overall rate constant of elimination of drug in normal patients.

Two methods can be used to determine K_{ri}, the overall rate constant of elimination of drug in the renally-impaired patient. These are: graphical method and non-graphical method.

Graphical Method

The graphical method for determination of rate constant of elimination of drug in the renallyimpaired patient uses equation (16-10), which is an equation of a straight line. In this equation of the straight line, the y-axis is $\%K_{ri}$, the x-axis is Cl_{cr}, the slope of the straight line is $\%K_r$ and the y-intercept is $\%K_{nr}$. Therefore, a plot of $\%K_{ri}$ as a function of Cl_{cr} should produce a straight line, and the y-intercept of this straight line will be $\%K_{nr}$.

The graphical use of equation (16-10) is illustrated in Figure 16-1. In this figure, the x-axis is creatinine clearance, Cl_{cr}, expressed as mL/min/1.73 m^2.

In the anuric patients, the value of the creatinine clearance = 0 mL/min/1.73 m^2 and in normal healthy adults, the value of creatinine clearance is taken as 100 mL/min/1.73 m^2. The y-axis in Figure 16-1 is the rate constant of elimination of drug in the presence of renal impairment, K_{ri}, expressed as a percentage of the normal rate constant of elimination, K and can range in value from 0% to 100%. The y-intercept is the rate constant of non-renal elimination of drug, K_{nr}, also expressed as a percentage of K and its value can also range from 0 to 100%.

To determine dosage adjustment in the renally-impaired patient using the graph shown in Figure 16-1, the first step is to determine the y-intercept. The value of the y-intercept, $\%K_{nr}$, is K_{nr} expressed as a percentage of overall rate constant of elimination of the drug, K. The values of the rate constants K, K_r and K_{nr} are generally available from the drug manufacturer or these values may be obtained from the published literature for the drug in question. The values of the rate constants K_r and K_{nr} expressed as a percentage of the overall rate constant of elimination, K are calculated as follows:

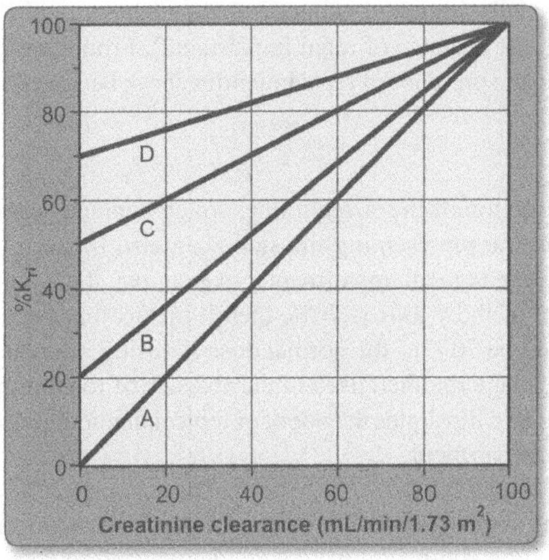

Fig. 16-1 Graphical method of determining K_{ri}.

$$\%K_r = \frac{K_r}{K} \times 100\% \tag{16-11}$$

and

$$\%K_{nr} = \frac{K_{nr}}{K} \times 100\% \tag{16-12}$$

A straight line is drawn to join the y-intercept, K_{nr}, with the top right-hand corner of the graph. The slope of this straight line represents K_{ri} (overall elimination rate constant of drug in the presence of renal impairment). The top right-hand corner of the graph represents creatinine clearance = 100 mL/min/1.73 m^2 (the value considered normal in healthy adults) and a y-value of $\%K_{nr}$ = 100%. A 100% value of $\%K_{nr}$ indicates that the drug is excreted solely by nonrenal elimination. Thus, the straight line drawn to connect the y-intercept on the x-axis with the top right-hand corner of the graph will represent K_{nr} which ranges in the creatinine clearance values of 0 mL/min/1.73 m^2 (completely anephric patient) to 100 mL/min/1.73 m^2 (the value considered normal in healthy adults). The graph in Figure 16-1 shows four straight lines having the y-intercepts marked as A, B, C and D, which are drawn to connect the top right-hand corner of the y-axis. Therefore, if in a given patient, K_{nr} is 0% of K, the straight line A in Figure 16-1 will be used and if K_{nr} is 20% of K, the straight line B in Figure 16-1 will be used. Similarly, if K_{nr} is 50% of K, the straight line C will be used, and if K_{nr} is 70% of K, then the straight line D in Figure 16-1 will be used.

The slope of the straight line (A, B, C or D) is used to read and interpret the graph in Figure 16-1. That is, this straight line is used for the determination of K_{ri}, the overall rate constant of elimination of drug in the presence of renal impairment and/or the new dose (as a percentage of the normal dose) that should be used in the presence of renal impairment. To read this graph, the value of creatinine clearance in the renally impaired patient is determined from the data obtained from clinical laboratory and this value is marked on the x-axis of the graph. A vertical line, parallel to the y-axis, is drawn to determine the point of intersection on the line representing the slope for drug in question. This point of intersection is now read on the right-hand side (y-axis) of the graph to obtain a value, which signifies the correction that must be made to obtain the new overall rate constant of elimination of drug (K_{ri}) in the presence of renal impairment. The value read on the y-axis on the right-hand side of the graph can also be used as a correction factor to calculate the new dose that should be used in the presence of renal impairment.

For example, if the point of intersection on the slope corresponds to a value of 70% on the y-axis on right-hand side of the graph, it means that the overall rate constant of elimination of the drug, K_{ri}, in the renally-impaired patient is 70% of the normal K (overall rate constant of elimination of drug in the absence of renal impairment). From this information, the biological half-life ($t_{1/2}$) of drug in the presence of renal impairment can be determined using the relationship:

$$t_{1/2} = \frac{0.693}{K_{ri}} \quad (16\text{-}13)$$

The point of intersection of the straight line, which connects patient's creatinine clearance value and the straight line representing the slope can also be used to calculate the necessary adjustment in the dose due to renal impairment. For example, if the point of intersection obtained on the right-hand side of the y-axis is 70%, then it means that the size of dose in the renally impaired patient should be 70% of the normal dose if dosing interval is based on the suggested dosage regimen, i.e. dosage regimen used in the absence of renal impairment.

The following example illustrates the use of graphical method for the determination of dosage regimen during renal impairment.

Example 16-1 The biological half-life of a tetracycline analog in healthy adults (having a creatinine clearance of 100 mL/min/1.73 m^2) is reported to be 6 h. If the dosage regimen suggested by the manufacturer of this analog in normal healthy adults is 500 mg administered every 6 hours, what dosage regimen would you suggest for a 35-year adult male patient, weighing 70 kg and having a creatinine clearance of 30 mL/min/1.73 m^2? According to the manufacturer of this tetracycline analog the rate constant of renal elimination of the analog was found to be 0.0462/h.

Solution

The half-life of the tetracycline analog is 6 h, therefore the overall rate constant of elimination, K of this analog is:

$$K = 0.1155/\text{h}$$

Since, $K = K_r + K_{nr}$ and $K_r = 0.0462/\text{h}$, therefore, K_{nr}, by difference, is:

$$K_{nr} = K - K_r = 0.1155/\text{h} - 0.0462/\text{h} = 0.0693/\text{h}.$$

The relative proportions (or percentages) of the renal and nonrenal rate constants of elimination of the drug, according to equations (16-11) and (16-12), are:

$$\%K_r = \frac{(0.0462/\text{hr})(100\%)}{0.1155/\text{h}} = 40\% \text{ and}$$

$$\%K_{nr} = \frac{(0.0693/\text{h})(100\%)}{0.1155/\text{h}} = 60\%$$

A plot of data in Example 16-1 is shown in Figure 16-2.

Since, the nonrenal rate constant of elimination, K_{nr}, of this drug is 60% of overall rate constant of elimination (K), therefore the y-intercept is 60%. A straight line is drawn from the 60% point on left-hand side of y-axis to the 100% point on the right-hand side of y-axis. This straight line represents the slope for new K (i.e. overall rate constant of elimination, K_{ri}, of the drug in the renally-impaired patient). This rate constant is based on creatinine clearance of the patient. A vertical line is now drawn (parallel to the y-axis) from the patient's creatinine clearance value to the straight line, which represents the slope.

If creatinine clearance in this patient was 100 mL/min/1.73 m^2 (i.e. if patient was not renally impaired) the vertical line drawn from the value of patient's creatinine clearance would be the right-hand side of the y-axis and it would intersect the straight line representing the slope at 100%, indicating the new K (or K_{ri}) to be equal to 100% of normal K. In this patient, creatinine clearance is 30 mL/min/1.73 m^2. The vertical line drawn parallel to the y-axis at a creatinine

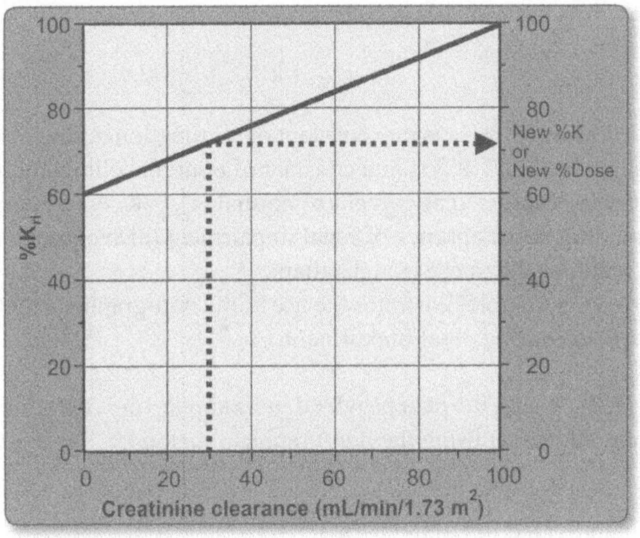

Fig. 16-2 Plot of data in Example 16-1.

clearance value of 30 mL/min/1.73 m^2 intersects the slope (K_r) at a point corresponding to 72% on the right-hand side of y-axis. This indicates that the overall rate constant of elimination of drug, K_{ri}, in this renally impaired patient is reduced to 72% of the normal K. This means that biological half-life of the antibiotic in this particular patient is, therefore,

$$t_{1/2} = \frac{0.693}{(0.72)(K)} = \frac{0.693}{(0.72)(1.1155/h)}$$

$$t_{1/2} = \frac{0.693}{0.08316/h} = 8.33\ h$$

The dosage regimen in this patient should therefore be based on biological half-life of 8.33 h instead of normal 6 hr reported for the tetracycline analog (500 mg every 8.33 h). Alternatively, the size of dose should be reduced considering the new overall rate constant of elimination, K_{ri}, in the patient is 72% of normal K. The dose in this patient (if the dosing interval is maintained at 6 hours) should therefore be 72% of the normal dose or 360 mg.

Non-graphical Method

The non-graphical method for determining dosage regimen uses an equation instead of the graph, but this method uses the same parameters that are used in the graphical method. In this method, the rate constant for overall elimination of drug from the body for the renally impaired (K_{ri}) is determined using equation (16-10) in its modified form. Equation (16-10) is:

$$\%K_{ri} = (\%K_r)(Cl_{cr}) + \%K_{nr}$$

This equation is modified so that creatinine clearance in the renally impaired patient is expressed as a fraction of normal creatinine clearance (creatinine clearance in the absence of renal impairment). Since the value of normal creatinine clearance is 100 mL/min/1.73 m^2, creatinine clearance in the renally impaired patient, expressed as a fraction of creatinine clearance in the absence of renal impairment, is:

$$Cl_{cr}\ \text{during renal impairment} = \frac{\text{patient's}\ Cl_{cr}}{\text{normal}\cdot Cl_{crr}} = \frac{Cl_{cr}}{100\%} \tag{16-14}$$

Therefore, equation (16-10) becomes:

$$\%K_{ri} = + \frac{(\%K_r)(Cl_{cr})}{100} + \%K_{nr} \tag{16-15}$$

In equation (16-15), $\%K_{ri}$ is rate constant of elimination during renal impairment (expressed as percent of normal K), $\%K_{nr}$ is rate constant of nonrenal elimination of drug in the absence of renal impairment (expressed as percent of normal K), $\%K_r$ is rate constant of renal elimination of unchanged drug in the absence of renal impairment (also expressed as percent of normal K) and Cl_{cr} is creatinine clearance of the patient.

The following Example illustrates the use of the non-graphical method for the determination of dosage regimen during renal impairment.

Example 16-2 Using the data provided in Example 16-1, determine dosage regimen for the renally impaired patient using the non-graphical method.

Solution

From the data provided in Example 16-1,

$$K = \frac{0.693}{6\text{ h}} = 0.1155/\text{h}$$

Since $K_r = 0.0462/\text{hr}$, therefore, K_{nr}, by difference is

$$K_{nr} = K - K_r = 0.1155/\text{h} - 0.0462/\text{h} = 0.0693/\text{h}.$$

Therefore, apparent rate constants of renal and nonrenal elimination of drug, K_{nr} and K_r, respectively, expressed as a percentage of normal K, are:

$$\%K_{nr} = \frac{K_{nr}}{K} \times 100\% = \frac{(0.0693/\text{h})(100\%)}{0.1155/\text{h}} = 60\%$$

$$\%K_r = \frac{K_r}{K} \times 100\% = \frac{(0.0462/\text{h})(100\%)}{0.1155/\text{h}} = 40\%$$

Using equation (16-15),

$$\%K_{ri} = \%K_{nr} + \frac{(\%K_r)(Cl_{cr})}{100} = 60\% + \frac{(40\%)(30)}{100} = 60\% + 12\% = 72\%$$

Thus, the overall rate constant of elimination (K) in this renally-impaired patient is 72% of the normal K. Therefore, the overall rate constant of elimination in the patient during renal impairment, K_{ri}, is:

$$K_{ri} = 72\% \text{ of the normal } K = (0.72)(0.1155/\text{h}) = 0.08316/\text{h}.$$

Using $K_{ri} = 0.08316/\text{hr}$ as the overall rate constant of elimination, the biological half-life of the drug in this renally impaired patient is:

$$t_{1/2} = \frac{0.693}{K_{ri}} = \frac{0.693}{0.08316/\text{h}} = 8.33\text{ h}$$

The dosage should be based on $K = 0.08316/\text{h}$ (not 0.1155/h) and $t_{1/2} = 8.33$ h (not 6 h).

This is the same answer as was obtained using the graphical method, suggesting that dosage in this renally impaired patient should be based on biological half-life of 8.33 h instead of the normal 6 h. That is, either the size of dose should be reduced considering the new overall rate constant of elimination or the dosing interval should be increased due to the reduced rate constant of elimination.

DOSAGE REGIMEN IN THE RENALLY IMPAIRED

Dosage regimen (size of each dose and interval between doses) in normal patients (patients with normal kidney function) is based on the size of maintenance dose, the dosing interval and biological half-life of the drug. Since biological half-life of the drug is a function of overall rate constant of elimination of the drug, the dosage regimen therefore depends on maintenance dose, dosing interval and overall rate constant of elimination of the drug. Because concentration of drug in plasma during multiple dosing depends on dosage regimen of the drug, therefore, dosage regimen of the drug may be equated to the concentration of drug in plasma during multiple dosing. The concentration of drug in plasma during multiple dosing is therefore a function of maintenance dose, dosing interval and overall rate constant of elimination of the drug. The relationship between concentration of drug in plasma (during multiple dosing) and the three factors, size of the maintenance dose, dosing interval and overall rate constant of elimination of the drug is as follows:

Dose

In the case of drugs, which follow linear pharmacokinetics, if the dosing interval between doses and the overall rate constant of elimination are held constant, then the concentration of drug in plasma during multiple dosing is directly proportional to the size of the drug dose, i.e. larger the size of maintenance dose (D), higher the concentration (C) of drug in plasma, i.e.

$$C \propto D \tag{16-16}$$

Dosing Interval

In the case of drugs which follow linear pharmacokinetics, if the size of maintenance dose and overall rate constant of elimination are held constant, then concentration of drug in plasma during multiple dosing is inversely proportional to the interval between the administration of each dose, i.e. larger the dosing interval (τ), lower the concentration of drug in the plasma, i.e.,

$$C \propto \frac{1}{\tau} \tag{16-17}$$

Elimination Rate Constant

In the case of drugs, which follow linear pharmacokinetics, if the size of each maintenance dose and the interval between the doses is held constant, then the concentration of drug in plasma during multiple dosing is proportional to biological half-life of the drug, i.e. longer the biological half-life of drug, longer the persistence of drug in the body. Since the rate constant of elimination of a drug is inversely related to biological half-life of the drug, it follows that concentration of drug in the plasma is inversely proportional to the overall rate constant of elimination of the drug, i.e. smaller the rate constant of elimination (K), higher the concentration of drug in the plasma. Therefore,

$$C \propto \frac{1}{K} \tag{16-18}$$

The effect of the three factors (maintenance dose, dosing interval and rate constant of elimination of the drug) on the concentration of drug in plasma can therefore be summarized into one equation by combining the three equations relating these three factors with the concentration of drug in plasma. Combining equations (16-16), (16-17) and (16-18) into one equation, one obtains the relationship:

$$C \propto \frac{D}{(\tau)(K)} \qquad (16\text{-}19)$$

In equation (16-19), since K appears in the denominator, it follows that in the renally-impaired patients, any reduction in the overall rate constant of elimination of drug can cause an increase in the concentration of drug in plasma, assuming that the maintenance dose and the dosing interval are not changed. As can be seen from equation (16-19), to maintain the levels of C (concentration of drug in the plasma) in the renally impaired patient similar to the levels of concentration obtained in patients with normal kidney function, either D (size of maintenance dose) or τ (dosing interval) or both D and τ, should be modified. This is because the practitioner can modify the size of maintenance dose and dosing interval, but has no control on the overall rate constant of elimination of drug during renal impairment. That is, to overcome the effect of reduced value of the rate constant of elimination of drug, K, a corresponding reduction must be made in the size of the maintenance dose, D and/or a corresponding increase must be made in the dosing interval, τ. In other words, one should maintain the following equality:

$$\frac{D}{(\tau_n)(K_n)} = \frac{D_{ri}}{(\tau_{ri})(K_{ri})} \qquad (16\text{-}20)$$

The terms D, τ and K with the subscript n, on the left-hand side of equation (16-20) refer to maintenance dose, dosing interval and the overall rate constant of elimination (K) of drug in normal patients (patients with normal kidney function). On the right-hand side of equation (16-20), the terms D, τ and K with the subscript 'ri' refer to maintenance dose, dosing interval, and overall rate constant of elimination of drug (K_{ri}) in patients with renal impairment.

For instance, in Example 16-1, the overall rate constant of elimination of drug in the renally impaired patient was found to be 72% of normal K, i.e. while the normal rate constant of elimination, K, in patients with normal kidney function is 0.1155/h, the rate constant of elimination in the patient during renal impairment, K_{ri}, became:

$$K_{ri} = 72\% \text{ of } 0.1155/h = (0.72)(0.1155/h) = 0.08316/h.$$

Hence, while the biological half-life of drug in patients with normal kidney function is:

$$t_{1/2} = \frac{0.693}{0.1155/h} = 6 \text{ h}$$

the biological half-life of drug during renal impairment changed to:

$$t_{1/2} = \frac{0.693}{0.08316/h} = 8.33 \text{ h}$$

Due to reduction in the overall rate constant of elimination of drug, there may be an increase in accumulation of drug during multiple dosing. Consequently concentration of drug in plasma at steady-state may be greater in the renally impaired patient than that observed in patients with normal kidney function. Therefore, dosage regimen in the renally impaired may have to be modified in order to compensate for the increase in concentration of drug in plasma at steady-state. To modify dosage regimen in order to meet this patient's needs, either the dose or the dosing interval or both can be adjusted.

A. Adjust Dose, Maintain Same Dosing Interval

To adjust dose while maintaining the same dosing interval, equation (16-20) is used to calculate the size of maintenance dose needed to attain concentration of drug in plasma during renal impairment (similar to the plasma concentration in the absence of renal impairment). According to equation (16-20),

$$\frac{D_n}{(\tau_n)(K_n)} = \frac{D_n}{(\tau_{ri})(K_{ri})}$$

For instance, in Example 16-1, a 500 mg dose was administered every 6 hours during normal kidney function. To calculate the size of maintenance dose during renal impairment (dosing interval to be maintained at 6 hours), when the overall rate constant of elimination changed from 0.1155/h to 0.08316/h, the relevant values are substituted into equation (16-20). Substitution yields:

$$\frac{500\text{ mg}}{(6\text{ h})(0.1155/\text{h})} = \frac{D_{ri}}{(6\text{ h})(0.08316/\text{h})}$$

$$D_{ri} = \frac{(500\text{ mg})(6\text{ h})(0.08316/\text{h})}{(6\text{ h})(0.1155/\text{h})} = 360\text{ mg}$$

Thus, a dose of 360 mg given every 6 hours would provide the same plasma levels of drug in this renally impaired patient as a dose of 500 mg given every 6 hours to the nonrenally impaired patient.

B. Adjust Dosing Interval, Maintain Same Dose

Sometimes, it may not be feasible or convenient to change maintenance dose. For example, the calculated maintenance dose may not be commercially available or the pharmacist may have difficulty in preparing the desired strength in a suitable dosage form. In such cases, one can use the same dose, but the dosing interval must be changed. Equation (16-20) can be used to calculate the dosing interval without changing the dose. For instance, in Example 16-1, the recommended maintenance dose was 500 mg administered every 6 hours. To calculate dosing interval during renal impairment (maintaining size of maintenance dose at 500 mg), when the overall rate constant of elimination of the drug changed from 0.1155/h to 0.08316/h, the relevant values are substituted into equation (16-20).

$$\frac{500\text{ mg}}{(6\text{ h})(0.1155/\text{h})} = \frac{500\text{ mg}}{(\tau_{ri})(0.08316/\text{h})}$$

$$\tau_{ri} = \frac{(500\text{ mg})(6\text{ h})(0.1155/\text{h})}{(500\text{ mg})(0.08316/\text{h})} = 8.33\text{ h}$$

A dose of 500 mg given every 8.33 hours would maintain the same plasma levels in this renally impaired patient as a dose of 500 mg given every 6 hours to the nonrenally impaired patient.

C. Adjust Both, Dose and Dosing Interval

Sometimes, it may not be convenient to change the size of maintenance dose (without changing dosing interval) to the calculated new dose or to change dosing interval (without changing the dose) to the dosing interval calculated for the renally-impaired patient. For example, the size of maintenance dose calculated in (A) above, may not be convenient because no such dosage strength may be available and the pharmacist may have great difficulty in preparing the required dosage strength in a suitable dosage form. Similarly, the calculated dosing interval in (B) shown above, may not be convenient because, e.g. the nursing staff may administer medications and treatments only at specific time intervals. In such cases, one can decide upon a suitable dose and calculate the corresponding dosing interval or a suitable dosing interval can be decided upon and the corresponding dose can be calculated. For example:

a. If it is decided to adjust the dose to 300 mg, then the dosing interval can be calculated using equation (16-20), by substituting the relevant values into this equation:

$$\frac{(500\text{ mg})}{(6\text{ h})(0.1155/\text{h})} = \frac{300\text{ mg}}{(\tau_{ri})(0.0.08316/\text{h})}$$

$$\tau_{ri} = \frac{(300\text{ mg})(6\text{ h})(0.1155/\text{h})}{(500\text{ mg})(0.08316/\text{h})}$$

$$\tau_{ri} = \frac{207.9\text{ mg}}{41.58\text{ mg/h}} = 5\text{ h}$$

i.e. a dose of 300 mg should be given every 5 hours.

b. If it is decided to adjust the dosing interval to 12 hours, then the maintenance dose can be calculated by substituting the relevant values into equation (16-20). Equation (16-20) is:

$$\frac{500\text{ mg}}{(6\text{ h})(0.1155/\text{h})} = \frac{D_{ri}}{(12\text{ h})(0.08316/\text{h})}$$

$$D_{ri} = \frac{(500\text{ mg})(12\text{ h})(0.08316/\text{h})}{(6\text{ h})(0.1155/\text{h})}$$

$$D_{ri} = \frac{498.96\text{ mg}}{0.693} = 720\text{ mg}$$

i.e. a dose of 720 mg should be given every 12 hours.

From the calculations shown above, it is evident that to maintain desired therapeutic plasma levels of drug in renally-impaired patients, the dosage regimen can be adjusted in a variety of ways. The practitioner has the option to adjust either maintenance of dose or dosing interval or both, to suit the needs of the patient under treatment. Some manufacturers indicate recommended dosage adjustments in renal failure (based on glomerular filtration rate of patient), in terms of new dosing interval and/or percentage of the maintenance dose suggested for patients with normal kidney function. Appendix C lists these values for some commonly used drugs.

Example 16-3 An adult, admitted into a hospital, was receiving an oral antibiotic at the recommended dose of 500 mg followed by 250 mg every 4 hours. After 1 week, the patient complained of symptoms typically associated with toxicity of the antibiotic. Clinical laboratory reported that in this patient the creatinine clearance had reduced from 100 mL/min/1.73 m^2 to 10 mL/min/1.73 m^2. According to the manufacturer's literature, the overall rate constant of elimination of this antibiotic in healthy adults is 0.173/h and the rate constant of nonrenal elimination of the antibiotic is 0.0346/h.

Calculate the following:

a. The dosage regimen, if dose is administered at the drug's new biological half-life intervals.
b. The size of maintenance dose, if the drug is administered every 4 hours.
c. The dosing interval if the size of maintenance dose is maintained at 250 mg.
d. The size of maintenance dose, if the interval between doses is increased to 12 hours.
e. Dosing interval, if the size of maintenance dose is changed to 100 mg.

Solution

The first step in this problem is to determine K_{ri}, the overall rate constant of elimination in the presence of renal impairment.

i. *Determination of K_{ri}:*

To determine the overall rate constant of elimination of drug in the presence of renal impairment, K_{ri}, one can use either the graphical method, as shown in Figure 16-1 or the non-graphical method, which involves using equation (16-15). Both methods should yield the same value of overall rate constant of elimination of drug in the presence of renal impairment. To determine K_{ri}, one needs to calculate the values of rate constants of renal and nonrenal elimination of drug, K_r and K_{nr}, respectively. Since, K = 0.173/h and K_{nr} = 0.0346/h, therefore, K_r by difference, is:

$$K_r = K - K_{nr} = 0.173/h - 0.0346/h = 0.1384/h.$$

The relative proportions of renal and nonrenal rate constants of elimination (expressed as % overall rate constant of elimination of drug, $\%K_r$ and $\%K_{nr}$, respectively), are calculated using equations (16-11) and (16-12). According to equation (16-11), renal rate constant of elimination, expressed as % overall rate constant of elimination, $\%_{Kr}$, of drug is:

$$\%K_r = \frac{(0.1384/h)(100\%)}{0.173/h} = 80\%$$

According to equation (16-12), $\%K_{nr}$, the nonrenal rate constant of elimination, expressed as percent of overall rate constant of elimination of the drug is: (0.0346/h)(100%)

$$\%K_{nr} = \frac{(0.0346/h)(100\%)}{0.173/h} = 20\%$$

a. *Non-graphical Method*

Equation (16-15) is used to determine K_{ri}, the overall rate constant of elimination of drug in the presence of renal impairment. Substituting the values of $\%K_{nr}$ and $\%K_r$ calculated above and creatinine clearance, Cl_{cr}, of the patient into equation (16-15):

$$\%K_{ri} = \%K_{nr} + \frac{(\%K_r)(Cl_{cr})}{100} = 20\% + \frac{(80\%)(10)}{100}$$

$$K_{ri} = 20\% + 8\% = 28\%$$

The overall rate constant of elimination (K) in this renally-impaired patient is 72% of the normal K. Therefore, K_{ri}, the overall rate constant of elimination in this patient during renal impairment is:

$$K_{ri} = 28\% \text{ of the normal } K = (0.28)(0.173/h) = 0.04844/h.$$

b. *Graphical Method*

A plot of the data is shown in Figure 16-3.

Since, the nonrenal rate constant of elimination, K_{nr}, of this drug is 20% of overall rate constant of elimination (K), therefore the y-intercept of this graph, K_{nr} is 20%. A straight line is drawn from the 20% point on left-hand side of the y-axis to the 100% point on right-hand side of the y-axis. This straight line now represents the slope, K_r, which is used to determine the new K (overall rate constant of elimination, K_{ri}, of drug

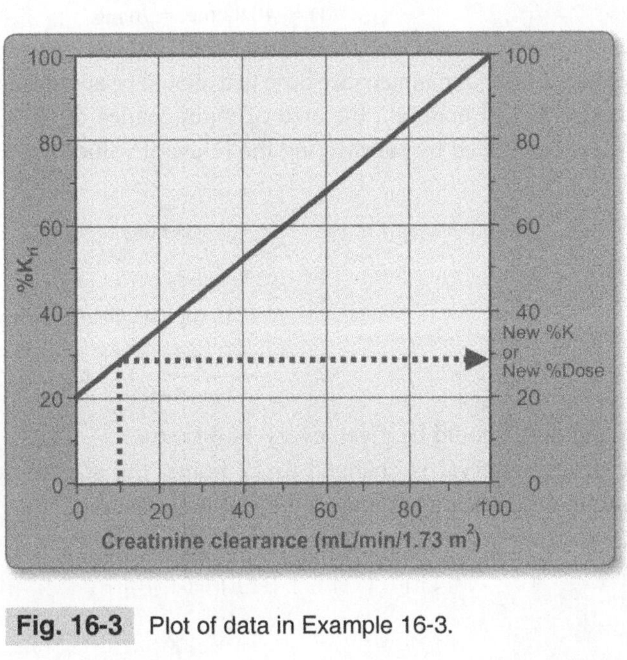

Fig. 16-3 Plot of data in Example 16-3.

in the renally-impaired patient), based on creatinine clearance of the renally-impaired patient. A vertical line is drawn (parallel to y-axis) from the patient's creatinine clearance value (10 mL/min/m^2 in this patient) to the slope. The vertical line at creatinine clearance of 10 mL/min/1.73 m^2 intersects the slope (K_r) at a point corresponding to 28% on the right-hand side of y-axis. This indicates that overall rate constant of elimination, K_{ri}, in this renally impaired patient is 28% of the normal K.

$$\text{Therefore, } K_{ri} = 28\% \text{ of the normal } K = (0.28)(0.173/h) = 0.04844/h$$

This is same answer as was obtained by the graphical method.

ii. *Determination of dosage regimen*

a. The size of dose that should be administered at the drug's new biological half-life intervals is determined based upon the dosage regimen of the patient before the patient suffered renal impairment:

The patient was receiving a maintenance dose of 250 mg every 4 hours. The biological half-life of the drug before renal impairment was:

$$t_{1/2} = \frac{0.693}{K} = \frac{0.693}{0.173/h} = 4\ h$$

This means that before suffering renal impairment, the patient was receiving a 250 mg dose at dosing intervals, which were equal to the biological half-life of the drug. The new biological half-life of the drug is calculated using the new overall rate constant of elimination of drug in this renally impaired patient (K_{ri} = 0.04844/h), as follows:

$$t_{1/2} = \frac{0.693}{K} = \frac{0.693}{0.04844/h} = 14.3\ h$$

Therefore, the 250 mg dose should be administered every 14.3 hours.

b. If it is decided to maintain the dosing interval at 4 hr, then the size of maintenance dose can be calculated by substituting the relevant values into equation (16-20): 250 *mg* D_{ri}

$$\frac{250\ mg}{(4\ h)(0.173/h)} = \frac{D_{ri}}{(4\ h)(0.04844/h)}$$

$$D_{ri} = \frac{(250\ mg)(4\ h)(0.04844/h)}{(4\ h)(0.173/h)}$$

$$D = \frac{48.44\ mg}{0.692} = 70\ mg$$

Therefore, the size of maintenance dose that should be administered every 4 hours is 70 mg.

c. If it is decided to maintain the size of maintenance dose at 250 mg, then the dosing interval is calculated by substituting the relevant values into equation (16-20):

$$\frac{250\ mg}{(4\ h)(0.173/h)} = \frac{250\ mg}{(\tau_{ri})(0.04844/h)}$$

$$\tau_{ri} = \frac{(250\ mg)(4\ h)(0.173/\ h)}{(250\ mg)(0.0484/h)}$$

$$\tau_{ri} = \frac{173\ mg}{12.11\ mg/h} = 14.3\ h$$

A 250 mg dose should be given every 14.3 hours.

d. If the dosing interval is changed to 12 hours, the size of dose can be calculated by substituting the relevant values into equation (16-20):

$$\frac{250\ mg}{(4\ h)(0.173/h)} = \frac{D_{ri}}{(12\ h)(0.04844/h)}$$

$$D_{ri} = \frac{(250\ \text{mg})(12\ \text{h})(0.04844/\text{h})}{(4\ \text{h})(0.173/\text{h})} = \frac{145.32}{0.692} = 210\ \text{mg}$$

A 210 mg dose should be given every 12 hours.

e. The dosing interval, if the size of dose is changed to 100 mg, is calculated by substituting the relevant values into equation (16-20):

$$\frac{250\ \text{mg}}{(4\ \text{h})(0.173/\text{h})} = \frac{100\ \text{mg}}{(\tau_{ri})(0.04844/\text{h})}$$

$$\tau_{ri} = \frac{(100\ \text{mg})(4\ \text{h})(0.173/\text{h})}{(250\ \text{mg})(0.04844/\text{h})}$$

$$\tau_{ri} = \frac{69.2\ \text{mg}}{12.11\ \text{mg/h}} = 5.7\ \text{h}$$

The patient should be given a 100 mg dose every 5.7 hours.

Example 16-4 The biological half-life of a drug (with creatinine clearance of 100 mL/min/1.73 m^2) is reported to be 12 hours, and the manufacturer's suggested dosage regimen of this drug in normal healthy adults is 300 mg administered every 12 hours. Calculate the biological half-life of the drug in a 50-year adult male patient, having a creatinine clearance of 30 mL/min/1.73 m^2. According to the manufacturer the rate constant of renal elimination for this drug is 0.03465/h.

Solution

The half-life of the drug is 12 h, therefore the overall rate constant of elimination, K is:

$$K = \frac{0.693}{12\ \text{h}} = 0.05775/\text{h}$$

Since, $K = K_r + K_{nr}$ and $K_r = 0.03465$/h, therefore, K_{nr}, by difference, is:

$$K_{nr} = K - K_r = 0.05775/\text{h} - 0.03465/\text{h} = 0.0231/\text{h}.$$

The relative proportions (or percentages) of the renal and nonrenal rate constants of elimination of the drug, according to equations (16-11) and (16-12), are:

$$\%K_r = \frac{(0.03465/\text{h})(100\%)}{0.05775/\text{h}} = 60\%$$

$$\%K_{nr} = \frac{(0.0231/\text{h})(100\%)}{0.05775/\text{h}} = 40\%$$

Using equation (16-15),

$$\%K_{ri} = \%K_{nr} + \frac{(\%K_r)(Cl_{cr})}{100} = 40\% + \frac{(40\%)(30)}{100} = 40\% + 18\% = 58\%$$

Thus, the overall rate constant of elimination (K) in this renally-impaired patient is 58% of the normal K. Therefore, overall rate constant of elimination in the patient during renal impairment, K_{ri}, is:

$$K_{ri} = 58\%\ \text{of the normal}\ K = (0.58)(0.05775/\text{h}) = 0.033495/\text{h}.$$

Using $K_{ri} = 0.033495$/h as the overall rate constant of elimination, the biological half-life of the drug in this renally impaired patient is:

$$t_{1/2} = \frac{0.693}{K_{ri}} = \frac{0.693}{0.033495/\text{h}} = 20.7\ \text{h}$$

Example 16-5 The biological half-life of a drug (with creatinine clearance of 100 mL/min/1.73 m^2) is reported to be 6 h, and the manufacturer's suggested dosage regimen of this drug in normal healthy adults is 100 mg administered every 6 hours. Calculate the biological half-life of the drug in a 45-year adult male patient, having a creatinine clearance of 40 mL/min/1.73 m^2. According to the manufacturer the rate constant of renal elimination for this drug is 0.0955/h.

Solution

The half-life of the drug is 12 hours, therefore overall rate constant of elimination, K is:

$$K = \frac{0.693}{6\ \text{h}} = 0.1155/\text{h}$$

Since, $K = K_r + K_{nr}$ and $K_r = 0.095/\text{h}$, therefore, K_{nr}, by difference, is:

$$K_{nr} = K - K_r = 0.1155/\text{h} - 0.0955/\text{h} = 0.02/\text{h}.$$

The relative proportions (or percentages) of the renal and nonrenal rate constants of elimination of the drug, according to equations (16-11) and (16-12), are given by the following relationships:

$$\%K_r = \frac{(0.0955/\text{h})(100\%)}{01155/\text{h}} = 82.68\%\ \text{and}$$

$$\%K_{nr} = \frac{(0.02/\text{h})(100\%)}{0.1155/\text{h}} = 17.32\%$$

Using equation (16-15),

$$\%K_{ri} = \%K + \frac{(\%K_r)(Cl_{cr})}{100}$$

$$\%K_{ri} = 17.32\% + \frac{(82.68\%)(40)}{100}$$

$$\%K_{ri} = 17.32\% + 33.07\% = 50.39\%$$

Thus, the overall rate constant of elimination (K) in this renally-impaired patient is 58% of the normal K. Therefore, overall rate constant of elimination in the patient during renal impairment, K_{ri}, is:

$$K_{ri} = 50.39\%\ \text{of the normal}\ K = (0.5039)(0.1155/\text{h}) = 0.0582/\text{h}.$$

Using $K_{ri} = 0.0582/\text{h}$ as the overall rate constant of elimination, the biological half-life of the drug in this renally impaired patient is:

$$t_{1/2} = \frac{0.693}{K_{ri}} = \frac{0.693}{0.0582/\text{h}} = 11.91\ \text{h}$$

DOSAGE ADJUSTMENT IN RENAL INSUFFICIENCY

Table 16-2 is a listing of dosage adjustments of some commonly used drugs during renal insufficiency. This is an alphabetical listing and it is intended to provide a quick reference guide to adjust either the dose or the dosing interval of these drugs during renal failure. The calculated suggested dose or dosing interval during renal insufficiency is based on the effect of glomerular filtration rate on elimination of the drug. For these calculations, a glomerular filtration rate of 100 mL/min or 0.6 L/h is considered as the normal filtration rate.

The meaning and explanation of various symbols and notations used in this listing are as follows:

GFR = glomerular filtration rate,
R = renal,
H = hepatic,
N = none,
% = percent of the normal dose,
A = should be avoided,
* = concentration of drug in the plasma should be used to determine exact dosing.

The information provided here is a result of compilation of data gathered from various sources of literature search. These include the following: Physician's Desk Reference, company literature and published reports from various sources, including the following:

GK McEvoy, ed., "American Hospital Formulary Service Drug Information," American Society of Hospital Pharmacists (1991)

RW Schrier and J. G. Gambertoglio (eds.), "Handbook of Drug Therapy in Liver and Kidney Disease," Little, Brown and Co., Boston (1991), and

WM Bennett, "Guide to Drug Dosing in Renal Failure," Clin Pharmacokinet, **15**, 3226 (1988).

Table 16-2 Dosage adjustment in renal insufficiency

Drug	*Route of elimination*	*Adjusted dosing interval (h) or %Dose for GFR (mL/min)*		
		>50	*10–50*	*<10*
Acetaminophen	H	4	6	8
Acetazolamide	R	6	12	A
Acetohexamide	H	12–24	A	A
Acyclovir (intravenous)	R	8	24	48
Acyclovir (oral)	R	N	12–24	24
Allopurinol	R	N	50%	10–25%
Alprazolam	H	N	N	N
Amantadine	R	12–24	24–72	72–168
Amikacin*	R	12	12–18	>24
Amiodarone	H	N	N	N
Amitriptyline	H	N	N	N
Amphotericin B	N	24	24	
Ampicillin	R,H	6	6–12	12–16
Aspirin	H,R	4	4–6	A
Atenolol	R	N	50%	25%
Aztreonam	R	N	50–75%	25%
Betaxolol	H,R	N	N	50%
Bretylium	R,H	N	25–50%	A
Bumetanide	R,H	N	N	N
Buspirone	H,R	N	N	25–50%
Captopril	R,H	N	N	50%
Carbamazepine*	H,R	N	N	75%
Carbenicillin	R,H	8–12	12–24	24–48
Cefamandole	R	6	6–8	8–12
Cefazolin	R	8	12	24–4
Cefixime	R	12–24	75%	50%
Cefoperazone	H	N	N	N
Cefotaxime	R,H	6–8	8–12	24

Contd...

Contd...

Cefotetan	R	12	24	24
Cefoxitin	R	8	8–12	24–4
Ceftazidime	R	8–12	24–28	48–7
Ceftriaxone	R,H	N	N	24
Ceftizoxime	R	8–12	36–48	48–7
Cefuroxime	R	N	12	24
Cephalexin	R	6	6	8–12
Cephalothin	R	6	6–8	12
Chloramphenicol	R,H	N	N	N
Chlordiazepoxide	H	N	N	50%
Chlorpromazine	H	N	N	N
Chlorpropamide	?	24–36	A	A
Cimetidine	R	6	8	12
Ciprofloxacin	R	N	12–24	24
Clindamycin	H	N	N	N
Clofibrate	H	6–12	12–24	24–48
Clonidine	R	N	N	N
Codeine	H	N	75%	50%
Colchicine (oral)	R,H	N	N	50%
Corticosteroids	H	N	N	N
Diazepam	H	N	N	N
Dicloxacillin	R,H	N	N	N
Digoxin*	R	24	36	48
Diltiazem	H	N	N	N
Dipyridamole	H	N	N	N
Disopyramide*	R,H	75%	25–50%	10–25%
Doxazosin	H	N	N	N
Doxepin	H	N	N	N
Doxycycline	R,H	12	12–18	18–24
Enalapril	H	N	N	50%
Encainide	H	N	N	N
Erythromycin	H	N	N	N
Ethambutol	R	24	24–36	48
Ethosuximide*	H,R	N	N	75%
Famotidine	R,H	N	N	50%
Flecainide*	R,H	N	50%	50%
Fluconazole	R,H	N	50%	25%
Flucytosine	R	6	24	24–48
Fluoxetine	H	N	N	N
Flurazepam	H	N	N	N
Fosinopril	R,H	N	N	N
Furosemide	R	N	N	N
Ganciclovir	R	12	24	24
Gemfibrozil	R,H	N	50%	25%
Gentamicin*	R	8–12	12	>24
Glipizide	H	N	N	N
Glucocorticoids	H	N	N	N
Glyburide	H	N	N	N
Guanfacine	H	N	N	N

Contd...

Contd...

Haloperidol	H	N	N	N
Heparin	H	N	N	N
Hydralazine(oral)	H	8	8	8–16
Ibuprofen	H	N	N	N
Imipenem	R	N	50%	25%
Imipramine	H	N	N	N
Indapamide	H	N	N	N
Indomethacin	H,R	N	N	N
Insulin	H	N	75%	50%
Isoniazid	H,R	N	N	N
Isradipine	H	N	N	N
Ketoconazole	H	N	N	N
Ketorolac (intramuscular)	H,R	N	N	50%
Labetalol	H	N	N	N
Lidocaine*	H,R	N	N	N
Lisinopril	R	N	50%	25%
Lithium*	R	N	50–75%	25–50%
Lorazepam	H	N	N	N
Lovastatin	H	N	N	N
Meperidine	H	N	75%	50%
Methyldopa	R,H	8	8–12	12–24
Metoclopramide	R,H	N	75%	50%
Metolazone	R	N	N	N
Metoprolol	H	N	N	N
Metronidazole	R,H	N	N	50%
Mexiletine	H,R	N	N	50–75%
Mezlocillin	R,H	4–6	6–8	8–12
Miconazole	H	N	N	N
Midazolam	H	N	N	50%
Minocycline	H	N	N	N
Minoxidil	H	N	N	N
Misoprostol	R	N	N	N
Moricizine	H	N	N	50–75%
Morphine	H	N	75%	50%
Nadolol	R	N	50%	25%
Naproxen	H	N	N	N
Netilmicin*	R	8–12	12	>24
Nicardipine	H	N	N	N
Nifedipine	H	N	N	N
Nitrates	H	N	N	N
Nitroprusside	N	N	N	N
Nizatidine	H	N	24	48
Norfloxacin	R	N	12–24	A
Nortriptyline	H	N	N	N
Ofloxacin	R	N	12–24	24
Omeprazol	H	N	N	N
Oxacillin	R,H	N	N	N
Penicillin G	R,H	N	75%	25–50

Contd...

Contd...

Pentamidine	?	N	N	24–48
Phenobarbital*	H,R	N	N	12–16
Phenytoin*	H	N	N	N
Pindolol	H,R	N	N	N
Piperacillin	R,H	4–6	6–8	8
Piroxicam	H	N	N	N
Prazosin	R,H	N	N	N
Primidone*	H,R	8	8–12	12–24
Probucol	?	N	N	N
Procainamide*	R,H	4	6–12	12–24
Propafenone	H	N	N	50–75%
Propranolol	H	N	N	N
Pyrazinamide	H,R	N	N	50%
Quinidine*	H,R	N	N	N
Ramipril	R,H	N	50%	50%
Ranitidine	R	N	18–24	24
Rifampin	H	N	N	N
Spironolactone	R	6–12	12–24	A
Sucralfate	N	N	N	N
Sulfamethoxazole	R,H	12	18	24
Sulfisoxazole	R	6	8–12	12–24
Sulindac	H,R	N	N	50%
Temazepam	H	N	N	N
Terbutaline	H,R	N	50%	A
Tetracycline	R,H	12	12–18	18–24
Theophylline	H	N	N	N
Thiazide	R	N	N	A
Ticarcillin	R	8	8–12	24
Timolol	H	N	N	N
Tobramycin*	R	8–12	12	>24
Tocainide*	R,H	N	N	50%
Tolazamide	H	N	N	N
Tolbutamide	H	N	N	N
Trazodone	H	N	N	N
Trimethoprim	R,H	12	18	24
Valproic acid*	H	N	N	75%
Vancomycin* (intravenous)	R	24–72	72–240	240
Verapamil	H	N	N	50–75%
Warfarin	H	N	N	N
Zidovudine	H	N	N	N

SUGGESTED READING

1. Evans WE, Schentag JJ and Jusko WJ. Applied Pharmacokinetics: Principles of Therapeutic Drug Monitoring, 3rd edition. Applied Therapeutics; 1995.
2. Gibaldi M and Perrier D. Pharmacokinetics, 2nd edition. Marcel Dekker; 1982.
3. Sadee W. Pharmacokinetics: Drug Level Monitoring. John Wiley & Son; 1980.
4. Wagner JG. Fundamentals of Clinical Pharmacokinetics. Drug Intelligence Publications; 1979.

PRACTICE PROBLEMS

16-1. The biological half-life of a drug in healthy adults is reported to be 5 h. The manufacturer has reported that the rate constant of renal elimination for this drug is 0.0462/h. Calculate the rate constant of nonrenal elimination of the drug.

16-2. The overall rate constant of elimination of an antibiotic is 0.099/h and the rate constant of nonrenal elimination is 0.0279/h. Calculate:

a. Rate constant of renal elimination expressed as a percentage of overall rate constant of elimination, and

b. Rate constant of nonrenal elimination expressed as percent of overall rate constant of elimination.

16-3. The biological half-life of an experimental antibiotic (maintenance dose = 300 mg, $\tau = 4$ h) in healthy adults (Cl_{cr} = 100 mL/min/1.73 m^2) is 4 h. What dosing interval would you recommend in the case of an adult who has a creatinine clearance of 70 mL/min/1.73 m^2 and it is decided that the patient should receive a maintenance dose of 300 mg. The reported K_r for this antibiotic is 0.1126/h.

16-4. The biological half-life of an experimental antibiotic (maintenance dose = 300 mg, $\tau =$ 4 h) in healthy adults (Cl_{cr} = 100 mL/min/1.73 m^2) is 4 h. Calculate the size of dose that should be administered every 4 hours to an adult who has creatinine clearance of 70 mL/min/1.73 m^2. The reported K_r for this antibiotic is 0.1126/h.

16-5. The biological half-life of an experimental antibiotic (maintenance dose = 300 mg) in healthy adults (Cl_{cr} = 100 mL/min/1.73 m^2) is 4 h. Calculate dosing interval if the dose is reduced to 200 mg in the case of an adult who has a creatinine clearance of 70 mL/min/1.73 m^2. The reported K_r for this drug is 0.1126/h.

16-6. The reported rate constant of renal elimination of a 400 mg dose of a drug having a biological half-life of 12 h is 0.04/h. Calculate the biological half-life of this drug in a patient who has a creatinine clearance of 20 mL/min/1.73 m^2.

16-7. The biological half-life of a drug in healthy adults is reported to be 10 h. The manufacturer has reported that the rate constant of non-renal elimination for this drug is 0.0462/h. Calculate the rate constant of renal elimination of the drug.

16-8. The biological half-life of a drug in healthy adults is reported to be 20 h. The manufacturer has reported that the rate constant of renal elimination for this drug is 0.01265/h. Calculate the rate constant of nonrenal elimination of the drug.

CHAPTER 17

THERAPEUTIC DRUG MONITORING

Therapeutic drug monitoring, as the term implies, involves monitoring concentration of drug in plasma for optimal drug therapy. In other words, therapeutic drug monitoring involves determination of concentration of drug in the plasma in order to optimize a patient's drug therapy. The primary objective of therapeutic drug monitoring is to attain rapid and safe concentration of drug in the plasma within the desired therapeutic range in order to provide, the safest approach to optimal drug therapy.

The usefulness of plasma drug concentration data in pharmacokinetic studies is based on the concept that pharmacologic response of a drug is closely related to concentration of drug at the receptor site (or the site of action). Therefore, the concentration of drug at the site of action must attain, a certain minimum level before the drug can elicit its therapeutic response. This minimum level of concentration has been popularly termed minimum effective concentration (MEC) or minimum therapeutic concentration (MTC). Also, the concentration of drug must be maintained below a certain level, termed minimum toxic concentration in order to exclude or minimize unwanted toxic response. It is expected that within this concentration range the drug will exhibit its therapeutic activity. Since, it is difficult, if not impossible, to measure concentration of drug at the specific receptor site or site of action and because the concentration of drug in plasma appears to correlate concentration of drug at the site of action, one determines concentration of drug in the plasma, as a measure of concentration of drug at the site of action (Fig. 17-1).

The pharmacokinetic data generated for a drug are usually based on studies conducted on a large patient population. These studies provide information on the range of plasma concentration

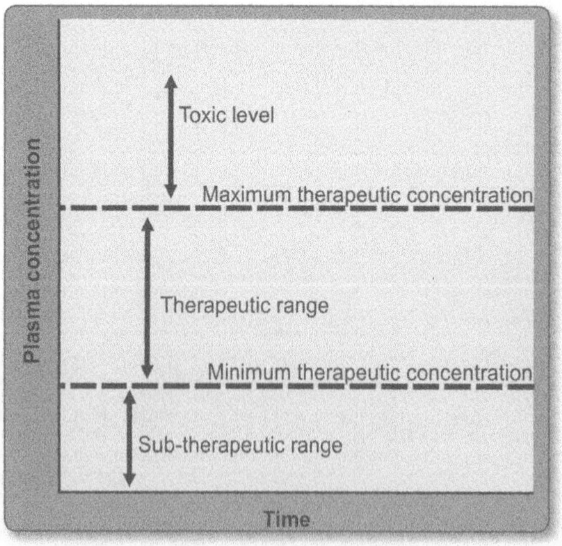

Fig. 17-1 Subtherapeutic, therapeutic and toxic levels of a drug

that is effective and safe in treating specific disease conditions. Within this range, termed the therapeutic range, the drug exhibits its desired effects, but below this range, called subtherapeutic range, the therapeutic effects are not seen. Plasma concentrations above the therapeutic range are generally termed as the toxic levels, because the drug may exhibit toxic effects at these concentrations.

It should be emphasized that since a large subject population is used in determining therapeutic and toxic concentrations of the drug, the data obtained in these studies reflect an average or mean value for these concentrations. It is a very well-known fact that individual patient response often plays an important role in the determination of therapeutic and toxic concentrations of a drug in the plasma. In most scientific studies, large differences have been reported in individual patient response to treatment with a given drug at a given dosage regimen. Therefore, the reported average values of therapeutic and toxic concentration of a drug are usually accompanied with a wide range. Hence, there may be substantial overlap in the values of these concentrations, that is, the therapeutic concentration of a drug in one individual may prove to be subtherapeutic concentration in another individual and toxic concentration in somebody else. Therefore, it should be realized that there is no fine line of demarcation, which separates subtherapeutic, therapeutic and toxic concentrations of a given drug and these concentrations are not necessarily divided by absolute boundaries.

HISTORICAL BACKGROUND

The most common example of overlap of subtherapeutic, therapeutic and toxic levels of a drug is seen in the case of salicylates. A recent review describing monitoring of salicylate concentration in the plasma reported that although plasma salicylate concentrations correlate with clinical and adverse effects of the drug, there is considerable overlap between the region of effective salicylate concentration and the region of salicylate concentration associated with adverse effects and toxicity. For example, symptoms of intoxication, such as central hyperventilation, nausea and vomiting may occur in adult patients, when the concentration of salicylate in the plasma approaches 300 mg/L and yet salicylate levels of 300 mg/L to 400 mg/L in plasma are frequently used to manage acute rheumatic fever. Similarly, the therapeutic plasma concentration range for the anti-inflammatory effects of salicylates is between 150 and 300 mg/L, but at this plasma concentration the drug may exhibit such side effects as hearing loss, vertigo, headaches and tinnitus.

An approximate relationship between the concentration of salicylate in the plasma and the pharmacodynamic effects of the drug is shown in Figure 17-2. The therapeutic concentrations of salicylate shown in this Figure are approximations, because some effects, for example, analgesic effect and anti-inflammatory effect of the drug in patients are subjective and cannot be measured objectively in a graded manner.

The assessment of a therapeutic concentration range for salicylates is somewhat complicated, due to the following reasons:

a. Binding of salicylate to plasma proteins depends on concentration of salicylate in plasma. At low therapeutic concentrations (about 100 mg/L) approximately 90 percent of salicylate is bound, but at high concentrations of salicylate in plasma (greater than 400 mg/L), only about 75 percent of salicylate is bound to the plasma proteins.
b. Changes in albumin levels in plasma affect plasma binding of salicylates.
c. The metabolism of salicylates is capacity-limited. Therefore, only about 10 percent of a small dose of salicylate (300 mg or less) is excreted unchanged in the urine, but the fraction excreted unchanged in the urine increases, when higher doses of salicylates are given.
d. The renal excretion of high levels of salicylates depends on the pH of urine. Alkaline urine favors rapid elimination due to increased dissociation of salicylates in alkaline medium,

necessitating larger doses or more frequent dosing to achieve higher plasma levels of salicylates. Patients with acidic urine require relatively smaller doses of salicylates to achieve the same plasma levels of salicylate, because dissociation of salicylates is decreased in acidic urine.

e. Concomitant therapy with other drugs also affects salicylate concentration in the plasma. For example:
   1. Administration of substances that increase the acidity of urine, such as ammonium chloride and/or ascorbic acid, may increase the plasma concentration of salicylates because of decreased urinary clearance.
   2. Co-administration of adsorbents, such as activated charcoal, can reduce absorption of salicylates from the gastrointestinal tract.
   3. Antacids may reduce the concentration of salicylates in plasma by either decreasing systemic absorption of salicylates or increasing clearance of salicylates.
   4. Administration of corticosteroids may cause increased renal clearance of salicylates.
   5. Concomitant administration of aspirin and caffeine may significantly increase the rate of appearance of aspirin in plasma, the maximum plasma concentration of aspirin and the bioavailability of aspirin.

Since the primary objective of therapeutic drug monitoring is to provide safest approach to optimal drug therapy, it is desirable to attain rapid and safe concentration of drug in the plasma within the desired therapeutic range of the drug in question. Interestingly, from a historical perspective, the progress in therapeutic drug monitoring can be traced back to the last 30 years or so. Before the concept of therapeutic drug monitoring gained popularity with the health professionals, drug dosage, as recently as until the 1960s, was largely a case of trial and error. For treatment with a given drug, most prescribers determined the therapeutic dose of the drug either based essentially on their own experience with the drug, or based on the suggested dosage range by the manufacturer, or based entirely on the word of mouth. The dosage range suggested by manufacturers was usually based on a study involving a large patient population, and the outcome of this study was an average dose range which was considered suitable for the majority of patients. Most prescribers gained experience in determining therapeutic dosage for their patients by initiating treatment at low dose levels, and increasing the dose until a therapeutic

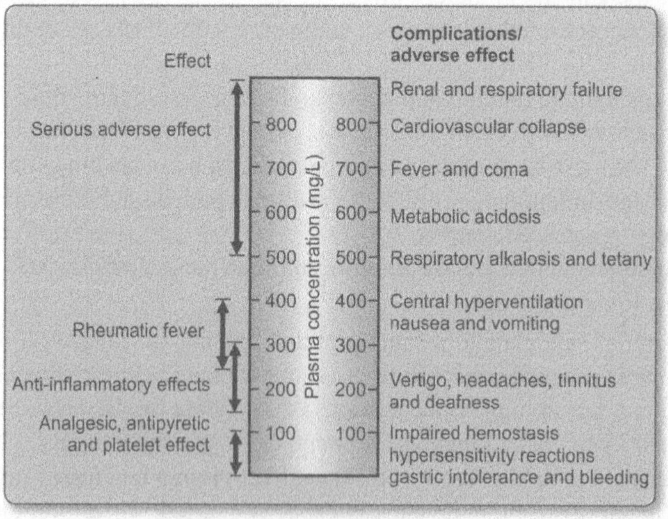

Fig. 17-2 Relationship between concentration of salicylate in plasma, effects and complications. (*Courtesy:* SH Dromgoole and DE Furst, 'Salicylates', in Applied Pharmacokinetics: Principles of Therapeutic Drug Monitoring, Evans, Schentag and Jusko, eds. 3rd ed, Applied Therapeutics, 1995).

effect was obtained or toxic reactions occurred. Some prescribers felt that the therapeutic dose of the drug was attained, as soon as therapeutic effects were observed (even with the smallest dose), while others felt that the therapeutic dose of the drug should be an amount that is slightly smaller than the amount that is capable of producing untoward or toxic symptoms. Thus, each prescriber had his/her own interpretation of what would be considered correct therapeutic dose.

Some early research in the 1950s had suggested that the concentration of drug in serum or plasma could be used as a measure to determine differences in the pharmacokinetics of various drugs and their analog, as well as the pharmacokinetic parameters of a drug in an individual patient. Therefore, researchers started to expand on this work and used this concept as leverage to advocate, as well as advance drug effectiveness and safety. Once the concept of drug effectiveness and safety gained momentum, it was followed, in the 1970s and early 1980s, by a period of extensive investigation and application of monitoring drug treatment and therapeutic, as well as toxic responses to treatment with drugs. Therapeutic drug monitoring became the hot subject predominantly, because of enthusiasm for using therapeutic plasma drug concentration ranges.

In therapeutic drug monitoring, a major assumption made by the practitioner is that concentration of drug in the plasma relates to therapeutic and/or toxic effects of the drug. This is because, for a large number of drugs, clinical studies have demonstrated that there is a therapeutically effective range of concentration of drug in the plasma. Therefore a sound knowledge of the plasma drug concentration may clarify, why a patient does not respond to the given drug therapy or why the drug exhibits an adverse effect. Table 17-1 lists range of therapeutic concentrations for some commonly used important drugs.

Table 17-1 Therapeutic concentration range (TCR) of some drugs

Drug	*TCR (mg/L)*	*Drug*	*TCR (mg/L)*
Acebutolol	0.5 – 2.0	Hetacillin	1.6 – 6.2
Acetaminophen	10 – 20	Hexobarbital	2 – 4
Acetazolamide	5 – 20	Hydrocortisone	0.05 – 0.250
Acetohexamide	20 – 60	Hydroxychloroquine	0.01 – 0.02
Acetylprocainamide	2 – 22	Ibuprofen	5 – 50
Acetylsalicylic Acid	20 – 300	Imipramine	0.15 – 0.5
Amantadine	0.2 – 0.9	Indomethacin	0.5 – 3
Amikacin	5 – 30	Isoniazid	0.5 – 15
p-Aminosalicylic Acid	0.6 – 4	Kanamycin	5 – 25
Amitriptyline	0.3 – 0.9	Levadopa	0.2 – 4
Amobarbital	1 – 8	Lidocaine	1.5 – 7
Amoxapine	0.2 – 0.4	Lincomycin	0.09 – 3
Amoxicillin	2 – 8	Lorazepam	0.02 – 0.05
Amphotericin B	0.2 – 2.0	Meperidine	0.2 – 0.6
Ampicillin	2 – 8	Meprobamate	5 – 15
Atenolol	0.2 – 1.3	Metformin	1 – 10
Azidocillin	0.01 – 0.8	Methacycline	1 – 10
Butobarbital	1 – 5	Methadone	0.3 – 1.1
Carbamazepine	4 – 12	Methicillin	1 – 6
Carbenicillin	10 – 125	Morphine	0.07 – 0.1
Cefamandole	0.5 – 5	Nadolol	0.025 – 0.275
Cefazolin	0.1 – 6.3	Nafcillin	0.03 – 1
Cefoperazone	0.2 – 8	Nalidixic Acid	5 – 50
Cefotaxime	0.2 – 8	Neomycin	5 – 10
Cefoxitin	1 – 10	Nitrazepam	0.03 – 0.06
Ceftizoxime	2 – 64	Nomifensine	0.025 – 0.075

Contd...

Contd...

Drug	*TCR (mg/L)*	*Drug*	*TCR (mg/L)*
Ceftriaxone	0.2 – 8	Nortriptyline	0.05 – 0.8
Cefuroxime	1 – 50	Oxacillin	5 – 6
Cephalexin	6 – 50	Oxazepam	1 – 2
Cephaloridine	0.1 – 16	Oxprenolol	0.04 – 0.1
Cephalothin	0.1 – 6.3	Oxytetracycline	0.05 – 3
Cephapirin	1 – 12	Papaverine	0.1 – 0.2
Cephradine	0.5 – 12	Penicillin G	1.5 – 3
Chloramphenicol	5 – 40	Penicillin V	3 – 5
Chlordiazepoxide	1 – 3	Pentazocine	0.03 – 0.1
Chloroquine	0.01 – 0.28	Pentobarbital	1 – 4
Chloropheniramine	0.005 – 0.01	Phenethicillin K	0.1 – 0.8
Chlorpromazine	50 – 300	Phenobarbital	10 – 50
Chlorpropamide	50 – 150	Phenylbutazone	40 – 150
Chlortetracycline	0.5 – 6	Phenytoin	10 – 20
Chlorthlidone	0.02 – 7.7	Polymyxin B	0.5 – 4
Cimetidine	0.25 – 1	Primidone	5 – 12
Clindamycin	0.002 – 0.5	Probenecid	100 – 200
Clofibrate	80 – 150	Procainamide	4 – 12
Clonazepan	0.01 – 0.07	Propoxyphene	0.2 – 0.8
Cloxacillin	7 – 14	Propranolol	0.05 – 0.1
Cytarabine	0.01 – 0.10	Quinidine	1 – 8
Dapsone	1 – 7	Rifampin	0.5 – 10
Desipramine	0.15 – 0.3	Salicylate	20 – 300
Dexamethasone	0.005 – 0.01	Secobarbital	1 – 15
Dextromethorphan	0.2 – 0.35	Streptomycin	20 – 25
Diazepam	0.1 – 1	Sulfadiazine	100 – 150
Deazoxide	15 – 25	Sulfadimethoxine	1 – 50
Dicloxacillin	15 – 18	Sulfaethidole	0.5 – 1
Dicumarol	5 – 10	Sulfamethazine	50 – 200
Dicyclomine	0.025	Sulfamerazine	50 – 200
Digitoxin	0.01 – 0.035	Sulfamethizole	50 – 200
Digoxin	0.001 – 0.002	Sulfamethoxazole	50 – 200
Diphenhydramine	0.01 – 0.1	Sulfisomidine	10 – 50
Disopyramide	2 – 8	Sulfisoxazole	90 – 150
Dopamine	0.01 – 0.1	Tetracycline	0.5 – 2
Doxepin	30 – 50	Theophylline	10 – 20
Erythromycin	0.5 – 2.5	Thyroxine	0.04 – 0.13
Ethchlorvynol	2 – 15	Timolol	0.005 – 0.01
Ethosuximide	50 – 100	Tolbutamide	50 – 250
Fenfluramine	0.04 – 0.12	Trimethoprim	0.5 – 12
Fentanyl	0.02 – 0.025	Tubocurarine	0.6
Flucytosine	35 – 70	Valproate	20 – 100
Furosemide	0.1 – 0.3	Vancomycin	5 – 40
Gentamicin	0.5 – 10	Verapamil	0.1 – 0.7
Griseofulvin	0.3 – 1.3	Viomycin	25 – 100
Haloperidol	0.001 – 0.015	Warfarin	1 – 10

CANDIDATES FOR THERAPEUTIC MONITORING

Although therapeutic drug monitoring is not essential for all drugs, the concept of therapeutic drug monitoring is so powerful that, if not all, at least a large number of drugs, for example, almost all potent drugs should be considered as prime candidates for therapeutic monitoring. Historically, however, therapeutic drug monitoring has been applied most commonly to a very few drugs only. These include the aminoglycosides, digoxin, phenytoin and theophylline. The application of therapeutic drug monitoring to a handful of drugs is a reflection of the routine use of these drugs in therapy. Not all drugs are monitored in all healthcare facilities. Some drugs are monitored only in specialized hospitals or clinics. These include cyclosporine, methotrexate and the psychotherapeutic agents. The lack of wide-spread use of therapeutic drug monitoring is due to many factors that mitigate against the application of subjecting, a drug to therapeutic monitoring. One of the major limitations to plasma monitoring of a drug is the occurrence of active metabolites of the drug. Procainamide, the antiarrhythmic agent, is one of the examples of a drug, which poses a special problem as far as therapeutic drug monitoring is concerned. Procainamide is acetylated and forms an active metabolite, N-acetylprocainamide, by a hepatic enzyme that shows genetic differences. Also, procainamide is partially excreted unchanged, while the metabolite is almost entirely handled by the kidneys. Thus, those patients who are rapid acetylators and who have a compromised renal function, the correlation between procainamide concentration in plasma and response of the drug is expected to differ from that observed in patients, who are slow acetylators and have normal renal function. Therefore, the concentration of both the drug and its metabolite should be monitored, especially in the presence of renal disease.

All drugs and dosage forms are not good candidates for therapeutic drug monitoring. Drugs and dosage forms that lend themselves to therapeutic monitoring must possess specific characteristics. Drugs that are currently subjected to therapeutic monitoring have at least the following common characteristics:

a. The intensity and probability of therapeutic or toxic effects of the drug correlate quantitatively with concentration of drug in the plasma, i.e. an increase in the dose of the drug or the presence of renal impairment will be expected to exhibit toxic or untoward effects.
b. The range of therapeutic and safe concentration of drug in the plasma is narrow, i.e. the drug is known to exhibit a narrow therapeutic index. Therapeutic index is defined as the ratio between the maximum and minimum plasma concentrations of the drug's therapeutic range. For example, if the maximum and minimum therapeutic concentrations of a drug are known to be 20 and 8 μg/mL, respectively, then the therapeutic index of the drug would be (20 μg/mL)/(8 μg/mL) = 2.5. Therapeutic index between a value of 2 to 3 is regarded as a narrow therapeutic index. Hence, a less than 2 therapeutic index means that the dose that commonly yields a subtherapeutic response is close to the dose of the drug that commonly produces some toxic reaction. Most drugs (except some antineoplastics) have a therapeutic index of 2 or more. Box 17-1 lists examples of drugs and dosage forms that are considered to possess narrow therapeutic range.
c. Toxicity or lack of effectiveness of the drug dose puts the patient at great potential risk. This situation is very common with potent drugs.
d. The pharmacologic effect observed persists for a relatively long time, because acute, short, or intermittent effects of the drug are not well-regulated by using plasma levels of the drug.
e. The concentration of drug in the plasma is the most practical intermediate end-point of the drug to be used, when there is no clearly observable therapeutic or toxic end-point of the drug. The distinction between therapeutic end-point and toxic end-point is that, while therapeutic end-point of the drug is prevention of a disease or condition (e.g. renal failure, pulmonary embolism, stroke, seizures, etc.), toxic end-point may be an arrhythmia or renal failure. The intermediate end point is an important parameter, because intermediate end-point is a measurable response and is an index of therapeutic range of the drug that relates to the toxic condition. Examples of intermediate end-point of the drug include concentration of drug in the plasma, prothrombin time for oral anticoagulants, blood or urine glucose concentration for hypoglycemic drugs, serum uric acid for uricosurics, rosette inhibition test for immunosuppressive agents and blood pressure for hypertensive drugs.

Box 17-1 Drugs and dosage forms having narrow therapeutic range

Aminophylline tablets
Aminophylline ER tablets
Carbamazepine tablets
Carbamazepine oral suspension
Clindamycin hydrochloride capsules
Clindamycin hydrochloride tablets
Clonidine transdermal patches
Dyphylline tablets
Disopyramide phosphate capsules
Disopyramide phosphate CR capsules
Ethinyl estradiol/progestin oral contraceptive tablets
Guanethidine monosulfate tablets
Isoetharine mesylate inhalation aerosol
Isoproterenol sulfate tablets
Lithium carbonate capsules
Lithium carbonate tablets
Lithium carbonate ER tablets
Metaproterenol sulfate tablets
Minoxidil tablets
Oxtriphylline tablets
Oxtriphylline delayed release (DR) tablets
Oxtriphylline ER tablets
Phenytoin sodium capsules
Phenytoin sodium ER capsules
Phenytoin sodium oral suspension
Prazosin hydrochloride capsules
Primidone tablets
Primidone oral suspension
Procainamide hydrochloride capsules
Procainamide hydrochloride tablets
Procainamide hydrochloride CR tablets
Quinidine sulfate capsules
Quinidine sulfate tablets
Quinidine sulfate ER tablets
Quinidine gluconate tablets
Quinidine gluconate ER tablets
Theophylline capsules
Theophylline ER capsules
Theophylline tablets
Theophylline ER tablets
Valproic acid capsules
Valproic acid syrup
Divalproex sodium DR capsules
Divalproex sodium DR tablets
Warfarin sodium tablets

f. There is no predictable dose-response relationship, that is, the dose of drug that produces a sub-therapeutic effect in one patient may produce a toxic reaction in another patient.
g. The availability of an assay procedure for the determination of concentration or the amount of drug in the plasma. Obviously, if the assay procedure for the determination of concentration of drug in the plasma is not available, it will be very difficult to monitor the drug for a given treatment or condition for which the drug is being used. The assay should, of necessity, possess the following characteristics: it should be precise, accurate, sensitive, specific, relatively easy and inexpensive. Also, it should require a small volume of sample and yield results quickly, enough to permit prudent therapeutic decisions.

From the above discussion it is evident that therapeutic drug monitoring is not essential for all drugs. Considering the time and expense involved in therapeutic drug monitoring, drugs which do not meet the criteria mentioned above are not routinely subjected to rigors of therapeutic monitoring. Table 17-2 lists drugs that are most frequently subjected to therapeutic monitoring.

As can be seen from Table 17-2, the list of drugs that are most frequently subjected to therapeutic monitoring is relatively short. This is because therapeutic monitoring for many drugs may not be necessary due to the following reasons:

a. Some drugs have a broad range of effective and safe dosage regimens. For these drugs effective plasma concentrations can be achieved and at the same time toxic concentrations can be avoided without having to determine the concentration of drug in plasma.
b. For some drugs it is not necessary to determine plasma concentrations, because more effective and less expensive intermediate measures of drug response are available to determine, whether the given dose of the drug should be increased, reduced or no change in dose is necessary. For example, measurement of blood pressure in therapy with drugs that affect blood pressure, blood coagulation time with anticoagulants, absence of seizures in antiepileptic therapy are good indicators of therapeutic dose of the drug.
c. Some drugs have such a narrow range of flexibility in their dosage that the relationship between plasma concentration of drug and its clinical response is not firmly established.
d. Therapeutic drug monitoring is an expensive proposition. It is costly in terms of equipment used in monitoring drug therapy, supplies needed for such monitoring and investment needed for the collection of necessary data, which can be used to correlate the concentration of drug in plasma versus response from the drug dose.

Individual variations in pharmacokinetics and pharmacodynamics make the design of dosage regimen different for different patients. Thus, the dosage regimen for a given patient has to be properly designed in order to achieve optimum concentration of drug at the site of action, so as to produce optimal therapeutic response with minimum or no side effects. Therefore, in the treatment with those drugs where the situation warrants close monitoring of concentration of drug in the plasma, it is important to consider not only the pharmacokinetic effects, but also the pharmacodynamic effects resulting from treatment with the drug.

Table 17-2 Drugs most frequently subjected to therapeutic monitoring

Antibiotics	Including the aminoglycosides (amikacin, gentamicin, netlimicin and tobramycin), chloramphenicol and vancomycin
Antiepileptics	Including carbamazone, phenytoin and valproic acid. Cardiac agents including digoxin and some antiarrythmics (amiodarone, lidocaine, procainamide and quinidine)
Psychotherapeutics	Including lithium and some tricyclic antidepressants (amitriptyline, imipramine and nortriptyline)
Miscellaneous Agents	Including cyclosporine, methotrexate and theophylline

In general, candidates for therapeutic drug monitoring are those drugs, which possess the following characteristics. A few of the criteria listed below are absolutely necessary, while some criteria may be only relatively important. However, most of these criteria must be met in order that the planned strategy is effective.

a. Drugs, which have a relatively narrow therapeutic index or narrow therapeutic window, i.e. the range of therapeutic concentration of drug is approximately equal to or less than two-fold (e.g. aminoglycoside antibiotics).
b. Drugs for which small changes in the concentration of drug in plasma are likely to exhibit large changes in drug response.
c. Drugs, which exhibit poor and erratic absorption. As a rule, the larger the variability in the absorption of the drug, the greater is the need for monitoring it.
d. Drugs, which exhibit relatively wide interindividual variations in the rate of metabolism, leading to marked differences in attaining steady-state plasma concentrations. These differences can be particularly important when children are being treated, because in children there are wide differences in body weight and metabolic rate.
e. Drugs, which exhibit saturation kinetics, thereby causing a steep relationship between dose and plasma levels within the therapeutic range (e.g. phenytoin).
f. Drugs whose signs of toxicity are difficult to recognize clinically or where signs of over-dosage or under-dosage are difficult to distinguish.
g. Drugs, which are administered in the presence of gastrointestinal, hepatic or renal disease, causing disturbance of drug absorption, metabolism or excretion.
h. When patients are receiving multiple drug therapy with the potential risk of drug interaction between the drugs.
i. When there is doubt about the patient's reliability in taking the dosage form as prescribed.

An important demonstration of potential benefits of monitoring plasma levels of drug is found in a report on digoxin toxicity from the Boston Collaborative Drug Surveillance Program. Adverse reactions to digoxin in hospitalized medical patients were monitored for 2 years at 2 hospitals in Boston. Both hospitals monitored approximately similar number of patients. One hospital monitored 272 patients and the other hospital monitored 291 patients. Dose-related adverse reactions were confirmed in 10 percent of 272 patients, but in only 4 percent of 291 patients. The only important differences between these studies were that serum digoxin concentrations were measured in more patients receiving digoxin at the second hospital than at the first hospital. Serum digoxin concentrations were measured in 40 percent of the patients receiving digoxin at the second hospital and in 12 percent of the patients in the first hospital. The mean digoxin concentrations were lower in the patients at the second hospital than in the patients at the first hospital.

FACTORS INFLUENCING DRUG VARIABILITY

As mentioned earlier, when a drug is administered to a large population, the concentration of drug in plasma achieved in the patients will undoubtedly vary. This variation is due to a wide interpatient variability, although the drug is administered at similar dose level and at a fixed dosage regimen to each patient. For most drugs, the interpatient variability results in plasma concentrations, which exhibit wide variations, i.e. the highest plasma concentration of drug attained differs greatly in each subject even though all subjects received the same dose of the same drug. For example, the highest plasma concentration (peak plasma concentration) of drug in some subjects may be as much as five or six fold the mean plasma concentration and the highest concentration of drug in the plasma of some subjects, may be as little as one-half or one-tenth of the mean plasma concentration. Figure 17-3 shows a typical example of variability in plasma drug concentration in subjects treated identically, i.e. all patients received the same dose of the same drug, administered in the same dosage form at the same time of the day and by the same route of administration.

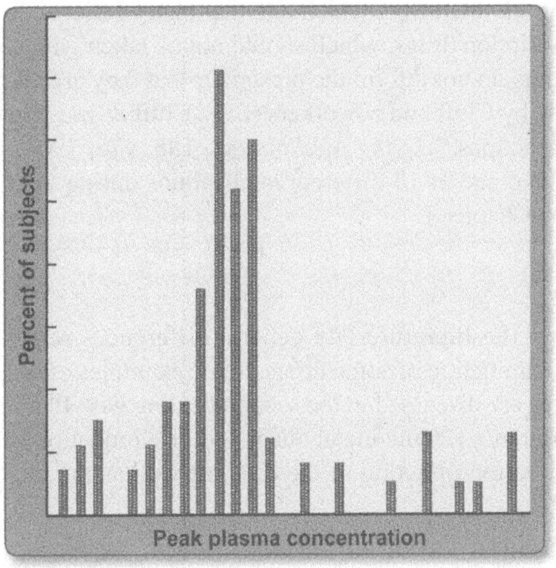

Fig. 17-3 Variability in plasma concentration in subjects receiving the same dose

Interpatient and intrapatient variability in the concentration of drug in plasma is caused by many factors. Some of the important factors, which have been shown to be responsible for interpatient variability include the following:

Variations in Drug Absorption

Variation in the rate and extent of absorption of a drug is seen not only in different patients receiving the same dose, but also in the same patient receiving the same drug dose in the same dosage form, but at different times of drug administration. This variation is caused by variability in the rate and extent of drug absorption and may be attributed to a variety of reasons. Many physicochemical factors and physiological factors are responsible for this variation. These factors include gastrointestinal motility, pH of the gastrointestinal tract, gastric emptying, gastrointestinal secretions, presence or absence of food in the gastrointestinal tract, presence or absence of food in the gastrointestinal tract, blood vessels serving the digestive system and presence of bacteria in the gastrointestinal tract. For a detailed description of these factors, the reader is referred to "Factors Influencing Drug Absorption" discussed in Chapter 4.

PRESENCE OF OTHER DRUGS

Concomitant administration of certain drugs or the presence of other drugs in the gastrointestinal tract may influence the rate of absorption, as well as the extent of absorption of some drugs and the elimination of a variety of drugs, thus influencing concentration of administered drug in the plasma. For example, concomitant administration of those drugs, which cause acidosis or alkalosis of urine could influence the elimination of weakly acidic and weak basic drugs. Some examples of these drugs are discussed in Chapters dealing with drug absorption and drug elimination.

Drug Interactions

Drug interaction is a phenomenon, which occurs when the effect of one drug is modified by the presence of another drug. One drug may alter the expected therapeutic response of another drug that has been administered just prior to, simultaneously or just after another drug. There are a number of reports in the literature, which cite that many patients, especially geriatric patients take some non-prescription drugs, which should not be taken with some prescription drugs. In most cases the patients do not inform the prescriber that they are taking these over-the-counter medications. A study by Cluff and coworkers (L. E. Cluff *et. al.*, "Studies on the Epidemiology of Adverse Drug Reactions," *J. Am. Med. Assoc.*, **188**, 976, 1964) reported that hospitalized patients receive an average of 14 different medications during their stay in the hospital. This study is described in Chapter 1.

Genetic Differences

Published reports in the literature cite genetic differences resulting in differences in the metabolism and/or elimination of some drugs. Some examples of drugs, which are affected due to genetic differences are discussed in the section dealing with Pharmacogenetics in Chapter 1. Therefore, such differences in the metabolism and/or elimination of these drugs would cause differences in the duration of action of the drug, as well as the biological half-life of drug in different individuals.

Disease States

Disease state in a patient can affect absorption, distribution, metabolism and elimination of the administered dose of the drug. Several disease states, which affect the emptying time of the stomach are cited in Chapter 4 in the section dealing with Gastric Emptying. The presence of these disease states may affect not only the rate and extent of absorption, but also the distribution of drug in various body fluids and tissues. Similarly, conditions which cause hepatic or renal failure (or insufficiency), may also affect elimination of some drugs.

Physiologic Differences

The term physiologic difference, as used here, refers to the age, gender, weight, nutritional status, etc. of the patient. There are several reports in the literature, which demonstrate that physiologic differences in patients can influence concentration of drug in the plasma. For example, drugs which have a strong affinity for lipids will have a tendency to bind to the lipids to a greater extent in an obese person than in a lean individual with very little fatty tissue. Such binding may necessitate administration of a larger dose of the drug to an obese person in order to achieve the desired therapeutic level of the free or unbound drug in plasma (see "Body Composition" discussed in Chapter 5). It should, however, be mentioned that since a larger fraction of the administered dose is bound to the fatty tissue in an obese individual (because of the larger adipose tissue mass in an obese person), the drug should be administered less frequently because the bound fraction acts as a depot for the drug and releases the drug for a longer period of time. Thus, obese patients may require larger doses of the drug administered less frequently and lean patients may need smaller doses of the drug, but administered more frequently.

The magnitude of interpatient variability differs in different drugs. Some drugs exhibit very small variability, while others may result in moderately to extremely high variability. The magnitude of variability *per se* may not be so important if the drug in question has a large therapeutic window with a broad range of safe dose, i.e. small changes in concentration of drug in the plasma do not result in significant changes in drug response. However, if therapeutic window of the drug is narrow (e.g. drugs such as aminoglycosides, digoxin, phenytoin, theophylline, quinidine, etc.) and/or small changes in concentration of drug in plasma exhibit large changes in drug response, then the interpatient variability becomes an important consideration for the clinical pharmacokineticist. The primary objective of dosage regimen for these drugs is to provide a safe and effective concentration of drug in the plasma that does not approach or exceed the minimum toxic concentration.

Figure 17-4 shows how the concentrations of phenytoin in the plasma vary among patients treated chronically with a daily dose of 300 mg. Although, plasma concentrations associated with optimal phenytoin therapy are normally between 10 mg/L and 20 mg/L, it is clear that there is a more than 50 percent incidence of concentrations for which subtherapeutic responses are probable and at the same time there is about a 16 percent incidence of concentrations at which toxic responses are probable.

Similarly, the range of therapeutic concentration of theophylline in the plasma is reported to be between 10 μg/mL and 20 μg/mL. This means that some patients will respond to theophylline treatment when concentration of drug in the plasma is approximately 10 μg/mL, whereas others will need as much as 20 μg/mL of theophylline concentration in the plasma before the drug shows therapeutic effect. For most patients, concentration of theophylline in plasma at levels less than 8 μg/mL is generally considered inadequate for the desired therapeutic effect and drug concentrations greater than 20 μg/mL are associated with such side effects as nausea vomiting, nervousness and tachycardia. Hence, administration of theophylline within the generally accepted 10 to 20 μg/mL concentration range may cause toxic symptoms in some patients even before the concentration of theophylline in plasma approaches 20 μg/mL.

Although most drugs follow linear pharmacokinetics, there are many drugs that do not follow linear pharmacokinetics. It should therefore be obvious that drugs that do not follow linear pharmacokinetics at the usual therapeutic concentrations of drug in the plasma pose a special problem. This is because, in these drugs, a small change in the dose of drug could possibly cause an extremely high increase in therapeutic response of the drug. The extremely high increase in therapeutic response of the drug could, in turn, lead to possible adverse effects of the drug. Phenytoin is an example of such a drug. Phenytoin is an example of a drug that does not follow linear pharmacokinetics at therapeutic concentrations and therefore a small change in the dose of phenytoin is likely to cause an extremely high increase in its therapeutic response, leading to potential adverse effects.

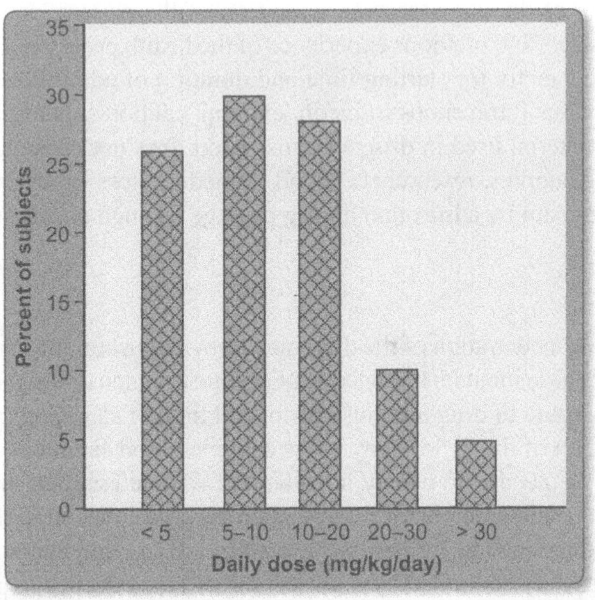

Fig. 17-4 Phenytoin plasma concentration among 100 ambulant patients chronically treated with a daily dose of 300 mg of phenytoin sodium

(*Courtesy:* TN Tozer and ME Winter, "Phenytoin," in "Applied Pharmacokinetics: Principles of Therapeutic Drug Monitoring, Evans, Schentag, and Jusko, eds. 3rd ed. Applied Therapeutics, 1995).

Therefore, in the treatment with those drugs where the situation warrants very close monitoring of concentration of drug in the plasma, it is important to consider not only the pharmacokinetic effects, but also the pharmacodynamic effects resulting from treatment with the drug in question.

PROCESS OF THERAPEUTIC DRUG MONITORING

Since the main objective of therapeutic drug monitoring is to provide the safest approach to optimal drug therapy in an individual patient, it is desirable to attain rapid and safe plasma concentrations within the desired therapeutic range. Therefore, the process of therapeutic drug monitoring in a given patient may be regarded as consisting of the following three important components:

1. Development of plasma profile in each patient
2. Observation of clinical effects of drug in the patient.
3. Interpretation and application of plasma concentration data in order to develop safe and effective dosage regimen.

Development of Plasma Profile

The development of plasma profile of the drug in a patient involves withdrawal of blood samples at predetermined time intervals. Before blood samples are taken from the patient, the practitioner should establish if there is indeed a need to measure concentration of drug in the plasma. In some cases patient's response may not be related to concentration of drug in the plasma, e.g. mild nausea or allergy may not be dose related. If the need for taking blood samples is justified, then the development of plasma profile of drug in a patient involves the following steps:

Administering a Predetermined Dose of the Drug

The amount of drug administered as the dose is usually based on the following factors: recommendation of the manufacturer, condition of the patient, presence of other conditions and/or disease states and previous experience of the health professional with the drug. All doses should be timed exactly for starting time and duration of administration. In administration of drugs by continuous intravenous infusion, extreme caution should be exercised to assure that any particular material used in drug administration does not cause loss of drug. In one of the most dramatic examples, researchers found immediate loss of about 50 percent of a dose of intravenous diazepam by adsorption during passage through plastic tubing of an infusion set.

Collection of Blood Samples

A single plasma concentration of the drug may not yield useful information unless other factors are considered. These include: knowledge of dosage regimen of drug, including size of dose and dosage interval, route of drug administration, and time of sampling (at peak, trough or steady-state concentration of drug). In many cases a single blood sample is not sufficient and several blood samples are needed to clarify adequacy of dosage regimen. In practice, trough plasma concentrations are easier to obtain than peak or average concentrations during a multiple-dose regimen. Also, there may be limitations to withdrawal of many blood samples, e.g. the number of blood samples may be limited by total volume of blood needed to perform drug analysis and time to assay each sample.

When the drug is administered through an extravascular route, blood sampling times for therapeutic drug monitoring should preferably be during the post-distributive phase for loading dose and maintenance dose, and at steady-state for maintenance doses. The reason for choosing this time frame is that after distribution equilibrium has been established, the concentration of drug in the plasma during the postdistributive phase is usually better correlated with the tissue concentration and presumably the concentration of drug at the site of action. For general development of plasma profile, when multiple samples of blood are collected to determine concentration of drug in the plasma at various time intervals, the time of collection of each blood sample is usually predetermined. However, in some emergency situations, the time of collection of blood samples may be dictated by the severity of condition, for example, sudden development of unwanted or toxic reaction. Ideally, blood samples should be collected by direct venipuncture in clean glass tubes without anticoagulant, because, presence of heparin can result in increased free fatty-acid concentrations, causing altered plasma-protein binding.

Determination of Drug Concentration in each Sample

Analyses of blood for concentration of the drug are usually performed by either a clinical chemistry laboratory or a clinical pharmacokinetics laboratory. Invariably there are a variety of analytical techniques and methods that may be used to determine concentration of drug in the plasma. For example, there are chromatographic methods (gas chromatography and high pressure liquid chromatography), fluorometry, spectrophotometry, immunoassay and radioisotopic methods. The assay used for the determination of concentration of drug in the plasma should be specific for the drug molecule rather than for the general structure of the drug, i.e. the assay should preferably be able to distinguish the drug, its metabolites and endogenous or exogenous substances, because interference from other materials may erroneously inflate the results. The specificity of the assay can usually be established rather easily, e.g. by simple chromatographic evidence.

In general, colorimetric and spectrophotometric assays are usually less specific. If a drug is administered in a small dose and its apparent volume of distribution is large, then the assay should also be sensitive enough to accurately determine the relatively small concentration of drug in the plasma. Sensitivity of the assay is the minimum detectable concentration of drug in the plasma and it should be at least 2 to 3 times the background noise. The method used for drug assay by the analytical laboratory may depend on several factors, e.g. instrumentation available in laboratory, physicochemical characteristics of the drug, the amount and nature of the biological specimen (blood and/or urine) available for assay, cost for each assay and analytical skills of the personnel responsible for performing assay in the laboratory. It is very desirable that the analytical laboratory has a standard operating procedure for the analytical technique for each drug, and it follows good laboratory practices.

As a general rule, all analytical methods used for the assay of drugs in the analytical laboratory should always be validated with respect to specificity, sensitivity, precision and accuracy of the drug being assayed. Since precision relates to reproducibility of the data, measurements of concentration of drug to establish precision should be obtained by replication of different concentrations of drug solutions prepared separately on different days. Accuracy refers to the difference between the value obtained by assay of drug and actual concentration of drug in the sample. To establish accuracy, known concentrations of drug in plasma (control) should be prepared by an independent technician to minimize any error in their preparation and checked against the samples being assayed.

Plasma Profile and Pharmacokinetic Model Development

A plot of concentration of drug in the plasma as a function of time provides a wealth of information concerning the drug in an individual patient. For example, the plasma profile could indicate whether the drug confers the characteristics of one-, two- or three-compartment model on the body. The biological half-life of the drug can usually be estimated directly from the plasma profile and an indication of apparent volume of distribution can also be obtained from the plasma profile. Plasma concentration data obtained following intravenous injection of a rapid bolus dose provides partial characterization of drug disposition properties (e.g. apparent volumes of distribution and clearance). Similarly, plasma concentration data obtained following oral administration of drug (whether in solution or in common dosage forms) provides additional pharmacokinetic parameters, which are related to absorption and intrinsic clearance of the drug.

Clinical Effects of the Drug

The second component of the process of therapeutic drug monitoring relates to the relationship between drug concentration at the site of action and the pharmacologic response in the patient. Therefore, therapeutic drug monitoring using plasma drug concentration data can be applied only when the plasma concentration of a drug exhibits a good correlation with the pharmacologic response, such as the one shown in Figure 17-5. This does not mean that the absence of a good correlation between the concentration of drug in plasma and the drug's pharmacologic response is absolutely essential for therapeutic drug monitoring. For those drugs, which do not exhibit a good correlation between the concentration of drug in plasma and clinical effects of the drug obtained after the administration of the drug dose, it may be possible to monitor some other pharmacodynamic parameters in order to optimize drug therapy. For example, adjustment of dose for each individual patient receiving cancer chemotherapy may depend upon the patient's ability to tolerate not only the size of dose, but also the drug itself. If the patient is able to tolerate the drug and the size of dose needs to be adjusted, this adjustment may be made based on severity of side effects of the drug. Similarly, for some drugs it may be easier to monitor an acute pharmacologic response, e.g. measuring clotting time in patients on anticoagulant therapy and monitoring blood pressure for hypertensive agents than determining concentration of drug in the plasma. In this context it should be mentioned that not all drugs are good candidates for therapeutic monitoring. Included in this category are drugs, which exhibit a sufficiently wide therapeutic window, drugs devoid of serious side effects and relatively inexpensive drugs with minimal or no side effects. Most antibiotics with relatively wide therapeutic window (e.g., cephalosporins, penicillins and tetracyclines) are usually not dose titrated, but the dosage is based on the judgment of the prescriber and his/her clinical experience with the drug.

Therapeutic monitoring is useful especially, where the drug has a narrow therapeutic index and/or wide intersubject variations in the concentration of drug in plasma are observed, when the

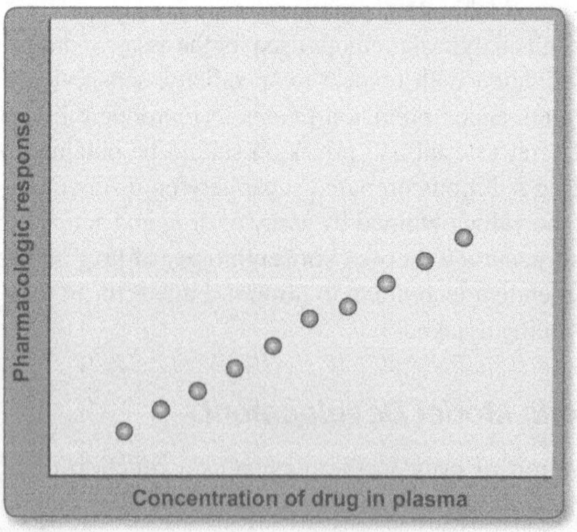

Fig. 17-5 Correlation of pharmacologic response with plasma drug concentration

same dose is administered to a large subject population. A number of drugs lend themselves to the concept of therapeutic drug monitoring based on concentration of drug in the plasma. Theophylline is an excellent example of a drug, whose pharmacodynamics and pharmacokinetics are fairly well-understood and concentration of theophylline in plasma correlates its pharmacologic effect. Thus, during an asthmatic attack, if the patient's theophylline level is below the therapeutic range, it will be wise to administer more theophylline to this patient.

If, on the other hand, the concentration of drug in plasma either does not correlate at all or correlates poorly to the pharmacologic response, then it is safe to assume that this drug does not lend itself to the determination of its plasma concentration for therapeutic monitoring. This assumption is based on the fact that when the drug does not exhibit a well-defined therapeutic range, it may exhibit toxic effects not only at high drug concentrations in plasma, but also at low concentrations in the plasma.

For some drugs, however, determination of plasma concentration for therapeutic monitoring may not be necessary if a simple physical measurement can be made. For example, in the treatment of hypertension with an antihypertensive drug, it is much easier to determine if there is a need for the adjustment of dosage by simply measuring the blood pressure of the patient, rather than determining the concentration of the antihypertensive drug in the plasma.

After concentrations of drug in the plasma are determined and reported by the laboratory, the practitioner must evaluate the data submitted by the laboratory carefully and properly. For instance, most laboratories report concentrations of total drug in the plasma rather than the concentration of free (unbound) drug. Total drug in the plasma includes the free drug (unbound drug) and drug bound to proteins and tissues, etc.). It is important to know the concentration of free drug in the plasma, because only the free (unbound) drug exhibits therapeutic activity and only the free drug undergoes elimination. The assay results from the laboratory might show that drug concentration in plasma is higher, lower or equivalent to the expected plasma levels. One should carefully evaluate these results, while considering the patient and the patient's pathophysiologic condition.

Often, other data might help verify high or low concentration of drug in the plasma, e.g. a complaint of overstimulation and insomnia by the patient might also collaborate the finding of higher than anticipated concentrations of theophylline in the plasma. Similarly, high serum creatinine and high blood urea nitrogen (BUN) values might indicate the reason that observed high concentration of drug in plasma in the patient was a result of slow renal drug clearance due to compromised kidney function. Therefore, therapeutic decisions should not be based solely on plasma drug concentrations, but the clinician should evaluate the data using sound medical and pharmacologic judgment and observation.

Box 17-2 lists some factors to consider, when interpreting the concentration of drug in the plasma.

Development of Dosage Regimen

The third component of therapeutic drug monitoring relates to development of dosage regimen based on concentration of drug in plasma. The concentration of drug in plasma can only be used as an indicator if the following assumptions are valid:

a. The concentration of drug in plasma is the only indicator that can be used to develop dosage regimen, because the pharmacologic effects of the drug cannot be assessed readily by other simple means, e.g. measurement of blood pressure during treatment with antihypertensive drugs.
b. Upon administration, the drug confers the characteristics of one-compartment pharmacokinetic model on the body.
c. The pharmacologic response of the drug is directly proportional to the concentration of drug in the plasma, at least over a limited concentration range (if not over the entire concentration range), i.e. the intensity of pharmacologic response of the drug is proportional to the concentration of drug in the plasma (Fig. 17-5).

Box 17-2 Pharmacokinetic evaluation of plasma concentration of drug

Plasma Concentration correct, but patient does not respond to therapy
Drug interaction at receptor site
Altered receptor sensitivity (e.g. tolerance)
Plasma concentrations higher than anticipated
Error in dosage regimen
Rapid bioavailability
Slow rate of drug elimination
Smaller than anticipated apparent volume of distribution
Wrong drug product (immediate release instead of controlled release)
Timing of blood sample
Incorrect assay methodology
Problem with patient compliance
Plasma concentrations lower than anticipated
Problem with patient compliance
Error in dosage regimen
Poor bioavailability
Rapid rate of drug elimination
Enlarged apparent volume of distribution
Steady-state not reached
Timing of blood sample
Wrong drug product (controlled or slow release instead of immediate release)
Incorrect assay methodology

Based on the assumption stated in (b) above, if upon administration the drug confers the characteristics of one-compartment pharmacokinetic model then the concentration of drug in plasma will be proportional to the size of the dose administered. Combining this rationale with the assumption stated in (c) above, if the pharmacologic response correlates with concentration of drug in the plasma (which, in turn, correlates with the size of dose administered), it follows that pharmacologic response observed in the patient would be proportional to the size of the dose administered.

Based on the assumptions stated above, if the drug in question lends itself to therapeutic monitoring, then a decision is made to formulate drug therapy regimen based upon clinical pharmacokinetic monitoring. The major steps involved in formulation of drug therapy regimen are as follows:

Diagnosis: As with any treatment, correct diagnosis plays an important role in therapeutic drug monitoring. However, since diagnosis of patient's ailment is more in the purview of the physician treating the patient, it is reasonable to assume that a proper diagnosis has been made by the attending physician and also that proper drug therapy has been selected by the attending physician.

Drug product selection: The selection of drug product for the treatment is usually the prerogative of the physician treating the patient. Sometimes the clinical pharmacist is part of the selection process. The clinician may choose one drug over another based on a number of factors, for example, presence or absence of pathophysiologic conditions, previous medical history of the patient, concurrent drug therapy, known allergies and physician's experience with the drug. The clinical pharmacist should remember, however, that some drugs with similar therapeutic indications may not necessarily exhibit similar pharmacokinetic parameters. For instance, they may exhibit differences in rates of metabolism, elimination and other pharmacokinetic parameters.

Dosage form selection: In many instances the prescriber has the option of choosing administration of drug from a variety of commercially available dosage forms. The choice of dosage form selected may affect clinical response, since bioavailability of a given drug often depends on the dosage form and the route of drug administration. Consequently, subsequent pharmacodynamics of drug in the patient will depend on the dosage form chosen for the treatment.

Dosage Regimen: A dosage schedule is now designed for the patient. This is generally based on the following considerations: recommendation of manufacturer concerning the size and frequency of administration of the drug dose, clinical experience of practitioner with the drug and patient's medical history (e.g. drug sensitivity, known allergies, concurrent drug therapy, drug interactions, patient compliance and presence of pathophysiologic conditions). When designing the therapeutic dosage regimen, the following factors must be considered:

a. The physiology of the patient. This includes the age, height, weight, gender, etc. of the patient under treatment.
b. The pathophysiologic condition of the patient (e.g. presence of renal impairment, hepatic disease, congestive heart failure), which may alter the normal pharmacokinetic profile of the drug.
c. Exposure of patient to other medication that may alter the usual pharmacokinetics of the drug being received by the patient.
d. Exposure of patient to environmental factors (such as smoking) that may affect the usual pharmacokinetics of the drug.
e. The absorption, distribution and elimination profile of the drug. Various published reports including review articles, monographs and references provide a listing of various selected pharmacokinetic parameters, such as clearance, bioavailability and elimination half-life of the drug. These pharmacokinetic parameters are often obtained from various clinical studies conducted by different researchers using a small patient population. Differences in the design of a clinical study, size of patient population and data analysis may lead to conflicting values for the same pharmacokinetic parameters. Therefore, it is difficult to determine, whether or not these reported pharmacokinetic parameters are reflected in the patient under treatment.
f. The target concentration of drug at the receptor site for the patient under treatment, including any change in receptor sensitivity to drug. Ideally, the target drug concentration and the therapeutic window for the drug should be obtained, if available. When using published target drug concentration in the development of a dosage regimen, the practitioner should verify if the reported target drug concentration is for the same condition as that of the patient and whether it represents an average steady-state concentration, a peak drug concentration or a trough drug concentration.
g. The choice of the drug dosage form. The route of drug administration and the desired onset and duration of clinical response will affect the choice of the drug dosage form. The dosage form chosen for treatment will affect the bioavailability of drug and therefore the subsequent pharmacodynamics of the drug in the patient.

Initiation of Therapy: Therapy is initiated based on the dosage form and dosage regimen selected for the patient. Along with the initiation of therapy, patient's clinical response to the treatment is monitored carefully.

Evaluation of Clinical Response: If the clinical response to patient's treatment is satisfactory, then an evaluation is made to determine whether the treatment should be continued with the existing dosage regimen that had been selected for the patient or the dosage regimen warrants some readjustment. If the clinical response is not satisfactory and/or unacceptable, then it may be necessary to revise the dosage regimen completely. Figure 17-6 shows various steps involved in the process for reaching dosage decisions with therapeutic drug monitoring.

If the clinical response is not satisfactory and/or unacceptable, a pharmacokinetic evaluation must be made. This decision may dictate the following:

1. Determination of concentration of drug in the plasma as a function of time.
2. Calculation of the various pharmacokinetic parameters in the individual patient.
3. Establishing a new dosage regimen.

New Dosage Regimen: Ideally the determination of new dosage regimen should be based upon pharmacokinetic parameters derived from plasma profile of the patient under treatment. When interpreting data dealing with the concentration of drug in plasma, the practitioner must consider pathophysiologic condition of the patient in order to accurately evaluate the dosage regimen. For example, higher than expected concentration of drug in the plasma may not necessarily be due to the dose of the drug, but may be resulting from slow renal clearance of drug due to compromised kidney function. This can be verified by other laboratory results, such as high serum creatinine and high blood urea nitrogen. Similarly, during treatment with theophylline, such symptoms as insomnia and over-stimulation might suggest higher than expected concentration of theophylline in the plasma. If, on the other hand, plasma levels of the drug are within the anticipated range, but the patient does not respond to therapy, it might indicate possible tolerance of the drug or perhaps drug interaction at the receptor site (or site of action). Similarly, lower than anticipated plasma levels of the drug are generally indicative of error in dosage regimen, poor bioavailability, rapid elimination or enlarged apparent volume of distribution.

Patient Compliance: Common problems associated with patient compliance may be due to neglect on the part of patient to follow instructions or actual difficulty in compliance. From various studies reported in the literature, there are many factors that may affect patient compliance. These include complicated instructions, multiple daily doses, forgetfulness on the part of the patient resulting either in skipping doses or taking more doses than prescribed, cost of medication, difficulty in swallowing the dosage form and adverse drug reaction. While some of these problems can be easily overcome once the specific problem is identified, there may be other factors that may not be as easy to resolve. Obviously, patient compliance is not a serious problem with institutionalized patients, because these patients have very little choice concerning the prescribed drug and drug dosage form and any compliance problem is identified very quickly. In these cases, problems with patient compliance are dictated by the fact that medication is provided by medical personnel; therefore, there is no skipping of the dose. In the case of ambulatory patients, the patient must remember to take medication as prescribed in order to obtain optimal clinical effect of the drug. Therefore it is very important that the clinician consider patient's life-style and needs when developing dosage regimen.

Special Recommendations: Sometimes it may be essential to give special instructions to a patient in order to achieve the desired goal. For example, the patient may be taking the drug after a meal instead of before a meal or the patient may not be adhering to a special diet (e.g. fat-free or low salt diet). In such cases the patient may not be responding to drug therapy as expected and may need special simple and easy to follow instructions.

INTRAVENOUS ADMINISTRATION

During multiple dosing, when fixed doses of the drug are administered at constant dosing intervals, if it is found that minimum concentration of drug in plasma at steady-state ($C_{min\ ss}$) in a particular patient is greater than the minimum therapeutic concentration of the drug, it implies that the patient may be receiving too much drug than is really necessary for the treatment. Obviously, in this patient, the maximum concentration of drug in plasma at steady-state ($C_{max\ ss}$) may possibly also approach toxic levels. Therefore, dosage regimen should be modified so as to reduce $C_{min\ ss}$ to a level that is approximately equal to or perhaps slightly higher than minimum

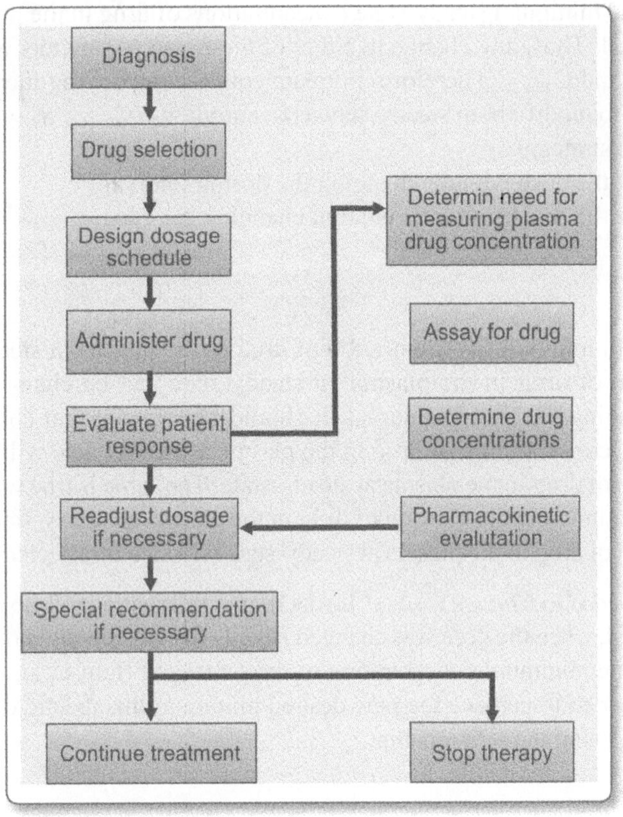

Fig. 17-6 Steps involved in the process of reaching dosage decisions with therapeutic drug monitoring

therapeutic concentration of the drug. Similarly, if in a patient, the minimum concentration of drug in the plasma at steady-state is less than the minimum therapeutic concentration of the drug, then the patient is obviously not receiving enough amount of drug for the treatment, because the plasma profile of the drug in this patient will exhibit periods of subtherapeutic concentration of the drug. If periods of subtherapeutic concentration of drug in the plasma are not desired in a given patient, then the concentration level of $C_{min\ ss}$ should be elevated so that the concentration of drug in the plasma remains equal to or perhaps slightly greater than the minimum therapeutic concentration of the drug. Thus, in the case of patients where the minimum concentration of drug in the plasma at steady-state is either less than or much greater than the minimum effective concentration of drug, the dosage regimen may need to be modified so as to adjust the levels of maximum and/or minimum concentration of drug in the plasma at steady-state, to match the minimum effective concentration of the drug.

For example, one may decide that $C_{min\ ss}$, the minimum concentration of drug at the steady-state, should be made equal to (or slightly greater than) the minimum effective concentration of the drug. From equations (13-30) and (13-29) it can be seen that for drugs, which exhibit linear pharmacokinetics and confer the characteristics of one-compartment model on the body, the steady-state maximum and minimum concentrations of drug in the plasma depend on the following three parameters: (i) The dose; (ii) The dosing interval; and (iii) The elimination rate constant of the drug. This is because both, $C_{max\ ss}$ and $C_{min\ ss}$ are a function of C_0 (which is a function of dose), the dosing interval, τ and the rate constant of elimination, K. Since the overall rate constant of elimination of a drug is assumed to be a fixed and constant quantity and if we assume that the overall rate constant of elimination of the drug does not change during the course of therapy in the patient under treatment, then the only other two variables that affect maximum and minimum steady-state concentrations of drug in the plasma are the dose and the dosing interval. Thus, any change in either of these two parameters would change the value of both, $C_{max\ ss}$ and $C_{min\ ss}$. Therefore, in treatments accompanying therapeutic drug monitoring, it is possible to modify both steady-state concentrations ($C_{max\ ss}$ as well as $C_{min\ ss}$,) by either of the following strategies:

a. Changing the dose without changing the dosing interval
b. Changing the dosing interval without changing the dose.

New Dose

The maximum minimum concentration of drug in the plasma at steady-state or the minimum concentration of drug in the plasma, at steady-state can be changed by changing the dose without changing the dosing interval. It should be realized that changing the dose to adjust the minimum concentration of drug in the plasma at steady-state will also affect the maximum concentration of drug in the plasma at steady-state. The same is true when the dose is changed to adjust the maximum concentration of drug in the plasma at steady-state, viz, now the minimum concentration of drug in the plasma at steady-state will also be affected due to change in the dose.

New Dose Needed to Change $C_{min\ ss}$: It was shown in equation (13-46) that without changing the dosing interval, when the dose was changed from D (usual recommended dose) to D″ (new dose), the steady-state minimum concentration of drug changed from $C_{min\ ss}$ to $C_{min\ ss''}$. Thus, the new Dose (D″) needed to achieve the new desired minimum therapeutic concentration ($C_{min\ ss''}$) can be calculated using the relationship,

$$\frac{C_{min\ ss}}{C_{min\ ss''}} = \frac{D}{D''}$$

therefore,

$$D'' = \frac{(D)(C_{min\ ss''})}{C_{min\ ss}} \tag{17-1}$$

Thus, without changing the dosing interval, the size of the new dose (D″) that should be used to attain the new desired minimum concentration of drug in the plasma at steady-state ($C_{min\ ss''}$) is calculated by multiplying the size of the conventionally recommended dose (D) and the ratio of new desired minimum concentration of drug in the plasma at steady-state ($C_{min\ ss''}$) to the minimum concentration of drug in the plasma at steady-state ($C_{min\ ss}$) attained by the conventionally recommended dose.

As mentioned above, the change in the dose will also affect the maximum concentration at steady-state. This is because $C_{max\ ss}$ is a function of C_0 and C_0 is a function of dose and apparent volume of distribution.

$$\text{Since, } C_0 = \frac{\text{dose}}{\text{apparent volume of distribution}},$$

Therefore, assuming that the apparent volume of distribution of the drug does not change due to a change in the size of the dose, it follows that when dose is changed, C_0 will also change proportionally, i.e.

$$\frac{\text{new } C_0}{\text{old } C_0} = \frac{\text{new dose}}{\text{old dose}} \tag{17-2}$$

$$\text{new } C_0 = \frac{(\text{old } C_0)(\text{new dose})}{\text{old dose}} \tag{17-3}$$

Example 17-1 The following data were obtained after administration of a single 300 mg intravenous bolus dose of an antibiotic: one-compartment pharmacokinetic model with C_0 = 30 μg/mL and K = 0.0866/h. Using these data calculate:

a. The size of dose that should be administered every 6 h in order to provide a minimum steady-state concentration of 27 μg/mL.
b. The maximum steady-state concentration with this dosage regimen.

Solution

a. If a 300 mg dose were administered every 6 hours, the minimum concentration achieved at steady-state can be calculated using the equation (13-30):

$$C_{min\ ss} = \frac{(C_0)(e^{-k\tau})}{1-e^{-kt}}$$

Here, $C_0 = 30$ μg/mL and $e^{-K\tau} = e^{-(0.0866)(6)} = e^{-0.5196} = 0.595$. Substituting these values into equation (13-30),

$$C_{min\ ss} = \frac{(30\ \mu g/mL)\left(e^{(-0.5196/h)(6\ h)}\right)}{1-e^{-(0.0866/h)(6\ h)}}$$

$$= \frac{(30\ \mu g/mL)(0.595)}{1-0.595}$$

$$= \frac{17.85\ \mu g/mL}{0.405} = 44.1\ \mu g/mL$$

That is, a 300 mg dose administered every 6 hours will give the minimum concentration of drug in the plasma at steady-state, $C_{min\ ss} = 44.1$ μg/mL. Since it is desired to attain a steady-state minimum concentration of drug in the plasma = 27 μg/mL and not 44.1 μg/mL, equation (17-1) is used to calculate the size of new dose (D″) that should be administered every 6 h to obtain the new desired minimum concentration of drug in plasma at steady-state ($C_{min\ ss''}$).

$$D'' = \frac{(D)(C_{min\ ss''})}{C_{min\ ss}}$$

$$= \frac{(300\ mg)(27\ \mu g/mL)}{44.1\ \mu g/mL} = 183.7\ mg$$

Therefore a 183.7 mg dose administered every 6 hours will provide the minimum steady-state concentration of 27 μg/mL.

b. To calculate the maximum concentration at steady-state attained with a dose of 183.7 mg, we need to calculate new C_0 because the observed $C_0 = 30$ μg/mL was obtained with a dose of 300 mg.

Equation (17-3) is used to calculate new C_0 (based on the new dose).

$$\text{new } C_0 = \frac{(\text{old } C_0)(\text{new dose})}{\text{old dose}}$$

$$= \frac{(30\ \mu g/mL)(183.7\ mg)}{300\ mg} = 18.37\ mg$$

Substituting the value of new C_0 (= 18.37 μg/mL) and $e^{-K\tau}$ (= $e^{-(0.0866)(6)} = 0.595$) into equation (13-29),

$$C_{max\ ss} = \frac{C_0}{1-e^{-K\tau}}$$

$$C_{max\ ss} = \frac{18.37\ \mu g/mL}{1-e^{-(0.0866/h)(6\ h)}}$$

$$= \frac{18.37\ \mu g/mL}{1-0.595}$$

$$= \frac{18.37\ \mu g/mL}{0.405} = 45.4\ \mu g/mL$$

From the calculations shown above, it is seen that in order to change the minimum concentration of drug in the plasma at steady-state from 44.1 μg/mL to 27 μg/mL, the dosage regimen is changed from a 300 mg dose administered very 6 h to a 183.7 mg dose administered every 6 hr. Due to the change in dose from 300 mg to 183.7 mg, the maximum concentration of drug in the plasma at steady-state will now be 45.4 μg/mL.

New dose needed to change $C_{max\ ss}$: From equation (13-45) it is seen that without changing dosing interval, when the usual dose, D, was changed to D″, the maximum concentration of drug in the plasma at steady-state changed from $C_{max\ ss}$ to $C_{max\ ss''}$.

Therefore, the new dose (D″) needed to achieve $C_{max\ ss''}$ can be calculated using the relationship:

$$\frac{C_{max\ ss}}{C_{max\ ss''}} = \frac{D}{D''}$$

$$D'' = \frac{(D)(C_{max\ ss''})}{C_{max\ ss}} \tag{17-4}$$

Thus, without changing the dosing interval, the size of the new dose (D″) that should be used to attain the new desired maximum concentration of drug in the plasma at steady-state ($C_{max\ ss''}$) is calculated by multiplying the size of the usually recommended dose (D) and the ratio of the new desired maximum concentration of drug in the plasma at steady-state ($C_{max\ ss''}$) to the maximum concentration of drug in the plasma at steady-state ($C_{max\ ss}$) achieved when the usually recommended dose (D) is used.

Just as was seen in the case of adjustment of dose (without changing the dosing interval) to achieve the desired minimum steady-state concentration of drug in the plasma, the change in dose to alter the maximum concentration of drug in the plasma at steady-state will also affect the minimum concentration of drug in the plasma at steady-state. This is because $C_{min\ ss}$ is also a function of C_0 and C_0 is a function of dose and the apparent volume of distribution.

Assuming that the apparent volume of distribution of the drug does not change with the change in dose, it follows that when the dose is changed, C_0 will also change proportionally according to the following relationship (which is the same as equation [17-3] described previously).

$$\text{new } C_0 = \frac{(\text{old } C_0)(\text{new dose})}{\text{old dose}}$$

Example 17-2 Using the data given in Example 17-1, calculate the following:

a. The size of dose that should be administered every 6 hours in order to provide a maximum steady-state concentration of 97 μg/mL.
b. The expected minimum concentration at steady-state with this dosage regimen.

Solution

a. If a 300 mg dose were administered every 6 hours, the maximum concentration of drug in the plasma at steady-state can be calculated using equation (13-29):

$$C_{max\ ss} = \frac{C}{1 - e^{-K\tau}}$$

Substituting the values of C_0 (= 30 μg/mL) and $e^{-K\tau}$ (= $e^{-(0.0866)(6)}$ = 0.595) from Example 17-1 into this equation,

$$C_{max\ ss} = \frac{30\ \mu g/mL}{1 - e^{-(0.0866/h)(6\ h)}}$$

$$= \frac{30\ \mu g/mL}{1 - 0.595}$$

$$= \frac{30\ \mu g/mL}{0.405} = 74.1\ \mu g/mL$$

That is, a 300 mg dose administered every 6 hours will provide the maximum concentration of drug in the plasma at steady-state, $C_{max\ ss}$ = 74.1 μg/mL.

Since it is desired to attain a maximum steady-state concentration of drug = 97 μg/mL, instead of 74.1 μg/mL, equation (17-4) is used to calculate the size of new dose (D″) that should be administered every 6 hours to give the new desired maximum concentration of drug in the plasma at steady-state ($C_{max\ ss''}$):

$$D'' = \frac{(D)(C_{max\ ss''})}{C_{max\ ss}}$$

$$= \frac{(300\ mg)(97\ \mu g/mL)}{74.1\ \mu g/mL} = 392.8\ mg$$

b. To calculate the new minimum steady-state concentration when the dose is changed from 300 mg o 392.8 mg, we need to know the new C_0 based upon the new dose. Using equation (17-3) to calculate

$$\text{new } C_0 = \frac{(\text{old } C_0)(\text{new dose})}{\text{old dose}}$$

$$= \frac{(30\ \mu g/mL)(392.8\ mg)}{300\ mg} = 39.28\ mg$$

Substituting the values of C_0 (= 39.28 μg/mL) and $e^{-K\tau}$ (= $e^{-(0.0866)(6)}$ = 0.595) into equation (13-30),

$$C_{min\ ss} = \frac{(C_0)(e^{-K\tau})}{1 - e^{-K\tau}}$$

$$C_{min\ ss} = \frac{(39.28\ \mu g/mL)(e^{-(0.0866/h)(6\,h)})}{1 - e^{-(0.0866/h)(6\,h)}}$$

$$= \frac{(39.28\ \mu g/mL)(0.595)}{1 - 0.595} = \frac{23.37\ \mu g/mL}{0.405} = 57.7\ \mu g/mL$$

From the calculations shown above, it is seen that to increase $C_{max\ ss}$ from 74.1 to 97 μg/mL, the dosage regimen should be changed from 300 mg every 6 hours to 392.8 mg every 6 hr. Because of the change in dose, the minimum concentration of drug in the plasma at steady-state will also increase from 44.1 μg/mL, as shown in Example 17-1, to 57.7 μg/mL.

New Dosing Interval

The maximum and minimum concentrations at steady-state can be modified by changing the dosing interval without changing the dose. The dosing interval can be calculated by rearranging equation (13-30) for the minimum concentration of drug in the plasma at steady-state or equation (13-29) for maximum concentration of drug in the plasma at steady-state.

New Dosing Interval to Change $C_{min\ ss}$

According to equation (13-30), the minimum concentration of drug in the plasma at steady-state is given by

$$C_{min\ ss} = \frac{(C_0)(e^{-K\tau})}{1 - e^{-K\tau}}$$

which upon cross-multiplication gives

$$(C_0)(e^{-K\tau}) = (C_{min\ ss})(1 - e^{-K\tau}) \tag{17-5}$$

Equation (17-5) may be written as

$$(C_0)(e^{-K\tau}) = (C_{min\ ss}) - (C_{min\ ss})(e^{-K\tau}) \tag{17-6}$$

Equation (17-6) can be rearranged as follows:
$-K\tau$

$$(C_0)(e^{-K\tau}) + (C_{min\ ss})(e^{-K\tau}) = C_{min\ ss} \tag{17-7}$$

Since the quantity ($e^{-K\tau}$) is common to both terms of the left-hand side of equation (17-7), equation (17-7) can be simplified to

$$(e^{-K\tau})(C_0 + C_{min\ ss}) = C_{min\ ss} \tag{17-8}$$

Dividing both sides of equation (17-8) with ($C_0 + C_{min\ ss}$), we have

$$e^{-K\tau} = \frac{C_{min\ ss}}{C_0 + C_{min\ ss}} \tag{17-9}$$

Equation (17-9) may be written as

$$\frac{1}{e^{K\tau}} = \frac{C_{min\ ss}}{C_0 + C_{min\ ss}} \tag{17-10}$$

Cross multiplication and rearrangement of equation (17-10) gives

$$e^{K\tau} = \frac{C_0 + C_{min\ ss}}{C_{min\ ss}} \tag{17-11}$$

Taking natural logarithms on both sides of equation (17-11) yields,

$$K\tau = \ln \frac{C_0 + C_{min\ ss}}{C_{min\ ss}} \tag{17-12}$$

Solving for τ, equation (17-12) becomes

$$\tau = \left(\frac{1}{k}\right) \ln \frac{C_0 + C_{min\ ss}}{C_{min\ ss}} \tag{17-13}$$

Thus, if the dose is not changed, the dosing interval needed to attain the new desired minimum concentration at steady-state ($C_{min\ ss''}$) is given by

$$\tau = \left(\frac{1}{k}\right) \ln \frac{C_0 + C_{min\ ss''}}{C_{min\ ss''}} \tag{17-14}$$

Example 17-3 Using the data provided in Example 17-1, calculate frequency of administration of a 300 mg dose if it is desired to maintain the minimum steady-state concentration of drug in the plasma at 27 μg/mL.

Solution

It was found in Example 17-1 that a 300 mg dose administered every 6 hours gave minimum steady-state concentration of drug in the plasma = 44.1 μg/mL. To calculate the frequency of administration of 300 mg dose to attain 27 mcg/mL as the minimum steady-state concentration, one substitutes the values of C_0, K and $C_{min\ ss''}$ found in Example 17-1 into equation (17-14)

$$\tau = \left(\frac{1}{k}\right) \ln \frac{C_0 + C_{min\ ss''}}{C_{min\ ss''}}$$

Substituting the values of C_0, K and the new desired $C_{min\ ss''}$ into equation (17-14),

$$\tau = \left(\frac{1}{0.0866/\text{h}}\right) \ln \frac{30\ \mu\text{g/mL} + 27\ \mu\text{g/mL}}{27\ \mu\text{g/mL}}$$

$$= \left(\frac{1}{0.0866/\text{h}}\right) \ln 2.1111$$

$$= \left(\frac{1}{0.0866/\text{h}}\right) (0.7472) = 8.637 \text{ h}$$

Thus, a dose of 300 mg administered every 8.63 hours (instead of 6 hours) will reduce the minimum steady-state concentration of drug in plasma from 44.1 μg/mL to the desired 27 μg/mL.

As indicated earlier, just as changing the dose for adjusting $C_{min\ ss}$ affected $C_{max\ ss}$, changing the dosing interval to adjust minimum concentration of drug in plasma at steady-state will also influence maximum concentration of drug in the plasma at steady-state. The maximum concentration of drug in plasma at steady-state can be calculated using equation (13-29)

$$C_{max\ ss} = \frac{C_0}{1 - e^{-K\tau}}$$

In this case, since the dose is not changed, the value of C_0 is remains unchanged. However, since dosing interval is changed, the value of $e^{-K\tau}$ must be recalculated.

$$(K)(\tau) = (0.0866/\text{h})(8.63 \text{ h}) = 0.7474 \text{ and } e^{-K\tau} = e^{-0.7474} = 0.4736.$$

Therefore,

$$C_{max\ ss} = \frac{30\ \mu\text{g/mL}}{1 - e^{-(0.0866/\text{h})(8.63\ \text{h})}}$$

$$= \frac{30\ \mu\text{g/mL}}{1 - 0.4736}$$

$$= \frac{30\ \mu\text{g/mL}}{0.5264} = 57\ \mu\text{g/mL}$$

Note that the value of $C_{max\ ss}$ found in this Example is greater than that found in Example 17-1 even though the $C_{min\ ss}$ values in both cases was identical. This is because the dose and dosing interval are different in the two Examples.

New dosing interval to change $C_{max\ ss}$: According to equation (13-29),

$$C_{max\ ss} = \frac{C_0}{1 - e^{-K\tau}}$$

Cross-multiplication of equation (13-29) gives

$$C_0 = (C_{max\ ss})(1 - e^{-K\tau}) \tag{17-15}$$

Equation (17-15) may be written as

$$C_0 = (C_{max\ ss}) - (C_{max\ ss})(e^{-K\tau}) \tag{17-16}$$

Rearranging equation (17-16),

$$(C_{max\ ss})(e^{-K\tau}) = C_{max\ ss} - C_0 \tag{17-17}$$

Solving for $e^{-K\tau}$, equation (17-17) becomes

$$e^{-K\tau} = \frac{C_{max\ ss} - C_0}{C_{max\ ss}} \tag{17-18}$$

Equation (17-18) may be written as:

$$\frac{1}{e^{K\tau}} = \frac{C_{max\ ss} - C_0}{C_{max\ ss}} \tag{17-19}$$

Cross multiplication and rearrangement of equation (17-19) yields:

$$e^{K\tau} = \frac{C_{max\ ss}}{C_{max\ ss} - C_0} \tag{17-20}$$

Taking natural logarithms on both sides,

$$K\tau = \ln \frac{C_{max\ ss}}{C_{max\ ss} - C_0} \tag{17-21}$$

$$\tau = \left(\frac{1}{K}\right) \ln \frac{C_{max\ ss}}{C_{max\ ss} - C_0} \tag{17-22}$$

Thus, the dosing interval needed to attain the new desired maximum concentration of drug in the plasma at steady-state ($C_{max\ ss''}$) is given by

$$\tau = \left(\frac{1}{K}\right) \ln \frac{C_{max\ ss''}}{C_{max\ ss''} - C_0} \tag{17-23}$$

Example 17-4 Using the data given in Example 17-1, calculate the dosing interval for the 300 mg dose if it is desired to maintain $C_{max\ ss}$ at 97 μg/mL.

Solution

It was found in Example 17-2 that when a 300 mg dose was administered every 6 hours, the maximum concentration of drug in the plasma at steady-state was 74.1 μg/mL. In order to calculate the frequency of administration of drug dose (dosing interval) without changing the size of dose, so as to increase the maximum concentration of drug in the plasma at steady-state to a level of 97 mcg/mL, equation (17-23) is used.

Substituting the values of C_0 (= 30 mcg/mL) and K (= 0.0866/h) from Example 17-1 and the desired $C_{max\ ss''}$ = 97 μg/mL, into equation (17-23) gives:

$$\tau = \left(\frac{1}{K}\right) \ln \frac{C_{max\ ss''}}{C_{max\ ss''} - C_0}$$

$$\tau = \left(\frac{1}{0.0866/h}\right) \ln \frac{97\ \mu g/mL}{97\ \mu g/mL - 30\ \mu g/mL}$$

$$= \left(\frac{1}{0.0866/h}\right) \ln \frac{97\ \mu g/mL}{67\ \mu g/mL}$$

$$= \left(\frac{1}{0.0866/h}\right) \ln 1.4478 = \frac{0.37}{0.0866/h} \ln 1.4478 == 4.27\ h$$

Thus, a 300 mg dose administered every 4.27 hours will provide the maximum steady-state concentration of drug in the plasma = 97 μg/mL. As was seen in Example 17-3, changing the dosing interval here will also influence the minimum steady-state concentration of drug in the plasma. In this particular case, the minimum concentration at steady-state can be calculated using equation (13-30)

$$C_{min\ ss} = \frac{(C_0)(e^{-Kgt})}{1 - e^{-K\tau}}$$

Since the size of the dose was not changed, the value of C_0 remains at 30 μg/mL (as given in Example 17-1). Since frequency of administration is now changed from 6 hours to 4.27 hours, the value of $e^{-K\tau}$ must be recalculated. (K)(τ) = (0.0866/h)(4.27 h) = 0.3698, $e^{-K\tau} = e^{-0.3698}$ = 0.6909. Therefore,

$$C_{min\ ss} = \frac{(30\ \mu g/mL)\left(e^{-(0.0866/h)(4.27\ h)}\right)}{1 - e^{-(0.0866/h)(4.27\ h)}}$$

$$= \frac{(30\ \mu g/mL)(0.6909)}{1 - 0.6909}$$

$$= \frac{20.707\ \mu g/mL}{0.3091} = 67.1\ \mu g/mL$$

Thus, changing the dosing interval (without changing the size of the dose) from 6 hours to 4.27 hours will increase the minimum concentration of drug in the plasma at steady-state from 47.1 μg/mL (as found in Example 17-1) to 67.1 μg/mL.

EXTRAVASCULAR ADMINISTRATION

In multiple dosing during extravascular administration, the difference between minimum therapeutic concentration and steady-state concentration (either $C_{min\ ss}$, the minimum concentration at steady-state or $C_{max\ ss}$, the maximum concentration at steady-state), may also have consequences similar to those indicated in the discussion dealing with the intravenous administration of the drug. Therefore, dosage regimen during extravascular administration may also require adjustments to suit the needs of the individual patient. The adjustment of the levels of maximum and/or minimum concentration of drug in the plasma at steady-state can be accomplished using the same rationale that was used for the adjustment of maximum and minimum steady-state concentrations during intravenous administration of the drug.

From a pharmacokinetic stand-point, the difference in the two routes of administrations is that during intravenous administration, both $C_{max\ ss}$ and $C_{min\ ss}$ depend on two factors:

i. C_0, which is a function of the apparent volume of distribution and size of the dose of the drug.
ii. $K\tau$, which is a function of the elimination rate constant and dosing interval.

During extravascular administration, on the other hand, while $C_{min\ ss}$ depends on B and $K\tau$, $C_{max\ ss}$ depends on B, $K\tau$ and the factor R as described in Chapter 13.

It will be recalled that the y-intercept B is the back-extrapolated y-intercept of the terminal linear portion of elimination phase of the plasma profile and B is a function of:

i. The dose of the drug administered
ii. The fraction of dose absorbed
iii. The apparent volume of distribution of the drug
iv. The rate constant of absorption of the drug
v. The rate constant of elimination of the drug.

The factor R, it will be recalled, is a function of rate constant of elimination and time of maximum absorption of the drug. For drugs, which follow linear pharmacokinetics and confer the characteristics of one-compartment model upon the body, the following four factors may be considered constant and not change during the course of therapy:

a. The apparent volume of distribution of the drug
b. The rate constant of absorption of the drug
c. The rate constant of elimination of the drug
d. The fraction of dose absorbed.

Since the time of maximum absorption (t_{max}) depends primarily on the absorption rate constant of the drug, this parameter may also be assumed to remain constant. Thus, there are only two variables, which may affect the maximum and minimum concentrations of drug in the plasma at steady-state during extravascular administration. These two variables are:

a. The size of maintenance dose of the drug
b. The dosing interval or the frequency of administration of the drug dose.

This is exactly what was found during intravenous administration of the drug. Therefore, a change in either the size of the dose or the dosing interval, would also change the value of $C_{max\ ss}$ and $C_{min\ ss}$.

New Dose

The effect of dose on steady-state concentrations of drug in plasma during extravascular administration of the drug is comparable to the effect of dose during intravenous administration. Similar to intravenous administration, the steady-state maximum and minimum concentrations of drug in the plasma during extravascular administration can be changed by changing the dose without changing the dosing interval. It should be realized, however, that if the dose is changed to adjust the minimum concentration of drug in the plasma at steady-state, the change in dose will also affect the maximum concentration of drug in the plasma at steady-state. Similarly, if the dose is changed to adjust the maximum concentration of drug in the plasma at steady-state, the change in dose will also affect the minimum concentration of drug in the plasma at steady-state.

New Dose Needed to Change $C_{min\,ss}$: It was shown in equation (13-45) that during extravascular administration, when the dose was changed from D to D″ (without changing the dosing interval), the minimum concentration of drug in the plasma at steady-state changed from $C_{min\,ss}$ to $C_{min\,ss''}$. Therefore, the new dose (D″) needed to achieve the new desired minimum therapeutic concentration ($C_{min\,ss''}$) can be calculated using the same relationship that was used to calculate the desired minimum therapeutic concentration of drug in the plasma during intravenous administration, i.e. equation (13-45) and equation (17-1):

$$\frac{C_{min\,ss}}{C_{min\,ss''}} = \frac{D}{D''}$$

$$D'' = \frac{(D)(C_{min\,ss''})}{C_{min\,ss}}$$

Thus, without changing the dosing interval, the size of the new dose (D″) that should be used to attain the new desired minimum concentration of drug in the plasma at steady-state ($C_{min\,ss''}$) during extravascular administration is calculated in the same manner that was used for the intravenous administration of the drug, i.e. by multiplying the size of the usually recommended dose (D) and the ratio of new desired minimum concentration of drug in the plasma at steady-state ($C_{min\,ss''}$) to the minimum concentration of drug in plasma at steady-state ($C_{min\,ss}$) attained by the conventionally recommended dose. Similar to intravenous administration, here also, due to the change in dose, maximum concentration of drug in the plasma at steady-state will change too.

New Dose Needed to Change $C_{max\,ss}$: From equation (13-46) it is seen that without changing the dosing interval, when the usual dose (D) is changed to the new dose (D″), the steady-state maximum concentration of drug in the plasma changed from $C_{max\,ss}$ to $C_{max\,ss''}$. Therefore, the new dose (D″) that will be needed to achieve the new desired $C_{max\,ss''}$ during extravascular administration of the drug can be calculated using the same relationship that was used for calculating the desired maximum concentration of drug in the plasma at steady-state during intravenous administration, i.e. equation (13-46) and equation (17-4):

$$\frac{C_{min\,ss}}{C_{min\,ss}} = \frac{D}{D''}$$

$$D'' = \frac{(D)(C_{min\,ss''})}{C_{min\,ss}}$$

Thus, the size of new dose (D″) that should be used to reach the new desired maximum concentration of drug in the plasma at steady-state ($C_{max\,ss''}$) can be calculated by multiplying the size of the usual recommended dose (D) with the ratio of the new desired maximum concentration of drug in the plasma at steady-state ($C_{max\,ss''}$) to the maximum concentration of drug at steady-state ($C_{max\,ss}$) achieved when the usually recommended dose (D) is used.

Example 17-5 The suggested dosage regimen of a drug is 500 mg tablet every 4 hr. According to the manufacturer, the drug, on administration, confers upon the body the characteristics of one compartment pharmacokinetic model with the following parameters: y-intercept, B = 30 mcg/mL, first-order rate constant of absorption, K_a = 1.5/h, and the first-order rate constant of elimination, K = 0.14/h. If it is desired that the maximum concentration of drug in the plasma at steady-state should not be less than 60 mcg/mL, calculate the size of dose, assuming F = 1.

Solution

If the manufacturer's recommended dosage regimen is followed, the maximum concentration of drug at steady-state will be calculated using equation (13-36):

$$C_{max\ ss} = \frac{(B)(e^{-R})}{1 - e^{-K\tau}}$$

To calculate $C_{max\ ss}$, we need to determine the values of $e^{-K\tau}$ and e^{-R}.

From the data provided: $e^{-K\tau} = e^{-(0.14)(4)} = e^{-0.56} = 0.5712$.

Since, $R = (K)(t_{max})$, we calculate the time of maximum concentration using equation (13-38):

$$t_{max} = \frac{\ln K_a - \ln K}{K_a - K}$$

$$= \frac{\ln 1.5/h - \ln 0.14/h}{1.5/h - 0.14/h} = \frac{2.37158}{1.36/h} = 1.7438\ h$$

Therefore, $R = (K)(t_{max}) = (0.14/h)(1.7438\ h) = 0.2441$, and $e^{-R} = e^{-0.2441} = 0.7834$

Substituting the values of B (= 30 μg/mL), e^{-R} (= 0.7834), and $e^{-K\tau}$ (= 0.5712) into equation (13-36):

$$C_{max\ ss} = \frac{(30\ \mu g/mL)\left(e^{-(0.14/h)(1.7438\,h)}\right)}{1 - e^{-(0.14/h)(4\,h)}}$$

$$= \frac{(30\ \mu g/mL)(0.7834)}{1 - 0.5712}$$

$$= \frac{23.50\ \mu g/mL}{0.4288} = 54.804\ \mu g/mL$$

Thus, extravascular administration of a 500 mg dose every 4 hours will provide a maximum steady-state plasma concentration of 54.804 μg/mL.

Since it is desired that the maximum concentration of drug in plasma at steady-state should not fall below 60 μg/mL, equation (17-4) is used to calculate the size of new dose (D″) that should be administered to the patient. Substituting the values of D = 500 mg, $C_{max\ ss}$ = 54.804 mcg/mL, and $C_{max\ ss''}$ = 60 mg into equation (17-4):

$$D'' = \frac{(D)(C_{max\ ss''})}{C_{max\ ss}}$$

$$= \frac{(500\ mg)(60\ \mu g/mL)}{54.804\ \mu g/mL} = 547.4\ mg$$

New Dosing Interval

The maximum and minimum concentrations of drug in the plasma at steady-state during extravascular administration of the drug can be modified by changing τ, the dosing interval without changing D, the size of the usually recommended maintenance dose. The new dosing interval (frequency of administration) can be calculated by rearranging equation (13-42) for the minimum concentration of drug in the plasma at steady-state and equation (13-36) for the maximum steady-state concentration of drug in the plasma.

New Dosing Interval to Change $C_{min\ ss}$: According to equation (13-42), the minimum steady-state concentration of drug in the plasma during extravascular administration is given by:

$$C_{min\ ss} = \frac{(B)(e^{-K\tau})}{1 - e^{-K\tau}}$$

Equation (13-42) is similar to equation (13-30), which is used for calculating steady-state minimum concentration of drug in the plasma during intravenous administration, with only one exception: the term C_0 in equation (13-30) is replaced by the term B in equation (13-42). It will be recalled that both, C_0 and B, are y-intercepts of the plasma profile. The y-intercept C_0 is obtained by back-extrapolating the linear plasma profile following intravenous administration of the drug, whereas y-intercept B is obtained by back-extrapolating the terminal linear portion of elimination phase of the plasma profile. This means that by using the same rationale that was used in rearranging equation (13-30) to develop equation (17-14), one should be able to rearrange equation (13-42) to arrive at an equation similar to equation (17-14) except that in equation (17-14), C_0 is replaced by B.

Therefore, the dosing interval needed to attain the new desired minimum concentration of drug in the plasma at steady-state ($C_{min\ ss''}$) is given by:

$$\tau = \left(\frac{1}{K}\right)\ln\frac{B + C_{min\ ss''}}{C_{min\ ss''}} \qquad (17\text{-}24)$$

where, $C_{min\ ss''}$ is the new desired minimum concentration of drug in the plasma at steady-state during extravascular administration.

Example 17-6 The following data were obtained after the administration of a 500 mg oral dose of an antibiotic: one-compartment pharmacokinetic model with y-intercept, B = 40 μg/mL, first-order rate constant of absorption, K_a = 1.757/h and first-order rate constant of elimination, K = 0.1732/h. If the minimum effective concentration of the drug is 15 μg/mL and it is desired to maintain $C_{min\ ss}$ at 16 μg/mL, calculate:

a. The dosing interval that should be used to provide desired minimum concentration of drug in the plasma at steady-state for a 500 mg dose.
b. The maximum steady-state concentration of drug in the plasma with this dosage regimen.

Solution

a. The frequency of administration (without changing the dose) to attain the desired minimum steady-state concentration of drug in the plasma = 16 μg/mL is calculated using equation (17-24)

$$\tau = \left(\frac{1}{K}\right)\ln\frac{B + C_{min\ ss''}}{C_{min\ ss''}}$$

Substituting B = 40 μg/mL, K = 0.1732/h, and $C_{min\ ss''}$ = 16 μg/mL into equation (17-24),

$$\tau = \left(\frac{1}{0.1732/\text{h}}\right)\ln\frac{40\ \mu\text{g/mL} + 16\ \mu\text{g/mL}}{16\ \mu\text{g/mL}}$$

$$= \left(\frac{1}{0.1732/\text{h}}\right)\ln\frac{56\ \mu\text{g/mL}}{16\ \mu\text{g/mL}}$$

$$= \left(\frac{1}{0.1732/\text{h}}\right)\ln 3.5 = \frac{1.2528}{0.1732/\text{h}} = 7.23\ \text{h}$$

Thus, administering the 500 mg dose every 7.23 hours will provide the desired 16 μg/mL minimum concentration of drug in the plasma at steady-state.

b. To calculate maximum concentration of drug in plasma at steady-state when a 500 mg dose is administered every 7.23 hours, following equation (13-36) is used.

$$C_{max\ ss} = \frac{(B)(e^{-R})}{1 - e^{-K\tau}}$$

Since the dose is not changed, the value of B remains the same (= 40 μg/mL). Also, because the rate constant of absorption, K_a and the rate constant of elimination, K, are not affected, therefore, the time of maximum concentration, t_{max}, remains unaffected (because time of maximum concentration is a function of rate constants of absorption and elimination). Similarly, the factor R is not changed because the factor R is a function of rate constant of elimination and time of maximum concentration. However, since the dosing interval is changed, the value of $e^{-K\tau}$ must be recalculated.

First, we calculate the time of maximum concentration. From equation (13-38),

$$t_{max} = \frac{\ln K_a - \ln K}{K_a - K}$$

$$= \frac{\ln 1.757/h - \ln 0.1732/h}{1.757/h - 0.1732/h}$$

$$= \frac{2.3169}{1.5838/h} = 1.4629 \text{ h}$$

The factor, $R = (K)(t_{max}) = (0.1732/h)(1.4629 \text{ h}) = 0.2534$, therefore, $e^{-R} = e^{-0.2534} = 0.7762$
$(K)(\tau) = (0.1732/h)(7.23 \text{ h}) = 1.2522$, therefore, $e^{-K\tau} = e^{-1.2522} = 0.2859$.

Substituting the values of B, e^{-R} and $e^{-K\tau}$ into equation (13-36), we have:

$$C_{max\ ss} = \frac{(40\ \mu g/mL)\left(e^{-(0.1732/h)(1.4629\ h)}\right)}{1 - e^{-(0.1732/h)(7.23\ h)}}$$

$$= \frac{(40\ \mu g/mL)(0.7762)}{1 - 0.2859}$$

$$= \frac{31.048\ \mu g/mL}{0.7141} = 43.48\ \mu g/mL$$

Thus, extravascular administration the 500 mg dose every 7.23 hours will provide maximum concentration = 43.48 μg/mL of drug in plasma at steady-state.

New Dosing Interval to Change $C_{max\ ss}$: According to equation (13-36), the maximum steady-state concentration of drug in the plasma during extravascular administration is given by:

$$C_{max\ ss} = \frac{(B)(e^{-R})}{1 - e^{-K\tau}}$$

This equation is similar to equation (13-29), which is used for calculating maximum concentration of drug in plasma during intravenous administration, except that the term C_0 in equation (13-29) is replaced by the term Be^{-R} in equation (13-36). This means that using the same rationale that was used in rearranging equation (13-29) to solve for τ in order to develop equation (17-14), one should be able to rearrange equation (13-36) to arrive at an equation that can be used to determine dosing interval for the desired steady-state maximum concentration of the drug in plasma. Equation (13-36) may be written as

$$(C_{max\ ss}) - (C_{max\ ss})(e^{-K\tau}) = (B)(e^{-R}) \tag{17-25}$$

or

$$-(C_{max\ ss})(e^{-K\tau}) = (B)(e^{-R}) - (C_{max\ ss}) \tag{17-26}$$

Equation (17-26) may be written as

$$(C_{max\ ss})(e^{-K\tau}) = (C_{max\ ss}) - (B)(e^{-R}) \tag{17-27}$$

$$e^{-K\tau} = \frac{(C_{max\ ss}) - (B)(e^{-R})}{C_{max\ ss}} \tag{17-28}$$

Equation (17-28) may be written as:

$$\frac{1}{e^{K\tau}} = \frac{(C_{\max ss}) - (B)(e^{-R})}{C_{\max ss}} \tag{17-29}$$

cross multiplication and rearrangement of equation (17-29) gives

$$e^{K\tau} = \frac{C_{\max ss}}{(C_{\max ss}) - (B)(e^{-R})} \tag{17-30}$$

Taking natural logarithms on both sides of equation (17-30) yields,

$$K\tau = \ln\frac{C_{\max ss}}{(C_{\max ss}) - (B)(e^{-R})} \tag{17-31}$$

$$\tau = \ln\left(\frac{1}{K}\right)\ln\frac{C_{\max ss}}{(C_{\max ss}) - (B)(e^{-R})} \tag{17-32}$$

Thus, the dosing interval needed to attain the new desired maximum concentration of drug in the plasma at steady-state ($C_{\max ss''}$) is given by

$$\tau = \left(\frac{1}{K}\right)\ln\frac{C_{\max ss''}}{(C_{\max ss''}) - (B)(e^{-R})} \tag{17-33}$$

Example 17-7 From the data given in Example 17-6, if it is desired to attain the maximum concentration of drug in plasma at steady-state at 65 mcg/mL, calculate:

a. The frequency of administration of the 500 mg dose.
b. The minimum steady-state concentration of drug in the plasma at this dosage regimen.

Solution

a. Equation (17-33) is used to calculate the frequency of administration.

From the data in Example 17-6, $K = 0.1732/\text{h}$ and. $e^{-R} = e^{-(0.1732)(1.4629)} = 0.7762$

Substituting these values into equation (17-33) for the new desired maximum steady-state concentration of drug in the plasma ($C_{\max ss''}$) of 65 µg/mL,

$$\tau = \left(\frac{1}{0.1732/\text{h}}\right)\ln\frac{65\ \mu\text{g/mL}}{65\ \mu\text{g/mL} - (40\ \mu\text{g/mL})\left(e^{-(0.1732/\text{h})(1.4629\,\text{h})}\right)}$$

$$= \left(\frac{1}{0.1732/\text{h}}\right)\ln\frac{65\ \mu\text{g/mL}}{65\ \mu\text{g/mL} - (40\ \mu\text{g/mL})(0.7762)}$$

$$= \left(\frac{1}{0.1732/\text{h}}\right)\ln\frac{65\ \mu\text{g/mL}}{33.952\ \mu\text{g/mL}}$$

$$= \left(\frac{1}{0.1732/\text{h}}\right)\ln 1.9145$$

$$= \frac{0.6694}{0.1732/\text{h}} = 3.86\ \text{h}$$

That is, a 500 mg dose administered every 3.75 hours will attain maximum steady-state concentration of 65 µg/mL.

b. With this dosage regimen, the expected minimum steady-state concentration of drug in the plasma can be calculated using equation (13-42).
Since the dose is not changed, the value of *B* remains at 40 mcg/mL.
The value of the persistence factor (when $\tau = 3.75$ h), is calculated as follows:

$$e^{-K\tau} = e^{-(0.1732)(3.75)} = e^{-0.6495} = 0.5223.$$

Substituting the values of B and $e^{-K\tau}$ into equation (13-42),

$$C_{min\ ss} = \frac{(40\ \mu g/mL)\left(e^{-(0.1732/h)(3.75\ h)}\right)}{1 - e^{-(0.1732/h)(3.75\ h)}}$$

$$= \frac{(40\ \mu g/mL)(0.5223)}{1 - 0.5223}$$

$$= \frac{20.89\ \mu g/mL}{0.4777} = 43.73\ \mu g/mL$$

That is, administration of the 500 mg dose every 3.75 hours to attain the maximum steady-state concentration of drug in plasma at 65 μg/mL will provide the minimum concentration of drug in plasma at steady-state = 43.73 μg/mL.

Example 17-8 The following data were obtained after the administration of a 400 mg oral dose of an antibiotic: one-compartment pharmacokinetic model with *y*-intercept, B = 30 μg/mL, first-order rate constant of absorption, K_a = 1.757/h and first-order rate constant of elimination, K = 0.1732/h. If it is desired to attain the maximum concentration of drug in plasma at steady-state at 50 μg/mL, calculate:

a. The frequency of administration of the 500 mg dose
b. The minimum steady-state concentration of drug in the plasma at this dosage regimen.

Solution

$$K = 0.1732/h \text{ and.} e^{-R} = e^{-(0.1732)(1.4629)} = 0.7762$$

Substituting these values into equation (17-33) for the new desired maximum steady-state concentration of drug in the plasma ($C_{max\ ss''}$) of 50 mcg/mL,

$$\tau = \left(\frac{1}{0.1732/h}\right) \ln \frac{50\ \mu g/mL}{50\ \mu g/mL - (30\ \mu g/mL)\left(e^{-(0.1732/h)(1.4629\ h)}\right)}$$

$$= \left(\frac{1}{0.1732/h}\right) \ln \frac{50\ \mu g/mL}{50\ \mu g/mL - (30\ \mu g/mL)(0.7762)}$$

$$= \left(\frac{1}{0.1732/h}\right) \ln \frac{50\ \mu g/mL}{26.714\ \mu g/mL}$$

$$= \left(\frac{1}{0.1732/h}\right) \ln 1.8717 = \frac{0.6268}{0.1732/h} = 3.62\ h$$

That is, a 400 mg dose administered every 3.62 hours will attain the maximum steady-state concentration of 50 μg/mL.

b. With this dosage regimen, the expected minimum steady-state concentration of drug in the plasma can be calculated using equation (13-42).
Since the dose is not changed, the value of B remains at 30 μg/mL.
The value of the persistence factor (when τ = 3.62 h), is calculated as follows:

$$e^{-K\tau} = e^{-(0.1732)(3.62)} = e^{-0.627} = 0.5342.$$

Substituting the values of B and $e^{-K\tau}$ into equation (13-42),

$$C_{min\ ss} = \frac{(30\ \mu g/mL)\left(e^{-(0.1732/h)(3.62\ h)}\right)}{1 - e^{-(0.1732/h)(3.62\ h)}}$$

$$= \frac{(30\ \mu g/mL)(0.5342)}{1 - 0.5342}$$

$$= \frac{16.026\ \mu g/mL}{0.4658} = 34.41\ \mu g/mL$$

That is, administration of the 400 mg dose every 3.62 hours to attain the maximum steady-state concentration of drug in plasma at 50 μg/mL will provide the minimum concentration of drug in plasma at steady-state = 34.41 μg/mL.

SUGGESTED READING

1. Applied Pharmacokinetics: Principles of Therapeutic Drug Monitoring. In: Evans WE. Schentag JJ, Jusko WJ. eds., 3rd ed. Applied Therapeutics; 1995.
2. Katzung BG. Basic and Clinical Pharmacology, 5th edition. Appleton and Lange, Norwalk, CT: Appleton and Lange; (1982).
3. Madan PL. Optimum Therapy Through Drug Monitoring. U. S. Pharmacist. 1996;21(5):HS5-HS27.
4. Richens A, Warrington S. When should Plasma Drug Levels be Monitored?. Drugs. 1979;17:488.
5. Therapeutic Drug Monitoring, Schumacker, ed. Appleton and Lange; 1995.

PRACTICE PROBLEMS

17-1. Following the administration of a single 250 mg intravenous bolus dose an antibiotic every 6 hours in a patient produced maximum steady-state plasma concentration of 20 μg/mL. If it is desired to attain maximum steady-state plasma concentration of the antibiotic in this patient at 16 μg/mL and the drug is known to confer the characteristics of one-compartment model, calculate the size of dose needed to change the maximum steady-state concentration.

17-2. Intravenous bolus administration of a single 250 mg dose of an antibiotic every 6 hours in a patient produces a 10 μg/mL minimum steady-state concentration of drug in the plasma. If the desired minimum concentration of drug at steady-state in this patient is 16 μg/mL and the drug is known to confer the characteristics of one-compartment model, calculate the size of dose needed to change the minimum steady-state concentration.

17-3. A single dose administration of a 30 mg intravenous bolus injection of a drug gave the following data: the characteristics of one-compartment pharmacokinetic model with C_0 = 2.5 mg/L and rate constant of elimination, K = 0.125/h. If the desired minimum steady-state concentration of the drug is 2 mg/L, calculate the following:

a. The dose that should be administered every 6 hours.

b. The expected maximum steady-state concentration at this dosing schedule.

17-4. A single dose administration of a 30 mg intravenous bolus injection of a drug exhibited one-compartment pharmacokinetic model with C_0 = 2.5 mg/L and the rate constant of elimination, K = 0.125/h. If the desired minimum steady-state plasma concentration of the drug is 2 mg/L, calculate the following:

a. The dosing interval if it is desired to administer a 30 mg dose, and

b. The expected maximum steady-state concentration at this dosing schedule.

17-5. Oral administration of a 250 mg dose of an antibiotic every 6 hours in a patient produces maximum steady-state concentration of 20 μg/mL. If the desired maximum steady-state concentration in this patient is 14.4 μg/mL and the drug is known to confer the characteristics of one-compartment model, calculate the size of dose needed to change the maximum steady-state concentration.

17-6. The following data were obtained after administration of a single 300 mg intravenous bolus dose of an antibiotic: one-compartment pharmacokinetic model with C_0 = 10 μg/mL and K = 0.0866/h. Using these data calculate:

a. The size of dose that should be administered every 6 hours in order to provide a minimum steady-state concentration of 27 μg/mL.
b. The maximum steady-state concentration with this dosage regimen.

17-7. The following data were obtained after administration of a single 300 mg intravenous bolus dose of an antibiotic: one-compartment pharmacokinetic model with C_0 = 10 μg/mL and K = 0.0866/h. Using these data calculate:

a. The size of dose that should be administered every 6 hours in order to provide a minimum steady-state concentration of 97 μg/mL.
b. The maximum steady-state concentration with this dosage regimen.

17-8. The following data were obtained after administration of a single 300 mg intravenous bolus dose of an antibiotic: one-compartment pharmacokinetic model with C_0 = 15 μg/mL, and K = 0.0866/h. Calculate the size of dose that should be administered every 6 h in order to provide a minimum steady-state concentration of 27 μg/mL.

17-9. The following data were obtained after administration of a 500 mg oral dose of an antibiotic: one-compartment pharmacokinetic model with y-intercept, B = 40 μg/mL, first-order rate constant of absorption, K_a = 1.757/h, and first-order rate constant of elimination, K = 0.1732/h. If the minimum effective concentration of the drug is 20 μg/mL and it is desired to maintain the minimum concentration at steady-state at 21 μg/mL, calculate the dosing interval that should be used to provide the desired minimum concentration of drug in the plasma at steady-state for the 500 mg dose.

17-10. The following data were obtained after administration of a 500 mg oral dose of an antibiotic: one-compartment pharmacokinetic model with y-intercept, B = 40 μg/mL, first-order rate constant of absorption, K_a = 1.757/h and first-order rate constant of elimination, K = 0.1732/h. If the minimum effective concentration of the drug is 15 μg/mL and it is desired to maintain the maximum concentration of drug at steady-state at 40 μg/mL, calculate the dosing interval that should be used to provide the desired maximum concentration of drug in the plasma at steady-state for the 500 mg dose.

CHAPTER 18

NON-COMPARTMENTAL METHODS

In recent years, a different type of pharmacokinetic analysis has become popular. This analysis is based on the observed data and statistical moment theory. Hence no particular model is assumed in this type of analysis. However, there are similarities in the compartment models and non-compartmental methods. Both techniques are based on the data derived from concentration of drug in the plasma as a function of time. To develop pharmacokinetic parameters using compartment models, one must fit the data to a particular compartment model. In non-compartmental methods, the data are not fitted to a compartment model, because no particular model is assumed. The compartment models represent a simplified kinetic approach to describe drug absorption, drug distribution and drug elimination. The non-compartmental methods are also used to calculate absorption, distribution and elimination parameters of a drug, but the parameters derived from these methods include such values as mean residence time (following intravenous, extravascular or infusion administration), mean absorption time, rate constant of absorption, rate constant of elimination and total body clearance of the drug. Non-compartmental methods are based on the theory of statistical moments. The simplicity and flexibility of these models is the principle reason for their wide application.

ADVANTAGES OF COMPARTMENT MODELS

1. The major advantage of compartment models as that the time course of drug in the body may be monitored quantitatively with a limited amount of data. Generally, only plasma drug concentrations and urinary drug excretion data are available and both of these data are usually adequate to monitor the time course of drug in the body.
2. Compartment models have been successfully applied to the prediction of the pharmacokinetics of the drug and the development of dosage regimens for many drugs.
3. Compartment models have been very useful in relating plasma drug levels to pharmacodynamic and toxic effects of drug in the body.
4. Compartment models may be used to extract some information about the underlying physiologic mechanism through model testing of the data.
5. Compartment analysis may lead to a more accurate description of the underlying physiologic processes and the kinetics involved in various processes.
6. The compartment model is particularly useful when several therapeutic agents are compared.
7. In the clinical pharmacokinetic literature, drug data comparisons are based on compartment models, even though alternative pharmacokinetic models have been available for a couple of decades.
8. The simplicity of the compartment model allows for easy tabulation of parameters such as the apparent volume of distribution and the half-lives of rate constants of the linear segments (α and β) of a biphasic plasma profile.

DISADVANTAGES OF COMPARTMENT MODELS

1. Compartmental models are sometimes misunderstood, overstretched and even abused. For example, the tissue levels of the drug predicted by a compartment model represent only a composite pool for drug equilibrium between all tissues and the circulatory system (plasma compartment). Naturally, any extrapolation to drug concentration in a specific tissue is inaccurate and is analogous to making predictions without any experimental data.
2. Although specific tissue drug concentration data are missing, many investigators may make predictions about tissue drug levels. Fundamentally, the principal use of the compartment model is to account for the mass balance of the drug in plasma and in the tissue pool and the amount of drug eliminated after drug administration.
3. The pharmacokinetic compartmental model is generally regarded as somewhat empirical and lacking physiologic relevance.
4. Disease-related changes in the physiologic processes are more readily related to the changes in the pharmacokinetics of the drug.
5. Many pharmacokinetic changes related to the disease state are essentially the result of physiologic changes, such as impairment of blood flow to the specific tissues or organs or a change in the mass of a specific organ. Experience has sown that these physiologic changes are better evaluated when a physiologic model is used rather than using a pharmacokinetic compartmental model. The physiologic pharmacokinetic model is much more realistic, because the physiologic pharmacokinetic model accounts for the processes involved in drug distribution, drug binding, drug metabolism and drug flow to the body organs.
6. Another advantage of the pharmacokinetic physiologic model is that the physiologic pharmacokinetic model may be modified to include the specific nature of a drug. For example, for an antitumor agent that penetrates inside the cell, the drug level in the interstitial water as well as the drug level in the intracellular water may be considered in the pharmacokinetic model. Blood flow and tumor size may even be included in the pharmacokinetic model to study any change in the drug uptake at that site.

NON-COMPARTMENTAL METHODS

The principle of non-compartmental analysis is based on the statistical theory, called the moments of a random variable. This theory is useful because the passage of a drug through the body can be considered a conjectural and imaginary process subject to some random fluctuations. These fluctuations cause the measurements of the variables, for example, the concentration of drug in the plasma as a function of time, to be basically repeatable from one dose to the next dose, but the measurements vary from one dose to the next dose.

In statistics, two parameters are used most frequently. These are 'average' or 'mean' and 'standard deviation.' Mean and standard deviation are meaningful numerical descriptive measures, because these two parameters describe the range or spread of values around the average value. The mean is a measure of central tendency and identifies the center of a set of observations, similar to an average value. The standard deviation is a measure of distribution and identifies the spread of a set of observations and their distribution about the mean.

A small standard deviation relative to the mean value is indicative of narrow spread of individual measurements and exhibits good consistency and reproducibility of the measurements. A large standard deviation relative to the mean value indicates poor consistency and data fluctuations. Obviously, one may have entirely different sets of observations that are very different from one another, but may possess the same mean and the same standard deviation. That is, just because two sets of observations have the same mean and the same standard deviation; it does not signify that the two sets are always similar. For example, consider the two sets of observations in Table 18-1:

Table 18-1 Results of two sets of observations

SET # 1		*SET # 2*	
Time	*Concentration*	*Time*	*Concentration*
1	10	1	34
2	20	2	36
3	30	3	38
4	40	4	40
5	50	5	42
6	60	6	44
7	70	7	46
	Mean = 40		Mean = 40

Although the average (mean) concentration in both sets of data is 40 units, one can see that these two sets of observation are entirely different sets of observations. In set # 1, the concentration range is relatively large (the range is 70 – 10 = 60 units) and in set # 2, the concentration range is much narrow (the range is 46 – 34 = 12 units).

In theory, a set data describing the concentration of drug in the plasma as a function of time may be considered a statistical distribution. In statistics, the equation of observations that defines the distribution is called the probability density function and a probability density function is characterized by the statistical moments of the function. A major use of the moments is to approximate the probability distribution of a random variable.

Moment Curve

The moment curve is a plot of $(C) \times (t^n)$ versus t (where, C is the concentration of drug in plasma and t is the time). When the value of the exponent n in the term $(C) \times (t^n)$ is equal to zero, the moment curve is called the zero-moment curve. This curve is a plot of $(C) \times (t^0)$ versus time or C versus time). When the value of the exponent n in the term $(C) \times (t^n)$ is equal to 1, the moment curve is called the first-moment curve. This curve is a plot of $(C) \times (t^1)$ versus time or $(C) \times (t)$ versus time. When the value of the exponent n in the term $(C) \times (t^n)$ is equal to 2, the moment curve is called the second-moment curve. This curve is a plot of $(C) \times (t^2)$ versus time. When the value of the exponent n in the term $(C) \times (t^n)$ is equal to 3, the moment curve is called the third-moment curve. This curve is a plot of $(C) \times (t^3)$ versus time.

The zero-moment curve describes area under the zero-moment curve and the first-moment curve represents the area under the first-moment curve. The second-moment about the mean is called the variance of distribution of the random variable and reflects the spread of distribution of a random variable, the third-moment determines the symmetry or lack of symmetry (skewness) of the distribution and the fourth-moment determines the extent to which a distribution is peaked or flat (kurtosis) of the distribution.

In pharmacokinetic studies, only the zero moment about the mean and the first-moment about the mean are used to plot the data representing concentration of drug in the plasma as a function of time curve. Estimates of zero-moment about the mean (AUC) are also useful for calculating such parameters as bioavailability and drug clearance.

Listed below are some of the statistical moments about the mean.

1. Area Under the Zero-Moment Curve

The area under the zero-moment plasma concentration versus time curve is the total area under the drug plasma concentration versus time curve from time zero to time infinity. This area is referred to as $AUC_{0-\infty}$ or simply AUC.

It will be recalled that the total area under the curve is the sum total of area under the curve from time zero to time t (AUC_{0-t}) and area under the curve from time t to time infinity ($AUC_{t-\infty}$). The area under the zero-moment curve from time zero to time t (AUC_{0-t}) is most commonly calculated according to the trapezoidal rule and the terminal area under the curve (from time t to time infinity, $AUC_{t-\infty}$) is calculated using the following relationship:

$$AUC_{t-\infty} = \frac{C_t}{K} \tag{18-1}$$

In equation (18-1) C_t is the last concentration point available in the data and K is the rate constant of elimination of the drug.

It will also be recalled that during intravenous bolus administration, for drugs that follow one-compartment pharmacokinetic model, $AUC_{0-\infty}$ is calculated using the relationship:

$$AUC_{0-\infty} = \frac{C_0}{K} \tag{18-2}$$

where, C_0 is concentration of drug in plasma immediately after administration of the intravenous bolus dose and K is the rate constant of elimination of the drug. Estimation of AUC_{0-t} and $AUC_{0-\infty}$ has been discussed previously. The trapezoidal rule is the most commonly used method for estimating AUC_{0-t}.

2. Area Under the First-Moment Curve

The area under the first-moment plasma concentration versus time curve from time zero to time infinity is represented by $AUMC_{0-\infty}$ or simply AUMC.

To estimate the area under the first-moment curve (AUMC), the observed plasma concentrations are multiplied by the corresponding time points and the product (C) × (t) is then plotted against the same time points. The most commonly used method of estimation of area under the first-moment curve from time zero to time t ($AUMC_{0-t}$) is the trapezoidal rule and the terminal area of the first-moment curve (from time t to time infinity, $AUMC_{t-\infty}$) is calculated using the following relationship:

$$AUMC_{t-\infty} = \frac{C_t(t)}{K} + \frac{C_t}{K^2} \tag{18-3}$$

where,

C_t = Last concentration point available in the data

t = The last time point available in the data and

K = Rate constant of elimination of the drug.

It should be realized that:

1. The area under the first-moment curve will always be greater than the area under the zero-moment curve, because area under the first-moment curve is represented not by concentration versus time (C) versus (t), but by the product of concentration and time versus time (C × t) versus (t). Thus, while in the case of the zero-moment curve, the area of each trapezoidal segment is a result of concentration multiplied by time (C × t), the area of each trapezoidal segment in a first-moment curve is a result of concentration multiplied by the square of time $(C \times t) \times (t) = C \times t^2$. This means that the areas of each of the trapezoidal segments would increase as the time of data collection increases.
2. Similarly, the terminal area (from the last data point at time *t* to time infinity) would be much greater in the first-moment curve than in the zero-moment curve, because, as can be seen from equation (18-3), the terminal area in the first-moment curve is a result of an additional term. This additional term is the last concentration point divided by the square of the rate constant of elimination. Hence, this additional term would have relatively significant value.
3. If the data are collected for a sufficiently long period of time, the terminal area under the zero-moment curve (from time *t* to time infinity) is only a fraction of the total area under the

zero-moment curve. But, the terminal area under the first-moment curve (from time *t* to time infinity) is not a small fraction of the total area under the first-moment curve, because the additional term in the equation is divided by the square of the rate constant of elimination..

3. Area Under the Second-Moment Curve

The area under the second-moment plasma concentration versus time curve from time zero to time infinity is represented by $AUM_2C_{0-\infty}$ or simply AUM_2C. The subscript 2 in the letter M represents the second-moment. To estimate area under the second-moment curve (AUM_2C), the observed concentrations of drug in plasma are multiplied by the square of the corresponding time points $\{(C)\times(t^2)\}$. A graph is then constructed by plotting $(C) \times (t^2)$ versus t, where, C is the plasma concentration of drug at any time t and t is the time. The most popular method of estimation of area under the second-moment curve from time 0 to time t, i.e. AUM_2C_{0-t} is the trapezoidal rule.

In most pharmacokinetic studies, the second-moment about the mean is rarely used, because the variance of distribution of the random variable (the spread of distribution of the random variable) is usually of little or no interest. The same is true for the third moment about the mean and the fourth-moment about the mean, because determination of the symmetry or lack of symmetry (skewness) of the distribution (area under the third moment) and the extent to which a distribution is peaked or flat (kurtosis) are rarely investigated.

Table 18-2 lists the equations used to calculate the total area under the curve (from time zero to time infinity) when the data are plotted according to the zero- or the first-moment about the mean.

MEAN RESIDENCE TIME

The term mean residence time (usually abbreviated as MRT) describes the average time for all the drug molecules to reside in the body. To understand the concept of mean residence time, consider the simplest case of a dose of drug administered intravenously. After the administration of an intravenous bolus dose, a large number of drug molecules distribute throughout the body. The number of molecules of drug in the drug dose may be calculated by converting the dose (in mg) into the number of moles of drug in the drug dose and multiplying the number of moles by

Table 18-2 Equations used to calculate total area under the curve

Route of administration	*Equations*	
	Zero-moment	*First-moment*
One-compartment Model		
Intravenous bolus dose	$\frac{C_0}{K}$	$\frac{C_0}{K^2}$
Extravascular bolus dose	$\frac{B}{\beta} - \frac{A}{\alpha}$	$\frac{B}{\beta^2} - \frac{A}{\alpha^2}$
Two-compartment Model		
Intravenous bolus dose	$\frac{B}{\beta} + \frac{A}{\alpha}$	$\frac{B}{\beta^2} + \frac{A}{\alpha^2}$
Extravascular bolus dose	$\frac{B}{\beta} + \frac{P}{\pi} - \frac{A}{\alpha}$	$\frac{B}{\beta^2} + \frac{P}{\pi^2} - \frac{A}{\alpha^2}$

the Avogadro number (6.022×10^{23}). For example, even a dose as small as 0.25 mg for a drug with a molecular weight of 250 will contain a very large number of molecules (as shown below).

$$\text{Number of molecules} = (\text{Number of moles})(\text{Avogadro number})$$

$$\text{Number of moles} = \frac{\text{Weight of substance in g}}{\text{Molecular weight}}$$

$$\text{Number of moles in 0.25mg of drug} = \frac{0.25\ \text{mg}}{250} = 1 \times 10^{-6}$$

$$\frac{1\ \text{mole}}{6.022 \times 10^{23}\ \text{molecules}} = \frac{1 \times 10^{-6}\ \text{moles}}{\text{'x' molecules}}$$

$$x = 6.022 \times 10^{17}\ \text{molecules}$$

Thus, a very small quantity of drug (0.25 mg) will contain approximately 6×10^{17} molecules. Upon administration, these molecules will stay (reside) in the body for different time periods. Some of the drug molecules will leave the body (eliminated from the body) almost immediately after entering (residence time of near zero, for example, 0.01, 0.03 or 0.07 seconds, etc.) and some other drug molecules will leave the body at later time periods. For example, some molecules will reside for 100, 500 or 1,000 seconds, while some molecules will reside for much longer time periods (residence time of 1,000, 10,000 or more than 50,000 seconds, etc.). The average time of residence of all of the drug molecules is the mean residence time.

Instantaneous Administration

The mean residence time is determined more readily after instantaneous administration of the drug dose (e.g. following an intravenous bolus dose), than after the administration of drug by any other mode. Following administration of an intravenous bolus dose, all molecules of the dose start their residence in the body at the same time (immediately after administration of the dose). None of the molecules is eliminated at time zero and at infinite time practically all of the molecules are eliminated. The summation of the residence time of each molecule and division of this summation by the total number of molecules estimates the mean residence time of the drug molecules for the administered dose.

Therefore, the mean residence time may be expressed in the form of the following equation:

$$\text{Mean residence time} = \frac{n_1 \times t_1 + n_2 \times t_2 + n_3 \times t_3 \times n_4 \times t_4 + n_5 \times t_5 + \ldots}{n_1 + n_2 + n_3 + n_4 + n_5 \ldots} \quad (18\text{-}4)$$

In this equation, n is the number of molecules introduced in the body and t is the residence time of these molecules.

Thus, n_1 is the number of molecules with an average time t_1 in the body, n_2 is the number of molecules with an average time t_2 in the body, n_3 is the number of molecules with an average time t_3 in the body, etc.

Equation (18-4) may be written as

$$\text{Mean residence time} = \frac{\text{Total residence time for all drug molecles in the body}}{\text{Total number of molecules ad min istred to the body}} \quad (18\text{-}5)$$

Irrespective of the distribution characteristics of a drug in the body, the mean residence time represents the time required for 63.2 percent of an intravenous dose to be eliminated. As such, it may be possible to determine mean residence time from urinary excretion data alone by determining the time required to excrete 63.2 percent of that amount, which is ultimately excreted as the unchanged drug. Since drug elimination follows first-order kinetics, elimination of 50 percent of the intravenous dose does not constitute mean residence time.

Non-instantaneous Administration

The mean residence time is a function of the method of drug administration, i.e. whether the drug is administered as an intravenous bolus injection, continuous intravenous infusion, oral administration, subcutaneous injection or by other extravascular means of routes of administration. The mean residence time values for non-instantaneous administration, e.g. zero-order constant rate infusion or first-order absorption, will always be greater than the mean residence time following intravenous bolus administration, because the drug spends additional time in at the site of drug administration, e.g. the gastrointestinal tract (oral administration), the muscle tissue (intramuscular injection) or the subcutaneous tissue (subcutaneous injection).

Following the extravascular administration of a drug solution, the mean residence time of the drug solution is the total of mean residence time of the drug after intravenous bolus dose plus the mean absorption time for drug the drug to be absorbed from the solution. Thus, in cases other than intravenous bolus injection, the mean residence time of the drug is equal to the mean residence time of the drug for the bolus injection plus the mean input time of the drug, i.e. the mean infusion time or the mean absorption time. In the case of drugs administered as a solid dosage form, the mean input time includes the time for the disintegration of the dosage form, de-aggregation of the granules or powder, dissolution of the drug (from the de-aggregated granules or powder) in the fluid at the site of administration and absorption of the drug solution.

Thus, for a drug administered as a continuous infusion, the mean residence time can be estimated using the following relationship:

$$MRT_{infusion} = MRT_{bolus} + 0.5T \tag{18-6}$$

In equation (18-6) $MRT_{infusion}$ is the mean residence time during continuous infusion, MRT_{bolus} is the mean residence time for intravenous bolus administration (instantaneous administration of the dose), T is the length of time of infusion and therefore, 0.5T is the mean infusion time.

Similarly, for a drug administered as an oral bolus dose, the mean residence time is given by the following equation:

$$MRT_{oral} = MRT_{bolus} + \frac{1}{K_a} \tag{18-7}$$

In equation (18-7),

MRT_{bolus} = Mean residence time for intravenous bolus administration (instantaneous administration of the dose) and

K_a = Rate constant of absorption of the drug.

METHODS OF DETERMINING MEAN RESIDENCE TIME

I. Mean Residence Time after Intravenous Bolus Injection

Several methods can be used to estimate mean residence time of a drug in the body. Some of the more commonly used methods are described here:

A. From the First-moment Curve

Using differential calculus and integral calculus, equation (18-4) can be simplified in the following form:

$$MRT = \frac{AIMC}{AUC} \tag{18-8}$$

In this equation,

AUMC is the area under the first-moment versus time curve from time zero to time infinity ($AUMC_{0-\infty}$) and AUC is the area under the zero-moment versus time curve from time zero to time infinity ($AUC_{0-\infty}$).

When the data are collected (and assayed for drug concentration) for a long period of time, the last concentration point will have a very small numerical value, because after five half-lives, about 97 percent of the drug has been eliminated. After six half-lives about 98.4 percent of the drug has been eliminated, and after seven half-lives more than 99 percent of the drug has been eliminated from the body. Since, less than 1 percent of the administered dose remains in the body after seven half-lives, collecting the data for more than seven half-lives assures that only an insignificant fraction of the administered dose is remaining to be eliminated from the body. Therefore, when the data are collected for a sufficiently long period of time (six to seven biological half-lives and beyond), both, the AUC (area under the zero-moment versus time curve) and the AUMC (area under the first-moment versus time curve) from time zero to time t may be used in equation (18-8) without extrapolating the areas for the terminal portions of the curves, i.e.

$$MRT_{bolus} = \frac{AUMC_{0-t}}{AUC_{0-t}} \quad (18\text{-}9)$$

where, $AUMC_{0-t}$ is area under the first-moment versus time curve from time 0 to time t and AUC_{0-t} is area under the zero-moment versus time curve from time 0 to time t.

It should be pointed out that when a model-independent approach is used in estimating the mean residence time, one should not use extrapolation beyond the data because all data extrapolation will be subject to error. This is because the real rate process is determined from the experimental data and should not be assumed. Therefore, one should collect additional data (data at least up to six or seven half-lives), rather than having to depend on extrapolation of the data.

Example 18-1 Calculate the mean residence time from the following plasma concentration versus time data obtained after the administration of a 200 mg intravenous bolus dose of a drug (time is in hour and plasma drug concentration is in mg/L):

Time	*Concentration*	*Time*	*Concentration*	*Time*	*Concentration*	*Time*	*Concentration*
0	20.0	5	7.0	10	2.0	15	0.6
1	16.0	6	5.0	11	1.5	16	0.5
2	13.0	7	4.0	12	1.2	17	0.4
3	10.0	8	3.0	13	1.0	18	0.3
4	8.0	9	2.4	14	0.8	19	0.2

Solution

Area Under the Zero-Moment Curve (AUC_{0-t}): To calculate area under the zero-moment curve (AUC_{0-t}), each drug plasma concentration is plotted as a function of its corresponding time. The data are plotted on a rectilinear graph paper and then each plasma concentration point is connected to the next adjacent plasma concentration point with a straight line. A perpendicular is drawn on the x-axis from each plasma concentration point to obtain the various geometric figures (segments) that comprise the curve from time 0 hr to 19 hours. This divides the plot into geometric figures whose area can be determined individually using an appropriate geometric formula for each figure.

The data, plotted in Figure 18-1, yield 19 segments (segments A to S). Each segment in Figure 18-1 is a trapezoid. The area of each trapezoid is calculated as follows:

$$\text{Area of trapezoid} = (0.5) \times (\text{Sum of two parallel sides}) \times (\text{Base})$$

The calculation of area under the zero-moment curve is tabulated in Table 18-3.

Area Under the First-Moment Curve ($AUMC_{0-t}$): The plasma concentrations are multiplied by corresponding time points and plotted against the same time points. Table 18-4 shows the calculations to obtain the data for plotting the graph of (concentration) × (time) versus time.

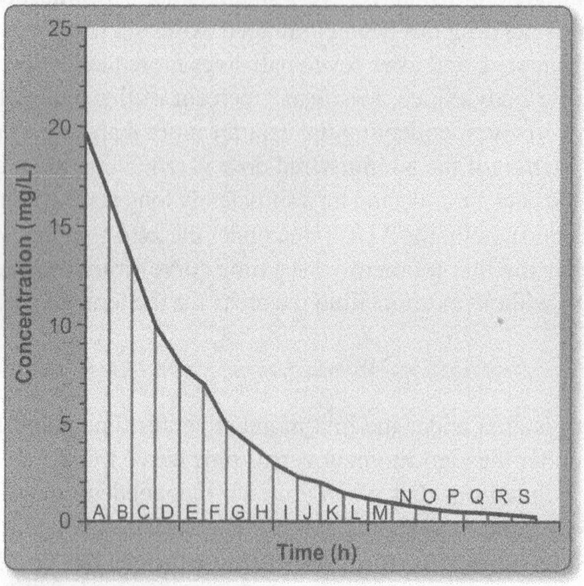

Fig. 18-1 Area under the zero-moment curve

Table 18-3 Calculation of area under the zero-moment curve

Segment	*Time Interval (h)*	*Area (mg x h/L)*	
A	0 - 1	0.5 × (20.0 + 16.0)	= 18.0
B	1 - 2	0.5 × (16.0 + 13.0)	= 14.5
C	2 - 3	0.5 × (13.0 + 10.0)	= 11.5
D	3 - 4	0.5 × (10.0 + 8.0)	= 9.0
E	4 - 5	0.5 × (8.0 + 7.0)	= 7.5
F	5 - 6	0.5 × (7.0 + 5.0)	= 6.0
G	6 - 7	0.5 × (5.0 + 4.0)	= 4.5
H	7 - 8	0.5 × (4.0 + 3.0)	= 3.5
I	8 - 9	0.5 × (3.0 + 2.4)	= 2.8
J	9 - 10	0.5 × (2.4 + 2.0)	= 2.2
K	10 - 11	0.5 × (2.0 + 1.5)	= 1.75
L	11 - 12	0.5 × (1.5 + 1.2)	= 1.35
M	12 - 13	0.5 × (1.2 + 1.0)	= 1.1
N	13 - 14	0.5 × (1.0 + 0.8)	= 0.90
O	14 - 15	0.5 × (0.8 + 0.6)	= 0.70
P	15 - 16	0.5 × (0.6 + 0.5)	= 0.55
Q	16 - 17	0.5 × (0.5 + 0.4)	= 0.45
R	17 - 18	0.5 × (0.4 + 0.3)	= 0.35
S	18 - 19	0.5 × (0.3 + 0.2)	= 0.25
		AUC_{0-19}	= 86.9

Figure 18-2 is a plot of $(C_p)(t)$ versus time. There are 19 segments in this plot. The first segment is a triangle and the remaining 18 segments are trapezoids. The area of each segment is calculated using the relevant formula for the geometric figure.

The calculations involved in calculating the area of each segment are tabulated in Table 18-5:

Mean Residence Time: Since the data were collected for a sufficiently long period of time, the areas under the zero- and the first-moment curves from time zero to time t may be used to estimate the mean residence time.

The mean residence time is estimated by substituting the values of AUC_{0-t} and $AUMC_{0-t}$ into equation (18-9)

$$MRT_{bolus} = \frac{AUMC_{0-t}}{AUC_{0-t}}$$

$$= \frac{368 \text{ mg} \times \text{h}^2/\text{L}}{86.9 \text{ mg} \times \text{h/L}} = 4.24 \text{ h}$$

Table 18-4 Calculations to plot the first-moment curve

t (h)	*C_p (mg/L)*	*(t)(C_p) (mg × h/L)*	*t (h)*	*C_p (mg/L)*	*(t)(C_p) (mg × h/L)*
0	20.0	0.0	10	2.0	20.0
1	16.0	16.0	11	1.5	16.5
2	13.0	26.0	12	1.2	14.4
3	10.0	30.0	13	1.0	13.0
4	8.0	32.0	14	0.8	11.2
5	7.0	35.0	15	0.6	9.0
6	5.0	30.0	16	0.5	8.0
7	4.0	28.0	17	0.4	6.8
8	3.0	24.0	18	0.3	5.4
9	2.4	21.6	19	0.2	3.8

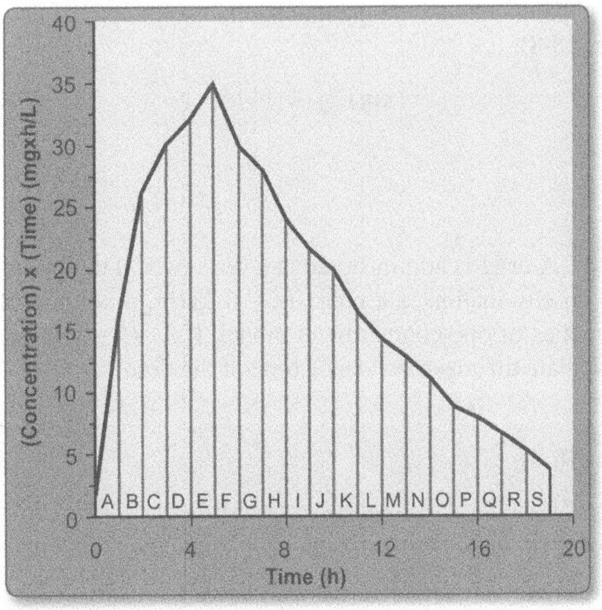

Fig. 18-2 Area under the first-moment curve

Table 18-5 Area under the first-moment curve

Segment	*Time interval (h)*	*Area (mg × h²/L)*	
A	0 – 1	0.5 × (16.0)	= 8.0
B	1 – 2	0.5 × (16.0 + 26.0)	= 21.0
C	2 – 3	0.5 × (26.0 + 30.0)	= 28.0
D	3 – 4	0.5 × (30.0 + 32.0)	= 31.0
E	4 – 5	0.5 × (32.0 + 35.0)	= 33.5
F	5 – 6	0.5 × (35.0 + 30.0)	= 32.0
G	6 – 7	0.5 × (30.0 + 28.0)	= 29.0
H	7 – 8	0.5 × (28.0 + 24.0)	= 26.0
I	8 – 9	0.5 × (24.0 + 21.6)	= 42.8
J	9 – 10	0.5 × (21.6 + 20.0)	= 20.8
K	10 – 11	0.5 × (20.0 + 16.5)	= 18.2
L	11 – 12	0.5 × (16.5 + 14.4)	= 15.45
M	12 – 13	0.5×(14.4 + 13.0)	= 13.7
N	13 – 14	0.5 × (13.0 + 11.2)	= 12.1
O	14 – 15	0.5 × (11.2 + 9.0)	= 10.1
P	15 – 16	0.5 × (9.0 + 8.0)	= 8.5
Q	16 – 17	0.5 × (8.0 + 6.8)	= 7.4
R	17 – 18	0.5 × (6.8 + 5.4)	= 6.1
S	18 – 19	0.5 × (5.4 + 3.8)	= 4.6
		$AUMC_{0-19}$	= 368.8

Example 18-2 Administration of a 500 mg dose of a drug, which follows the kinetics of one-compartment model, yielded the following data: AUC = 85 mg × h/L and AUMC = 450 mg × h²/L, calculate the mean residence time.

Solution

Using equation (18-8),

$$MRT_{bolus} = \frac{AUMC}{AUC}$$

$$= \frac{450 \text{ mg} \times \text{h}^2/\text{L}}{85 \text{ mg} \times \text{h/L}} = 5.3 \text{ h}$$

Example 18-3 A drug is administered at a dose of 500 mg by intravenous bolus injection. The drug has an elimination rate constant = 0.231/h, a volume of distribution = 20 L and follows the kinetics of one-compartment model. If AUC = 110 mg × h/L and AUMC = 470 mg × h²/L, calculate the mean residence time of the drug.

Solution

Using equation (18-8),

$$MRT_{bolus} = \frac{AUMC}{AUC}$$

$$= \frac{470 \text{ mg} \times \text{h}^2/\text{L}}{110 \text{ mg} \times \text{h/L}} = 4.27 \text{ h}$$

B. From Elimination Rate Constant

The mean residence time may also be calculated using the compartmental approach. As shown in Table 18-2, for intravenous bolus administration in one-compartment pharmacokinetic model, the AUC and AUMC are given by:

$$AUC = \frac{C_0}{K} \text{ and } AUMC = \frac{C_0}{K^2}$$

Substituting the values of AUC and AUMC into equation (18-8),

$$MRT_{bolus} = \frac{AUMC}{AUC} = \frac{C_0/K^2}{C_0/K} \tag{18-10}$$

$$MRT_{bolus} = \frac{1}{K} \tag{18-11}$$

Similarly, for intravenous bolus administration in a two-compartment pharmacokinetic model, the AUC and AUMC are given by:

$$AUC = \frac{B}{\beta} + \frac{A}{\alpha}, \text{ and } AUMC = \frac{B}{\beta^2} + \frac{A}{\alpha^2}$$

Substituting the values of AUMC and AUC into equation (18-8),

$$MRT_{bolus} = \frac{AUMC}{AUC} = \frac{\frac{B}{\beta^2} + \frac{A}{\alpha^2}}{\frac{B}{\beta} + \frac{A}{\alpha}} \tag{18-12}$$

when α is much greater than β, equation (18 − 12) is approximately equal to:

$$MRT_{bolus} = \frac{1}{\beta} \tag{18-13}$$

Thus, mean residence time for a drug after an intravenous bolus injection is the reciprocal of the elimination rate constant, i.e. in this case the mean residence time is inversely related to the rate constant of elimination.

Example 18-4 A drug is administered at a dose of 500 mg by intravenous bolus injection. The drug has an elimination rate constant of 0.231/h, a volume of distribution = 20 L and follows the kinetics of one-compartment model. If area under the zero-moment curve is 110 mg × h/L and the area under the first-moment curve is 470 mg × h^2/L, calculate the mean residence time from elimination rate constant.

Solution

The data provided in this Example is identical to the data in Example 18-3 and the mean residence time needs to be calculated using elimination rate constant (not by using AUC and AUMC). From the data available, one can estimate the mean residence time using a variety of equations. Using equation (18-11), the mean residence time is:

$$MRT_{bolus} = \frac{1}{K}$$

$$= \frac{1}{0.231/h} = 4.33 \text{ h}$$

Example 18-5 A drug is administered at a dose of 500 mg by intravenous bolus injection. The drug has a volume of distribution = 20 L, a half-life of 4 h and follows the kinetics of one-compartment model. Calculate the mean residence time.

Solution

From the data available, one can estimate the mean residence time using a variety of equations. However, if one wanted to use equation (18-11) to estimate the mean residence time, one would need to know the elimination rate constant of the drug. Since the biological half-life is 4 hr, therefore, the rate constant of elimination is:

$$K = \frac{0.693}{t_{1/2}} = \frac{0.693}{4\ h} = 0.17325/h$$

Substituting the value of rate constant of elimination into equation (18-11), 11

$$MRT_{bolus} = \frac{1}{K} = \frac{1}{0.17325/h} = 5.77\ h$$

C. By the Area Method

Another method of estimating the mean residence time is the relationship between AUC and C_0. According to this relationship:

$$MRT_{bolus} = \frac{AUC}{C_0} \tag{18-14}$$

Example 18-6 A drug is administered at a dose of 500 mg by intravenous bolus injection. The drug has an elimination rate constant of 0.231/h, a volume of distribution of 20 L and follows the kinetics of one-compartment model. If area under the zero-moment curve is 110 mg × h/L and the area under the first-moment curve is 470 mg × h^2/L, calculate the mean residence time by the area method.

Solution

In this Example also, the data provided is identical to the data given in Example 18-3, but the mean residence time should be determined using the area method.

From the data provided:

$$C_0 = \frac{Dose}{V_d} = \frac{500\ mg}{20\ L} = 25\ mg/L$$

Therefore, using equation (18-14), the mean residence time is:

$$MRT_{bolus} = \frac{AUC}{C_0}$$

$$= \frac{110\ mg \times h/L}{25\ mg/L} = 4.40\ h$$

Example 18-7 A drug is administered at a dose of 500 mg by intravenous bolus injection. The volume of distribution of the drug 25 L and the drug follows the kinetics of one-compartment model. If area under the zero-moment curve is 100 mg × h/L, calculate the mean residence time.

Solution

From the data provided:

$$C_0 = \frac{Dose}{V_d} = \frac{500\ mg}{25\ L} = 20\ mg/L$$

Since, C_0 = 20 mg/L and AUC = 100 mg × hr/L, equation (18-14) can be used to calculate the mean residence time. Substituting these values into equation (18-14):

$$MRT_{bolus} = \frac{AUC}{C_0} = \frac{100\ mg \times h/L}{20\ mg/L} = 5.0\ h$$

Comparison of Methods Used to Calculate MRT

The mean residence time calculated using different equations yields slightly different answers. In most cases this is due to approximation in the summation of the moment areas AUC and AUMC. For instance, in Example 18-3, the mean residence time calculated using the relationship between AUMC and AUC was estimated to be 4.27 hr. However, if the mean residence time was calculated using the elimination rate constant in Example 18-4 and the relationship between AUC and C_0 in Example 18-6, one obtains a mean residence time of 4.33 hr and 4.40 hr, respectively. Similarly, if one calculated the mean residence time in another Example using a different equation (assuming that the information needed for a different equation was available in the given Example), one may obtain a different value for the mean residence time. Table 18-6 lists the mean residence time calculated using different equations for some of the Examples shown above

Example 18-8 A drug is administered at a dose of 300 mg by intravenous bolus injection. If the area under the zero-moment curve is 125 mg × hr/L, the volume of distribution of the drug is 20 L and the drug follows the kinetics of one-compartment model, calculate the mean residence time.

Solution

From the data provided:

$$C_0 = \frac{\text{Dose}}{V_d} = \frac{300\text{ mg}}{20\text{ L}} = 15\text{ mg/L}$$

Therefore, using equation (18-14), the mean residence time is:

$$MRT_{\text{bolus}} = \frac{AUC}{C_0} = \frac{125\text{ mg} \times \text{h/L}}{15\text{ mg/L}} = 8.33\text{ h}$$

Example 18-9 A drug is administered at a dose of 500 mg by intravenous bolus injection. If the area under the zero-moment curve is 225 mg × h/L, the volume of distribution of the drug is 25 L and the drug follows the kinetics of one-compartment model, calculate the mean residence time.

Table 18-6 Mean residence time calculated using different equations

Example	*Equation*	*Mean residence time (h)*
18-1	18-9	4.24
	18-14	4.35
18-3	18-8	18-11
	18-14	4.27
	4.33	4.40
18-4	18-11	18-8
	18-14	4.33
	4.27	4.40
18-5	18-11	18-8
	18-14	5.77
	5.67	5.60
18-6	18-14	18-8
	18-11	4.40
	4.27	4.33

Solution

From the data provided:

$$C_0 = \frac{\text{Dose}}{V_d} = \frac{500\ \text{mg}}{25\ \text{L}} = 20\ \text{mg/L}$$

Therefore, using equation (18-14), the mean residence time is:

$$\text{MRT}_{\text{bolus}} = \frac{\text{AUC}}{C_0}$$

$$= \frac{225\ \text{mg} \times \text{h/L}}{20\ \text{mg}} = 11.25\ \text{h}$$

Example 18-10 A drug is administered at a dose of 500 mg by intravenous bolus injection. The drug follows the kinetics of one-compartment model. If AUC = 110 mg × h/L and AUMC = 470 mg × h²/L, calculate the rate constant of elimination of the drug.

Solution

Using equation (18-8),

$$\text{MRT}_{\text{bolus}} = \frac{\text{AUMC}}{\text{AUC}} = \frac{470\ \text{mg} \times \text{h}^2\text{/L}}{110\ \text{mg} \times \text{h/L}} = 4.27\ \text{h}$$

According to equation (18-11),

$$\text{MRT}_{\text{bolus}} = \frac{1}{K}\text{, therefore, } K = \frac{1}{\text{MRT}_{\text{bolus}}} = \frac{1}{4.27\ \text{h}} = 0.234\text{/h}$$

Example 18-11 A drug is administered at a dose of 500 mg by intravenous bolus injection. The drug follows the kinetics of one-compartment model. If AUC = 100 mg × h/L and AUMC = 500 mg × h²/L, calculate the biological half-life of the drug.

Solution

Using equation (18-8),

$$\text{MRT}_{\text{bolus}} = \frac{\text{AUMC}}{\text{AUC}} = \frac{500\ \text{mg} \times \text{h}^2\text{/L}}{100\ \text{mg} \times \text{h/L}} = 5.0\ \text{h}$$

According to equation (18-11),

$$\text{MRT}_{\text{bolus}} = \frac{1}{K}\text{, therefore, } K = \frac{1}{\text{MRT}_{\text{bolus}}} = \frac{1}{5.0\ \text{h}} = 0.2\text{/h and}$$

$$t_{1/2} = \frac{0.693}{K} = \frac{0.693}{0.2\text{/h}} = 3.465\ \text{h}$$

II. Mean Residence Time During Continuous Infusion

The mean residence time of a drug during continuous infusion is calculated using equation (18-6):

$$\text{MRT}_{\text{infusion}} = \text{MRT}_{\text{bolus}} + 0.5\text{T}$$

Example 18-12 Administration of a 1,000 mg intravenous bolus dose of a drug yielded the following data: area under the zero-moment curve = 225 mg × h/L, volume of distribution = 25 L and the drug follows the kinetics of one-compartment model. Calculate the mean residence time if the drug were administered as a continuous infusion over a 10 hours period.

Solution

From the data provided: Dose 1,000 mg

$$C_0 = \frac{\text{Dose}}{V_d} = \frac{1000 \text{ mg}}{25 \text{ L}} = 40 \text{ mg/L}$$

Therefore, using equation (18-14), the mean residence time during intravenous bolus injection is:

$$MRT_{bolus} = \frac{AUC}{C_0} = \frac{225 \text{ mg} \times \text{h/L}}{40 \text{ mg/L}} = 5.625 \text{ h}$$

The mean residence time of drug during continuous infusion is calculated using equation (18-6):

$$MRT_{infusion} = 5.625 \text{ h} + 0.5(10 \text{ h}) = 10.625 \text{ h}$$

Example 18-13 A drug follows the kinetics of one-compartment model. The mean residence time in an individual following administration of an intravenous bolus dose, an intravenous infusion and a bolus oral dose, on separate occasions, was 6, 10 and 12 h, respectively. Calculate the duration of infusion, assuming a constant-rate input.

Solution

The mean residence time of a drug during continuous infusion is calculated using equation (18-6):

$$MRT_{infusion} = MRT_{bolus} + 0.5T$$

Substituting the values of mean residence time during intravenous bolus injection and continuous intravenous infusion into equation (18-6), one gets:

Therefore, the duration of infusion, T = 2(10 h − 6 h) = 8 h

Example 18-14 A drug follows the kinetics of one-compartment model. Administration of a 500 mg intravenous dose yielded the following data: C_0 = 20 mg/L and area under the zero-moment curve = 120 mg × h/L. Calculate the mean residence time of the drug, if the drug were administered as a continuous infusion over a 4 hours period.

Solution

The mean residence time during intravenous bolus injection is given by equation (18-14):

$$MRT_{bolus} = \frac{AUC}{C_0} = \frac{225 \text{ mg} \times \text{h/L}}{40 \text{ mg/L}} = 6 \text{ h}$$

The mean residence time of the drug during continuous infusion is calculated using equation (18-6):

$$MRT_{infusion} = 6 \text{ h} + 0.5(4 \text{ h}) = 8 \text{ h}$$

Example 18-15 A drug follows the kinetics of one-compartment model. The mean residence times in an individual following administration of an intravenous bolus dose and an intravenous infusion, on separate occasions, were found to be 10 hours and 12 hours, respectively. Calculate the duration of infusion, assuming a constant-rate drug input.

Solution

The mean residence time of a drug during continuous infusion is calculated using equation (18-6):

$$MRT_{infusion} = MRT_{bolus} + 0.5T$$

Substituting the relevant values into equation (18-6), one gets:

$$12\text{ h} = 10\text{ h} + 0.5T$$

Therefore, duration of infusion, $T = 2(12\text{ h} - 10\text{ h}) = 4\text{ h}$

III. Mean Residence Time During Oral Administration

The mean residence time of a drug following the administration of an oral dose is equal to the mean residence time of drug in the body (mean residence time for intravenous bolus administration, i.e. instantaneous administration), plus the additional time the drug spends at the site of administration (e.g. in the gastrointestinal tract after oral administration). It has been shown that for immediate-release dosage forms the mean additional time the drug spends at the site of administration is approximately equal to the reciprocal of the rate constant of absorption of the drug. Therefore, the mean residence time after oral administration can be estimated using equation (18-7) and adding to this equation, the additional time the drug spends at the site of administration (the gastrointestinal tract). Therefore, the equation to estimate the mean residence time of a drug following the administration of an oral dose is as follows:

$$MRT_{oral} = MRT_{bolus} + \frac{1}{K_a}$$

Since, $MRT_{bolus} = \dfrac{1}{K}$

Therefore, equation (18-7) may be written as:

$$MRT_{oral} = \frac{1}{K} + \frac{1}{K_a} \qquad (18\text{-}15)$$

Example 18-16 Administration of a 1,000 mg intravenous bolus dose of a drug yielded the following data: area under the zero-moment curve = 200 mg × h/L, volume of distribution = 25 L and the drug follows the kinetics of one-compartment model. Calculate the mean residence time if a 1,000 mg dose of the drug were administered orally. The rate constant of absorption of the drug is 0.987/h.

Solution

From the data provided:

$$C_0 = \frac{Dose}{V_d} = \frac{1000\text{ mg}}{25\text{ L}} = 40\text{ mg/L}$$

Therefore, using equation (18-14), the mean residence time during intravenous bolus injection is:

$$MRT_{bolus} = \frac{AUC}{C_0} = \frac{200\text{ mg} \times \text{h/L}}{40\text{ mg/L}} = 5.0\text{ h}$$

and the mean residence time during oral administration is given by equation (18-7): 1

$$MRT_{oral} = MRT_{bolus} + \frac{1}{K_a}$$

$$= 5\text{ h} + \frac{1}{0.987/\text{h}}$$

$$= 5\text{ h} + 1.01\text{ h} = 6.01\text{ h}$$

Example 18-17 Calculate the mean residence time of a 500 mg dose of the drug administered orally. The rate constant of elimination of the drug is 0.1/h and the rate constant of absorption of the drug is 0.95/h.

Solution

Using equation (18-15), $MRT_{oral} = \frac{1}{K} + \frac{1}{K_a} = \frac{1}{0.1/h} + \frac{1}{0.95/h} = 10\ h + 1.05\ h = 11.05\ h$

Example 18-18 Administration of a 500 mg intravenous bolus dose of a drug yielded the following data: area under the zero-moment curve = 100 mg × h/L, volume of distribution = 25 L and the drug follows the kinetics of one-compartment model. Calculate the mean residence time if a 500 mg dose of the drug were administered orally. The rate constant of absorption of the drug is 0.87/h.

Solution

From the data provided:

$$C_0 = \frac{Dose}{V_d} = \frac{500\ mg}{25\ L} = 20\ mg/L$$

Therefore, the mean residence time during intravenous bolus injection is estimated using equation (18-14) as follows:

$$MRT_{bolus} = \frac{AUC}{C_0} = \frac{100\ mg \times h/L}{20\ mg/L} = 5.0\ h$$

and the mean residence time during oral administration is given by equation (18-7): 1

$$MRT_{oral} = MRT_{bolus} + \frac{1}{K_a}$$

$$= 5\ h + \frac{1}{0.87/h}$$

$$= 5\ h + 1.15\ h = 6.15\ h$$

Example 18-19 Calculate the mean residence time of a 500 mg dose of the drug administered orally. The rate constant of elimination of the drug is 0.01/h and the rate constant of absorption of the drug is 0.85/h.

Solution

According to equation (18-15): 11

$$MRT_{oral} = \frac{1}{K} + \frac{1}{K_a}$$

Substituting the values of K and Ka into equation (18-15), one gets:

$$MRT_{oral} = \frac{1}{K} + \frac{1}{K_a} = \frac{1}{0.1/h} + \frac{1}{0.85/h} = 10\ h + 1.18\ h = 11.18\ h$$

MEAN ABSORPTION TIME

The term mean absorption time (MAT) describes the average time for all the drug molecules to be absorbed from the site of administration. Mean absorption time applies only to drugs administered extravascularly, because the rate of systemic drug absorption after intravenous bolus dose is zero due to the fact that the drug is placed directly into the systemic circulation.

The concept of mean absorption time is similar to the concept of mean residence time. After the administration of an extravascular bolus dose of a drug in a solution, a large number of drug molecules are available for absorption. The number of molecules of the drug dose may be calculated by converting the dose in mg into the number of moles and multiplying moles by Avogadro number (6.023×10^{23}). The molecules will be absorbed into the systemic circulation at different time periods. Some of the drug molecules will be absorbed almost immediately (absorption time of near zero, e.g. 0.01, or 0.03, etc.) and some other drug molecules will be absorbed at later time periods (absorption time of 100, 5000 or 10,000, etc.). The average time of absorption of all of the drug molecules is the mean absorption time. Summation of the absorption time of each molecule and division by the total number of molecules absorbed estimates the mean absorption. Therefore, mean absorption time may be expressed in the form of the following equation:

$$\text{Mean Absorption Time} = \frac{n_1 \times t_1 + n_2 \times t_2 + n_3 \times t_3 + n_4 \times t_4 + n_5 \times t_5 + \ldots}{n_1 + n_2 + n_3 + n_4 + n_5 \ldots} \tag{18-16}$$

where, n is the number of molecules absorbed and t is the absorption time of these molecules. Thus, n_1 is the number of molecules with an average absorption time t_1, n_2 is the number of molecules with an average absorption time t_2, n_3 is the number of molecules with an average absorption time t_3, etc.

Equation (18-16) may be written as

$$\text{Mean Absorption Time} = \frac{\text{Total absorption time for all drug molecules}}{\text{Total number of molecules absorbed}} \tag{18-17}$$

The mean residence time calculated for a drug after intravenous bolus dose basically reflects the elimination rate processes in the body. After extravascular administration, e.g. oral administration, the mean residence time is the result of both drug absorption and drug elimination. Therefore, mean residence time after oral administration is the total of the mean residence time after intravenous bolus administration plus the mean absorption time for the extravascular dose, i.e.

$$MRT_{oral} = MRT_{bolus} + MAT \tag{18-18}$$

Equation (18-18) may be rearranged as:

$$MAT = MRT_{oral} - MRT_{bolus} \tag{18-19}$$

Thus, the mean absorption time for an oral dose is equal to the difference in the mean residence time of the orally administered dose and intravenously administered bolus dose. Substituting the value of mean residence time after intravenous bolus dose from equation (18-11) into equation (18-19),

$$MAT = MRT_{oral} - \frac{1}{K} \tag{18-20}$$

Similarly, substituting the value of mean residence time after extravascular administration from equation (18-7) into equation (18-19), 1

$$MAT = \left(MRT_{bolus} + \frac{1}{K_a}\right) - MRT_{bolus} \tag{18-21}$$

which, upon simplification gives:

$$\text{Mean Absorption Time} = \frac{1}{K_a} \tag{18-22}$$

It should be pointed out that equation (18-22) has certain limitations. From a practical standpoint, the most important limitation of equation (18-22) is concerned with the extravascular bioavailability of the drug. If the bioavailability of the drug from an oral dosage form is 100 percent, or approximately 100 percent, then equation (18-22) represents a true value of the mean absorption time. However, if the bioavailability of the drug is much less than 100 percent, then the mean absorption time obtained using equation (18-22) is not a true value, but may be considered only an apparent value. The reduced bioavailability of the oral dose may be due to a variety of reasons, e.g., because of presystemic metabolism, decomposition of drug at the site of absorption, etc.

Example 18-20 The following data were obtained after administration of single 1,000 mg of a drug orally and intravenously, on separate occasions, in a crossover design: oral bolus dose: $AUC_{0-\infty}$ = 125 mg × h/L and $AUMC_{0-\infty}$ = 280 mg × h^2/L, intravenous dose: $AUC_{0-\infty}$ = 200 mg × h/L and $AUMC_{0-\infty}$ = 410 mg × h^2/L. Calculate the mean absorption time for the orally administered dose from the data provided.

Solution

Using equation (18-8),

$$MRT_{oral} = \frac{AUMC}{AUC} = \frac{280 \text{ mg} \times h^2/L}{125 \text{ mg} \times h/L} = 2.24 \text{ h}$$

Using equation (18-8),

$$MRT_{bolus} = \frac{AUMC}{AUC} = \frac{410 \text{ mg} \times h^2/L}{200 \text{ mg} \times h/L} = 2.05 \text{ h}$$

The mean absorption time for the oral dose is estimated using equation (18-19):

$$MAT = MRT_{oral} - MRT_{bolus}$$
$$= 2.24 \text{ h} - 2.05 \text{ h} = 0.19 \text{ h}$$

Example 18-21 The mean residence time after administration of a 500 mg intravenous dose of a drug was 2.5 h and the mean residence time following administration of a 500 mg oral dose of the same drug was 2.75 h. Calculate the mean absorption time for the orally administered dose.

Solution

The mean absorption time for the orally administered dose is estimated using equation (18-19):

$$MAT = MRT_{oral} - MRT_{bolus}$$
$$= 2.75 \text{ h} - 2.5 \text{ h} = 0.25 \text{ h}$$

Example 18-22 The mean residence time following administration of a 500 mg oral dose of a drug was 5.5 h. If the rate constant of elimination of the drug is 0.231/h, calculate the mean absorption time.

Solution

The mean absorption time is estimated using equation (18-20): 1

$$MAT = MRT_{oral} - \frac{1}{K}$$
$$= 5.5 \text{ h} - \frac{1}{0.231/\text{h}}$$
$$= 5.5 \text{ h} - 4.33 \text{ h} = 1.17 \text{ h}$$

Example 18-23 The rate constant of absorption of a drug following administration of a 500 mg oral dose was found to be 0.533/h, calculate the mean absorption time of the drug.

Solution

The mean absorption time is estimated using equation (18-22): 11

$$\text{MAT} = \frac{1}{K_a} = \frac{1}{0.533/\text{h}} = 1.88 \text{ h}$$

Example 18-24 The rate constant of absorption of a drug following administration of a 500 mg oral dose was found to be 0.63/h, calculate the mean absorption time of the drug.

Solution

The mean absorption time is estimated using equation (18-22):

$$\text{MAT} = \frac{1}{K_a} = \frac{1}{0.63/\text{h}} = 1.59 \text{ h}$$

RATE CONSTANT OF ELIMINATION

The non-compartmental analysis is used to estimate elimination rate constant as follows:

Intravenous Bolus Dose

1. One-compartment Model

As shown in Table 18-2, for intravenous bolus administration in one-compartment pharmacokinetic model, the AUC and AUMC are given by:

$$\text{AUC} = \frac{C_0}{K} \text{ and AUMC} = \frac{C_0}{K^2}$$

Dividing AUC by AUMC gives:

$$\frac{\text{AUC}}{\text{AUMC}} = \frac{C_0 \times K^2}{C_0 \times K} \qquad (18\text{-}23)$$

therefore,

$$\frac{\text{AUC}}{\text{AUMC}} = K \qquad (18\text{-}24)$$

2. Two-compartment Model

Similarly, for intravenous bolus administration in a two-compartment pharmacokinetic model, as shown in Table 18-2, the AUC and AUMC are given by:

$$\text{AUC} = \frac{B}{\beta} + \frac{A}{\alpha} \text{ and AUMC} = \frac{B}{\beta^2} + \frac{A}{\alpha^2}$$

Dividing AUC by AUMC gives:

$$\frac{\text{AUC}}{\text{AUMC}} = \frac{\frac{B}{\beta} + \frac{A}{\alpha}}{\frac{B}{\beta^2} + \frac{A}{\alpha^2}} \qquad (18\text{-}25)$$

Equation (18-25) may be written as:

$$\frac{\text{AUC}}{\text{AUMC}} = \frac{\frac{\alpha B + \beta A}{(\beta)(\alpha)}}{\frac{\alpha^2 B + \beta^2 A}{(\beta^2)(\alpha^2)}} \qquad (18\text{-}26)$$

Equation (18-26) is simplified to:

$$\frac{\text{AUC}}{\text{AUMC}} = \frac{\alpha B + \beta A}{(\beta)(\alpha)} \times \frac{(\beta^2)(\alpha^2)}{\alpha^2 B + \beta^2 A} \tag{18-27}$$

When α is much greater than β, the term αB + βA approaches αB and the term $\alpha^2B + \beta^2A$ approaches α^2B. Equation (18-27) then becomes:

$$\frac{\text{AUC}}{\text{AUMC}} = \frac{\alpha B}{(\beta)(\alpha)} \times \frac{(\beta^2)(\alpha^2)}{\alpha^2 B} \tag{18-28}$$

equation (18-28) then reduces to:

$$\frac{\text{AUC}}{\text{AUMC}} = \beta \tag{18-29}$$

Thus, for a drug that exhibits a two-compartment model, the rate constant of elimination of drug from the body following intravenous bolus dose can be approximated from the ratio of AUC and AUMC, as long as α is much greater than ß, i.e. the distribution of drug in the tissue compartment is relatively rapid and the drug has a relatively long biological half-life.

Example 18-25 The area under the zero-moment curve following a 50 mg intravenous bolus dose of a drug was found to be 40 mg/h/L. If the area under the first-moment curve is 190 mg × h^2/L, calculate the rate constant of elimination of the drug.

Solution

According to equation 18-24,

$$K = \frac{\text{AUC}}{\text{AUMC}} = \frac{44 \text{ mg} \times \text{h/L}}{190 \text{ mg} \times \text{h}^2/\text{L}} = 0.232/\text{h}$$

Example 18-26 The area under the zero-moment curve following a 100 mg intravenous bolus dose of a drug was found to be 85 mg/h/L. If the area under the first-moment curve is 200 mg × h^2/L, calculate the rate constant of elimination of the drug.

Solution

According to equation 18-24,

$$K = \frac{\text{AUC}}{\text{AUMC}} = \frac{85 \text{ mg} \times \text{h/L}}{200 \text{ mg} \times \text{h}^2/\text{L}} = 0.425/\text{h}$$

Example 18-27 A drug follows the pharmacokinetics of a two-compartment model. The area under the zero-moment curve following a 100 mg intravenous bolus dose of the drug was found to be 160 mg/h/L. If the area under the first-moment curve is 200 mg × h^2/L, calculate the rate constant of elimination of drug from the body.

Solution

According to equation 18-29,

$$\beta = \frac{\text{AUC}}{\text{AUMC}} = \frac{160 \text{ mg} \times \text{h/L}}{200 \text{ mg} \times \text{h}^2/\text{L}} = 0.08/\text{h}$$

Extravascular Bolus Dose

As shown in Table 18-2, during extravascular bolus administration of a drug, which confers upon the body the characteristics of one-compartment pharmacokinetic model, the areas under the moment curve (AUC and AUMC) are given by:

$$AUC = \frac{B}{\beta} - \frac{A}{\alpha} \text{ and } AUMC = \frac{B}{\beta^2} - \frac{A}{\alpha^2}$$

For immediate-release dosage forms, which do not exhibit lag-time, the two intercepts A and B and are equal. When A = B, the AUC and AUMC are given by:

$$AUC = \frac{B}{\beta} - \frac{B}{\alpha} \text{ and } AUMC = \frac{B}{\beta^2} - \frac{B}{\alpha^2}$$

Dividing AUC by AUMC gives:

$$\frac{AUC}{AUMC} = \frac{\frac{B}{\beta} - \frac{B}{\alpha}}{\frac{B}{\beta^2} - \frac{B}{\alpha^2}} \quad (18\text{-}30)$$

$$\frac{AUC}{AUMC} = \frac{\frac{B(\alpha - \beta)}{\alpha\beta}}{\frac{B(\alpha^2 - \beta^2)}{\alpha^2\beta^2}} \quad (18\text{-}31)$$

For drugs that have a long half-life and are rapidly absorbed, α is usually much greater than β and in these cases (α – β) approaches α and ($\alpha^2 - \beta^2$) approaches α^2. Equation (18-31) is then approximately equal to:

$$\frac{AUC}{AMUC} = \frac{B\alpha}{\alpha\beta} \times \frac{\alpha^2\beta^2}{B\alpha^2} \quad (18\text{-}32)$$

$$\frac{AUC}{AUMC} = \beta \quad (18\text{-}33)$$

Thus, the rate constant of elimination of a drug from the body following extravascular administration can be estimated from the ratio of AUC and AUMC.

Example 18-28 The area under the zero-moment curve following administration of a 50 mg oral dose of a drug was found to be 11 mg/h/L. If the area under the first-moment curve is 81 mg × h²/L, calculate the rate constant of elimination of the drug.

Solution

According to equation 18-33,

$$\beta = \frac{AUC}{AUMC} = \frac{11 \text{ mg} \times \text{h/L}}{82 \text{ mg} \times \text{h}^2\text{/L}} = 0.136/\text{h}$$

Example 18-29 The AUC and AUMC following a 250 mg oral dose of a drug were 60 mg/h/L and 400 mg × h²/L, respectively. Calculate the rate constant of elimination of the drug.

Solution

According to equation 18-33,

$$\beta = \frac{AUC}{AUMC} = \frac{60 \text{ mg} \times \text{h/L}}{400 \text{ mg} \times \text{h}^2\text{/L}} = 0.15/\text{h}$$

RATE CONSTANT OF ABSORPTION

In the compartmental analysis of plasma profile, the rate constant of absorption of the drug is determined by feathering of the plasma profile obtained after the administration of a single bolus dose. The method of residuals (also known as the feathering technique) is used to resolve the biphasic plasma profile into linear segments in order to obtain the rate constant of absorption and the rate constant of elimination of the drug.

The simplest method of estimating the rate constant of absorption of a drug using the non-compartmental analysis is from the mean absorption time of the extravascularly administered dose. The relationship between mean absorption time of a drug following its oral administration and the rate constant of absorption of the drug is given by the following equation (18-22):

$$MAT = \frac{1}{K_a}$$

This equation can be rearranged to:

$$K_a = \frac{1}{MAT} \tag{18-34}$$

Example 18-30 The mean absorption time of a drug following the administration of a 500 mg dose is 3.75 h. Calculate the rate constant of absorption of the drug.

Solution

According to equation (18-34),

$$K_a = \frac{1}{MAT} = \frac{1}{3.75\ h} = 0.267/h$$

TOTAL BODY CLEARANCE

Of all the concepts in pharmacokinetics, the concept of clearance has the greatest potential for clinical applications. This is because the clearance of a drug is the most useful parameter for the evaluation of an elimination mechanism of the drug. Not only this, a sound knowledge of clearance of a drug can be used to determine various other pharmacokinetic parameters associated with the drug. For example, clearance of a drug determines the maintenance dose that is required to achieve a given steady-state plasma concentration of the drug during multiple dosing. If one knows the clearance of a drug and one wants to achieve a certain steady-state plasma concentration of the drug, it is easy to compute the required maintenance dose.

It will be recalled that clearance is defined as the volume of drug-containing plasma that is cleared of the drug per unit time. Therefore, clearance is a ratio of excretion rate of the drug to the concentration of drug in the plasma. Thus, clearance is a proportionality factor, which relates the rate of elimination of the drug to the concentration of drug in plasma. Since concentration of drug in the plasma is a function of concentration of drug in the apparent volume of distribution, therefore, clearance may also be viewed from a physiologic approach as the loss of drug across an organ of elimination. Looking at clearance from a physiologic approach has many advantages. The most important advantage lies in predicting the effects of various factors on the elimination of a drug and in evaluating the effects of various factors on the elimination of a drug. Some of these factors are:

i. Changes in blood flow
ii. Changes in plasma protein binding
iii. Changes in enzyme activity or
iv. Changes in the secretory activity.

Determination of Clearance

The total body clearance in non-compartmental analysis is estimated using an equation, which is independent of compartmental analysis, i.e., the data are not fitted to compartmental analysis. This model-independent equation is:

$$Cl = \frac{(F)(Dose)}{AUC_{0-\infty}} \tag{18-35}$$

where,

Cl = Total body clearance

F = The fraction of dose absorbed

Dose = Amount of drug administered and

$AUC_{0-\infty}$ = Area under the zero-moment curve from time zero to time infinity.

It will be recalled that total body clearance is the sum of the clearance values by each of the eliminating organs, i.e. clearance of drug through kidneys, liver, lungs, etc. Obviously, during intravenous administration, the value of *F* is always equal to 1, because the dose is placed directly into systemic circulation.

Intravenous Bolus Administration: When a drug is administered intravenously as a bolus injection, the value of F in equation (18-35) is equal to 1 and equation (18-35) becomes

$$Cl = \frac{Dose}{AUC_{0-\infty}} \tag{18-36}$$

For drugs that exhibit one-compartment pharmacokinetic model, equation (18-36) can take several forms. Some of these are given here:

1. Based on Dose, MRT and AUMC

According to equation (18-8):

$$MRT = \frac{AUMC}{AUC}$$

Therefore, AUC is equal to:

$$AUC = \frac{AUMC}{MRT} \tag{18-37}$$

Substituting the value of AUC from equation (18-37) into equation (18-36), one gets:

$$Cl = \frac{(Dose)(MRT)}{AUMC} \tag{18-38}$$

2. Based on Dose, MRT and C_0

Similarly, according to equation (18-14):

$$MRT = \frac{AUC}{C_0}$$

which upon rearrangement gives,

$$AUC = (MRT)(C_0) \tag{18-39}$$

Therefore, substituting the value of AUC from equation (18-39) into equation (18-36), one gets:

$$Cl = \frac{Dose}{(MRT)(C_0)} \tag{18-40}$$

3. Based on MRT and V_d

It will be recalled that,

$$\frac{Dose}{C_0} = V_d \tag{18-41}$$

Therefore, equation (18-40) becomes

$$Cl = \frac{V_d}{MRT} \tag{18-42}$$

4. Based on K and V_d

According to equation (18-11):

$$MRT = \frac{1}{K} \tag{18-36}$$

Therefore, equation (18-42) becomes

$$Cl = (K)(V_d) \tag{18-43}$$

It should be pointed out that determination of total body clearance following intravenous bolus dose is not limited to the equations presented here. It is possible to develop other equations from equation (18-36), which can estimate total body clearance.

Example 18-31 The area under the zero-moment curve from time zero to time infinity ($AUC_{0-\infty}$) after the administration of a 500 mg oral dose of a drug was computed to be 200 mg × h/L. If the fraction of dose absorbed is 0.8, calculate clearance of the drug.

Solution

According to equation (18-35),

$$Cl = \frac{(F)(Dose)}{AUC_{0-\infty}}$$

Substituting the values of F, dose and AUC into equation (18-35),

$$Cl = \frac{(0.8)(500\ mg)}{200\ mg \times h/L} = 2\ L/h = 33.3\ mL/min$$

Example 18-32 The following data were obtained after administration of a single 200 mg intravenous dose of a drug: $C_0 = 20$ mg/L, $V_d = 10$ L, $AUC_{0-\infty} = 87$ mg × h/L and $AUMC_{0-\infty} = 375$ mg × h^2/L. Calculate the clearance of the drug.

Solution

The data provided in this Example lend themselves to calculate clearance in many different ways.

1. Using equation (18-36):

$$Cl = \frac{Dose}{AUC_{0-\infty}} = \frac{200\ mg}{87\ mg \times h/L} = 2.3\ L/h = 38\ mL/min$$

2. Using equation (18-38):

According to equation (18-38):

$$Cl = \frac{(Dose)(MRT)}{AUMC}$$

If one wanted to use equation (18-38), one would need the value of mean residence time. According to equation (18-8):

$$MRT = \frac{AUMC}{AUC} = \frac{375\ mg \times h^2/L}{87\ mg \times h/L} = 4.31\ h$$

Substituting the value of mean residence time into equation (18-38):

$$Cl = \frac{(200\text{ mg})(4.31\text{ h})}{375\text{ mg} \times \text{h}^2/\text{L}} = 2.3\text{ L/h} = 38\text{ mL/min}$$

3. *Using equation (18-40):*
According to equation (18-40):

$$Cl = \frac{\text{Dose}}{(\text{MRT})(C_0)}$$

If one wanted to use equation (18-40), one would need the value of mean residence time. The value of mean residence time, according to equation (18-8) was found to be 4.31 hr. Substituting the relevant values into equation (18-40):

$$Cl = \frac{200\text{ mg}}{(4.31\text{ h})(20\text{ mg/L})} = 2.32\text{ L/h} = 39\text{ mL/min}$$

4. *Using equation (18-42):*
According to equation (18-42):

$$Cl = \frac{V_d}{\text{MRT}}$$

Substituting the values of mean residence time (calculated in # *2* above) and volume of distribution (given in the data) into equation (18-42),

$$Cl = \frac{10\text{ L}}{4.31\text{ h}} = 2.32\text{ L/h} = 39\text{ mL/min}$$

5. *Using equation (18-43):*
According to equation (18-43):

$$Cl = (K)(V_d)$$

If one wanted to use equation (18-43), one would need the value of rate constant of elimination of the drug. The rate constant of elimination of the drug, according to equation (18-2) is: C_0 20 mg/L

$$K = \frac{C_0}{\text{AUC}} = \frac{20\text{ mg/L}}{87\text{ mg} \times \text{h/L}} = 0.23\text{/h}$$

Substituting the relevant values into equation (18-43):

$$Cl = (0.23\text{/h})(10\text{ L}) = 2.3\text{ L/h} = 38\text{ mL/min}$$

Example 18-33 The area under the zero-moment curve from time zero to time infinity ($AUC_{0-\infty}$) following administration of a single 1,000 mg intravenous bolus dose of a drug was computed to be 400 mg × h/L. Calculate clearance of the drug.

Solution

Using equation (18-36):

$$Cl = \frac{\text{Dose}}{AUC_{0-\infty}}$$

$$= \frac{1{,}000\text{ mg}}{400\text{ mg} \times \text{h/L}} = 2.5\text{ L/h} = 42\text{ mL/min}$$

Example 18-34 The area under the zero-moment curve from time zero to time infinity ($AUC_{0-\infty}$) after the administration of a 250 mg oral bolus dose of a drug was computed to be 100 mg × h/L. If the fraction of dose absorbed is 0.6, calculate clearance of the drug.

Solution

According to equation (18-35),

$$Cl = \frac{(F)(Dose)}{AUC_{0-\infty}}$$

substituting the values of F, dose and AUC into equation (18-35),

$$Cl = \frac{(0.6)(250 \text{ mg})}{100 \text{ mg} \times \text{h/L}} = 1.5 \text{ L/h} = 25 \text{ mL/min}$$

SUGGESTED READING

1. Bialer M, Look ZM and Siber M. The relationship between drug input and mean residence time in the body. Biophram Drug Dispos. 1986;7:577.
2. Chan KK and Gibaldi M. Estimation of statistical moments and steady-state volume of distribution for a given drug by intravenous infusion. J Pharmacokinet Biopharm. 1982;10:551.
3. Cutler DJ. Theory of mean absorption time. J Pharm Pharmacol. 1978;30:476.
4. Wagner JG. Types of mean residence times. Biophram Drug Dispos. 1988;9:41.
5. Yamaoka K, Nakagawa T and Uno T. Statistical moments in pharmacokinetics. J Pharmacokinet Biopharm. 1978;6:547.

PRACTICE PROBLEMS

18-1. The equation $C = 40e^{-0.2t}$ describes the plasma profile of a drug, which upon intravenous bolus injection of a 1 g dose, confers the characteristics of one-compartment pharmacokinetic model upon the body. If concentration is in mg/L and time is in hr, calculate the area under the zero- and the first-moment curves.

18-2. The equation $C = 40e^{-0.2t}$ describes the plasma profile of a drug which, upon intravenous bolus injection of a single 1 g dose, confers the characteristics of one-compartment pharmacokinetic model upon the body. If concentration is in mg/L and time is in hr, calculate the mean residence time of the drug (a) from the moment curve, (b) from the elimination rate constant and (c) by the area method.

18-3. The following data were obtained following 1 g bolus dose of a drug. Time is in hr and concentration is in mg/L. Calculate: (a) AUC_{0-t} and (b) $AUMC_{0-t}$.

Time	*Concentration*	*Time*	*Concentration*	*Time*	*Concentration*
0	60.0	5	19.7	10	6.6
1	48.0	6	15.7	11	5.1
2	38.4	7	12.6	12	4.1
3	30.7	8	10.1	13	3.3
4	24.6	9	8.0	14	2.6

18-4. A 600 mg bolus dose of a drug gave the following data (concentration is in mg/L and time is in hour). Calculate (a) AUC_{0-t} and (b) $AUMC_{0-t}$.

Time	*Concentration*	*Time*	*Concentration*	*Time*	*Concentration*
0	60.0	3	12.9	6	2.8
1	36.0	4	7.8	7	1.7
2	21.6	5	4.7	8	1.0

18-5. A 500 mg bolus dose of a drug administered orally gave the following data (The fraction of dose absorbed is 1, there is no lag time, time is in hr and concentration is in mg/L). Calculate (a) AUC_{0-t} and (b) $AUMC_{0-t}$.

Time	Concentration	Time	Concentration	Time	Concentration
0	0	5	23.19	10	11.16
1	23.70	6	20.16	11	9.60
2	29.56	7	17.46	12	8.26
3	28.98	8	15.03	13	7.11
4	27.09	9	12.96	14	6.12

18-6. After an intravenous bolus 500 mg dose of a drug, plasma drug concentrations were determined as a function of time. The area under the zero-moment curve was found to be 20 mg × h/L and area under the first-moment curve was computed to be 100 mg × h^2/L. Calculate the mean residence time of this drug.

18-7. A drug is administered at a dose of 500 mg by rapid intravenous bolus injection. The drug has an established elimination rate constant of 0.1155/hr and the volume of distribution of this drug is known to be 12 L and the drug follows the kinetics of one-compartment pharmacokinetic model. If area under the zero-moment curve is 200 mg × h/L and area under the first-moment curve is 900 mg × h^2/L, calculate the mean residence time: (a) by the first-moment curve and (b) by the area method.

18-8. Following the administration of a single 1,000 mg intravenous bolus dose of a drug, the following pharmacokinetic parameters were determined: C_0 = 100 µg/mL, area under the zero-moment curve = 1 mg × h/mL, area under the first-moment curve = 10 mg × h^2/mL, V_d = 10 L and K = 0.1/h. Calculate mean residence time:

a. By the first-moment curve,
b. By the area method and
c. From elimination rate constant.

18-9. Following a single 1 g intravenous bolus dose of a drug, the following pharmacokinetic parameters were determined: C_0 = 100 mg/L, area under the zero-moment curve = 500 mg × hr/L, area under the first-moment curve = 2,500/mg × h^2/L, volume of distribution = 10 L and rate constant of elimination = 0.2/h. Calculate the mean residence time:

a. By the first-moment curve,
b. By the area method and
c. From the elimination rate constant.

18-10. The following data were obtained after administration of a 200 mg intravenous bolus dose of a drug (time is in hour and plasma drug concentration is in mg/L). Calculate the mean residence time:

a. By the first-moment curve and
b. By the area method.

Time	Concentration	Time	Concentration	Time	Concentration	Time	Concentration
0	20.0	4	3.0	8	0.47	12	0.07
1	13.0	5	1.9	9	0.29	13	0.04
2	7.8	6	1.2	10	0.18	14	0.03
3	4.9	7	0.75	11	0.11	15	0.02

18-11. Administration of a single 1,000 mg intravenous bolus dose of a drug yielded the following data: area under the zero-moment curve (AUC) = 225 mg × h/L, apparent volume of distribution = 40 L and the drug follows the kinetics of one-compartment pharmacokinetic model. Calculate the mean residence time if 1,000 mg of this drug were administered as a continuous infusion over an 8 hours period.

18-12. Administration of a single 1,000 mg intravenous bolus dose of a drug yielded the following data: area under the zero-moment curve = 200 mg × h/L, apparent volume of distribution = 25 L and the drug follows the kinetics of one-compartment pharmacokinetic model. Calculate the mean residence time, if a 1,000 mg dose of the drug were administered orally. The rate constant of absorption of the drug is 0.80/h.

18-13. Following the administration of a single 200 mg intravenous bolus dose of a drug, the following parameters were determined: total area under the zero moment curve ($AUC_{0-\infty}$) = 14 mg × h/L and total area under the fist moment curve ($AUMC_{0-\infty}$) = 125 mg × h^2/L. Calculate the mean residence time of the drug.

18-14. The following data were obtained after the administration of a 500 mg dose of a drug (time is in hour, concentration is in mg/L), the fraction of dose absorbed = 1, rate constant of absorption = 0.95/h, rate constant of elimination = 0.15/h and apparent volume of distribution = 11.875 L. Calculate the mean residence time for the orally administered dose of the drug.

Time	Concentration	Time	Concentration	Time	Concentration
0	0	5	23.19	10	11.16
1	23.70	6	20.16	11	9.60
2	29.56	7	17.46	12	8.26
3	28.98	8	15.03	13	7.11
4	27.09	9	12.96	14	6.12

18-15. Following the administration of a single 300 mg rapid intravenous bolus dose of a drug, the area under the zero-moment curve (AUC) was computed to be 100 mg × h/L. Calculate clearance of the drug.

18-16. Following the administration of a 200 mg intravenous bolus dose of a drug, the area under the zero-moment curve was computed to be 100 mg × h/L and the area under the first-moment curve was computed to be 1,000 mg × h^2/L. Calculate clearance of the drug.

18-17. Following the administration of a 150 mg rapid intravenous bolus dose of a drug, C_0 was found to be 10 mg/L and the mean residence time of the drug was estimated to be 10 hours. Calculate clearance of the drug.

18-18. The volume of distribution of a drug administered as an intravenous bolus dose is 30 L and its mean residence time is 10 hours. Calculate total clearance of the drug.

18-19. The area under the zero-moment curve from time zero to time infinity ($AUC_{0-\infty}$) after the administration of a 1,000 mg oral dose of a drug was computed to be 250 mg × h/L. If the fraction of dose absorbed is 0.75, calculate clearance of the drug.

ANSWERS

CHAPTER 2

2-1. (a) $r = 0.998$ (b) $m = 0.519$ %/month (c) $b = -0.528$ % (d) $y = 0.519x - 0.528$
2-2. (a) $r = -0.986$ (b) $m = -1.1786$ μg/L/h (c) $b = 9.1251$ μg/L (d) $y = 9.1251 - 1.1786x$
2-3. 0.58
2-4. 3.747
2-5. –1.715
2-6. –0.886
2-7. 1.096
2-8. 6.7455
2-9. 128.424 mg
2-10. (a) 94.517 μg/L (b) 6 hours
2-12. (a) –0.992 (b) –5.446 μg/L per month (c) 103.57 μg/L (d) $y = 103.57 - 5.4464x$
2-13. 2.175 mg
2-14. 259.83 μg/L
2-15. 6.67 hours
2-16. 4.643 mg/week
2-17. (a) 0.9190 (b) 0.5 units/month (c) 998 units
2-18. $y = 494.5 - 3.5856t$
2-19. 196.4 mg
2-20. 18.25 mg
2-21. 1002 mg
2-22. 299 μg/L
2-23. 300 μg/L
2-24. 6 hours

CHAPTER 3

3-1. (a) first-order (b) 9 mg/mL (c) 5.5 months (d) 0.44 mg/mL
3-2. (a) zero-order (b) 802 mg (c) 11.2 mg/day (d) 35.8 days (e) 746 mg
3-3. $C_0 = 320$ mg/L, $K = 0.00243$/day, $t_{130\ mg/L}$ = about 1 year
3-4. 0.15 μg/L
3-5. 20.6 μg/mL
3-6. $C_0 = 133$ mg, $K = 3.007$ mg/week, $t_{1/2} = 22.12$ weeks
3-7. About 22 weeks
3-8. (a) 27.78 months (b) 176 mg
3-9. 12 months
3-10. 40 months

3-11. 697 mg per fluid ounce
3-12. 12 months
3-13. 40 days
3-14. 315 mg/tablet
3-15. 1.34 mg/5 mL/day
3-16. 9 months
3-17. 2.772 years
3-18. 317.5 mg/tablet
3-19. C_0 = 12.5 μg, K = 1 μg/h, $t_{1/2}$ = 6.25 h
3-20. (a) 40 μg/mL (b) 0.1/h (c) 6.93 h (d) 1.99 μg/mL
3-21. 12.71 months
3-22. (a) 104 μg/L (b) 5.45 μg/L/h (c) 9.5 h
3-23. 37 days
3-24. 39.35%
3-25. 0.01161/day
3-26. 46.78 mg/mL
3-27. 58.67 mg/mL
3-28. 189 mg
3-29. 10.16 months

CHAPTER 4

4-1. 9.1%
4-2. 5.9%
4-3. 75.97%
4-4. 9.1%
4-5. 8.4
4-6. 7.6 mg/min
4-7. 0.09
4-8. 0.8882
4-9. 3.5
4-10. 5.0
4-11. 24%

CHAPTER 5

5-1. 86.4 mg
5-2. 93.75 L
5-3. 300 mg
5-4. 2.93 mg/L
5-5. 14.7 L
5-6. 88.8 mg
5-7. 4.62 mg
5-8. 27 mg
5-9. 0.75 μg/mL
5-10. 13.51 μg/mL
5-11. 0.2 mg/L
5-12. 1 mg/L
5-13. 150%

CHAPTER 6

6-1. (a) 14% (b) 0.6%
6-2. (a) 0.4% (b) 56%
6-3. 0.25
6-4. 0.25
6-5. 0.2

CHAPTER 7

7-1. (a) 8 mL/min (b) glomerular filtration with extensive reabsorption
7-2. (a) 17.2 mL/min (b) glomerular filtration with extensive reabsorption (c) 8 hours
7-3. 64 min
7-4. 320 min
7-5. About 6 hours
7-6. About 12 hours
7-7. 21 min
7-8. 62.4 min
7-9. 82.5 mL/min
7-10. 79.86 mL/min
7-11. 54 mL/min
7-12. 73 mL/min
7-13. 0.2
7-14. 43.83%

CHAPTER 8

8-1. 93% or 465 mg
8-2. 79.4%
8-3. 631.4 mcg × h/mL
8-4. Onset of action = 0.4 hour, intensity of action = 36.0 mg/L, duration of action = 12.2 hours, AUC_{0-14} = 325.6 mg × h/L, AUC_{total} = 397.8 mg × h/L
8-5. AUC_{0-14} = 124.8 mg × h/L, AUC_{total} = 194.1 mg × h/L, onset of action = 1.4 hours intensity of action = 12 mg/L, duration of action = 10.2 h
8-6. 430 mg × h/L
8-7. 120 mg × h/L
8-8. 0.25 h, 4.25 mg/L, 6.75 h, 25.9 mg × h/L
8-9. 1151.1 μg × h/mL
8-10. 108.8%
8-11. 0.4 hour, 18.8 mg/L, 10.1 h, 154.4 mg × h/L
8-12. AUC_{0-7}: intravenous = 34.9 mg × h/L, tablet = 20.55 mg × h/L, capsule = 22.425 mg × h/L (a) 43.56 mg × h/L (b) tablet = 58.9%, capsule = 64.3% (c) the onset of action (in h), intensity of action (in mg/L) and duration of action (in h) from each of the three dosage forms is as follows:

Dosage form	Onset of action	Intensity of action	Duration of action
Intravenous	0	10.0	5.3
Tablet	1.0	3.9	3.7
Capsule	0.5	4.1	4.61

8-13. 87 μg × h/L

CHAPTER 9

9-1. None of the tablet formulations are pharmaceutically equivalent
9-2. Formulations A, E are pharmaceutical alternatives and B, D are pharmaceutical alternatives
9-3. Calculated value of t-statistic for 11 DF is: ratios = 2.8793, differences of the logarithms = 2.9668.
9-4. Calculated value of t-statistic for 11 DF is: ratios = 3.5786, differences of the logarithms = 3.5649.
9-5. Formulations A and D are pharmaceutical alternatives
9-6. Calculated value of t-test on ratios is 14.433. Published value of t-statistic is 2.2. Since calculated value is greater than published value, the AUC is not similar, i.e. products are not bioequivalent. Calculated value of t-test on differences is 2.385. Published value of t-statistic is 2.2. Since the calculated value is greater than published value, the AUC is not similar, i.e. the two products are not bioequivalent.
9-7. Calculated value of t-test on ratios is 8.66. Published value of t-statistic is 2.2. Since calculated value is greater than published value, the AUC is not similar, i.e. products are not bioequivalent. Calculated value of t-test on differences is 2.3485. Published value of t-statistic is 2.2. Since the calculated value is greater than published value, the AUC is not similar, i.e. the two products are not bioequivalent.
9-8. Calculated value of t-test on ratios is 2.825. Published value of t-statistic is 2.2. Since calculated value is greater than published value, the AUC is not similar, i.e. products are not bioequivalent. Calculated value of t-test on differences is 2.682. Published value of t-statistic is 2.2. Since the calculated value is greater than the published value, the AUC is not similar, i.e. the two products are not bioequivalent.

CHAPTER 11

11-1. Equation: $C = 60\ e^{-0.6t}$, Biological half-life = 1.155 h

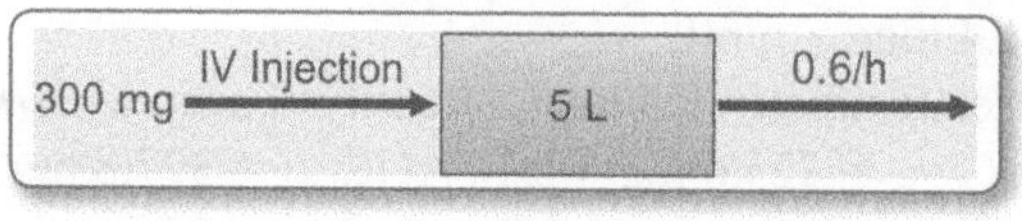

11-2. 1.386 h, 0.044 μg/mL, 0.5/h, 6.25 L
11-3. 3.4 h, 41.7 L
11-4. $C = 20\ e^{-0.17t} + 50\ e^{-0.7t}$

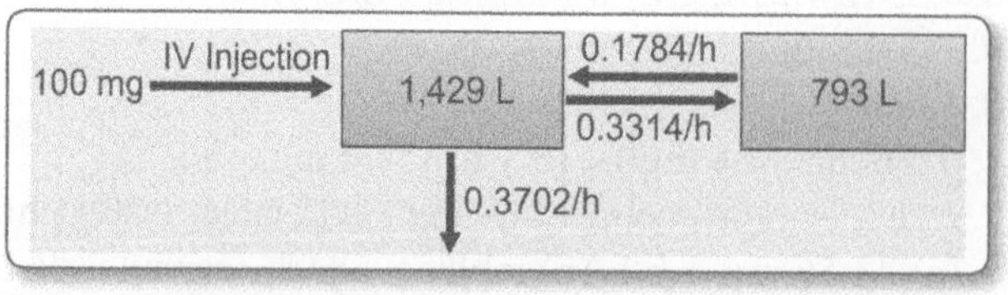

11-5. $C = 20\ e^{-0.27t} + 60\ e^{-1.32t}$

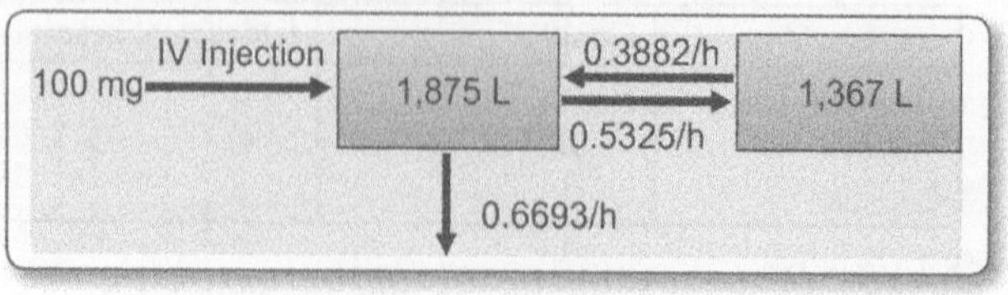

11-6. $C = 10\ e^{-0.23t} + 40\ e^{-1.18t}$

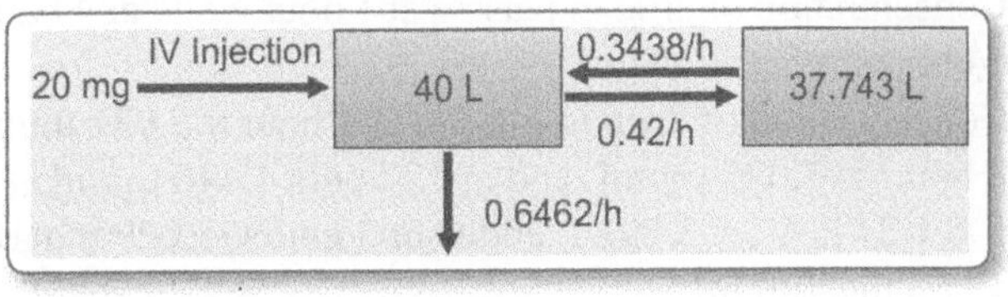

11-7. $C = 17\ e^{-0.189t} + 70\ e^{-0.559t}$

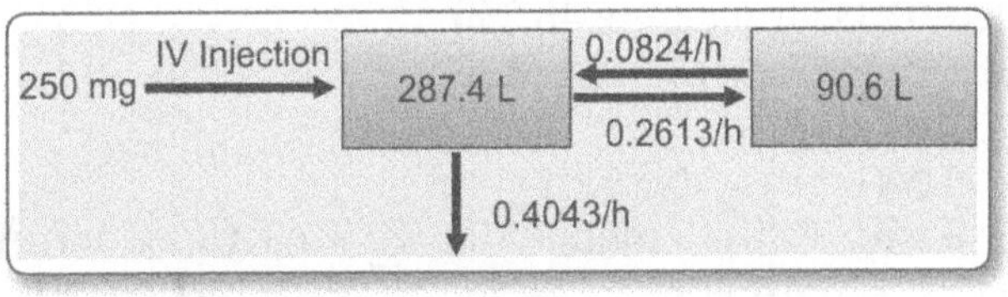

11-8. 50, 23.7, 18, and 145 L
11-9. $K_{12} = 0.04375/h$, $K_{21} = 0.05625/h$, $K_{10} = 0.08/h$, and $t_{½} = 23.1$ h
11-10. 200 L
11-11. (a) 1.98 hours (b) 32.609 L (c) 1.13 mg/L
11-12. (a) 4.62 hours (b) 4.1667 L (c) 0.268 mg/L
11-13. (a) 12.5 L (b) 0.832 mg/L (c) 1.98 h
11-14. (a) 6 μg/mL (b) 4.62 h (c) 24.7 L (d) 0.6649 mg/L
11-15. 7.5 L
11-16. (a) 5.33 hours (b) 500 μg/L (c) 10 L (d) 1806.206 μg × h/L
11-17. (a) 4.62 hours (b) 220 μg/L (c) 227 L (d) 392.041 μg × h/L
11-18. 2.5 mg/L
11-19. (a) 6.93 h (b) 150 μg/L (c) 333.33 L
11-20. 5 mg/L
11-21. (a) 60 mg/L (b) 6.03 h (c) 6.536 μg/mL (d) 167.924 mg × h/L
11-22. 1 mg/L
11-23. (a) 69.3 hours (b) 150 μg/L (c) 666.667 L

CHAPTER 12

12-1. $C = 36\ e^{-0.271t} - 36\ e^{-0.641t}$, 3.369 L
12-2. $C = 50\ e^{-0.17t} - 50\ e^{-0.72t}$
12-3. $C = 35\ e^{-0.153t} - 35\ e^{-0.613t}$
(B = 35 μg/mL, A = 35 μg/mL, $\beta = K = 0.153/h$, $\alpha = K_a = 0.613/h$)
$t_{1/2} = 4.53$ h, $V_d = 22.845$ L and L = 0 h
12-4. $C = 20\ e^{-0.17t} - 50\ e^{-0.7t}$
(B = 20 mg/L, A = 50 mg/L, $\alpha = Ka = 0.7/h$, $\beta = K = 0.17/h$)
$t_{1/2} = 4.1$ h and L = 1.729 h. The corrected y-intercepts are: $B^* = A^* = 14.91$ mg/L and the new equation in the presence of lag time is: $C = 14.91\ e^{-(0.17)(t-1.729)} - 14.91\ e^{-(0.7)(t-1.729)}$, $V_d = 35.433$ L
12-5. 12.97
12-6. $C = 70(e^{-0.139t} - e^{-0.708t})$
12-7. $C = 20(e^{-0.049t} - e^{-0.428t})$, $K_a = 0.428/h$, $K = 0.049/h$, $t_{1/2} = 14.1$ h and $V_d = 45.736$ L
12-8. $C = 20e^{-0.15t} + 30e^{-0.40t} - 50e^{-1.19t}$
12-9. $C = 25e^{-0.11t} + 40e^{-0.35t} - 65e^{-1.1t}$
12-10. 14.64
12-11. $t_{max} = 13.4$, $C_{max} = 22.84$, and concentration at 2 hours = 8.580, at 4 hours = 14.433, at 8 hours = 20.728 and at 10 hours = 22.105

12-12. (a) 9.14 hours (b) 6.69 mg/L (c) 5.87 mg/L
12-13. Concentration of drug in plasma at 1 hour = 5.9, at 4 hours = 11.6, at 10 hours = 8.6 and at 14 hours = 5.9
12-14. Concentration of drug in plasma at 1 hour = 5.031 μg/mL, at 2 hours = 7.675 μg/mL, at 8 hours = 7.025 μg/mL and at 12 hours 4.446 μg/mL
12-15. L = 1.21 h, V_d = 3.291 L and C at 2 hours = 3.29 mg/100 mL
12-16. 13.63 mg/100 mL
12-17. K_a = 1.133/h and $t_{1/2}$ = 4.589 h
12-18. K_a = 0.335/h and $t_{1/2}$ = 46.2 h
12-19. K_a = 0.15/h and $t_{1/2}$ = 34.65 h
12-20. 63.105 μg/L
12-21. $C = 20(e^{-0.3\,t}) - 40(e^{-1.3\,t})$
12-22. $C = 50(e^{-0.15\,t}) - 100(e^{-0.65\,t})$, K_a = 0.65/h, K = 0.15/h, $t_{1/2}$ = 4.62 h, L = 1.386 h, $t_{max\,L}$ = 4.319 h, $C_{max\,L}$ = 20.12 μg/mL, corrected B = corrected A = 40.625 μg/mL, V_d = 16 L, AUC = 208.3 mg × h/mL
12-23. (a) 0.35/h (b) 34.65 h
12-24. $C = 30(e^{-0.15\,t}) - 60(e^{-0.65\,t})$
12-25. $C = 105(e^{-0.239t} - e^{-0.71t})$, K_a = 0.71/h, K = 0.139/h, $t_{1/2} \approx 5$ h and V_d = 5.92 L, t_{max} = 2.86 h AUC = 607.5 μg × h/mL
12-26. $C = 70(e^{-0.278\,t} - e^{-1.42\,t})$, K_a = 1.42/h, K = 0.278/h, $t_{1/2} \approx 2.5$ h, and V_d = 8.88 L, t_{max} = 1.43 h AUC = 202.5 μg × h/mL
12-27. 1050 mg×h/L
12-28. 1683 mg×h/L
12-29. 4.62 hours

CHAPTER 13

13-1. (a) 0.44 (b) 0.19
13-2. (a) 0.65 (b) 0.87
13-3. (a) 1.35 (b) 1.48 (c) 1.52 (d) 1.54 (e) 1.55
13-4. (a) 5.52 mg/L (b) 4.18 mg/L
13-5. (a) 2.91 mg/L (b) 2.21 mg/L
13-6. (a) 5.12 mg/L (b) 3.87 mg/L
13-7. (a) 0.14 mg/L and 1.14 mg/L (b) 0.33 mg/L and 1.33 mg/L (c) 1.00 mg/L and 2.00 mg/L
13-8. (a) 22 μg/mL and 622 μg/mL (b) 200 μg/mL and 800 μg/mL (c) 1.17 mg/mL and 1.77 mg/mL
13-9. (a) 4 mg/L and 6.7 mg/L (b) 1.3 mg/L and 4.5 mg/L (c) 0.57 mg/L and 3.85 mg/L
13-10. $C_{max\,ss}$ = 1.8 mg/L and $C_{max\,ss}$ = 0.96 mg/L
13-11. (a) 26.4 μg/mL, 746.4 μg/mL (b) 240 μg/mL, 960 μg/mL (c) 1.44 mg/mL, 2.16 mg/mL
13-12. (a) 0.224 mg/L and 1.824 mg/L (b) 0.528 mg/L and 2.128 mg/L (c) 1.6 mg/L and 3.2 mg/L
13-13. (a) 0.196 mg/L and 1.596 mg/L (b) 0.462 mg/L and 1.862 mg/L (c) 1.4 mg/L and 2.8 mg/L
13-14. (a) 0.252 mg/L and 2.052 mg/L (b) 0.594 mg/L and 2.394 mg/L (c) 1.8 mg/L and 3.6 mg/L

CHAPTER 14

14-1. (a) 15.47 mg (b) 20 mg
14-2. (a) 55.32 mg (b) 37.5 mg
14-3. (a) 732 mg (b) 378 mg
14-4. 1198 mg

14-5. 883 mg
14-6. 1108 mg
14-7. 487 mg
14-8. 486 mg
14-9. (a) 15.48 mg (b) 20 mg
14-10. (a) 9.3 mg (b) 12 mg
14-11. (a) 15.48 mg (b) 20 mg

CHAPTER 15

15-1. (a) 0.012 mg (b) 0.012 min
15-2. 3.15 mg/L
15-3. (a) 1.18 mg/L (b) 3.169 mg/L (c) 5.41 mg/L (d) 6.527 mg/L
15-4. 4.8 mg/L
15-5. (a) 2.7 mg/L (b) 4.8 mg/L (c) 5.7 mg/L
15-6. (a) 1.012 mg/L (b) 3.432 mg/L (c) 4.639 mg/L (d) 5.594 mg/L
15-7. 13.468 mg/L
15-8. 38.98 mg/h
15-9. 374.22 mg
15-10. (a) 5.947 mg/L (b) 7.799 mg/L
15-11. 420 mg
15-12. 41.58 mg/h
15-13. 45.87 hours
15-14. (a) 736 mg/h (b) 32 mg/h
15-15. (a) 612 mg/h (b) 23 mg/h
15-16. (a) 617.5 mg/h (b) 34.65 mg/h
15-17. (a) 926.3 mg/h (b) 51.975 mg/h
15-18. (a) 772.5 mg/h (b) 64.1 mg/h
15-19. (a) 692 mg/h (b) 58.212 mg/h
15-20. 51.975 mg/h
15-21. 44.55 mg/h
15-22. 360 mg
15-23. 370 mg
15-24. 48.1 mg/h
15-25. 33.29 h
15-26. (a) 490 mg/h (b) 20.79 mg/h

CHAPTER 16

16-1. 0.0924/h
16-2. (a) 70% (b) 30%
16-3. 5 hours
16-4. 241.5 mg
16-5. 3.3 hours
16-6. 27 hours
16-7. 0.0231/h
16-8. 0.022/h

CHAPTER 17

17-1. 200 mg every 6 hours
17-2. 400 mg every 6 hours
17-3. (a) 26.8 mg (b) 4.23 mg/L
17-4. (a) 6.5 hours (b) 4.5 mg/L
17-5. 180 mg every 6 hours
17-6. (a) 551.1 μg/mL (b) 45.4 μg/mL
17-7. (a) 1178.4 mg (b) 57.5 mg
17-8. 367 mg
17-9. 6.16 hours
17-10. 6.76 hours

CHAPTER 18

18-1. AUC = 200 mg × h/L, AUMC = 1,000 mg × h^2/L
18-2. (a) 5 hours (b) 5 hours (c) 5 hours
18-3. (a) 256 mg × h/L (b) 947.35 mg × h^2/L
18-4. (a) 119 mg × h/L (b) 205.3 mg × h^2/L
18-5. (a) 237.555 mg × h/L (b) 1325.88 mg × h^2/L
18-6. (a) 237.555 mg × h/L (b) 1325.88 mg × h^2/L
18-6. 5 h
18-7. (a) 4.5 hours (b) 4.8 hours
18-8. (a) 10 hours (b) 10 hours (c) 10 hours
18-9. (a) 5 hours (b) 5 hours (c) 5 hours
18-10. (a) 2.05 hours (b) 2.16 hours
18-11. 13 hours
18-12. 6.25 hours
18-13. 8.93 hours
18-14. 7.72 hours
18-15. 3 L/h = 50 mL/min
18-16. 2 L/h = 33 mL/min
18-17. 1.5 L/h = 25 mL/min
18-18. 3 L/h = 50 mL/min
18-19. 3 L/h = 50 mL/min

APPENDIX A

GLOSSARY OF TERMS

Listed below are terms and their definitions, which are frequently used in biopharmaceutics and pharmacokinetics. It should be pointed out, however, that these terms are defined in their broadest sense and convey a general idea about the meaning of these terms.

Absolute Bioavailability is the total amount of drug absorbed into the general circulation from a given route of administration.

Absorption of drugs is the process of uptake of the compound from the site of administration into the systemic circulation.

Accumulation is the increase of drug concentration in the blood and tissues upon multiple dosing until steady state is reached.

Agonist is a substance that combines with a receptor to initiate a response.

Antagonist is a substance, which has the capability to antagonize the agonist.

Area Under the Curve is the area bounded by the drug blood level versus time curve.

Area Under the Zero Moment Curve is the area bounded by the plasma concentration versus time curve.

Area Under the First Moment Curve is the area bounded by the (plasma concentration × time) versus time curve.

Biliary Excretion is the removal of intact drug molecules or their metabolites in the bile.

Biliary Recycling (see Enterohepatic Recirculation).

Bioavailability is the rate and extent of absorption of drug from an administered dosage form which enters the systemic circulation.

Bioequivalence (see Bioequivalent Drug Products)

Bioequivalence Requirement is the requirement imposed by the Food and Drug Administration (FDA) for *in vitro* and/or *in vivo* testing of specified drug products.

Bioequivalent Drug Products are those pharmaceutical equivalents whose rates and extends of absorption do not show a significant difference when administered at the same molar dose.

Biological Half-Life of a drug is the time necessary for the amount of drug in the body to be reduced to 50 percent.

Biopharmaceutics deals with the availability of the drug and/or drug product to the human or animal body from a given dosage form.

Biophase is the actual site of drug action in the body.

Blood Flow Rate is the rate of blood perfusion in an organ and is usually expressed in mL per 100 g of the organ weight per minute.

Blood Levels denote the concentration of drug in blood after administration of a dosage form.

Bolus Dose is the dose administered rapidly.

A **Brand Product** is a drug product labeled with the registered trade mark of a single company.

Central Compartment is the sum of all body regions (organs and tissue) in which the drug concentration is in instantaneous equilibrium with the concentration in blood or plasma.

Chemical Equivalents are those multiple-source drug products, which contain essentially identical active ingredient(s) and meet existing physicochemical standards of official compendia.

Chronopharmacology is the study of drug action as affected by the time of day or a specific cycle of time-dependent physiology.

Circadian Rhythm is the biological clock controlling rhythms of processes during a twenty four hour cycle, i.e. a twenty four hour cycling of events.

Clearance (Total Clearance) is the hypothetical volume of distribution (in mL) of the un-metabolized drug, which is cleared per unit time (minute) by any pathway of drug removal (see also, creatinine clearance, hepatic clearance, intrinsic clearance, non-renal clearance and renal clearance).

Clinical Pharmacokinetics is the application of pharmacokinetic principles in the safe and effective treatment of individual patients and in the optimization of drug therapy.

A **Compartment** (in pharmacokinetics) is an entity, which can be described by a definite volume and a concentration of drug contained in that volume.

Competitive Antagonist is a substance, which competes for the receptors and occupies a significant proportion of the receptors, thereby pre-empting them from reacting maximally with an agonist.

Competitive Binding is the binding of drug molecules to various elements of the body, e.g. plasma proteins, where two molecules compete for the same binding site.

Complexation is the physical binding of drug molecules and formulation components with physiological components, e.g. mucin.

Concentration Gradient is the difference in the concentration in two phases usually separated by a membrane.

Continuous Infusion is intravenous administration of a large volume of drug solution administered continuously over a relatively large period of time.

Creatinine Clearance is the ratio of rate of creatinine excreted in urine to the concentration of creatinine in plasma.

Deep Tissue Compartment is the pharmacokinetic compartment where distribution of drug is very slow, e.g. very poorly perfused tissues, adipose tissues, etc.

Dispersion is a liquid preparation containing relatively large solute particles suspended in a vehicle.

Disposition is the loss of drug from the central compartment due to distribution into other compartments and/or elimination and metabolism.

Dissociation Constant expresses the degree of dissociation of a chemical compound in a given solvent at a given temperature.

Diurnal Variation (see Circadian Rhythm).

Dosage Form is the pharmaceutical form containing the active ingredient(s) and excipients necessary in formulating the desired product.

Dosage Regimen is the systematized dosage schedule for therapy, required to maintain a therapeutic concentration in the body.

Dose-Response Curve is the graphical presentation of response (pharmacological or clinical effectiveness, or toxicity) versus dose.

Dose Size is the amount of drug to be administered.

Dosing Interval is the time period between administration of maintenance doses.

A **Drug** is a chemical compound (of synthetic, semisynthetic, natural or biological origin), which interacts with human or animal cells to produce a response.

A **Drug Product** (see Dosage Form).

A **Drug Substance** is a physiologically active agent used in the diagnosis, cure, prevention or treatment of disease.

Drug-Receptor Interaction is the combining of a drug molecule with the receptor for which it has affinity and the initiation of a pharmacologic response by its intrinsic activity.

Drug Release is the release or dissolution of the active ingredient from a dosage form into solution.

Elimination Half-Life (see Biological Half-Life).

Endogenous substances are those substances, which belong to the body naturally, e.g. amino acids, sugars, etc.

Enteral Routes are routes of administration, which directly involve the gastrointestinal tract.

Enterohepatic Recirculation is the emptying of drugs into small intestines via bile and their reabsorption form the intestinal lumen into systemic circulation.

Enterohepatic Recycling (see Enterohepatic Recirculation).

Enzyme Induction is the increase in enzyme content or rate of enzymatic processes resulting in faster metabolism of a compound.

Enzyme Inhibition is the decrease in the rate of metabolism of a compound usually by competition for an enzyme system.

Excretion of drug is the final elimination of drug from the body's systemic circulation.

Excretion Ratio is the ratio of organ clearance of the total drug to the rate of blood flow.

Exogenous describes something foreign to the body.

Extraction Ratio is the fraction of drug removed from plasma by the liver. The term extraction ratio is usually used in relation to first-pass effect.

Extravascular Administration is the administration of a drug by all routes except those where the drug is directly introduced into the bloodstream.

Fast Disposition is the term used to describe drugs having a biological half-life of 4 hours or less.

Feathering (Method) is the graphical method used for resolving a non-linear profile into its linear segments, e.g. separating the absorption rate constant from the elimination rate constant, or the α-slope from the β-slope.

First-Pass Effect generally refers to metabolism (biotransformation, not chemical degradation) in the liver upon oral administration before the drug reaches systemic circulation.

Flip-Flop Model is a pharmacokinetic model in which the rate constant of the input function is smaller than the rate constant of the output function.

The Gastrointestinal Tract is the part of the alimentary canal consisting of stomach, small intestine and large intestine.

A **Generic Product** is a drug product marketed under the non-proprietary name of a drug.

Glomerular Filtration is filtration of drugs in the glomeruli with plasma water.

Half-Life (see Biological Half-Life).

Hepatic Clearance is the hypothetical volume of distribution in mL of the unmetabolized drug, which is cleared in one minute via the liver.

Hybrid Rate Constants are composite rate constants consisting of two or more microconstants.

Infusion Rate is the rate (volume per unit time) at which a drug is infused into systemic circulation.

Initial Dose is the size of the dose used in initiating therapy.

Instantaneous Distribution is the attainment of equilibrium immediately after the introduction of drug into the system.

Interstitial Space is the space between cellular elements of a structure or part.

Intravascular Administration is all routes of administration where the drug is directly introduced into the bloodstream.

Intrinsic Clearance is the theoretical unrestricted maximum clearance of the unbound drug by an elimination process.

Infusion Rate is the rate of drug infusion (usually expressed in mg/h)

Lag Time is the period of time, which elapses between the time of administration and the time of drug in the blood.

Lean Body Weight is a patient's body weight minus the fat mass.

Loading Dose (see Initial Dose).

Maintenance Dose is the size of the dose (after the Initial Dose) required maintaining the clinical effectiveness or therapeutic concentration according to the dosage regimen.

Mean Absorption Time is the average time for all the drug molecules to be absorbed from the site of administration.

Mean Residence Time is average time for all the drug molecules to reside in the body.

Michaelis-Menten Kinetics is saturation kinetics used to characterize such phenomena as protein binding, adsorption and non-linear or saturation processes often observed with increasing the size of the dose.

Microconstants are those constants, which are part of the hybrid constants. For example, K_{10}, K_{12}, K_{21}, K_{13}, K_{31}, etc. are microconstants.

A **Model** (in pharmacokinetics) is a mathematical description of a biologic system, which can be used to simulate the rate processes describing the movement of drug in the body.

Moderate Disposition is the term used to describe drugs having a biological half-life of between 4 and 8 hours.

Multiple Dose Administration is the repeated administration of a drug at intervals shorter than those required for virtually complete elimination of the previous dose.

Nomogram is a graphic method of calculation from two or more given parameters.

Non-competitive Antagonist is a substance, which reacts with the receptor in such a way as not to prevent agonist-receptor combination but to prevent the combination from initiating a response.

Non-enteral Routes are routes of administration, which do not directly involve drug administration, through the gastro-intestinal tract.

Non-linear Pharmacokinetics is the kinetics of drug absorption, distribution, biotransformation and elimination, which is dependent on the administered dose.

Non-renal Clearance is the hypothetical plasma volume in mL, which is cleared in 1 minute via the non-renal route.

Oral Administration includes buccal and sublingual administration and swallowing of the drug so that the drug is absorbed from the mouth cavity or from the gastrointestinal tract.

Parameters (in pharmacokinetics) are the rate constants, volumes of distribution, clearance, etc.

Partial Agonist is a substance, which can elicit some but not a maximal effect and which antagonizes an agonist.

Partition Coefficient expresses the ratio of concentration of drug in each phase of a system consisting of two or more immiscible liquids.

Perfusion Model is a pharmacokinetic model based on blood flow to various organs and the rate of drug equilibration between various organs.

Peripheral Compartment (see Tissue Compartment).

Pharmaceutical Alternatives are drug products that contain the identical therapeutic moiety or its precursor, but not necessarily in the same amount, dosage form or as the same salt or ester.

Pharmaceutical Equivalents are drug products that contain identical amounts of the identical active drug ingredient in identical dosage forms, but not necessarily containing the same inactive ingredients.

Pharmacodynamics deals with the relationship between concentration of drug at the site of action and the magnitude of effect produced by the drug.

Pharmacogenetics deals with unusual drug responses that have a genetic or a hereditary basis.

Pharmacokinetics deals with the time course of drug and its metabolites in the body and the kinetics of absorption, distribution, metabolism and elimination of the drug.

Placebo is an inert substance, identical in appearance to material being tested in experimental research and indistinguishable from the test material.

Plasma Levels (or concentration) denote the concentration of drug in the plasma after administration of a dosage form.

Plateau Concentration is the accumulated concentration of a drug in the plasma or tissue after chronic dosing when a plateau level (steady state) is reached between intake and elimination of the drug.

Polymorphic Form of a drug, referred to as the metastable form, usually differs in its physico-chemical properties as compared to the thermodynamically stable form.

Priming Dose (see Initial Dose).

Prolonged Infusion is constant intravenous infusion carried over a long period of time.

Protein Binding is the phenomenon, which occurs when a drug combines with the protein of the plasma or tissue to form a reversible complex.

Rate Constant is a parameter, which governs the rate of transfer of drug per unit of time.

Rate Limiting Step is the process with the slowest rate constant in a system of simultaneous kinetic processes.

A **Receptor** is a substance to which the drug molecule binds in order to exhibit its pharmacological effect.

Receptor Site is a site in the biophase to which a drug molecule can bind.

Relative Bioavailability is the extent of absorption from a test preparation relative to the extent of absorption from the reference preparation.

Renal Clearance is the hypothetical plasma volume in mL, which is cleared in 1 minute via the kidney.

Residual Method (see Feathering Method).

Serum-Levels denote the drug concentration in serum after administration of a dosage form.

Shallow Tissue Compartment is the pharmacokinetic compartment where distribution of drug is slow, e.g. tissues with less than high perfusion or proteins, etc.

Slow Disposition is the term used to describe drugs having a biological half-life of between 8 and 24 hours.

Steady State is a level of drug concentration in blood and tissue upon multiple dosing when input and output are at equilibrium, i.e. the system attains a dynamic equilibrium.

Therapeutic Index is the ratio of the toxic dose to the minimally effective dose.

Tissue Compartment(s) are pharmacokinetic compartment(s) where distribution of drug is slow, e.g. poorly perfused tissues, proteins, adipose tissues, etc. In multicompartment models, tissue compartments may be further subdivided into *shallow tissue compartment, deep tissue compartment*, etc.

Total Area Under the Curve is the area under the plasma concentration versus time curve from time zero to infinity.

Total Clearance (see Clearance).

Toxicokinetics is the study of kinetics of absorption, distribution and excretion of drugs at high doses.

Trapezoid Rule is the method of calculating the area under the curve by breaking up a curve into a large number of trapezoids.

Truncated Area Under the Curve is the area under the plasma concentration versus time curve from time zero to time t.

Ultra-Fast Disposition is the term used to describe drugs having a biological half-life less than 1 hour.

Urinary Recycling is the phenomenon that occurs when drugs filtered through the glomeruli are reabsorbed from the tubules into systemic circulation.

Very Slow Disposition is the term used to describe drugs having a biological half-life greater than 24 hours.

Volume of Distribution is a hypothetical volume of body fluid that would be required to dissolve the total amount of drug at the same concentration as that found in the blood, plasma or serum.

APPENDIX B

NOMENCLATURE AND SYMBOLS

The reading and understanding of pharmacokinetic publications is sometimes made difficult because not everybody uses the same nomenclature and symbols. The use of two or more different symbols for the same parameter or expression can be very confusing. Everyone realizes that defining each symbol in every publication not only consumes printing space, but is also unnecessarily time consuming for the reader. Until a uniform nomenclature is accepted and practiced, these difficulties will continue. However, in order to minimize these problems at this time, every effort has been made to adhere to the symbols, which are not only easy to write and communicate, but are also accepted by major publications. The nomenclature and symbols used in this book are defined in the text where they first appear, but for the convenience of the reader these are defined here once again.

In the scientific literature, some symbols have been used to mean more than one quantity. For example, the symbol A has been used to signify a variety of terms, including surface area of particles, the y-intercept (compartment models), surface area of the absorbing membrane (passive diffusion) and the surface area of the pores (convective transport). However, since the context in which the symbol is used is different in each case, it is expected that there will be no confusion due to multiple meaning of a given symbol.

SYMBOL	EXPLANATION
A	Back-extrapolated y-intercept of the residual concentration points obtained after first feathering of the drug-plasma concentration profile
A	Surface area of the absorbing membrane
A	Surface area of the pores
A*	Corrected value of A in the presence of lag-time
α	Fraction of drug not bound to plasma proteins
α	Hybrid constant obtained from the slope of the feathered line having y-intercept = A
A_{cr}	Rate of excretion of creatinine
AD	Adult dose
ANDA	Abbreviated new drug application
ANOV	Analysis of variance
A_t	Amount of drug in the body at time t
AUC	Area under the plasma concentration versus time curve
AUC_{ref}	Area under the plasma concentration versus time curve from the reference preparation
AUC_{test}	Area under the plasma concentration versus time curve from the test preparation
AUC_{0-t}	Area under the plasma concentration versus time curve from time zero to time t

$AUC_{0-\infty}$	Area under the plasma concentration versus time curve from time zero to virtual elimination of the drug
$AUC_{t-\infty}$	Area under the plasma concentration versus time curve from time t to the virtual elimination of the drug
AUC_{total}	Total area under the plasma concentration versus time curve
AUMC	Area under the first moment-time curve
AW	Adult weight
B	Back extrapolated y-intercept of the terminal points of the drug-plasma concentration profile
B*	This code is used for therapeutic equivalence evaluations and includes those drug products that require further FDA investigation and review to determine therapeutic equivalence
B*	Corrected value of B (the back-extrapolated y-intercept of the terminal linear phase of drug plasma concentration profile) in the presence of lag-time
BSA	Body surface area
β	Hybrid constant obtained from the slope of line obtained from the terminal data points and having y-intercept = B
C	Concentration of drug in plasma
C_A	Arterial plasma drug concentration entering the liver
C_{cr}	Serum creatinine concentration
C_{max}	Maximum concentration of drug in plasma following a single dose
$C_{max\ (L)}$	Maximum concentration of drug in plasma in the presence of lag-time
$C_{max\ n}$	Maximum concentration of drug in the plasma following the nth dose
$C_{max\ ss}$	Maximum concentration of drug in the plasma at steady state
$C_{max\ ss''}$	New desired maximum concentration of drug in the plasma at steady state
C_{min}	Minimum concentration of drug in the plasma following a single dose
$C_{min\ n}$	Minimum concentration of drug in the plasma following the nth dose
$C_{min\ ss}$	Minimum concentration of drug in the plasma at steady state
$C_{min\ ss''}$	New desired minimum concentration of drug in the plasma at steady state
C_{ss}	Concentration of drug in the plasma at steady state
C_t	Concentration of drug in the plasma at time t
C_p	Concentration of drug in plasma
C_u	Concentration of drug in urine
C_u	Concentration of creatinine in urine
C_V	Venous plasma drug concentration exiting the liver
C_0	Concentration of drug in the plasma at time zero
C_0	Concentration of drug in the plasma immediately following intravenous injection
CA	Age of the child next birthday
CD	Child's dose
Cl	Total body clearance
Cl_{cr}	Creatinine clearance
Cl_h	Hepatic clearance
Cl_{nr}	Non-renal body clearance
Cl_r	Renal body clearance
Cl_T	Total body clearance
CW	Child's weight

ΔC	Concentration gradient
D	Diffusion coefficient of the drug
D	Dose
D"	The size of new dose needed to attain the desired concentration of drug in the plasma
D*	Loading or priming dose
D_n	Maintenance dose in patients with normal kidney function
D_{ri}	Maintenance dose in patients during renal impairment
dc	Change in concentration
DF	Degrees of freedom
dt	Change in time
dc/dt	Change in concentration with change in time
dc/dt	Rate of reaction
$(dc/dt)_{max}$	Maximal rate of transport at high drug concentration
E	Loss factor
ER	Excretion ratio
ER	Extraction ratio
ERPF	Effective renal plasma flow
$e^{-K\tau}$	Persistence factor
F	Fraction of the administered dose absorbed
FDA	The US Food and Drug Administration
FR	(glomerular) Filtration rate
G	Factor which takes into account the delay in accumulation during extravascular administration
GFR	Glomerular filtration rate
h	Thickness of the absorbing membrane
K	Affinity constant of drug for the carrier
K	Apparent first-order rate constant of elimination
K	Apparent first- or zero-order rate constant
K	Partition coefficient
K_a	Apparent first-order rate constant of absorption
K_e	Apparent first-order rate constant of elimination
K_m	Apparent first-order rate constant of metabolism
K_n	Apparent first-order rate constant of elimination in patients with normal kidney function
K_{nr}	Apparent first-order rate constant of non-renal elimination
K_o	Zero-order rate of drug input during continuous intravenous infusion (infusion rate)
K_r	Apparent first-order rate constant of renal elimination
K_{ri}	Apparent first-order elimination rate constant during renal impairment.
K_{10}	Apparent first-order rate constant of elimination of drug from central compartment
K_{12}	Apparent first-order rate constant of transfer of drug from the central compartment into the second compartment
K_{12}	Apparent first-order rate constant of transfer of drug from the central compartment into the tissue compartment (two compartment model)

K_{13}	Apparent first-order rate constant of transfer of drug from the central compartment into the third compartment
K_{13}	Apparent first-order rate constant of transfer of drug from the central compartment into the deep tissue compartment (three compartment model)
K_{21}	Apparent first-order rate constant of transfer of drug from the second compartment into the central compartment
K_{21}	Apparent first-order rate constant of transfer of drug from the tissue compartment into the central compartment (two compartment model)
K_{23}	Apparent first-order rate constant of transfer of drug from the second compartment into the third compartment
K_{23}	Apparent first-order rate constant of transfer of drug from the peripheral tissue compartment into the deep tissue compartment (three compartment model)
K_{31}	Apparent first-order rate constant of transfer of drug from the third compartment into the central compartment
K_{31}	Apparent first-order rate constant of transfer of drug from the deep tissue compartment into the central compartment (three compartment model)
K_{32}	Apparent first-order rate constant of transfer of drug from the third compartment into the second compartment
K_{32}	Apparent first-order rate constant of transfer of drug from the deep tissue compartment into the peripheral tissue compartment (three compartment model)
L	Lag-time
LBM	Lean body mass
LBW	Lean body weight
MAT	Mean absorption time
MEC	Minimum effective concentration
MRT	Mean residence time
MTC	Minimum therapeutic concentration
MTC	Mean toxic concentration
N	Number of pores
n	Order of reaction
η	Viscosity of fluid in the pores
P	Persistence factor
P	Back-extrapolated y-intercept of the residual concentration points obtained after the second feathering of the drug-plasma concentration profile
PD	Pharmacodynamics
PK	Pharmacokinetics
π	Hybrid constant obtained from the slope of the feathered line having y-intercept = P
Q	Blood flow
Q_H	Hepatic blood flow
R	A factor used in calculating maximum concentration of drug in the plasma at steady state during extravascular multiple dosing. This factor has a value = (K) (t_{max})
R	Radius of pores
RR	Reabsorption rate
S	Accumulation factor
S*	Accumulation factor due to absorption

SD	Standard deviation
SR	(active) Secretion rate
τ	Dosing interval
t	The t statistic
t	Time
t_{inf}	Infusion period
t_{max}	Time of maximum concentration of drug in the plasma
$t_{max(L)}$	Time of maximum concentration of drug in plasma (t_{max}) in the presence of lag-time
τ_n	Dosing interval in patients with normal kidney function
t_p	Time of peak concentration (see t_{max})
τ_{ri}	Dosing interval in patients during renal impairment
$t_{1/2}$	Biological half-life
USP	United States Pharmacopeia
V	Volume of urine excreted
V_c	Apparent volume of central compartment
V_d	Apparent volume of distribution
V_{max}	Maximal rate of transport at high drug concentration
V_t	Apparent volume of tissue compartment

INDEX

Page numbers followed by *f* and *t* refer to figure and table, respectively.

A

B

C

D

E

F

G

H

I

Q

R

S

U

V

W

Y

Z